THE PATHOLOGY OF INCIPIENT NEOPLASIA

DONALD EARL HENSON, M.D., F.A.C.P.

Division of Cancer Prevention and Control
National Cancer Institute,
Bethesda, Maryland

JORGE ALBORES-SAAVEDRA, M.D.

Professor of Pathology and
Director, Division of Anatomic Pathology
University of Miami, School of Medicine
Miami, Florida

1986   W. B. SAUNDERS COMPANY
Philadelphia   London   Toronto   Mexico City
Rio de Janeiro   Sydney   Tokyo   Hong Kong

W. B. Saunders Company: West Washington Square
                           Philadelphia, PA   19105

Library of Congress Cataloging in Publication Data
Main entry under title:

The Pathology of incipient neoplasia.

1. Precancerous conditions.   I. Henson, Donald
   Earl.   II. Albores-Saavedra, Jorge. [DNLM: 1.
   Neoplasms—pathology. 2. Precancerous
   Conditions—pathology. QZ 200 P2965]

RC262.P38 1986   616.99′207   85–22050

ISBN 0–7216–1144–3

Editor: Suzanne Boyd
Designer: Bill Donnelly
Production Manager: Bob Butler
Illustration Coordinator: Peg Shaw
Page Layout Artist: Meg Jolly

The Pathology of Incipient Neoplasia   ISBN   0–7216–1144–3

Last digit is the print number: 9   8   7   6   5   4   3   2   1

Contributors

JORGE ALBORES-SAAVEDRA, M.D.
> Professor of Pathology, University of Miami School of Medicine; Professor and Director, Division of Anatomic Pathology, University of Miami Jackson Memorial Medical Center, Miami, Florida
> *Introduction; Gallbladder and Extrahepatic Bile Ducts; Soft Tissue*

KEVIN E. BOVE, M.D.
> Professor of Pediatrics and Pathology, University of Cincinnati College of Medicine; Associate Director, Department of Pathology, Childrens Hospital Medical Center, Cincinnati, Ohio
> *Wilms' Tumor*

B. E. BUCK, M.D.
> Assistant Professor of Clinical Surgery and Pathology, University of Miami School of Medicine; Attending Staff, Departments of Surgery and Pathology, Jackson Memorial Medical Center, Miami, Florida
> *Wilms' Tumor*

PELAYO CORREA, M.D.
> Professor of Pathology, Lousiana State University Medical Center; Attending Staff, Charity Hospital of New Orleans, New Orleans, Louisiana
> *Stomach*

JOHN D. CRISSMAN, M.D.
> Professor of Pathology, School of Medicine, Wayne State University; Director of Anatomic Pathology, Harper-Grace Hospitals, Detroit, Michigan
> *Upper Aerodigestive Tract*

ANTONIO L. CUBILLA, M.D.
> Professor of Pathology, Facultad de Ciencias Médicas, National University of Asunción; Chairman, Director of Pathology, Instituto Nacional del Cáncer, Asunción, Paraguay
> *Pancreas*

RONALD A. DeLELLIS, M.D.
> Professor of Pathology, Tufts University School of Medicine; Pathologist, New England Medical Center, Boston, Massachusetts
> *Multisystem Neuroendocrine Neoplasms*

KATHERINE DeSCHRYVER-KECSKEMETI, M.D.

Associate Professor of Pathology, Washington University Medical School; Associate Pathologist, Barnes Hospital, St. Louis, Missouri
Small Intestine; Large Intestine

MICHAEL J. DROLLER, M.D.

Professor and Chairman, Department of Urology, Mount Sinai Medical Center; Chairman, Department of Urology, Mount Sinai Hospital, New York; Consultant in Urology, Bronx Veterans Administration Hospital, Bronx; Acting Director, Urology, City Hospital Center, at Elmhurst, New York
Prostate Gland

PATRICK J. FITZGERALD, M.D.

Visiting Professor, Department of Pathology, Cornell University Medical College, New York, New York
Pancreas

GILBERT H. FRIEDELL, M.D.

Professor of Pathology and Director, Lucille Parker Markey Cancer Center, University of Kentucky, Lexington, Kentucky
Urinary Bladder

EDWIN GOULD, M.D.

Assistant Professor, Department of Pathology, University of Miami School of Medicine and Jackson Memorial Medical Center, Miami, Florida
Breast

PHILIP M. GRIMLEY, M.D.

Professor, Department of Pathology, F. Edward Hébert School of Medicine, Uniformed Services University of the Health Sciences, Bethesda, Maryland
Multisystem Neuroendocrine Neoplasms

ILEANA R. HAWKINS, M.D.

Chief, Department of Pathology, Alaska Native Medical Center, Anchorage, Alaska
Urinary Bladder

DONALD EARL HENSON, M.D.

Program Director, Community Oncology and Rehabilitation Branch, Division of Cancer Prevention and Control, National Cancer Institute, Bethesda, Maryland
Introduction; Gallbladder and Extrahepatic Bile Ducts

ELAINE S. JAFFE, M.D.

Chief, Hematopathology Section, Laboratory of Pathology, and Deputy Chief, Laboratory of Pathology, National Cancer Institute, Bethesda, Maryland
Lymphoid System

A. B. JENSON, M.D.

Associate Professor, Georgetown University Schools of Medicine and Dentistry; Staff Pathologist, Georgetown University Hospital, Washington, D.C.
Uterine Cervix

ROBERT J. KURMAN, M.D.

Associate Professor of Pathology and Obstetrics and Gynecology, Georgetown University Schools of Medicine and Dentistry, Washington, D.C.
Endometrium

KAROLY LAPIS, M.D.

Director, Institute of Pathology and Experimental Cancer Research, Semmelweis Medical University, Budapest, Hungary; former Fogarty Scholar in Residence, National Cancer Institute, Bethesda, Maryland
Liver

AZORIDES R. MORALES, M.D.

Professor and Chairman, Department of Pathology, University of Miami School of Medicine; Chief, Pathology Services, University of Miami Jackson Memorial Medical Center, Miami, Florida
Breast

GEORGE K. NAGY, M.D.

Pathologist, St. Vincent Hospital, Worcester, Massachusetts
Urinary Bladder

HENRY J. NORRIS, M.D.

Chairman, Department of Gynecologic and Breast Pathology, Armed Forces Institute of Pathology, Washington, D.C.
Endometrium

JUAN E. OLVERA-RABIELA, M.D.

Professor of Pathology, National University of Mexico, School of Medicine; Chief, Autopsy Service, General Hospital of Mexico City, Mexico, D.F., Mexico
Central Nervous System

BRUCE D. RAGSDALE, M.D.

Associate Professor of Pathology, Georgetown University Schools of Medicine and Dentistry; Surgical Pathologist, Georgetown University Hospital, Washington, D.C.
Bone

DANIEL J. SANTA CRUZ, M.D.

Associate Professor of Pathology, Washington University School of Medicine; Associate Pathologist, Barnes Hospital, St. Louis, Missouri
Skin

ZSUZSA SCHAFF, M.D.

Associate Professor of Pathology, Institute of Pathology and Experimental Cancer Research, Semmelweis Medical University, Budapest, Hungary; former Eleanor Roosevelt Fellow, International Union Against Cancer, at Hepatitis Branch, Food and Drug Administration, Bethesda, Maryland
Liver

ROBERT E. SCULLY, M.D.

Professor of Pathology at the Massachusets General Hospital, Harvard Medical School; Pathologist, Massachusetts General Hospital, Boston, Massachusetts
Ovary; Testis

DONALD E. SWEET, M.D.
> Chairman, Department of Orthopedic Pathology, Armed Forces Institute of Pathology, Washington, D.C.
> *Bone*

MYRON TANNENBAUM, M.D., Ph.D.
> Professor of Pathology and Professor of Urology, Mount Sinai Medical School; Attending Pathologist, Mount Sinai Hospital; Chief of Surgical Pathology and Cytopathology, Bronx Veterans Administration Hospital, New York, New York
> *Prostate Gland*

LEWIS B. WOOLNER, M.D., C.M.
> Professor of Pathology (Emeritus), Mayo Medical School and Mayo Clinic, Rochester, Minnesota
> *Lung*

Preface

The fact that many malignant tumors have a morphologically recognizable precursor lesion has important implications for the diagnosis and control of cancer. Because these lesions usually do not cause symptoms, their presence is often unsuspected clinically. Early diagnosis, however, is important because it provides the best opportunity for cure. As a result, efforts to find these lesions by screening, by careful examination of individuals known to be at high risk, and by sophisticated diagnostic techniques are reasonable. Already, pathologists seem to sense that the number of early lesions has increased. Unfortunately, a lack of experience with these lesions and a lack of uniform histologic criteria for the precursors in many organs can make diagnostic interpretation difficult. Even after a diagnosis has been made, problems may remain because in many cases therapeutic strategies are empiricial and even controversial.

It seems evident that physicians need a better understanding of the early phases of neoplasia both in humans and in experimental animals to provide optimal treatment and patient care. So far, experimental models for the study of early cancer have not provided sufficient data that pathologists can use to solve the diagnostic problems caused by these lesions in humans.

As long as the etiology of human malignant neoplasms remains unknown and effective preventive measures continue to be unavailable, the most practical method of reducing morbidity and mortality will be the detection of early lesions. It is therefore reasonable to assume that in the future more early cancers will be discovered and treated. Pathologists and clinicians should be prepared to meet this increase.

In this book, we have attempted to bring together the information available on the clinicopathologic features of early lesions in most human tissues and organs. Needless to say, because the field is broad and controversial, such a task cannot be accomplished by only one person. We have asked highly qualified pathologists who have had an interest in these lesions to summarize their knowledge and experience. It is our hope that pathologists, oncologists, and all physicians interested in the diagnosis, natural history, and treatment of the early stages of cancer will find this book useful and stimulating.

DONALD EARL HENSON, M.D.

JORGE ALBORES-SAAVEDRA, M.D.

DEDICATION

To all residents with whom we have worked
and shared knowledge and friendship.

D.E.H.
J.A.-S.

Contents

DONALD EARL HENSON
JORGE ALBORES-SAAVEDRA

1 Introduction

As new methods for the early detection of cancer are developed, especially for screening, it seems reasonable to expect that many lesions will be found that surgeons will biopsy. Thus, in the future, pathologists will be called on to deal more with the early or incipient lesions of invasive cancer. These lesions, which traditionally have included hyperplasia, metaplasia, various forms of dysplasia, and carcinoma-in-situ, have always presented diagnostic problems. They occur not only along epithelial surfaces, such as in the breast and uterine cervix, but also as complications of other lesions, such as polyps, benign tumors, and even chronic inflammatory conditions (Riddell, 1976). Conversely, some lesions, such as papillomatosis of the bile ducts, which histologically show complex papillary patterns, are often difficult to separate from papillary carcinomas. Other lesions—for instance, the epithelial atypia of repair, which is entirely benign—may be confused with in-situ cancer histologically.

In this book, the term "incipient" refers to the earliest stages of malignant neoplastic transformation that are visible with the light microscope. The definition therefore considers all lesions that are thought to be possible precursors of invasive cancer. These lesions are all included because with our present knowledge it is uncertain at which stage the neoplastic change is reached or at what point it is no longer reversible (Bajardi, 1984). Although most pathologists would probably agree that these lesions follow the sequence of hyperplasia to dysplasia to carcinoma-in-situ to invasive carcinoma, there is evidence that not all lesions complete the sequence and that some may even reverse direction with the result that the epithelial surface returns to its normal appearance. Furthermore, with some malignant tumors, the sequence may not start with hyperplasia but instead follow the routes of adenoma to carcinoma-in-situ to invasive carcinoma or dysplasia to invasive carcinoma. Regardless of the sequence, the same problems continue to confront pathologists in the histologic interpretation of these lesions.

In humans, our knowledge about the pathology of malignant tumors is largely based on the invasive forms of cancer. Less is known about the early or preclinical stages of tumor development. Most of our information about early cancer is limited to those sites in which the preclinical stages can be detected by laboratory means, such as cytology. The most thoroughly studied precursor lesions are those found in the uterine cervix, although other sites are also coming under study (Deschner, 1982; Albores-Saavedra et al., 1984). The situation, however, has become more complex, even in the well-studied sites. For example, recent work on papilloma virus, which is discussed in the chapter on the uterine cervix, indicates that these agents may also have an influence on the histology of early lesions.

Furthermore, questions arise about the nature of these early lesions—questions that do not always apply to the corresponding invasive cancers. These questions include the morphologic and biochemical determinants of progression, regression, dormancy, invasiveness, and so forth, all of which have a bearing on treatment and prognosis. Invasive cancers ordinarily do not regress, but the factors that preclude invasion in the early or incipient lesions are unknown. All pathologists have seen atypical hyperplastic lesions in the breast, but with our present knowledge we cannot predict with confidence the future growth potential or invasive capacity of such lesions. In some sites, especially the uterine cervix, the chance of regression inversely correlates with the extent of the histologic abnormality. Indeed, our experience seems to tell us that dysplastic lesions, compared with in-situ-carcinomas, are more apt to regress or at least not progress to invasive cancer. Again, however, the comparison is not always clear because dysplasias often form a continuum, and the more severe forms of dysplasia may be biologically equivalent to in-situ carcinoma.

For some sites, such as soft tissues, brain, and salivary glands, the precursors of malignant tumors are practically unknown. In other sites, embryonal rests may play an important role as precursors. For

1

example, Wilms' tumors seem to arise from hamartomatous remnants in the kidney (Bove and McAdams, 1976). In fact, the kidney appears to be one of the few organs in which embryonal rests have been morphologicaly documented to give rise to malignant tumors.

Also falling into this area of incipient neoplasia is the concept of minimal cancer. Introduced originally for small breast cancers less than 0.5 cm, this concept nonetheless expresses some uncertainty about the behavior and treatment of small cancers and in-situ lesions. In the liver, small cancers less than 4 cm in size are referred to as "minute." In the lung, certain small neoplasms are designated as "tumorlets." The term "minimal" as applied to small carcinomas can be vague and even misleading because it can refer to either size or behavior. It would be ideal to replace vague terms with more precise terminology that clearly refers to the biologic potential and not to appearance, size, or other characteristics. For example, some cancers of the skin can reach large size and never metastasize. In this regard, these cancers are also minimal, at least from a biologic point of view.

In practice, many diagnostic terms have been used for these early lesions. Often conveying a mixture of descriptive and prognostic meanings, these terms include "benign atypical hyperplasia," "mild or severe dysplasia," "epithelial atypias," "borderline changes," "grade one-half carcinoma," "intraepithelial neoplasia," and "minimal cancer." Most of these terms simply express our inability to relate the morphologic change to the biologic potential. However, they all reflect some concern on the part of pathologists about the future growth of these lesions and their danger for the patient. There is lack of agreement not only about the meaning and interpretation of existing terminology but also about new definitions, which can lead to confusion as well. For example, the term "dysplasia" as used in cases of inflammatory bowel disease has recently been defined as an unequivocal neoplastic alteration of the colonic epithelium (Riddell et al., 1983).

Although it would be helpful to have a uniform nomenclature for all precursor lesions, it is apparent to us that the terminology is too complex. For instance, the same term may have different meanings for different sites. Furthermore, in some organs, such as the kidney and liver, many traditional terms, such as "carcinoma-in-situ," cannot be applied as in some of the other sites. Moreover, the precursor lesions of many tumors have not been described. In some sites—for example, breast—the terminology is so variable that a pathologist who attempts to describe the precursor lesions becomes so bogged down in definitions and in the infinite interpretations of previous work that he or she can never really approach the description. Perhaps the terminology of some breast lesions should be defined in terms of the risk for subsequent cancer arising in the breast.

Furthermore, the time that is required to complete the sequence of hyperplasia to invasive cancer is variable. In some patients, lesions seem to take years to progress, whereas in others only a short time is needed. In fact, the full sequence may not even be evident morphologically, and for some lesions the evidence supporting the full sequence is weak. We all have seen invasive cancers arising directly from histologically normal epithelium. Further, it is well documented that early carcinoma can be superimposed on atypical epithelial proliferations. This is seen, for example, in solar keratosis of the skin and with atypical lesions of the mucous membranes.

It is possible that the two sequences—hyperplasia to invasive cancer and adenoma to invasive cancer—are only the morphologic signs of a multistep process that is required for neoplastic development. Reasons for such a process do not rest on histologic observations but on studies of chemical carcinogenesis from which the concept of tumor initiation and promotion developed. Based on results in laboratory animals, we can only assume that in humans tumor initiation also occurs before the histologic changes are evident. In contrast, hyperplasia and dysplasia may be regarded as the visible signs of promotion. In fact, it has been suggested that the terminology of premalignant lesions should be based on the multistep theory of carcinogenesis (Rywlin, 1984).

One purpose of this book, in addition to providing guidance for pathologists, is to foster development of generalized concepts for the sequential stages that must occur prior to the start of invasive cancer. Because early lesions are found along many epithelial surfaces, certain changes common to all sites must occur that signal invasion. These could include the production of specific embryonic substances, extent of dedifferentiation, extent of heterogeneity, antigenic variation, and other changes.

Above all, it is important that we determine whether the sequence is a stepwise discontinuous process or a smooth continuum because this will influence our concepts of progression. At the morphologic level, many of these lesions form a continuum, which is why it is so difficult for pathologists to separate benign lesions from malignant ones. It is also important to know, especially for therapeutic purposes, whether the ultimate biologic potential is predetermined in the incipient lesion, or whether it unfolds over time owing to chance or random processes. If the incipient lesion is cancer from the beginning, this information must be taken into account in any therapeutic strategy. Correct diagnosis and proper treatment of these precursor lesions should reduce the prevalence of invasive cancer.

Because it is not possible in many cases to predict whether these incipient lesions will actually complete the sequence, these lesions as a group are often considered potential precursors for invasive cancer. In fact, it is often on the basis of this potential alone, rather than on solid histologic criteria, that pathologists often advise surgeons about treatment and follow-up.

In recent years, pathologists have recognized that these lesions are often multifocal, which is important for the design of treatment and even follow-up strategies. Furthermore, the fact that these lesions are multifocal supports the concept of the field theory of cancer, which we studied in our pathology courses. We can only assume, however, that multifocal tumors result from a common carcinogenic stimulus. In fact, we suggest that pathologists, in dealing with early lesions, also think in terms of field changes as well as in terms of limited or focal changes. Pathologists should bear in mind that precursor lesions are often found in the vicinity of malignant tumors, especially those of epithelial origin. For example, one of the more recent and important contributions to our understanding of the origin of germ cell tumors was achieved by a careful study of testes removed from patients with minimally invasive lesions. Intratubular germ cell neoplasia, which is found in a high proportion of testes with invasive cancer, is now considered to be a true precursor lesion.

In some sites, metaplasia seems to presage cancer. For example, intestinal metaplasia often precedes invasive cancer of the stomach. Although metaplasia is often considered to be a response to injury, its position in the sequence is uncertain. Nonetheless, metaplasia, at least in some sites, is regarded as a precancerous lesion. In fact, it may even influence the histologic type of invasive cancer. In the gallbladder, for instance, intestinal metaplasia is thought to give rise to intestinal-type carcinomas, and in the uterine cervix and the lung, squamous metaplasia can give rise to squamous cell carcinomas. As pathologists, we are often led to the conclusion, based on experience, that metaplastic epithelium is more susceptible to malignant transformation than is normal epithelium.

In general, the histologic type of cancer does not reflect the etiology. Although some etiologic agents, such as vinyl chloride, are associated with distinct histologic types, in this case angiosarcomas of the liver, it is not possible to infer the etiology from the histology of the tumor. In fact, a single carcinogen, such as ionizing radiation, may give rise to a wide variety of malignant tumors. However, it seems reasonable to conclude that the rate of progression from hyperplasia to invasive cancer may reflect the intensity of the neoplastic stimulus or the susceptibility of the tissue to neoplastic development. The stronger the stimulus, the faster the progression; the weaker the stimulus, the slower the progression (Foulds, 1969).

Even though the terms "dysplasia" and "carcinoma-in-situ" refer to changes occurring along surface epithelium, analogous changes that precede neoplasia probably occur in non-epithelial sites, such as lymph nodes and soft tissues. Little is known, however, about these changes. It seems reasonable to assume that every cancer has its own precancer. Presumably, the lesions in the non-epithelial sites also follow a similar sequence from hyperplasia to early cancer. For instance, in the chapter on early bone tumors, the concept of sarcoma-in-situ is introduced, which is analogous to the concept of carcinoma-in-situ. In soft tissue, chronic lymphedema may lead to the proliferation of small lymphatic channels, which in turn may progress to lymphangiosarcoma. In some cases, the precursor turns out to be a benign tumor. For example, some adenocarcinomas of the colon originate from papillary adenomas. In the chapter on soft-tissue tumors, neurofibromatosis, a condition that may give rise to malignant schwannomas, is discussed in detail. Chondrosarcomas have been known to arise in benign cartilaginous tumors.

In animals, early lesions have been studied, especially those occurring in the liver during experimental carcinogenesis. These animal studies have focused on hepatocellular changes in enzyme content, ability to take up iron, and histologic staining variations. However, we can only presume that the early changes seen in animals also occur in humans. Nonetheless, in the liver in humans, dysplasia seems to be an important premalignant change, as it is in other sites.

In addition to morphology, there are other differences between precancerous lesions and the corresponding invasive tumors. Precancerous lesions are often multiple and may occupy wide areas of the surface mucosa, especially in hollow organs such as the urinary bladder and gallbladder. Although no statistical data are available, these lesions seem to be more common than invasive cancers. In Gardner's syndrome, for instance, the colon contains hundreds of polyps, but only one or, at the most, several evolve into invasive cancer, although given time, all may progress to malignancy. In the skin, pigmented nevi are certainly more common than malignant melanomas. For these reasons, incipient lesions, wherever they occur, often seem to represent a separate disease category, distinct from the invasive forms of cancer. As suggested in the chapter on the uterine cervix, the incipient lesions may represent a heterogeneous group of diseases, of which only some are precancerous.

Important contributions to our understanding of the histology of early lesions have come from studies on genetically determined cancers. Usually inherited as an autosomal dominant character, these cancers have largely been identified through the work of epidemiologists who have followed families, often for many generations, in which there is a high prevalence of malignant tumors. Surveillance of these families and biopsy of suspicious lesions have provided the opportunity for pathologists to observe many malignant tumors in their early or incipient stages. C cell hyperplasia, the precursor lesion for genetically determined medullary carcinoma, was first recognized by a study of thyroid glands removed from patients at high risk for this tumor (Wolfe et al., 1973). These asymptomatic patients had only elevated levels of serum calcitonin, which prompted surgeons to perform prophylactic thryoidectomies. Hyperplasia of the adrenal medulla, the precursor of pheochromocytoma, was described in patients with the multiple endocrine neoplasia syndrome Type II and is now considered the earliest recognizable morphologic abnormality in the adrenal gland of these patients. Pheochromocytomas may only represent extreme degrees of nodular hyperplasia of the adrenal medulla (DeLellis et al., 1976). Other genetically determined lesions—for instance familial polyposis coli, the dysplastic nevus syndrome, Wilms' tumor, and von Recklinghausen's neurofibromatosis—have been studied and characterized by pathologists.

Heterogeneity is considered a property of malignant neoplastic cells, but to what extent heterogeneity occurs in the precursor or early lesions remains to be determined. Most studies on heterogeneity have been done on the invasive forms of cancer (Henson, 1982; Hand et al., 1983; Albino et al., 1981). However, the extent of heterogeneity may prove a better marker for early neoplasia than histologic appearance. In this regard, efforts to phenotype these incipient lesions more precisely are needed.

From a clinical perspective, these early lesions can have consequences that go beyond the everyday work of diagnostic pathologists. These lesions involve treatment regimens that include extent of surgery, medicolegal controversies, and the cost of patient care, including that of follow-up, as well as occupational cancer and early exposure to carcinogens. Space limitation does not allow us to discuss these issues in detail. In practical terms, though, knowledge of the biology and extent of these lesions clearly relates to the question of whether the cancer can be treated by local means alone, such as limited resection, or whether it requires extensive, mutilating surgery.

The purpose of this book is to describe these early lesions and to provide criteria for their progression and their differential diagnosis. Most likely, problems of diagnosis will remain until histologic markers are found that correlate with progression. In the meantime, pathologists, as consultants in patient management, must still provide some estimate about the natural history of these lesions and their propensity for invasion, based on traditional staining and histologic criteria.

The chapters in this book are not all uniform or comprehensive, but of necessity they reflect the interests, experience, and concerns of the authors as well as the amount of information available for each site.

Nonetheless, it is through such diversity that these incipient lesions will eventually be approached as a whole. Although this book is primarily designed to call attention to these early lesions, it contains other information that we believe is important for pathologists—for instance what information the pathologist should convey in tissue reports and what additional clinical data the pathologist should specifically request from the surgeon or primary physician about the patient after the lesion has been examined.

Finally, we want to acknowledge the work of all the contributors and to thank them for their time and creative efforts. This book is essentially their collective work.

References

Albino, A. P., Lloyd, O. K., Houghton, A. N., Oettgen, H. F., Old, L. J.: Heterogeneity in surface antigen and glycoprotein expression of cell lines derived from different melanoma metastases of the same patient. J. Exp. Med. 154:1764–1778, 1981.

Albores-Saavedra, J., Angeles-Angeles, A., Manrique, J. J., Henson, D. E.: Carcinoma in situ of the gallbladder. A clinicopathologic study of 18 cases. Am. J. Surg. Pathol. 8:323–333, 1984.

Bajardi, F.: Histogenesis of spontaneous regression of cervical intraepithelial neoplasias. Cancer 54:616–619, 1984.

Bove, K. E. and McAdams, J.: The Nephroblastomatosis Complex and Its Relationship to Wilms' Tumor: A Clinicopathologic Treatise. In Rosenberg, H. S., Bolande, R. P. (eds.): Perspectives in Pediatric Pathology. Vol. 3. Chicago, Year Book Medical Publishers, 1976, pp. 185–223.

DeLellis, R. A., Wolfe, H. J., Gagel, R. F., Feldman, Z. T., Miller, H. H., Gang, D. L., Reichlin, S.: Adrenal medullary hyperplasia. Am. J. Pathol. 83:177–196, 1976.

Deschner, E. E.: Early proliferative changes in gastrointestinal neoplasia. Am. J. Gastroenterol. 77:207–211, 1982.

Foulds, L.: Neoplastic Development. London, Academic Press, 1969.

Hand, H. P., Nuti, M., Colcher, D., Schlom, J.: Definition of antigenic heterogeneity and modulation among human mammary carcinoma cell populations using monoclonal antibodies to tumor-associated antigens. Can. Res. 43:728–735, 1983.

Henson, D. E.: Heterogeneity in tumors (editorial). Arch. Pathol. Lab. Med. 106:597–598, 1982.

Riddell, R. H.: The precarcinomatous phase of ulcerative colitis. Curr. Top. Pathol. 63:179–219, 1976.

Riddell, R. H., Goldman, H., Ransohoff, D. F., et al.: Dysplasia in inflammatory bowel disease. Standardized classification with provisional clinical applications. Hum. Pathol. 14:931–968, 1983.

Rywlin, A. M.: Terminology of premalignant lesions in light of the multistep theory of carcinogenesis. Hum. Pathol. 15:806–807, 1984.

Wolfe, H. J., Melvin, K. E. W., Cervi-Skinner, S. J., Al Saadi, A. A., Juliar, J. F., Jackson, C. E., Tashjian, A. H., Jr.: C-Cell hyperplasia preceding medullary thyroid carcinoma. N. Engl. J. Med. 289:437–441, 1973.

2 Skin

The skin is a very complex structure composed of the epidermis, adnexal structures, and dermis. It is a highly differentiated tissue that is ideally suited to its function as a protective barrier between humans and their environment.

The epidermis is composed of at least four well-documented cell types. They exist in a perfectly balanced symbiotic relationship. Keratinocytes of ectodermal origin and melanocytes of neuroectodermal origin are found, as well as Langerhans cells, which are probably of mesodermal origin, and the still mysterious Merkel cells. A population of wandering cells foreign to the epidermis is also present.

A wide variety of hyperplastic, benign, and malignant growths occur in the epidermis. Owing to the great frequency of these lesions and the ease with which they can be sampled, a very complex nomenclature has been developed The entire concept of cutaneous neoplasia, however, rests on a paucity of knowledge regarding the biologic potential of the morphologic lesions described. This has occurred in part because complete study of a lesion requires excision and precludes study of its natural history. Scientific conclusions with respect to the biologic potential of preinvasive lesions are further hampered by descriptive terms such as "carcinoma-in-situ," "dysplasia," and "dystrophy," which are not uniformly defined.

For the sake of simplicity, this chapter reviews current dermatopathologic concepts and terminology regarding cutaneous neoplasia in light of the fact that some of these terms are controversial and may be inexact. The serious limitations in concepts and terms are emphasized. It is hoped that the long overdue consensus in standardization of nomenclature can be reached in the near future.

Lesions of Keratinocytes

The biology of malignant lesions of cutaneous keratinocytes is poorly understood. Little is known about the sequence of events from the oncogenic transformation of a keratinocyte to the development of invasive properties, or metastatic potential. These intraepidermal lesions are described with names that imply age ("senile keratosis"), etiology ("solar keratosis" "actinic keratosis," "erythema ab igne," "arsenical keratosis"), or biologic potential ("carcinoma-in-situ"). Whether they have similar or different abilities to become invasive is unknown, as is their individual malignant potential.

It has been widely believed that these lesions go through a sequence, starting from a few atypical cells and eventually filling the epidermis (carcinoma-in-situ, intraepidermal neoplasia). It is, however, widely known that actinic keratosis does not need to follow this progression to become invasive. Some actinic keratoses have only basal cell layer atypia yet are associated with early dermal invasion. Bowen's disease, however, is rarely seen in association with dermal invasion, despite the full-thickness epidermal atypia that is characteristic of this lesion.

Extrapolation of concepts regarding other visceral sites such as the uterine cervix has further complicated our understanding of these skin lesions. In fact, the natural history of these morphologically similar lesions may be quite different. One positive trend in gynecologic pathology, however, has been the introduction of the concept of intraepithelial neoplasia (IEN) to replace carcinoma in situ (Crum, 1982).

Both terms "dysplasia" and "dystrophy" have been applied to the changes that often precede the development of IEN. "Dysplasia" is a misnomer for preneoplasia, although it is widely used. At times it is wrongly used interchangeably with the term "atypia." For example, the term "cellular dysplasia" is sometimes incorrectly used to describe "cellular atypia." However, the word "dysplasia" has a well-established place in medical nomenclature used to indicate faulty growth: renal dysplasia, ectodermal dysplasia.

The word "dystrophy" later replaced dysplasia" to

describe those otherwise unclassified lesions of the vulva that exhibited disorderly growth. Although the change was justified in view of the highly confusing lexicon, the terminology was not accurate. The word "dystrophy" already has an established meaning for conditions such as muscular dystrophies.

Although the concept of "vulvar dystrophies" has proved popular among gynecologic pathologists, parallel between this group of conditions and equivalent cutaneous disorders cannot be drawn (New nomenclature for vulvar disease, 1978).

The problems in cutaneous pathology are compounded by the fact that the same precursor lesions can give rise to very different types of lesions. Actinic keratoses can evolve into squamous cell carcinomas, basal cell carcinomas, and keratoacanthomas, tumors with clearly different biologic behavior. However, the same lesion can originate from different precursors. Squamous cell carcinoma originates from actinic keratosis, Bowen's disease, arsenical keratosis, epidermodysplasia verruciformis, and other lesions.

Although the etiology and evolutionary sequence of keratinocytic tumors are not well known, several conditions could serve as models that may help investigators solve this puzzling problem. Epidermodysplasia verruciformis is being used as a model for the study of viral carcinogenesis (Lutzner, 1978; Jablonska et al., 1979; Yabe et al., 1978). Xeroderma pigmentosum offers researchers a unique possibility to study the effect of tumor induction by light (Clendenning, 1971). The nevoid basal cell carcinoma syndrome could provide clues to the role of genetics in the development of basal cell carcinoma (Howell, 1984).

The definition of neoplasia has been based on several criteria, including the irreversibility of tumor growth. This concept is weak because "premalignant" lesions may become stable and progress no further. In addition, inflammatory changes can produce involution and even disappearance of neoplastic growths, as can be seen in carcinoma-in-situ and basal cell carcinomas. Interestingly, the lack of evolution of some "premalignant" lesions into invasive carcinoma has been used as a proof that these conditions are not always classifiable as malignant precursors. Using this logic, one could not consider an aborted first trimester fetus a pregnancy because it did not result in the live birth of a child! It is therefore undeniable that in some early neoplastic growths the malignant "neoplasia-to-be" may suffer host responses that abort its biologic potential without denying its real identity as a true early neoplastic growth. The issue raised, however, is whether the cellular and histologic changes used to diagnose these conditions are reliable indicators of such potential or actually reflect nonspecific cellular changes.

Because of these issues, few terms are more difficult to define than "premalignant." Is a premalignant condition benign but invariably destined to become a malignant neoplasm? Will transformation occur always, often, or sometimes? Is "premalignant" really synonymous with "preinvasive"?

In this chapter, premalignant lesion" will be defined as a benign condition that is often associated with the development of malignant tumors. "Preinvasive conditions" are those tumors that share most of the cytologic features of malignant neoplasms but are circumscribed to the epithelium and are therefore non-invasive.

The concept of "microinvasion" is also a very difficult one. Most tumors of the epidermis grow both exophytically and endophytically, regardless of whether they are benign or malignant. The penetration of the dermis by keratoacanthomas is deep, reaching to the lower portions of the reticular dermis, yet the tumor is considered benign.

Superficial basal cell carcinomas do not invade beyond the superficial dermis, have wide epidermal contact, and may be best interpreted as basal cell carcinomas-in-situ (Fig. 2–1). This concept, however, is often not clinically appreciated, so these tumors are treated like other variants of basal cell carcinoma.

We define "microinvasive epidermal tumors" on the basis of three criteria: These neoplasms have penetrated beyond superficial (papillary) dermis, they have independent nests of tumor cells detached from the surface component, and the keratinization process becomes independent of surface keratinization (Fig. 2–2).

Despite these criteria, the evaluation of early invasion often remains a personal, subjective matter (Jones, 1984). Fortunately, early invasive epidermal neoplasms behave in a "benign" fashion. Complete excision is curative most of the time, and metastatic spread from cutaneous microinvasive squamous cell carcinomas is extremely rare.

A review of common epidermal neoplasms that emphasizes pathologic findings follows.

ACTINIC KERATOSIS (SENILE KERATOSIS, SOLAR KERATOSIS)

This very common lesion has multiple morphologic variations. It can be defined most simply as a circumscribed growth of cytologically atypical keratinocytes with associated changes in the keratinization process.

Several morphologic variations of actinic keratosis are described (Woringer, 1961). In the "atrophic" form, the epidermis is thin and limited to three or four cell layers. The basal cells are replaced by continuous single layers of atypical keratinocytes that are interrupted only by the entrance of adnexal structures in the epidermis. The "acantholytic" form has similar features. In addition, the neoplastic cells of this variant have a pronounced lack of cohesiveness among themselves, with the adjacent normal keratinocytes forming large "clefts" and lacunae in which rounded, acan-

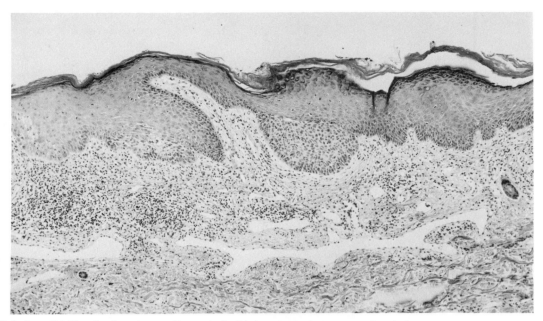

Figure 2–1. Superficial basal cell carcinoma. Conceptually this is an in-situ lesion, since the whole tumor is connected to the epidermis.

tholytic cells appear (Carapeto and Garcia Perez, 1974).

Some forms of actinic keratosis may display a massive keratin layer that appears clinically as a cutaneous horn. These variants are known as *hyperplastic* or *hyperkeratotic actinic keratoses* (Fig. 2–3). The keratinization pattern contrasts with that of the adnexal structures, giving the keratin a vertical alter-

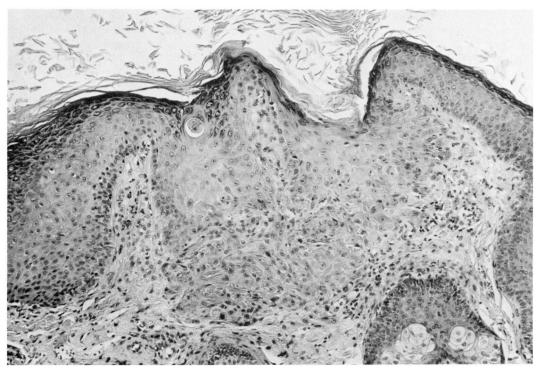

Figure 2–2. Microinvasive squamous cell carcinoma. Although the mass of the tumor cells is anatomically within the epidermal domain, the lower part of the lesion is beginning to invade the dermis.

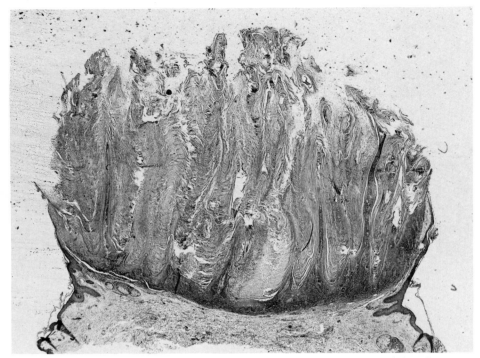

Figure 2–3. Hypertrophic actinic keratosis. There is a large keratin build-up. The lesion presented clinically as a cutaneous horn.

nation of parakeratosis from the actinic epidermis and orthokeratosis from the adnexa (Figs. 2–4 and 2–5). Occasionally, cellular atypism is not impressive, and the epidermis may have a general pallor and an associated parakeratotic surface keratinization. The diagnosis becomes evident only when the actinic epidermis is compared with surrounding normal epidermis or the merging of adnexal structures. A more pronounced, full-thickness cellular atypia with marked dyskeratosis and atypical mitoses can be seen in the form known as "bowenoid actinic keratosis." Its distinction from Bowen's disease is extremely difficult and probably meaningless because differences in biological behavior do not appear significant.

An interesting variant that causes clinical confusion is the "spreading pigmented actinic keratoses." They appear clinically as heavily pigmented macular lesions. Histologically, a proliferation of atypical keratinocytes

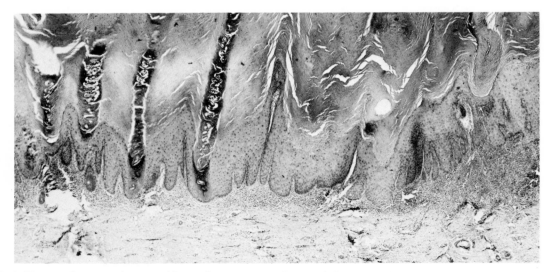

Figure 2–4. Hypertrophic actinic keratosis. Massive keratinization with vertical alternation of ortho- and parakeratosis, corresponding to normal adnexal and deranged epidermal keratinization, respectively.

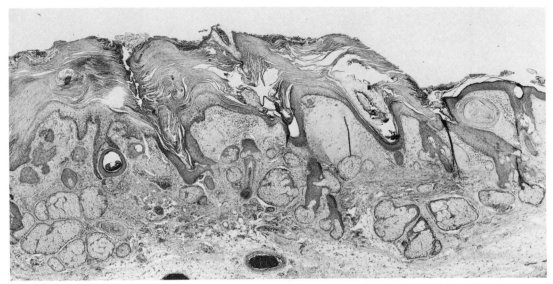

Figure 2–5. Hypertrophic actinic keratosis. Changes are similar to those in Figure 2–4 in hair-bearing skin. Note the sharp right lateral margin of the lesion.

and heavily pigmented dendritic melanocytes is seen (James et al., 1978). An unusual variant of actinic keratosis is the "epidermolytic" form. Epidermolytic hyperkeratosis is a typical histologic change characterized by vacuolar changes of keratinocytes at the upper spinous and granular layers with coarse keratohyalin granules and compact hyperkeratosis. These changes are found in a variety of non-neoplastic conditions. Of course, epidermolytic actinic keratosis has the associated atypical cytologic changes required for the diagnosis of actinic keratosis in addition to the epidermolytic changes (Ackerman and Reed, 1973).

A very curious variant is "lichenoid actinic keratosis." This lesion presents with, in addition to the typical epidermal changes, a dense band-like infiltrate in the dermis that penetrates and obscures the dermal-

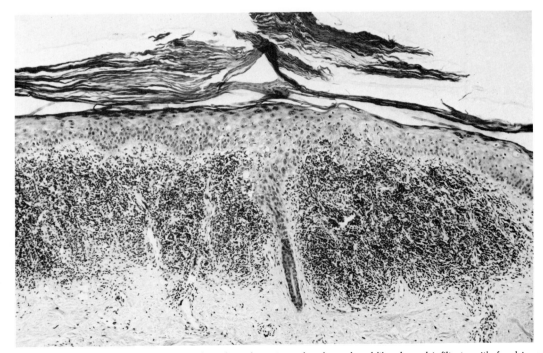

Figure 2–6. Lichenoid actinic keratosis. Pronounced epidermal atypia and a dense band-like dermal infiltrate with focal invasion of the epidermis.

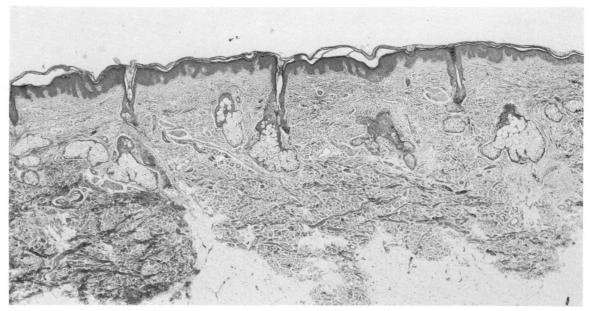

Figure 2–7. Large cell acanthoma. The entire lesion is excised and is very inconspicuous.

epidermal junction (Fig. 2–6). The basal keratinocytes show marked cytoplasmic vacuolization. This lesion can easily be mistaken for an inflammatory condition rather than being diagnosed as a true neoplastic process of keratinocytes (Hirsch and Marmelzat, 1967; Tan and Marks, 1982).

It is not clear whether these morphologic variants have different biologic potential. It is tempting to assume that their invasive potential correlates with the degree of cytologic atypia. Based on our experience, this assumption is not necessarily correct. Controlled clinical pathological studies are needed to evaluate this point.

LARGE CELL ACANTHOMA

This curious cutaneous lesion was described by Pinkus in 1969. It appears clinically as a macular light tan to dark brown lesion on sun-exposed skin, usually the forehead. Histologically, the epidermal changes vary from atrophic to acanthotic, although verrucous changes also can be seen. The basal layer often is hyperpigmented, and the rete ridges may show a rounded contour. The cytology of the keratinocytes initially appears unremarkable (Fig. 2–7), but careful examination reveals that the keratinocytes are much larger than usual, with both nuclei and cytoplasm being enlarged (Fig. 2–8). This abnormality becomes more evident when the keratinocytes of this lesion are compared with those of adjacent normal epidermis or with the smaller adnexal keratinocytes (Fig. 2–9). There is no cellular atypism, but photocytometry shows that the nuclei are hyperploid (Fand and

Pinkus, 1970). Although this lesion appears benign it has been classified as one of the keratinocytic dysplasias (Rahbari and Pinkus, 1978).

CARCINOMA-IN-SITU

Few topics in pathology are as controversial as carcinoma-in-situ. Authors disagree on the terminology, definitions, and biologic behavior of this lesion. Numerous terms coined to replace "carcinoma-in-situ" have failed to accomplish a unifying effect: They have been enthusiastically adopted by some and rejected by others. The term "intraepithelial neoplasia" may be the most appropriate replacement but is not yet widely accepted (Crum, 1982; Callen and Headington, 1980).

The nomenclature and concept of progressive cellular atypia leading to invasive carcinoma were first developed for certain tumors of the uterine cervix and then extrapolated to legions of other epithelia. Two important problems appeared as this concept was applied to other organs:

1. The progression from mild atypia to severe atypia to carcinoma-in-situ to invasive carcinomas has been challenged owing to insubstantial evidence of the "inevitable," required steps.

2. Lesions with similar histologic changes behave differently in different parts of the body. It is clear that an actinic keratosis may become invasive after having only one single layer of atypical keratinocytes. Conversely, Bowen's disease, which has all the features of carcinoma-in-situ, seldom becomes invasive. The mucosal counterpart in the glans penis and vulva is

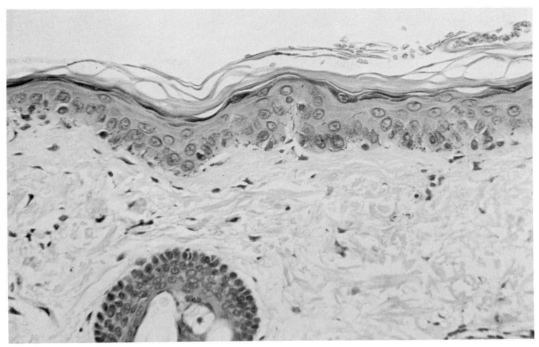

Figure 2–8. Large cell acanthoma. Large keratinocytes which appear unremarkable at first glance. Compare their size with the adnexal keratinocytes in the hair follicle.

associated with more aggressive behavior, as are other carcinomas-in-situ that are located in mucosal sites adjacent to the skin (Degos et al., 1976). In a 1978 report, Smith challenged the whole concept of carcinoma-in-situ and judged the histologic diagnosis as non-specific and unverifiable. However, in 1979 Ackerman defended the diagnosis of carcinoma-in-situ as a histological entity.

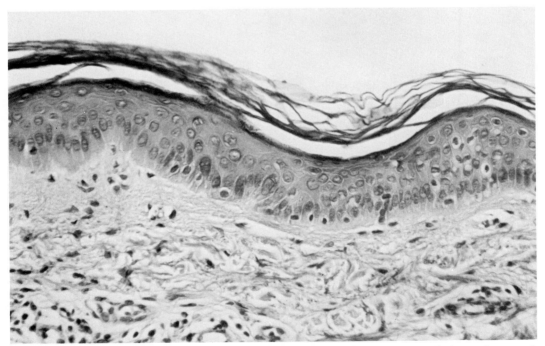

Figure 2–9. Large cell acanthoma. Edge of the lesion. The larger keratinocytes on the left contrast with the smaller normal ones to the right.

If "carcinoma-in-situ" is defined as full-thickness keratinocytic atypia, quite a few entities with different natural history, etiology, and biologic behavior can be identified with this term.

The most characteristic is Bowen's disease. The term "Bowen's disease" is usually used as a synonym of carcinoma-in-situ, but it more precisely describes a particular clinical presentation of a large erythematous plaque that is often located on the trunk. Similar lesions located on the vulva, glans penis, and oral cavity have been known as "erythroplasia." Chronic ingestion of arsenic may produce histologic changes that are indistinguishable from those of Bowen's disease. Most "leukoplakias" of mucosal lining are simply hyperkeratosis. Occasionally, carcinoma-in-situ may have similar keratin build-up and present as a white lesion (leukoplakia). Some forms of actinic keratosis may have extensive cellular atypism throughout the thickness of the lesion. Those variants are known as "bowenoid actinic keratosis." Although they might be histologically identical with other carcinomas-in-situ, their clinical presentation is different from that of Bowen's disease.

Perhaps one of the most fascinating entities of this group is the so-called "bowenoid papulosis" (Wade et al., 1978; Ulbright et al., 1982). These are often multiple papular lesions located in the anogenital area. They clinically resemble condyloma acuminata but have all the histologic features of carcinoma-in-situ.

Until recently, none of the lesions of bowenoid papulosis has been reported to become invasive, and, in fact, some lesions have regressed spontaneously. Papillomavirus common antigens have been demonstrated in 13 of 18 cases studied by Penneys and coworkers in 1984.

The histologic changes of carcinoma-in-situ vary greatly. A single histologic description will not accurately reflect its morphologic spectrum (Strayer and Santa Cruz, 1980). The general aspect of the epidermis varies from atrophic (Fig. 2–10), to acanthotic (Fig. 2–11), to frankly verrucous (Fig. 2–12). Although by definition carcinoma-in-situ requires full-thickness keratinocytic atypism, few lesions have a distinct intraepidermal nesting pattern of atypical keratinocytes separated by septa of normal keratinocytes (Fig. 2–13).

The cytology shows a high degree of cellular and nuclear variation, numerous mitotic figures (many of them atypical), and abundant apoptosis (dyskeratosis). Some lesions, however, show a regular cytologic appearance that is not striking at first glance. The diagnosis can be made on the basis of lack of upward maturation, cytologic atypia, and high-level mitoses with associated apoptosis. Some lesions of carcinoma-in-situ, especially those in dark-skinned individuals, show varying degrees of melanin pigmentation. In some cases, the melanin is limited to the basal layer of the epidermis; in others, numerous pigmented

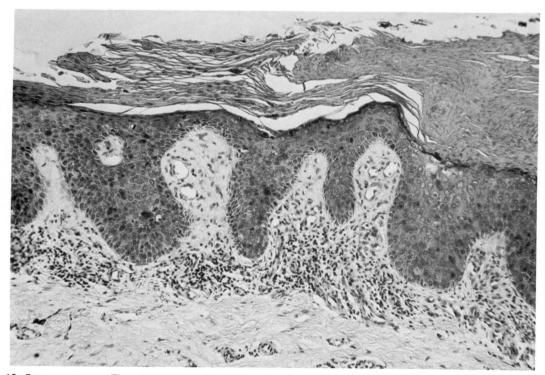

Figure 2–10. Carcinoma-in-situ. There is pronounced full-thickness epidermal atypia. However, the maturation process is preserved with presence of granular layer and orthokeratotic horny layer. Vascular proliferation and an inflammatory infiltrate are present in the dermis.

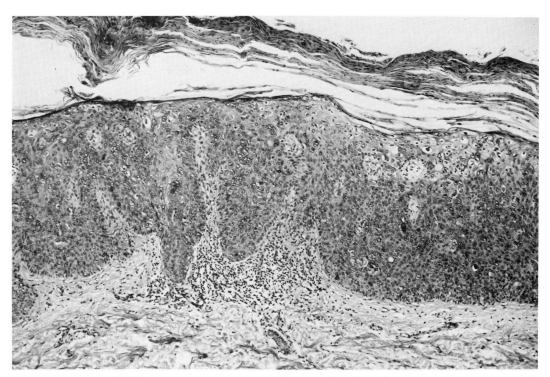

Figure 2–11. Carcinoma-in-situ. Highly atypical cytologic features with giant multinucleated keratinocytes and parakeratotic horny layer.

dendritic melanocytes are present through the epidermis.

The stromal reaction to carcinoma-in-situ varies from nothing at all to dense lymphocytic infiltrates with intense lichenoid features. Occasionally, the stromal reaction produces partial regression of the lesion. Under some carcinomas-in-situ there is a dense vascular proliferation that is almost hemangiomatous. Amyloid globules can be seen in the dermal papilla in some cases (Fig. 2–14). Some lesions of carcinoma-in-situ may have adnexal differentiation (Fulling et al., 1981).

The histology of bowenoid papulosis, although essentially identical to that of regular carcinoma-in-situ, may have some unique features. The general architecture of the lesion is of a localized acanthosis similar to condylomata. In fact, some lesions of bowenoid papulosis share the benign cytologic features of condyloma and the atypism of carcinoma-in-situ in the same lesion (Fig. 2–15). Although there is widespread cytologic atypism in bowenoid papulosis, the lesion has a more uniform appearance, and the low-power view has a "salt and pepper" look given by the dark nuclei and clear vacuolar changes of the keratinocytes. The involvement of pilosebaceous units characteristic of carcinoma-in-situ is absent in bowenoid papulosis. These histologic changes—in addition to the papular, multicentric clinical presentation—allow one to make the correct diagnosis most of the time.

NEVOID BASAL CELL CARCINOMA SYNDROME (NBCCS)

The NBCCS is an autosomal, dominantly inherited disorder characterized by development of multiple basal cell carcinomas early in life. The syndrome is also characterized by palmar and plantar pits, jaw cysts, ovarian tumors, fibrosarcoma of the jaws, medulloblastomas, and other developmental abnormalities and tumors.

The syndrome is an ideal model for genetically induced basal cell carcinomas and allows the study of the development of this tumor from early stages. The penetrance of the gene is 97 percent, and approximately 75 percent of the patients experience early onset of carcinomas. The palmar pits are believed to be basal cell carcinomas-in-situ from which invasive basal cell carcinomas rarely develop (Howell, 1984).

EPIDERMODYSPLASIA VERRUCIFORMIS (EV)

Epidermodysplasia verruciformis is a disorder characterized by multiple flat warts that often appear in the first decade of life. Many of these warts undergo progressive malignant transformation, developing into squamous cell carcinomas.

Carcinomatous transformation occurs in 34 percent of the patients studied (Lutzner, 1978). Cancer may

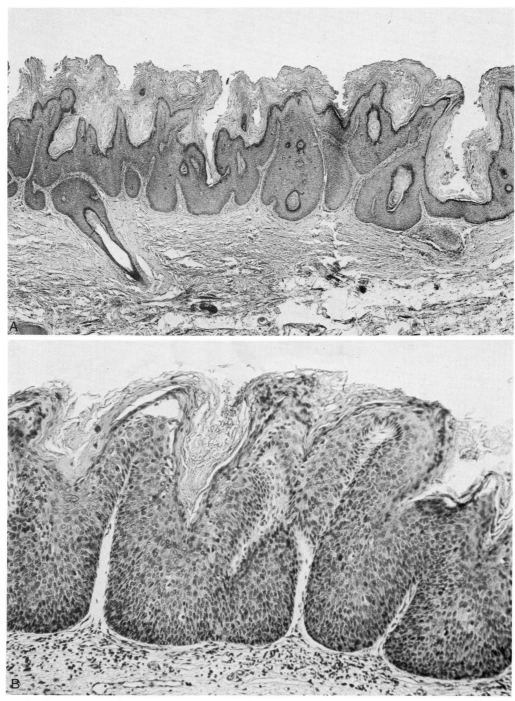

Figure 2–12. *A,* Carcinoma-in-situ. Note the verrucous pattern with preserved granular layer and orthokeratosis. *B,* Uniform atypism, lack of upward keratinocytic maturation, and high-level mitoses.

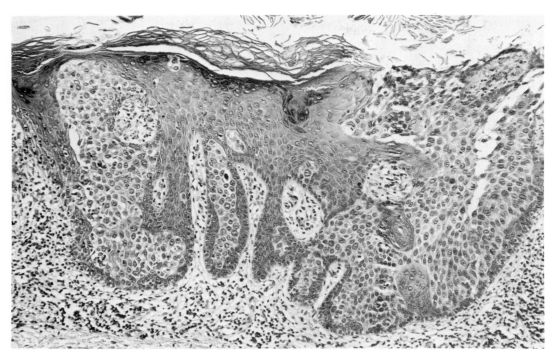

Figure 2–13. Carcinoma-in-situ. Nests of atypical cells are separated by septa of normal intervening epidermis.

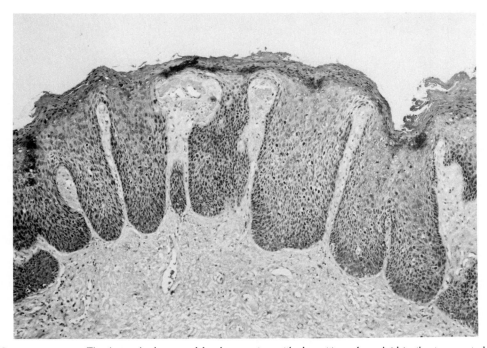

Figure 2–14. Carcinoma-in-situ. This lesion had areas of focal regression with deposition of amyloid in the two central dermal papillae. This amyloid material stained positively with antikeratin antibodies and represents involuted tumor keratinocytes.

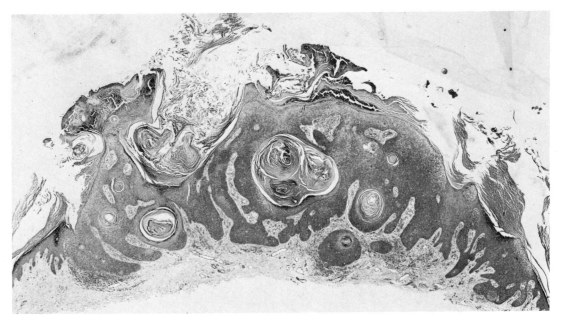

Figure 2–15. Bowenoid papulosis. The general architectural appearance of a condyloma with widespread keratinocytic atypia is characteristic of this condition.

appear in patients as young as 13 years of age, although the average age of onset is 31 years.

The pattern of genetic inheritance is uncertain. An autosomal recessive trait has been suggested by authors who have identified the lesion as a familial disorder (Lutzner, 1978). There may be regression of lesions in epidermodysplasia verruciformis (Jablonska et al., 1979).

Histologically, the verrucous growths undergo progressive transformation of the cell architecture, with faulty maturation and development of atypical cytologic changes.

The virus belongs to the human papillomavirus (HPV) group and is very similar to the common wart virus. The etiologic agent has been identified as HPV3 or HPV4. Malignancy has developed in only one family, whose members were infected with HPV4 (Jablonska et al., 1979). The virus has been identified in both benign and malignant lesions (Lutzner, 1978; Yabe et al., 1978).

References

Ackerman, A. B.: Carcinoma in situ. Hum. Pathol. 10:127–128, 1979.

Ackerman, A. B. and Reed, R. J.: Epidermolytic variant of solar keratosis. Arch. Dermatol. 107:104–106, 1973.

Callen, J. P., and Headington, J. T.: Bowen's and non-Bowen's squamous intraepidermal neoplasia of the skin. Arch. Dermatol. 116:422–426, 1980.

Carapeto, F. J. and Garcia Perez, A.: Acantholytic keratosis. Dermatologica 148:233–239, 1974.

Clendenning, W. E.: Xeroderma pigmentosum. Dermatology. In

Fitzpatrick, T. B., Arndt, K. A., Clark, W. H., et al. (eds.): General Medicine. McGraw Hill, New York, 1971.

Crum, C. P.: Vulvar intraepithelial neoplasia: The concept and its application. Hum. Pathol. 13:187–189, 1982.

Degos, R., Civatte, J., Belaich, S., et al.: Maladie de bowen cutanée ou muqueuse. Ann. Dermatol. Syph. 103:5–14, 1976.

Fand, S. B. and Pinkus, H.: Polypoidy in benign epidermal neoplasia. J. Cell Biol. 47:59A, 1970.

Fulling, K. H., Strayer, D. S., Santa Cruz, D. J.: Adnexal metaplasia in carcinoma in situ of the skin. J. Cut. Pathol. 8:79–88, 1981.

Hirsch, P. and Marmelzat, W. L.: Lichenoid actinic keratosis. Dermatol. Internatl. 6:101, 1967.

Howell, J. B.: Nevoid basal cell carcinoma syndrome. Profile of genetic and environmental factors in oncogenesis. J. Am. Acad. Dermatol. 11:98–104, 1984.

Jablonska, S., Orth, G., Jarzabek-Chorzelska, M., et al.: Twenty-one years of follow-up studies of familial epidermodysplasia verruciformis. Dermatologica 158:309–327, 1979.

James, M. P., Wells, G. C., Whimster, L. W.: Spreading pigmented actinic keratoses. Br. J. Dermatol. 98:373–379, 1978.

Jones, R. E., Jr.: Questions to the editorial board and other authorities. Am. J. Dermatopathol. 6:301–306, 1984.

Lutzner, M. A.: Epidermodysplasia verruciformis. An autosmal recessive disease characterized by viral warts and skin cancer. A model for viral oncogenesis. Bull. Cancer 65:169–182, 1978.

New nomenclature for vulvar disease. Int. J. Gynaecol. Obstet. 13:237–239, 1978.

Penneys, N. S., Mogollon, R. J., Nadji, M., et al.: Papilloma virus common antigens. Papillomavirus antigen in verruca benign papillomatous lesions, trichilemmoma, and bowenoid papulosis: An immunoperoxidase study. Arch. Dermatol. 120:859–861, 1984.

Pinkus, H.: Epidermal mosaic in benign and precancerous neoplasia (with special reference to large cell acanthoma). Acta Dermatol. 64, 65:53–59, 1969–1970.

Rahbari, H. and Pinkus, H.: Large cell acanthoma. One of the actinic keratoses. Arch. Dermatol. 114:49–52, 1978.

Smith, C.: Carcinoma in situ. Hum. Pathol. 9:373–374, 1978.

Strayer, D. S. and Santa Cruz, D. J.: Carcinoma in situ of the skin: A review of histopathology. J. Cut. Pathol. 7:244–259, 1980.

Tan, C. Y. and Marks, R.: Lichenoid solar keratosis prevalence and immunologic findings. J. Invest. Dermatol. 79:365–367, 1982.

Ulbright, T. M., Stehman, F. B., Roth, L. M., et al.: Bowenoid dysplasia of the vulva. Cancer 50:2910–2919, 1982.

Wade, T. R., Kopf, A. W., Ackerman, A. B.: Bowenoid papulosis of the penis. Cancer 42:1890–1903, 1978.

Woringer, F.: De la kératose sénile à l'épithélioma. Dermatologica 122:349–359, 1961.

Yabe, Y, Yasui, M., Yoshino, N., et al.: Epidermodysplasia verruciformis: Viral practicles in early malignant lesions. J. Invest. Dermatol. 71:225–228, 1978.

Lesions of Melanocytes

In the past, little was known about malignant melanoma except that it was characterized by distinctive brownish-black tumors located on the skin and that it had a progressive, fatal course. There has been, however, a tremendous increase in the awareness and understanding of this lesion since the 1960s. Early lesions have been increasingly recognized in the macular stage, and the precursor lesions are now more clearly defined. Epidemiologic studies have emphasized the role of genetics, sun exposure, and other factors related to the development of melanoma. As knowledge accumulates, however, the clinician and the pathologist are under more pressure to classify patients appropriately so that the prognosis can be determined and proper treatment initiated (Kopf, Rodriguez-Sains, Rigel, et al., 1982). Early detection and treatment of small melanomas have resulted in a dramatic decrease in mortality from this disease, and the reputation of melanomas as an invariably fatal neoplasm is fading.

Several methods are available for the classification of malignant melanomas. Clark and coworkers have created the modern rational basis for understanding the natural history of melanomas (Clark et al., 1969). Their concept of melanoma subtypes, as defined by radial and vertical growth phase, includes lentigo maligna, superficial spreading melanoma, and nodular melanomas. This has been challenged by Ackerman, who suggests that these "different" types are actually morphologic variants of the same disease (Ackerman, 1980). Another step forward was represented by the development of a microstaging system that allowed the treating physician to compare therapeutic modalities rationally and to offer more precise prognostic information. Popularized by Clark, the level system staged primary lesions of melanoma in progressive "levels of invasion." It considered cutaneous anatomic structures as points of reference. Level I melanoma is entirely confined to the epidermis, whereas Level V invades deeply into subcutaneous fat. Intermediary dermal levels are classified as Levels II to IV (Clark et al., 1959). Breslow more recently developed a simple system in which the depth of invasion is measured through the eyepiece of the microscope and expressed in millimeters (Breslow, 1970, 1980). Because it was soon realized that this microstaging system was a more powerful predictor of prognosis than Clark's system, the latter is seldom used today (Balch et al., 1978).

MELANOCYTIC HYPERPLASIAS AND DYSPLASIAS

The progression from an innocent-looking melanocytic lesion to an aggressive melanoma has not been properly documented. There is, however, abundant indirect evidence suggesting that malignant melanomas often evolve from precursor lesions. These precursor lesions lie at the dermal-epidermal junction, where the vast majority of melanomas originate. The rare melanomas that begin in the dermis are not considered here.

Normal melanocytes are interspersed in the basal layer of the epidermis over the entire cutaneous surface and are also seen in some mucosal linings. They are rather inconspicuous and are characterized by a clear perinuclear halo. Their primary function is to produce melanin. Nevi and other neoplasms of melanocytes are common and are recognized by their coloration, which is imparted by this pigment. However, not every clinically or histologically pigmented lesion is a pure lesion of melanocytes. In fact, many non-melanocytic conditions have an increased number of melanocytes in addition to the proliferating keratinocytes. Examples include lentigo senilis, seborrheic keratosis, actinic keratosis, Bowen's disease, large cell acanthoma, basal cell carcinoma, and squamous cell carcinoma. None of these diseases is associated with malignant proliferation of melanocytes, although clinically they all can pose differential diagnostic problems with true melanocytic lesions.

The word "lentigo" is applied to lesions that are clinically flat and hyperpigmented. Lentigo simplex, the simplest pigmented lesion, is a localized hyperpigmentation of the epidermal basal layer, not necessarily accompanied by melanocytic proliferation. The other lesions that will be discussed are grouped as "melanocytic hyperplasias" and are by definition accompanied by a proliferation of melanocytes.

Two morphologically distinct types of melanocytic proliferations are recognized histologically: lentiginous and epithelioid. There is a range of findings between the two ends of this spectrum, although some authors believe that there are enough differences to constitute two distinct, parallel systems: melanocytic (lentiginous proliferations) and nevocytic (epithelioid proliferations) (Mishima, 1960; Mishima and Matsunaka, 1975). All these lesions can also be classified by their degree and amount of cellular atypia.

LENTIGINOUS MELANOCYTIC HYPERPLASIA

Clinically, lentiginous melanocytic hyperplasia presents as a heavily pigmented macule. The histopathologic correlate of this lesion must be defined by both cytologic and growth-pattern criteria. Histologically, the melanocytes are rather inconspicuous, with small pyknotic nuclei surrounded by scant cytoplasm and with prominent artifactual perinuclear halos. The cells are arranged along the basal layer in the fashion of a "picket fence." The melanocytes are often spindle-shaped or dendritic with long emissions of cytoplasm that arborize through the lower half of the epidermis. Pigment production is abundant, but most is found in the dendritic projections and adjacent keratinocytes. Occasionally, overabundant production of pigment "drops" into the dermis and is captured by numerous macrophages. This appearance may be confused with early dermal invasion by melanocytes. The coarseness of the intracytoplasmic pigment will, however, differentiate macrophages from intradermal melanocytes.

In early stages, the melanocytic proliferation is very unimpressive, and keratinocytic hyperpigmentation is usually the most notable finding. As the number of melanocytes increases, the lesion becomes more evident, with numerous basal melanocytes demonstrating clear perinuclear halos. Cytologic atypia and mitotic figures are not present. In more advanced proliferations, the melanocytes are arranged in bundles and fascicles of spindle cells disposed along the dermal-epidermal junction parallel to the epidermal surface. The epidermis generally remains little changed. However, the epidermis is relatively thin in lentiginous hyperplasias of the face, commonly seen in elderly patients. Also, in acral areas, the epidermis may be slightly acanthotic. Hyperplastic melanocytes may grow around adnexal structures, especially hair follicles, but do not extend beyond the confines of the superficial dermis.

Lentiginous hyperplasias commonly occur on sun-exposed parts of the body, namely, the face, neck, scalp, and external parts of the arms. This is also the typical growth pattern of melanocytic hyperplasias and dysplasias of the oral cavity, vagina, glans penis, anus, and visceral sites such as the esophagus. When located on the lip, these lentiginous hyperplasias are termed "oral melanotic macules." They are usually asymptomatic and measure 2 to 3 mm in diameter. These lesions are seen with increasing frequency with age and are especially common in blacks. The macules of the Peutz-Jeghers syndrome cannot be distinguished histologically from the isolated oral melanotic macules. Similar lesions presenting on the palms and soles are termed "volar melanotic macules." The dark pigmentation in these lesions causes clinical difficulties in distinguishing benign hyperplasias from early acral lentiginous melanomas. Cytologically benign-appearing lentiginous hyperplasias are sometimes seen in areas adjacent to invasive acral lentigi-

nous melanomas. Whether benign volar lentiginous hyperplasias are in fact premalignant remains to be settled. We have seen rather large lesions on the sole that appear very innocent histologically but that would appear to represent early melanocytic dysplasias because of the patient's age as well as the lesion's size and rapid progression. Small plantar macules that are histologically indistinguishable from these larger lesions are commonly present for long periods of time and appear to have negligible malignant potential, if any.

Similar problems are encountered in macular facial lesions in elderly people. These are very common and are associated with fair skin and with a history of sun exposure. Most of these macules appear similar clinically. Histologically, solar lentigines vary from lentigo simplex to lentigo senilis, large cell acanthomas, pigmented actinic keratoses, and sometimes lentigo maligna.

LENTIGINOUS MELANOCYTIC DYSPLASIAS
(Table 2–1)

The passage from hyperplasia to dysplasia cannot be documented either clinically or histologically with certainty. If hyperplasia and dysplasia represent two distinct processes, they certainly do not differ significantly either histologically or morphologically. A spectrum exists in which histologic features of hyperplasia blend into dysplastic changes. The problems this creates are illustrated by lentigo maligna (Hutchinson's melanotic freckle, Dubreuilh's melanosis circumscripta preblastomatosa). Lentigo maligna frequently appears on the faces of elderly people as a flat, irregularly shaped pigmented macule. The diameter of these macules often exceeds 2 cm. When the entire lesion is examined histologically, it becomes evident that there is a considerable variation in the morphology of melanocytic proliferations. Areas of simple basal cell layer hyperpigmentation alternate with extensive atypical melanocytic proliferation. Whether this represents extremes in a spectrum or a coincidental association is not clear. It does underscore the difficulty of diag-

Table 2–1. Lentiginous (Spindle Cell) Melanocytic Dysplasias

Diffuse melanocytic hyperplasia along epidermal and follicular basal layers
Dendritic melanocytes
Shrinking artifact (melanocytic nuclei surrounded by "lacunae")
Hyperpigmentation of keratinocytes and melanocytes
Atrophy (lentigo maligna) or hypertrophy (acrolentiginous) of rete ridges
Fasciculated, horizontal nests
Variable host response
Mild to moderate cellular atypia

(Reproduced with permission from Brodell, R. T. and Santa Cruz, D. J.: Semin. Diag. Pathol. 2:63–86, 1985.)

nosing large facial macular lesions with small biopsy specimens.

The dysplastic changes in early lentiginous lesions are very subtle. Cytologic atypism is often only mild to moderate. The significant changes are usually of growth pattern rather than of atypical cellular features.

Cytologically, lentiginous dysplasias are characterized by slight to moderate nuclear and cytoplasmic size variation. The nuclei may become more vesicular and often have visible nucleoli, not present in lentiginous hyperplasias. The cells are spindled, with more ample cytoplasm and less tendency to form dendritic emissions. The perinuclear halo is less prominent. The cells have a propensity to form nests that are rounded or fasciculated along the lower layers of the epidermis. Upward migration of melanocytes is infrequent when compared with the epithelioid proliferations and often seen only when a high degree of cellular atypism is present. The stromal reaction is also very sparse or non-existent in early stages of lentiginous dysplasias. This is particularly notable in lentigo maligna, in which moderate to severe melanocytic atypia is sometimes seen with total absence of stromal reaction. Conversely, small lentiginous melanocytic proliferations may display little cytologic atypia with pronounced stromal response.

Stromal reactions in lentiginous melanocytic dysplasias are characterized by fibrosis and a lymphocytic inflammatory infiltrate in the superficial dermis. The fibrosis is found as layers of dense collagenous tissue that follow the lower epidermal contour. This lamellar fibrosis eventually becomes confluent and expands the superficial dermis.

The lymphocytic component is often associated with a mild to moderate vascular proliferation. The inflammatory infiltrate may be seen alone or in addition to dermal fibrosis. Some junctional nevi seen in childhood may have a similar lentiginous pattern of growth with associated lamellar fibrosis. These are normal evolutionary steps in the life history of nevi, but owing to the increased awareness of dysplastic nevi they are often overdiagnosed. These junctional nevi do not have cellular atypism, and the associated stromal reaction does not have an abundant inflammatory component.

Nevi of recent onset in people over 40 years of age are always viewed with suspicion. It must be remembered, however, that regular junctional nevi do occur in all age groups, albeit more rarely in older people.

Lentiginous melanocytic dysplasias can be seen in different clinical contexts.

Facial Lentiginous Melanocytic Dysplasias

These dysplasias of melanocytes are commonly known as "lentigo maligna" or "Hutchinson's mela-

notic freckle" (McGovern et al., 1980; Mishima, 1960). These are often large macular lesions occurring commonly on the face of elderly patients. The histologic changes range from simple melanin hyperpigmentation to melanoma-in-situ. Sometimes, the entire histologic spectrum can be seen in the same lesion. In later stages, areas of regression are seen and lesions may become invasive in a multifocal fashion. When lentigo maligna invades the dermis, it is known as "lentigo meligna melanoma." The invasive portion is often spindle-shaped and occasionally produces an intense desmoplastic reaction that may mask the melanocytic nature of the dermal component (desmoplastic melanoma).

Volar Lentiginous Melanocytic Dysplasias

This lesion occurs on palms, on soles, and in subungual regions (Arrington et al., 1977; Feibleman et al., 1980; Paladugu et al., 1983; Patterson and Helwig, 1980). Although they are morphologically similar to the facial dysplasias, they are modified by local factors. The epidermis, which is naturally thick in these areas, may be truly acanthotic. The dendritic nature of the melanocytes is very evident in volar lesions. Palmar and plantar lesions have a tendency to develop rounded, epithelioid melanocytes in invasive stages in addition to the spindle cell component. In very early stages, the cytologic features of volar lentiginous dysplasias can look deceptively benign. In those cases, the size of the lesion, the time of onset, and the age of the patient play an important role in making the correct diagnosis.

Truncal Lentiginous Melanocytic Dysplasias

These lesions may be found in any site but are most common in the trunk, upper arms, and thighs. They are often smaller than the facial and volar dysplastic lesions, measuring 1 centimeter or less. The natural history of truncal lesions is less well documented than that of facial and volar lesions. Diagnosis is often made after full excision. The presence of lentiginous dysplasia adjacent to invasive melanoma has been noted in more than 20 percent of 225 cases of melanomas, excluding lentigo maligna melanomas (Rhodes et al., 1983). Whether this means that the dysplastic changes are precursors to the melanoma or that these dysplastic changes merely represent the advancing border of the melanoma is not yet clear. Solitary lesions may either appear at the dermal-epidermal junction of pre-existing dermal nevi or appear de novo.

An interesting form of lentiginous melanocytic dysplasia is the pigmented spindle cell nevus, originally described by Reed and coworkers in 1975. This nevus

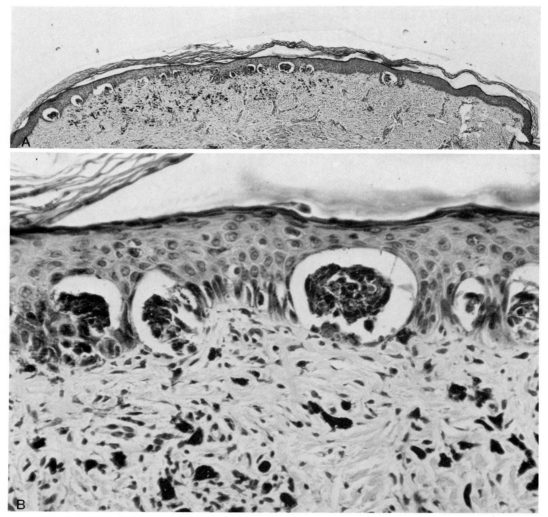

Figure 2–16. Pigmented spindle cell nevus. *A,* Small lesion on the thigh of a 28-year-old woman. *B,* The lesion is composed of rounded nests with scattered single melanocytes intraepidermally. Dermal fibrosis and numerous pigment-loaded macrophages are present.

is found as a heavily pigmented lesion measuring less than 6 mm and is often located on proximal extremities in young adults. In a recent study of 90 patients, 30 patients were men and 60 were women, with an average age of 25 years (Sagebiel et al., 1984). Histologically, pigmented spindle cell nevi present as densely packed, heavily pigmented bundles of spindled melanocytes located in the lower half of the epidermis (Figs. 2–16 to 2–19). The melanocytes have prominent nucleoli, and mitotic figures are rarely seen. There is a variable dermal host response that sometimes may closely resemble the radial growth phase of melanoma (Reed et al., 1975). Conservative complete excision is curative, with no recurrences or metastasis seen in 38 patients followed after surgical excision (Sagebiel et al., 1984). The pigmented spindle cell nevus has many features in common with the nonpigmented spindle and epithelioid cell nevus (Spitz nevus). Although most lesions have rather uniform

cytologic features, some spindle melanocytic dysplasias may present with increasing degrees of cellular atypia (Figs. 2–20 and 2–21).

EPITHELIOID MELANOCYTIC HYPERPLASIA

Although lentiginous hyperplasias are common, pure epithelioid hyperplasias of melanocytes are relatively rare, and most of them fall in the spectrum of epithelioid cell nevus. Epithelioid melanocytes are rounded cells with ample pale cytoplasm and fine "powdery" cytoplasmic melanin. Their nuclei are vesicular with finely dispersed chromatin and prominent nucleoli. The epithelioid melanocytes have a tendency to form nests that are located at the tips of the epidermal rete ridges.

Although benign lesions of epithelioid melanocytes are infrequent, malignant melanomas with epithelioid

Text continued on page 25

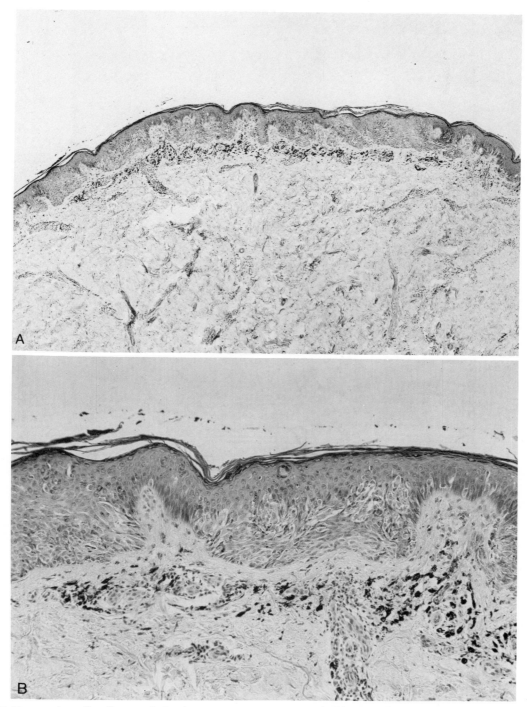

Figure 2–17. Pigmented spindle cell nevus. *A,* Another small lesion on the chest of a 32-year-old man. *B,* Fasciculated bundles of relatively amelanotic melanocytes in the lower half of the epidermis. A sprinkling of lymphocytes and macrophages is present in the dermis.

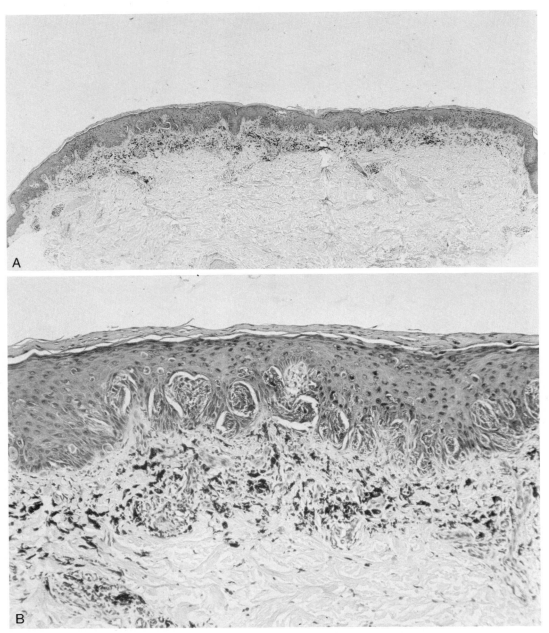

Figure 2–18. Pigmented spindle cell nevus. *A,* A 6-mm pigmented lesion on the shoulder of a 43-year-old man. *B,* Rounded nests of spindle melanocytes with associated intense lymphocytic reaction, vascular proliferation, and dermal macrophages.

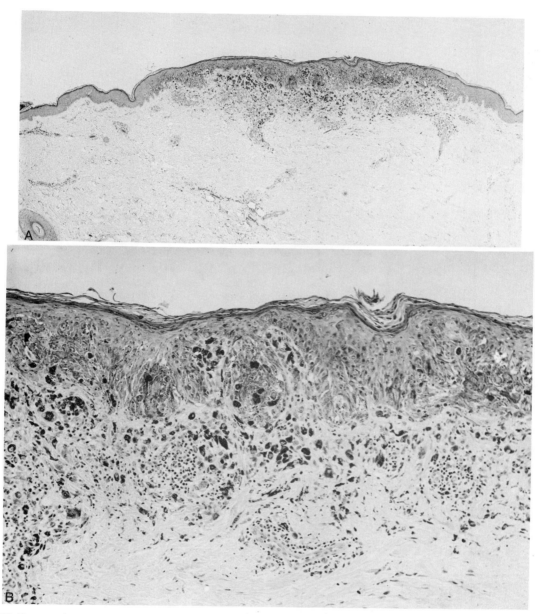

Figure 2–19. Pigmented spindle cell nevus. *A,* An intensely pigmented lesion measuring 4-mm on the thigh of a 38-year-old woman. *B,* Diffuse proliferation of pigmented dendritic melanocytes with dense dermal inflammatory response.

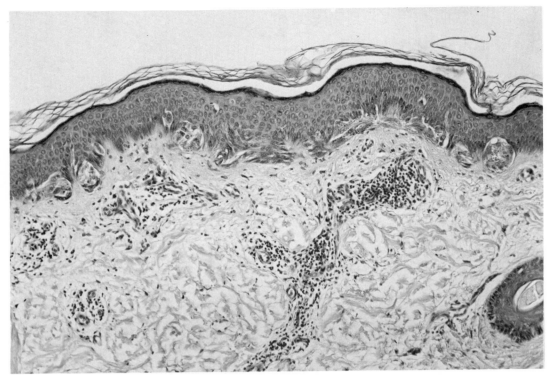

Figure 2–20. Lentiginous melanocytic dysplasia. *A,* A 15-mm lesion on the back of a 45-year-old man. The melanocytes are spindly and arranged in bundles or nests. The inflammatory reaction is perivascular and has no contact with the atypical melanocytes.

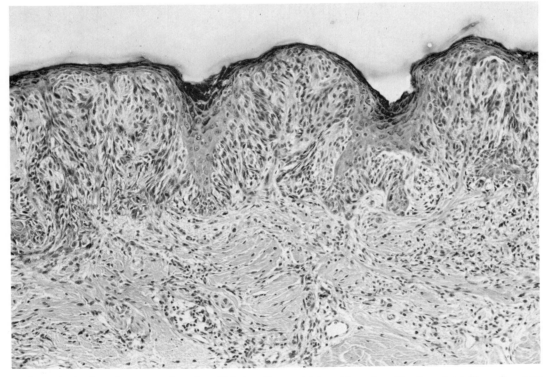

Figure 2–21. Severely dysplastic lentiginous (spindle cell) lesion. Compact intraepidermal proliferation of spindle melanocytes. Note the dermal lamellar fibrosis and inflammatory response.

features are common. Nodular and superficial spreading melanomas are often composed of large rounded melanocytes (Price et al., 1976).

The epithelioid cell nevus is characterized by large, often pleomorphic epithelioid melanocytes. Because of the cytologic features and frequent presence of a lymphocytic stromal response, epithelioid cell nevi pose considerable diagnostic problems to the pathologist, but they do not have any malignant potential.

EPITHELIOID MELANOCYTIC DYSPLASIA
(Table 2–2)

Atypical proliferations of epithelioid melanocytes are seen less commonly than lentiginous dysplasias. They share most of the features of the benign hyperplasias. In addition, pronounced cytologic atypism can be seen in most lesions. The stromal response is often intense, with more lymphocytic component but less mesenchymal reaction than demonstrated by the average lentiginous dysplasia. Epithelioid dysplasias have a tendency to produce a "pagetoid" invasion of the epidermis that in advanced stages has a "buck-shot" appearance. Because of this feature, the diagnosis of melanoma-in-situ is made much more frequently for epithelioid dysplasias than for comparable lentiginous dysplasias.

In some cases, the stromal reaction may have all the morphologic features of the radial growth phase

Table 2–2. Nevocytoid Epithelioid Melanocytic Dysplasias

Rounded epithelioid melanocytes
Pale cytoplasm with "powdery" melanin
Tendency to form rounded nests with random, irregular
  appearance
Brisk host response
Frequent cellular atypia
Single cell invasion of the upper layers of the epidermis

(Reproduced with permission from Brodell, R. T. and Santa Cruz, D. J.: Semin. Diag. Pathol. 2:63–86, 1985.)

of melanoma. Those lesions should be studied very carefully because microinvasion may be present (Fig. 2–22) (Weedon, 1982).

Single atypical epithelioid melanocytes are often associated with lesions that are otherwise classified as "lentiginous dysplasias." This is particularly common in the dysplastic nevus syndrome.

DYSPLASTIC NEVUS

The significance and use of the term "dysplastic" has been discussed elsewhere. The term "dysplastic nevus" has gained wide acceptance and has good practical value. It was first described in the context of a heritable condition in which patients have numerous large moles and a family history of similar lesions resulting in multiple melanomas (Clark et al., 1978:

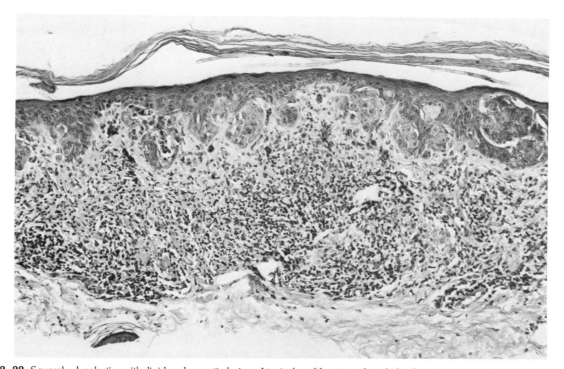

Figure 2–22. Severely dysplastic epithelioid melanocytic lesion. Atypical proliferation of epithelioid melanocytes with a dense lymphocytic reaction.

Elder et al., 1982; Greene and Fraumeni, 1979; Reimer et al., 1978). It was found later that a similar clinical and histologic presentation could be seen in patients without a significant family history (Elder et al., 1980; Rahbari and Mehregan, 1980). Once the histologic and clinical appearances had been defined, the concept of dysplastic nevus was extended to isolated single lesions (Rhodes et al., 1983).

In the definition of dysplastic nevi, Elder and co-workers require a cytologically atypical melanocytic proliferation with lymphocytic host response and fibroplasia (Elder et al., 1982).

Isolated Dysplastic Nevus

The life story of melanocytic nevi suggests that most lesions start as a junctional proliferation of melano-

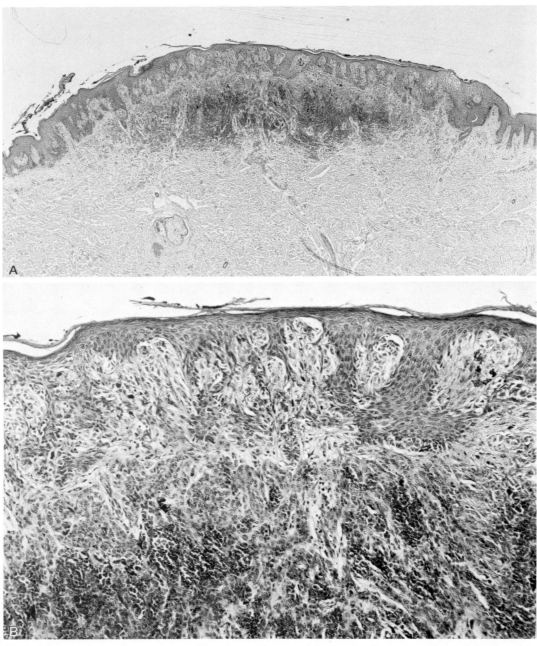

Figure 2–23. A, A longstanding melanocytic nevus. Note the proliferation of the junctional component beyond the dermal aggregates of melanocytes. B, Close-up showing a benign dermal nevus and a densely packed atypical proliferation of spindle melanocytes. Note the absence of stromal reaction.

cytes at a young age (junctional nevus). The junctional melanocytes will eventually "drop" into the superficial dermis, which has both intraepidermal and dermal components (coumpound nevus). Finally, most lesions will evolve into purely dermal nevi by the time an individual is 40 years of age. Because new nevi may develop throughout life, regular nevi in early stages of evolution can be found in persons in their fifties and sixties.

A "new" junctional proliferation of melanocytes may develop later in life in a small number of pre-existing intradermal melanocytic nevi. This proliferation can be either lentiginous or epithelioid (Fig. 2–23). There may be degrees of cellular atypism varying from simple basal cell layer hyperpigmentation (lesions that qualify morphologically as lentigo simplex) to exuberant intraepithelial atypia with brisk host response (melanoma-in-situ). This "new" proliferation is often separated from the pre-existing nevus by the stromal reaction, which consists of fibrosis, vascular proliferation, and a chronic inflammatory infiltrate.

Whether these atypical changes are truly premalignant has not been settled. However, these findings parallel those seen in other dysplastic melanocytic lesions. The fact that a sizable number of melanomas appear to rise in pre-existing nevi suggests a close relationship between dysplastic changes in nevi and the development of melanomas (McGovern, 1983; Rhodes et al., 1983; Sagebiel, 1979).

The pathologic reporting of these isolated dysplastic nevi should be done with utmost care. The number of "isolated" dysplastic nevi that a patient is permitted to have, before being classified as having the dysplastic nevus syndrome, has not been determined (Elder et al., 1982).

Dysplastic Nevus Syndrome

Synonyms and related terms include B-K mole syndrome; familial atypical multiple mole-melanoma syndrome; large atypical mole syndrome, familial and sporadic; nevoid melanoma syndrome; atypical mole-familial melanoma syndrome; and atypical intraepidermal melanocytic hyperplasia.

Patients with dysplastic nevus syndrome present at an early age with melanocytic lesions that vary from few to hundreds. These melanocytic lesions appear mostly during adolescence and continue to occur through life. Individual lesions will enlarge and sometimes undergo dramatic morphologic changes.

Some patients have a family history of similar lesions or history of familial melanomas. This is the so-called "familial dysplastic nevus syndrome" (Clark et al., 1978; Greene and Fraumeni, 1979; Reimer et al., 1978). Recently, it has been determined that sporadic patients may have numerous dysplastic moles and yet lack a family history of similar lesions. This is recognized as the "sporadic dysplastic nevus

Table 2–3. Clinical Features of Dysplastic Nevi

Macular component	
Size:	Larger than 5 mm
Color:	Variable—tan, brown, red
Outline:	Irregular
Number:	Variable—from 10 to more than 200
Distribution:	Trunk, upper limbs, buttocks, groin, scalp, breasts
Time of appearance:	Acquired; lesions start in adolescence and continue to appear in adulthood

(Reproduced with permission from Brodell, R. T. and Santa Cruz, D. J.: Semin. Diag. Pathol. 2:63–86, 1985.)

syndrome" (Elder et al., 1980; Rahbari and Mehregan, 1980).

The familial and sporadic forms of the syndrome have no morphologic differences either clinically or histologically and will be described together.

Clinical Presentation (Table 2–3)

Dysplastic nevi range in number from a few to hundreds in afflicted patients. The lesions are mostly located in the trunk and proximal extremities. They start to appear after puberty, and the patients continue to develop new lesions through their lifetime. Individual lesions also enlarge and change in color and shape.

Although the patients have a wide range of lesions including numerous macular, freckle-like lesions, the typical dysplastic nevus often measures more than 5 mm. The lesions have an irregular outline and variegated pigmentation with tan, brown, or red coloration. Most lesions are macular with preserved skin markings. Some are centrally papular with an irregular macular periphery.

Table 2–4. Histology of Dysplastic Nevi

Common to most lesions
Melanocytic nuclear pleomorphism and hyperchromasia
Perivascular lymphocytic infiltrates
Fibroplasia
Dermal nevus cells

Lentiginous melanocytic dysplasia
Irregular, non-nested basal melanocytes
Prominent cytoplasmic retraction artifact
Dark nuclei
Hyperpigmentation

Epithelioid melanocytic dysplasia
Epithelioid cells with powdery pigment
Vesicular nuclei with prominent nucleoli
Tendency to form nests with size variation and lateral fusion
Intraepidermal multinucleated melanocytes

(Reproduced with permission from Brodell, R. T. and Santa Cruz, D. J.: Semin. Diag. Pathol. 2:63–86, 1985.)

Histology (Table 2–4)

There is a wide range of histologic changes in dysplastic nevi. Small freckle-like macular lesions show very irregular variable basal cell layer pigmentation. Occasionally, prominent melanocytes may be seen. Cellular atypia and stromal reaction are as a rule absent. The larger, typical dysplastic nevi may have small, immature aggregates of dermal melanocytes with little melanin synthesis (Figs. 2–24 to 2–26). Many dysplastic nevi have only a junctional component. This component has two cytologic types, as described before in the discussion of melanocytic dysplasias: lentiginous and epithelioid.

Although all these small lesions belong to the spectrum of dysplastic nevi, features required for the histologic diagnosis of dysplastic nevus are nuclear atypia and lymphocytic and mesenchymal response

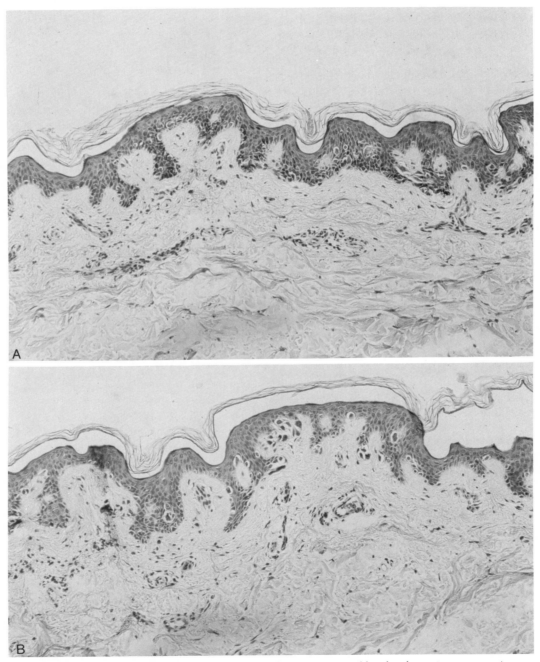

Figure 2–24. *A* and *B*, Dysplastic nevus syndrome. Numerous atypical basal melanocytes are present.

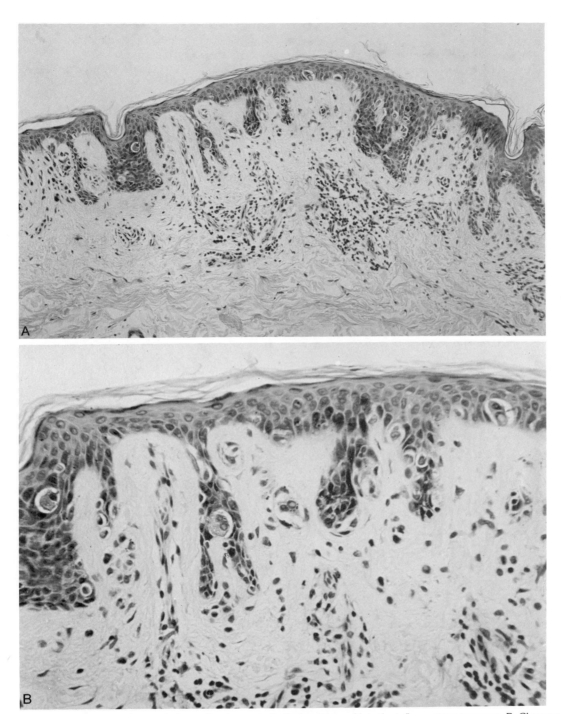

Figure 2–25. Dysplastic nevus syndrome. *A,* Atypical melanocytes in the basal layer. Note the inflammatory response. *B,* Close-up showing the variation of melanocyte sizes.

(Elder et al., 1982). The melanocytes display variable nuclear pleomorphism and hyperchromasia. Histologic sections may show isolated, very atypical melanocytes or clusters, often arranged horizontally between the epidermis and the dermis.

The stromal reaction is very prominent in some lesions as continuous lamellar and eosinophilic fibrosis that wraps around the rete ridges. This fibrosis, unlike normal papillary dermis, produces bright streaks under polarized light. This fibrotic reaction, although a highly characteristic stromal reaction in dysplastic melanocytic lesions, can be seen in other conditions. Some

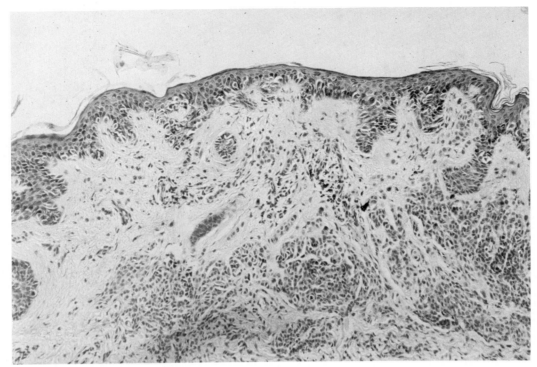

Figure 2–26. Dysplastic nevus syndrome. A dermal nevus has dysplastic junctional changes. Both components are separated by the stromal reaction.

early junctional nevi in childhood and adulthood may have similar changes and may cause the pathologist to misdiagnose this benign condition as dysplastic. Similar stromal reactions may be seen in inflammatory conditions unrelated to melanocytic lesions, such as senescent lichenoid reactions, and in the poikiloderma–parapsoriasis spectrum. This change is also commonly seen as a consequence of chronic rubbing and scratching of the skin.

Some dysplastic nevi may show increasing cytologic atypia, suggesting a progression to melanoma-in-situ. Dermal microinvasion is often very difficult to evaluate owing to the long-term evolutionary changes in the superficial dermis. Indirect evidence of possible microinvasion includes the presence of epidermal changes of melanoma-in-situ or evidence of regression.

EARLY MALIGNANT MELANOMA

Most malignant melanomas start intraepidermally. The sequence of events leading to dermal invasion and the development of a metastatic potential is largely speculative. Most authors agree that it requires a progressive multistep sequence. The major points of disagreement relate to imprecise nomenclature and definitions.

There is abundant indirect information suggesting that many cutaneous melanomas evolve through progressive phases, starting from rather unremarkable precursor lesions. Lesions in each of these phases may remain stable, progress to the next step, or involute (Table 2–5).

Melanocytic tumors are typically stable for long periods or are slowly progressive. Patients often remember a long-standing lesion that started to change only recently. Lesions of lentigo maligna may sometimes be present for more than 20 years with little, if

Table 2–5. **Histogenesis of Melanoma**

Phases of Development	Characteristics
Phase 1: melanocytic hyperplasia	Growth-pattern atypia; no cytologic atypia
Phase 2: melanocytic dysplasia	Atypical melanocytic hyperplasia (cytologic and growth-pattern atypia) Stromal reaction (lamellar fibrosis, vascular proliferation, lymphocytic infiltrate)
Phase 3: melanoma-in-situ	All the features of melanoma except dermal invasion
Phase 4: invasive melanoma	
Phase 5: metastatic melanoma	Satellite lesions Lymph node metastasis Visceral metastasis

(Reproduced with permission from Brodell, R. T. and Santa Cruz, D. J.: Semin. Diag. Pathol. 2:63–86, 1985.)

any, change. Therefore, there is no doubt that melanocytic lesions may be *stable*.

Progression also is well illustrated clinically and histologically. Nearly two thirds of 824 patients with melanoma stated that the tumor arose in a pre-existent skin lesion (Milton, 1972). The same group of researchers studied histologically 723 cases of melanoma with a superficial spreading component; there was evidence that 39 percent originated in a precursor lesion (McGovern et al., 1985). Similarly, Rhodes and coworkers documented that more than 20 percent of patients with melanomas have closely associated dysplastic nevi (Rhodes et al., 1983). Furthermore, cytologic changes may occur concurrently in a melanoma and in other benign nevi found in the same skin region (Tucker et al., 1980). Whether this represents a field effect of a local activating factor or actually multiple "hits" of the carcinogenic stimulus that initiated the melanoma is not clear.

Progression of a melanocytic lesion in the earlier stages is, however, a rare event. From the hundreds of lesions in a patient with dysplastic nevus syndrome, only a few may evolve into malignant melanomas. Similarly, although dysplastic changes in regular nevi are rather frequent, they are rare in relation to the total number of nevi found in these patients.

Atypical melanocytic proliferation is met by a host response characterized by lymphocytic and mesenchymal components. This phenomenon may produce partial or total *regression* of the lesion. Most melanomas have focal areas of regression as part of their evolution. Although partial regression of melanoma is very common, total regression is very rare. Well-documented cases of metastatic cutaneous melanoma with the primary lesion undergoing total regression have been reported (Milton et al., 1967; Smith and Stehlin, 1965). In as many as 4 percent of metastatic melanomas, no primary lesion can be found. A total regression of the cutaneous lesion may explain at least some of these cases.

Whether a significant number of dysplastic and malignant lesions of melanocytes regress without the patient's even being aware of the atypical lesion is not known. The disappearance of a small lesion could easily go unnoticed by the patient. Halo nevi are melanocytic nevi that spontaneously involute. The reason for this specific immunologic attack on a group of nevus cells remains a puzzle. Elucidation of the phenomenon of the halo nevus may explain many aspects of the regressive phenomenon of melanomas.

The inflammatory response may be a biologic "mistake." Alternatively, the nevus may be "confused" with an evolving melanoma because of changes in surface antigens. Although questions remain, the phenomenon of regression of melanomas was usually perceived as a protective defensive event. Studies have not, however, demonstrated any prognostic significance to the presence of regression (McGovern et al., 1980; Trau et al., 1983).

Even though the transformation of a benign melanocytic lesion into a malignant melanoma is not mandatory and is a rare event, many authors have proposed a multistep progressive phenomenon.

Sagebiel proposed the following sequence: The starting event is a proliferation of atypical melanocytes (atypical melanocytic hyperplasia) that is soon met by a host response characterized by superficial dermal fibrosis and chronic inflammatory reaction (atypical melanocytic hyperplasia with host response). The lesion further evolves by early dermal invasion (atypical melanocytic hyperplasia with host response and microinvasion) to acquire all the features of malignant melanoma (Sagebiel, 1979). In his study, the average age at which each of these steps occurred demonstrated a progressive chronologic order (mean incidence 36, 38, and 46 years of age, respectively). Furthermore, the same study showed that the average age for all forms of atypical hyperplasias was 6 years younger than that of a similar group of patients with low-risk melanoma (Sagebiel, 1979).

McGovern proposes similar conceptual ideas on the histogenetic development of melanomas (McGovern, 1983). He divides the process into four phases. The first two are equivalent to Sagebiel's steps. In Phase 3, "the nevus cells cease to resemble nevus cells and acquire the characteristics of melanoma cells." The definition of Phase 3 describes implicitly melanoma-in-situ. Phase 4 corresponds to invasive melanoma.

Interestingly, several authors—including Sagebiel, McGovern, and Reed—allow for dermal invasion at the stage of atypical melanocytic hyperplasia. Many pathologists will comfortably diagnose "atypical hyperplasia" as long as it is totally intraepidermal and use the term interchangeably with "melanoma-in-situ." However, they may hesitate to "undercall" a dysplastic lesion with dermal invasion. Although the histogenetic steps are arguable, there probably is very little, if any, clinical prognostic significance to the distinction. Lesions diagnosed as atypical melanocytic hyperplasia, melanoma-in-situ, and small melanomas with microinvasion will invariably be "cured" by conservative total excision.

A definition of "melanoma-in-situ" is not universally recognized. It is clear that somewhere along the progression of atypical melanocytic proliferations, the cells develop the ability to invade the dermis and develop the metastatic capabilities that are the hallmark of malignant melanoma. Whether this progression happens totally within the confines of the epidermis or requires an interaction with the dermal tissue is not known. Some authors define melanoma-in-situ as a totally intraepidermal lesion (Clark et al., 1975). Ackerman states that melanoma starts as an increased number of relatively normal-appearing single melanocytes in a small focus within the basal layer of the epidermis. The lesion then demonstrates the increasing cytologic atypia followed by a confluence of melanocytes to form nests (Ackerman, 1980).

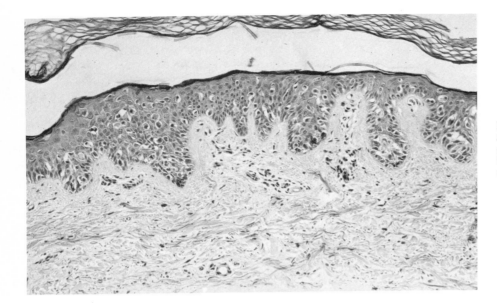

Figure 2–27. Melanoma-in-situ; atypical melanocytes arranged singly throughout the epidermis. Note the absence of an inflammatory reaction.

Weedon reviewed 66 cases diagnosed originally as melanoma-in-situ by multiple sectioning of the blocks. An invasive component was found in eight cases. He also noted that seven of the eight cases had focal areas of regression. None of his patients had recurrences or metastasis after a follow-up of more than 5 years (Weedon, 1982). This study emphasizes the shortcomings of the histologic diagnosis of melanoma-in-situ but does not invalidate the biologic concept (Figs. 2–27 and 2–28).

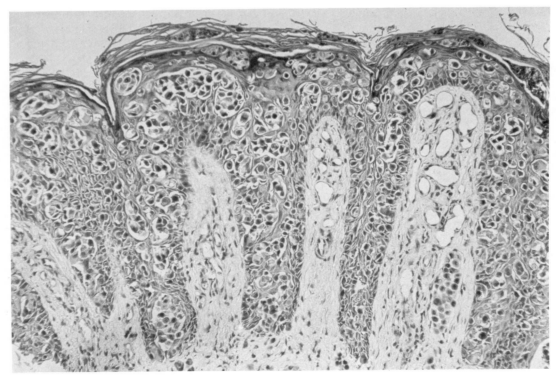

Figure 2–28. Single and nested epithelioid melanocytes throughout the epidermis. The lesion is mostly in-situ, but a focus of dermal invasion is present on the right.

Macular (Radial) and Nodular (Vertical) Growth Phases of Melanomas

Melanomas evolve through two main phases: the macular (radial) growth phase (Table 2–6) and the nodular (vertical) growth phase (Table 2–7). Clark and coworkers defined these concepts in their 1969 landmark study on melanoma and in successive publications. Although these growth phases are extremely useful for explaining the evolutionary steps of melanoma, they have been questioned because of their inaccurate geometric implications. Use of the terms "macular" and "nodular" for radial and vertical could remedy this situation without introducing much of the confusion often produced by new nomenclature.

Macular growth phase represents the early proliferation of malignant melanocytes and the corresponding stromal reaction. Implicitly included in this definition is the ability of the melanocytes to become invasive both upwards in the epidermis and into the superficial dermis. Areas of regression are frequently seen (Clark et al., 1975).

In the macular phase, the proliferation of melanocytes is largely intraepidermal but also incudes early dermal invasion. Single dermal melanocytes are often difficult to appreciate when there is a brisk inflammatory and mesenchymal response (Figs. 2–29 and 2–30). The melanocyte type will often impart to the lesion peculiar clinical, histologic, and biologic properties. Melanomas with macular growth phase composed of epithelioid melanocytes are known as "superficial spreading melanomas" (Clark et al., 1975; Kuhnl-Petzoldt, 1974; Mishima and Matsunaka, 1975; Price et al., 1976). Similarly, those composed of small dendritic or spindly melanocytes are called "lentigo maligna" (McGovern et al., 1980; Mishima, 1960)

Table 2–6. Macular Growth Phase

Poor circumscription of the lesion with lateral extension of atypical melanocytes.
Atypical intraepidermal melanocytic hyperplasia
  Marked variation in size and shape of the nests
  Marked variation in size and shape of melanocytes
  Nuclear atypia
  Mitosis
  Invasion of upper layer of the epidermis
  Invasion of adnexal epithelium
Focal dermal invasion by atypical melanocytes
Absence of vertical maturation of melanocytes
Lamellar and superficial dermal fibrosis
Vascular proliferation
Perivascular lymphocytic infiltrate with lichenoid features
Focal regression (senescent lichenoid reaction)
  Necrosis and degeneration of melanocytes
  Disappearance of tumor cells
  Flattening of rete ridges
  Dermal fibrosis with expansion of papillary dermis
  Melanin-containing dermal macrophages

(Reproduced with permission from Brodell, R. T. and Santa Cruz, D. J.: Semin. Diag. Pathol. 2:63–86, 1985.)

Table 2–7. Nodular Growth Phase

Nodular component in otherwise flat lesion
Pronounced cellular atypia (frequent)
Confluent masses of atypical dermal melanocytes
Absence of vertical maturation
Intralesional transformation
Depression of cellular immune response
Lymphatic and perineural invasion

(Reproduced with permission from Brodell, R. T. and Santa Cruz, D. J.: Semin. Diag. Pathol. 2:63–86, 1985.)

and acral lentiginous melanoma (Arrington et al., 1977; Feibelman et al., 1980; Paladugu et al., 1983; Patterson and Helwig, 1980).

Malignant melanomas without demonstrable macular growth phase are known as "nodular melanomas" (Clark et al., 1975). This is not to say that nodular melanomas did not go through similar evolutionary stages or that they never had a macular growth phase, although this is not apparent at the time the lesions are studied. Although the most valuable prognostic information is obtained from Breslow's measurement, these different types of melanomas have individual features that make them distinct. Intermediate forms do occur but do not invalidate the concepts we have reviewed.

Ackerman has challenged the classification of melanomas based on biologic types defined by differences in the macular (radial) growth phase (Ackerman, 1980; Ackerman, 1982).

This proposal has an appealing simplicity but disregards important concepts regarding the life history and biologic implications of the different types of melanomas. All melanomas may start from a single melanocyte, but the clinical situations in which they are encountered—such as dysplastic nevus syndrome, congenital hairy nevus, and nodular melanoma—are different enough to justify the preservation of biologic and clinical types of melanoma (Elder et al., 1982).

Although some melanomas arise from evolving dysplastic lesions, many appear to be arising in normal skin. It is sometimes difficult to differentiate between severe melanocytic dysplasias and small melanomas.

In their dermal invasion, melanocytic dysplasias may recapitulate the differentiation stages of regular nevi. The dermal melanocytes become smaller in both nuclei and cytoplasm and eventually become spindle-shaped, with more stromal component separating the individual melanocytes. The degree of maturation is often moderate and is inverse to the severity of the cytologic atypia (Reed, 1983). Some authors have identified some cytologic features that help identify early melanomas. McGovern observed that the proliferating melanocytes cease to resemble nevus cells and acquire cytologic characteristics of melanoma cells. These include variation of nuclear and cytoplasmic size and large clear cytoplasm with "powdery" pigment (McGovern, 1983). Also included are the lack

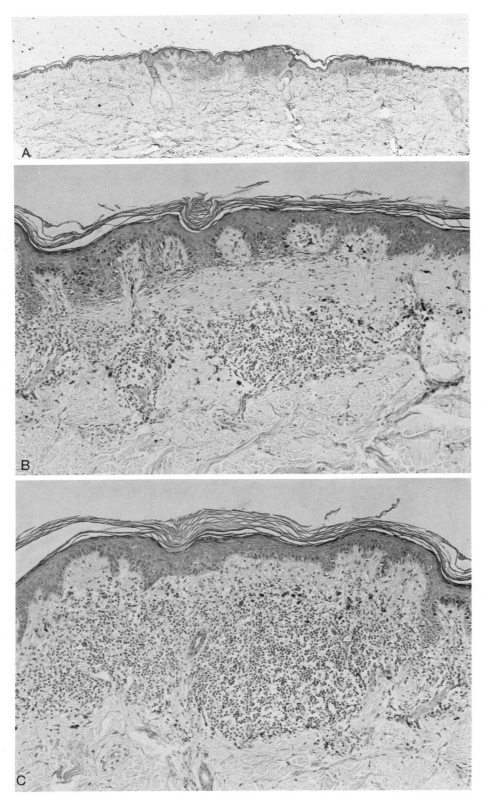

Figure 2–29. Small melanoma. *A,* A 7-mm lesion on the arm of a 55-year-old man. *B,* Close-up of the right lateral border. The cells are distributed in bundles parallel to the epidermal surface. Dense lamellar fibrosis and lymphocytic response are present. *C,* Area of partial regression in the center of the lesion. Few atypical melanocytes remain on the right. The inflammatory response is intense.

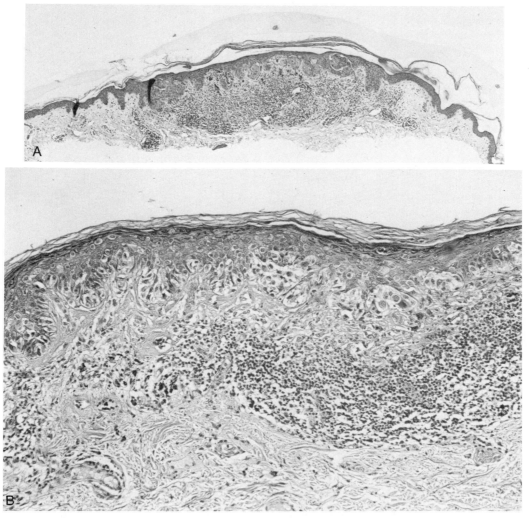

Figure 2–30. Small melanoma. *A*, A 5-mm papule present on the back of a 35-year-old woman. *B*, Proliferation of rounded melanocytes singly and in nests. Note the upward migration of single cells. The dermis is densely fibrotic with an intense inflammatory response.

of vertical maturation seen in benign nevi and some dysplastic melanocytic proliferations.

The concept of symmetry developed by Reed involves growth-pattern and cytologic features. The lesion is symmetric in the geometric sense: contour from side to side and from top to bottom. It also includes the vertical maturation of dermal melanocytes. There is progressive reduction in size of the cells from superficial rounded and plump cells organized in nests with abundant melanogenesis (Type A melanocytes) to small amelanotic melanocytes in the central portion of the lesion (Type B) to spindle amelanotic melanocytes widely separated by collagenous stroma at the deepest part of the lesion (Type C). The concept of symmetry also requires uniform nuclear and cytoplasmic characteristics (Reed, 1983). Benign lesions are symmetric, whereas malignant lesions are often asymmetric. Some melanomas may

have an expansive growth with symmetric features. These rare lesions are known as "minimal deviation melanomas" (Reed, 1983).

Melanomas enter the nodular growth phase in a variable period of time. Some melanomas appear to have an accelerated growth rate and brief or no demonstrable macular growth phase. These are known as "nodular melanomas." However, most melanomas have a macular component in addition to the nodular phase. This nodular component has serious prognostic significance. Most metastatic melanomas are associated with the nodular growth phase. Prognosis and the risk of metastasis are directly related to tumor size. The most valuable prognostic indication is the evaluation of tumor thickness, expressed in millimeters (Balch et al., 1978; Breslow, 1970). The histologic hallmark of nodular growth phase is the invasion of reticular dermis (Levels IV and V of Clark's

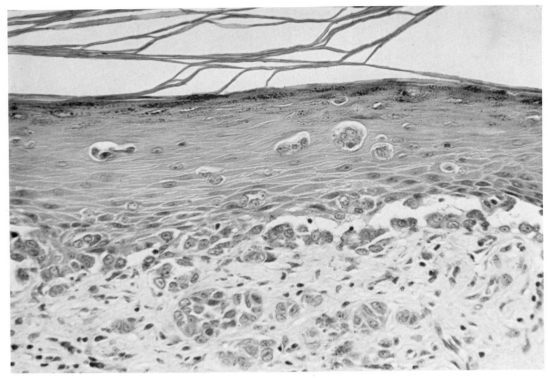

Figure 2–31. Invasive melanoma. The atypical melanocytes are invasive to both the upper layer of the epidermis and the dermis. The inflammatory response is mild and apparently ineffective.

system) (Fig. 2–31). Many melanomas are diagnosed today at Level III or earlier. These tumors fill and expand the papillary dermis without invading the reticular dermis. Some melanomas are polypoid in configuration and thick (more than 1.85 mm), yet do not invade the reticular dermis. The prognosis of these melanomas directly relates to the tumor thickness.

The melanomas in nodular growth phase present an expansive plaque or nodule with little intervening stroma. The host response is variable but often is sparse. The variegated appearance of the tumor cells in the nodular phase is known as "intralesional transformation." Although benign melanocytic lesions often display morphologic variation of cell types and melanin production, this occurs as an orderly transition. Symmetry is present in the lesion, with vertical arrangement of melanocytes (Types A, B, and C) and superficial melanogenesis. However, in intralesional transformation the nests of melanocytes vary greatly in size, cell type, and melanin production. Therefore, adjacent nests of melanoma cells with widely differing morphologic features are common. Nests of rounded melanocytes are found side by side with nests of spindle cells. Melanotic and amelanotic nodules are present. Some melanotic nodules can be seen at the deepest part of the melanoma (the opposite is seen in the vertical maturation of benign nevi).

In summary, melanoma remains a life-threatening disease for which early excision remains the best treatment. Successful treatment depends on early clinical detection of suspicious lesions by patients, confirmation by physicians, and pathologic recognition of precursor and early lesions. The pathologic diagnosis is particularly important, with recognition of melanoma-prone individuals and families who require close clinical follow-up so that future lesions can be excised in early stages. It is hoped that with this approach the difficulties in treatment of metastatic melanoma can be avoided in many cases.

The author thanks Dr. Robert T. Brodell for his assistance in the manuscript preparation.

References

Ackerman, A. B.: Malignant melanoma: A unifying concept. Hum. Pathol. 11:591–595, 1980.

Ackerman, A. B.: Disagreements about classification of malignant melanomas. Am. J. Dermatopathol. 4:447–452, 1982.

Arrington, J. H., Reed, R. J., Ichinose, H., et al.: Plantar lentiginous melanoma: A distinctive variant of human cutaneous malignant melanoma. Am. J. Surg. Pathol. 1:131–143, 1977.

Balch, C. M., Murad, T. M., Soong, S. J., et al.: A multifactorial analysis of melanoma: Prognostic histopathological features comparing Clark's and Breslow's staging lesions. Ann. Surg. 188:732–742, 1978.

Breslow, A.: Thickness, cross-sectional areas and depth of invasion in the prognosis of cutaneous melanoma. Ann. Surg. 172:902–908, 1970

Breslow, A.: Prognosis in cutaneous melanoma: Tumor thickness as a guide to treatment. Pathol. Ann. Part I:1–22, 1980.

Brodell, R. T., and Santa Cruz, D. J.: Borderline and atypical melanocytic lesions. Semin. Diag. Pathol. 2:63–86, 1985.

Clark, W. H., Ainsworth, A. M., Benardino, E. A., et al.: The developmental biology of primary human malignant melanomas. Semin. Oncol. 2:83–103, 1975.

Clark, W. H., Jr., From, L., Bernardino, E. A., Mihm, M. C., Jr.: The histogenesis and biological behavior of primary malignant melanoma of the skin. Cancer Res. 29:705–717, 1969.

Clark, W. H., Reimer, R. R., Greene, M., et al.: Origin of familial malignant melanomas from heritable melanocytic lesions. "The B-K Mole Syndrome." Arch. Dermatol. 114:732–738, 1978.

Elder, D. E., Goldman, L. I., Goldman, S. C., et al.: Dysplastic nevus syndrome: A phenotypic association of sporadic cutaneous melanoma. Cancer 46:1787–1794, 1980.

Elder, D. E., Green, M. H., Guerry, D., et al.: The dysplastic nevus syndrome. Our definition. Am. J. Dermatopathol. 4:455–460, 1982.

Elder, D. E., Jucovy, P. M., Clark, W. H.: Melanoma classification. A testable hypothesis. Am. J. Dermatopathol. 4:443–445, 1982.

Feibleman, C. E., Stoll, H., Maize, J. C.: Melanomas of the palm, sole and nailbed. A clinicopathologic study. Cancer 46:2492–2504, 1980.

Greene, M. H. and Fraumeni, J. F.: The hereditary variant of malignant melanoma. *In* Clark, W. H., Goldman, L. I., Mastrangelo, M. J. (eds.): Human Malignant Melanoma. New York, Grune and Stratton, 1979.

Kamino, H. and Ackerman, A. B.: Malignant melanoma in situ: The evolution of malignant melanoma within the epidermis. *In* Ackerman, A. B. (ed.): Pathology of Malignant Melanoma. New York, Masson Publishing Co., 1981, pp. 59–91.

Kopf, A. W., Rodriguez-Sains, R. S., Rigel, D. S., et al.: "Small" melanomas. Relation of prognostic variables to diameter of primary superficial spreading melanomas. J. Dermatol. Surg. Oncol. 8:765–770, 1982.

Kuhnl-Petzoldt, C.: Superficial spreading melanoma: Histological findings and problems of differentiation. Arch. Dermatol. Forsch. 250:309–321, 1974.

McGovern, V. J.: Melanoma; Histological Diagnosis and Prognosis. New York, Raven Press, 1983.

McGovern, V. J., Shaw, H. M., Milton, G. W.: Prognosis in patients with thin malignant melanoma: Influence of regression. Histopathology 7:673–680, 1983.

McGovern, V. J., Shaw, H. M., Milton, G. W., et al.: Is Malignant melanoma arising in a Hutchinson's melanocytic freckle a separate disease entity? Histopathology 4:235–242, 1980.

McGovern, V. J., Shaw, H. M., Milton, G. W.: Histogenesis of malignant melanoma with an adjacent component of the superficial spreading type. Pathology 17:251–254, 1985.

Milton, G. W.: The diagnosis of malignant melanoma. *In* McCarthy, W. H. (ed.): Melanoma and Skin Cancer. Sydney, Australia, S. Blight, 1972, pp. 163–174.

Milton, G. W., Lane Brown, M. M., Gilder, M.: Malignant melanoma with an occult primary lesion. Br. J. Surg. 54:651–658, 1967.

Mishima, Y.: Melanosis circumscripta (Dubreuilh). A non-nevoid premelanoma distinct from junctional nevus. J. Invest. Dermatol. 34:361–375, 1960.

Mishima, Y. and Matsunaka, M.: Pagetoid premalignant melanosis and melanoma: Differentiation from Hutchinson's melanotic freckle. J. Invest. Dermatol. 65:434–440, 1975.

Paladugu, R. R., Winberg, C. D., Yonemoto, R. H.: Acral lentiginous melanoma. A clinicopathologic study of 36 patients. Cancer 52:161–168, 1983.

Patterson, R. H., and Helwig, E. B.: Subungual malignant melanoma: A clinical-pathological study. Cancer 46:2074–2087, 1980.

Price, N. M., Rywlin, A. M., Ackerman, A. B.: Histologic criteria for the diagnosis of superficial spreading malignant melanoma: formulated on the basis of proven metastatic lesions. Cancer 38:2434–2441, 1976.

Rahbari, H. and Mehregan, A. H.: Sporadic atypical mole syndrome. A report of five nonfamilial BK mole syndrome-like cases and histopathologic findings. Arch. Dermatol. 117:329–331, 1980.

Reed, R. J.: The pathology of human cutaneous melanoma. *In* Contanzi, J. J. (ed.): Malignant Melanoma. The Hague, Martinus Nishoff Publishing, 1983, pp. 85–116.

Reed, R. J., Ichinose, H., Clark, H. H., Jr., Mihm, M. C., Jr.: Common and uncommon melanocytic nevi and borderline melanomas. Semin. Oncol. 2:119–147, 1975.

Reimer, R. R., Clark, W. H., Greene, M. H., et al.: Precursor lesions in familial melanoma. A new genetic preneoplastic syndrome. J.A.M.A. 239:744–746, 1978.

Rhodes, A. R., Harrist, T. J., Day, C. L., et al.: Dysplastic melanocytic nevi in histologic association with 234 primary cutaneous melanomas. J. Am. Acad. Dermatol. 9:563–574, 1983.

Sagebiel, R. W.: Histopathology of borderline and early malignant melanomas. Am. J. Surg. Pathol. 3:543–552, 1979.

Sagebiel, R. W., Chinn, E. K., Egbert, B. M.: Pigmented spindle cell nevus. Clinical and histological review of 90 cases. Am. J. Surg. Pathol. 8:645–653, 1984.

Smith, J. L. and Stehlin, J. S.: Spontaneous regression of primary malignant melanomas with regional metastases. Cancer 18:1399–1415, 1965.

Trau, H., Kopf, A. W., Rigel, D. S., et al.: Regression in malignant melanoma. J. Am. Acad. Dermatol. 8:363–368, 1983.

Tucker, S. B., Horstmann, J. P., Hertel, B., et al.: Activation of nevi in patients with malignant melanoma. Cancer 46:822–827, 1980.

Weedon, D.: A reappraisal of melanoma in situ. J. Dermatol. Surg. Oncol. 8:774–775, 1982.

JOHN D. CRISSMAN

3 Upper Aerodigestive Tract

The majority of the diagnostic problems dealing with premalignant intraepithelial neoplasia, carcinoma-in-situ (CIS), and "early" carcinomas of the upper aerodigestive tract occur in squamous mucosa. This chapter will address some of the author's experience in diagnosis of this relatively common but ill-defined group of diseases. The basis of this accumulated experience has been developed from a number of sources, including insight provided by important contributions from the literature. In addition, numerous discussions and sharing of patient material with fellow pathologists who are interested in head and neck disease have greatly helped me formulate ideas and opinions regarding intraepithelial and early invasive neoplasia of the upper aerodigestive tract mucosa. In this chapter I will attempt to define my understanding of the histologic characteristics of precursor changes and how they relate to the development of intraepithelial neoplasia and subsequent invasive carcinoma. The morphologic alterations presented will be drawn from personal experiences in conjunction with those of head and neck surgeons, initially at the University of Cincinnati and more recently at Wayne State University. It has been my privilege to work with surgeons who have had substantial curiosity and interest in pursuing the study of upper aerodigestive tract mucosa carcinogenesis and who have continued to stimulate my interest in this disease group. Key studies from the literature, which have been useful in the development of my understanding of carcinomas that arise in the upper aerodigestive tract, will be cited to help those pathologists interested in this perplexing and poorly understood group of diseases.

DEFINITIONS

In order to develop a common nomenclature, I will define the following terms. These are working definitions, interpreted in relation to head and neck diseases, and should help the reader better understand the text.

Leukoplakia. This is a mucosal alteration with a whitish appearance. There is no defined histopathologic counterpart for this gross observation. This term should be used only as a clinical description for mucosal alteration and should not be applied as a pathologic term or diagnosis. The appearance of leukoplakia is usually associated with mucosal thickening and is rarely accompanied by cellular and epithelial maturation abnormalities.

Erythroplakia. This is a mucosal alteration with a reddish appearance. It is usually easily traumatized with resultant bleeding. Although there is no specific histopathologic definition, the reddish appearance is usually associated with a thin mucosa, which demonstrates significant maturation abnormalities and cellular alterations. Again, this term should be reserved for clinical descriptions and should never be applied as a pathologic diagnosis.

Dysplasia. This is defined as an abnormal mucosal development. This term is commonly applied to mucosal maturation abnormalities, which are best defined in the uterine cervix. Grading of squamous mucosal dysplasia is a pathologist's interpretation of the extent of morphologic alterations (Table 3–1). These interpretations are commonly divided into three categories—mild, moderate, and severe—according to the degree of alteration present. It must be emphasized that the major rationale for grading dysplasia is to enable the pathologist to communicate to the surgeon his estimation of the probability of the mucosal change proceeding to invasive carcinoma (e.g., mild dysplasia—low probability; severe dysplasia—high probability).

Intraepithelial Neoplasia. This term is applied to the spectrum of epithelial alterations that precede invasive carcinoma and that are categorized as dysplasia/CIS. The major objective in classifying these epithelial alterations is to identify the morphologic expressions of neoplasia, usually an irreversible change. It is clear that many epithelial alterations are reactions to reversible injuries, not true neoplastic transformations. Identification of a lesion as a grade

Table 3–1. **Histologic Criteria for the Diagnosis of Intraepithelial Neoplasia in Upper Aerodigestive Tract Mucosa**

Cellular abnormalities
Nuclear pleomorphism, variation in size, shape, and staining characteristics

Increased mitoses in all portions of the mucosa, often with abnormal forms

Large, prominent nucleoli

Maturation abnormalities
Proliferation of basal or "uncommitted" cells composing all or a substantial portion of the epithelium

Abnormal formation of intracellular keratin (dyskeratosis) in the epithelium, occasionally with the development of intraepithelial keratin pearls

Loss of normal, orderly maturation with loss of cell polarity and alteration in nuclear/cytoplasmic ratios (loss of mosaic pattern)

of intraepithelial neoplasia rather than as dysplasia/CIS does not solve the pathologist's problem of differentiating reactive or reversible epithelial alterations from true neoplastic changes. It does, however, emphasize the goal of classifying epithelial maturation abnormalities and cytologic alterations as potentially reversible lesions or as neoplastic expressions. The latter invariably will persist or progress to invasive carcinoma.

Keratosis. Most definitively, keratosis is an increase in surface keratin commonly resulting in a leukoplakic clinical appearance. The term "keratosis" traditionally has been used to describe laryngeal glottic mucosal alterations and also has been used to describe mucosal changes in other upper aerodigestive tract sites, but it does not have a universally accepted histologic definition.

Carcinoma-in-Situ (CIS). This tumor, also referred to as "preinvasive carcinoma," connotes mucosal alterations that are so severe that they would almost always persist or progress to invasive cancer if left untreated. It should be noted that mucosal CIS is most commonly observed adjacent to invasive neoplasms. Whether this intimate association of CIS precedes the invasive cancer or represents intraepithelial spread cannot usually be determined. Isolated CIS is rare but may be encountered in the upper aerodigestive tract.

Early Carcinoma. This lesion is defined histologically as invasive carcinoma that has penetrated the basement membrane of the epithelium and has invaded the adjacent submucosal tissues. It is invariably associated with an intact epithelium demonstrating CIS. Although a definition of "early carcinoma" cannot be based on any absolute scale of depth of invasion, we will confine the use of the term in this chapter to microscopic invasion, which is usually not appreciated clinically as invasive carcinoma. Early carcinoma is intimately associated with overlying CIS and only focally infiltrates the submucosal tissue. This

finding is similar to the spectrum of features of microinvasion of the uterine cervix. To make a diagnosis of early or microinvasive carcinoma, the pathologist must know the clinical appearance of the mucosa and the relationship of the biopsy to the clinical findings. A biopsy of a small erythroplakic mucosal change may be diagnosed as microinvasive cancer, whereas a biopsy from the edge of a large ulcerative carcinoma obviously may not.

NEOPLASIA OF THE UPPER AERODIGESTIVE TRACT (UADT)

For many years, preneoplastic mucosal alterations of the upper aerodigestive tract have been considered curiosities by surgeons and pathologists. Affected patients often present with a history of heavy alcohol and cigarette abuse. When these "at risk" patients present with head and neck cancer, they usually do so with advanced-stage disease. Members of this patient population often fail to seek medical attention until a carcinoma has progressed sufficiently to result in functional symptoms.

Since the 1970s, surgery and radiotherapy have been developing as major therapy in head and neck oncology. More recently, improvements in medical oncology have contributed to the care of the affected patient population. Advances in nutrition and general medical support have improved survival. Progress in chemotherapy also has contributed to improved clinical responses. Response rates to chemotherapy, with a relief in symptoms, have improved so much that it may be difficult to convince some patients of a need for surgery. Probably one of the most important observations in the management of head and neck cancer patients is that they are now recognized as predisposed to develop carcinomas in all portions of the "at risk" upper aerodigestive tract mucosa. It is well established that in this group of patients there is a high incidence of multicentric neoplasms, now recognized as one of the causes for therapeutic failures in head and neck cancer patients (Cohn and Peppard, 1980; Gluckman and Crissman, 1983). At initial presentation, this group of patients may harbor a second or third silent neoplasm in some other anatomic site. Also, these predisposed patients often develop additional squamous cell carcinomas (which may or may not be recognized and treated) after treatment of their presenting symptomatic cancer.

The incidence of multiple squamous cell carcinomas arising in the upper aerodigestive tract is now accepted as being as high as 20 percent, with some reports of an even higher incidence (Gluckman et al., 1980). There are many reasons for this increased incidence. Most important, there now exists a greater awareness of this phenomenon, which has stimulated a more extensive search for these lesions. This includes thorough evaluation of the patient at the initial presentation and more careful long-term follow-up. Endoscopy has allowed clear visualization of the "at risk" mucosa of the upper aerodigestive tract, permitting identification and biopsy of a greater number of intraepithelial and early carcinomas.

Historically, multicentric squamous cell carcinomas of the upper aerodigestive tract have been classified by their temporal sequence in recognition. Simultaneously developing carcinomas are usually diagnosed at initial presentation. Synchronous carcinomas include those that present either simultaneously or within 6 months of the original tumor. The 6-month period is stipulated because those tumors are most likely to be present at the time of initial evaluation. With improvements in examination, this arbitrary distinction is probably invalid. Presently, neoplasms should be considered either synchronous or metachronous in their presentation. The histologic criterion for the diagnosis of multicentric neoplasms is that each neoplasm must be geographically separate and distinct, not connected by either submucosal or intraepithelial neoplastic change.

The diagnosis of anatomically separate squamous cell carcinomas is usually not a problem, even when these neoplasms are close together. The use of multiple biopsies, including sampling of the mucosa intervening between the two clinically evident malignancies, is usually sufficient. Many surgeons tend to sample multiple sites in evaluating head and neck cancer patients. Multiple biopsies are often used to define the extent of the presenting carcinoma and to identify multicentric sites. The most important histologic observation of a separate "early" primary infiltrating carcinoma is identification of its origin from the overlying epithelium. Although this is often a difficult observation, biopsy of an early neoplasm will demonstrate the pattern of invasion arising from the overlying intraepithelial carcinoma, a key histologic feature (Fig. 3–1). With advancing cancer, the infiltrating tumor may obliterate the intraepithelial changes. In this instance, the important pattern of carcinoma originating from the surface mucosa will be lost.

Diagnosis of early carcinomas by the pathologist reinforces the surgeon's ability to diagnose multiple primary carcinomas. Also, these observations are extremely important in biopsies from the sites of previously treated carcinomas, which are easily confused with persisting carcinoma. The distinction is extremely important because the therapy for persisting squamous cell carcinoma is usually more radical than that utilized for a subsequently developing metachronous "early" carcinoma in adjacent anatomic site. Figure 3–2 demonstrates a biopsy from the soft palate adjacent to a previously treated carcinoma of the tonsillar pillar. The diagnosis of squamous cell carcinoma in this case was interpreted by the surgeon as persisting disease, and a radical resection was planned as a salvage procedure. In a review of the pathology, it was stressed that the neoplasm appeared to represent a second primary arising from a minor salivary gland duct. A wide excision was performed, and the patient remains free of disease at 2 years post surgery. Careful choice of the biopsy site with proper orientation is of paramount importance. It is usually recommended that biopsy specimens of any malignant neoplasm be obtained from the junction of normal and abnormal mucosa or from the edge of an ulcer. This allows for evaluation of the pattern of invasion and the relationship of the cancer to adjacent squamous mucosa.

The full clinical significance of multiple primary neoplasms in the upper aerodigestive tract is only now being appreciated. Recognition of simultaneously

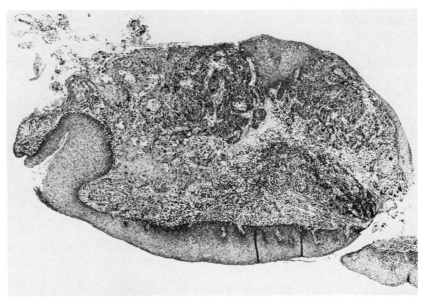

Figure 3–1. A typical biopsy, using the cut forceps, from the upper aerodigestive tract mucosa. This technique often results in a hemisphere of tissue covered by mucosa; on section the circumference is often covered by mucosa. This biopsy represents an early or microinvasive carcinoma. The diagnosis can be made only in the context of the gross findings. In this case, the biopsy was from a focal area of erythroplakia on the anterior tonsillar pillar.

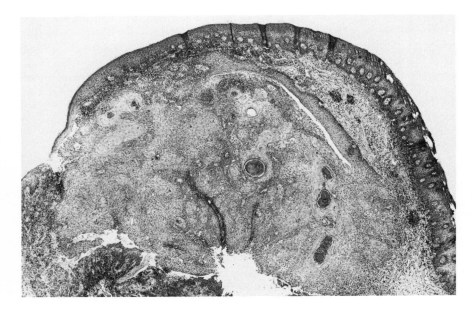

Figure 3–2. This biopsy is from the soft palate of a patient previously treated for a moderately differentiated squamous cell carcinoma of the tonsil. Because of the well-differentiated appearance, with only early invasion and the impression of arising from a minor salivary gland duct, this neoplasm was interpreted as a second primary cancer. As a result, a simple excision was performed, and the patient continues to do well.

presenting cancers profoundly affects the treatment strategy. The possibility of a second metachronous neoplasm has altered the concept of a "5-year cure." The effect of multiple cancers on survival is not well documented but unquestionably compromises longevity. In a community tumor registry study of 5337 patients with squamous cell carcinoma of the upper and aerodigestive tract mucosa, 736 had additional second and third primary tumors of either the upper aerodigestive tract, esophagus, or lung (Gluckman and Crissman, 1983). The 5-year survival rates of 548 patients with second upper aerodigestive tract cancers and sufficient follow-up were 22.3 percent, compared with 35 percent for patients without second cancers. Head and neck cancer surgeons now recognize the importance of identification of second and subsequent carcinomas of the affected mucosa, and pathologists will be faced with increased numbers of mucosal biopsies for interpretation in the future. Many of the biopsies of endoscopic identified neoplasms will unquestionably consist of "preinvasive" carcinomas and "early" carcinomas (Weaver et al., 1979).

CLINICAL PRECURSORS TO SQUAMOUS CELL CARCINOMA: LEUKOPLAKIA AND ERYTHROPLAKIA

The reaction of squamous mucosa to various forms of injury, including carcinogenic influences, depends in part on the anatomic site of injury. The common reaction of squamous mucosa to injury invariably includes cellular proliferation, or hyperplasia, either reactive (reversible) or neoplastic (irreversible). The pathologist's goal is to identify which of these changes is truly neoplastic and are most likely to persist or

progress. Mucosal hyperplasia is reflected by epithelial thickening (acanthosis) and varying degrees of accumulation of surface keratin (hyperkeratosis), regardless of the type of injury. These changes are most commonly encountered in the buccal mucosa, alveolar ridge, hard palate, dorsal tongue, and laryngeal glottis. When epithelial thickening and accumulation of surface keratin are sufficient, the clinical appearance of these mucosal changes is often leukoplakic. The histologic counterpart is usually an orderly progression, or maturation, of the cells from the basilar layer to the anucleated surface keratin. Despite this observation, there have been numerous references to leukoplakia as one of the "premalignant," or percursor, stages in the development of squamous cell carcinoma. However, a number of patient series in which there has been careful documentation of both the gross appearance and well-defined histologic criteria for epithelial abnormalities, including dysplasias and carcinoma-in-situ, do not appear to support this concept (Waldron and Shafer, 1975). Long-term follow-up of patients with clinical leukoplakic changes demonstrates an extremely low frequency of transformation to invasive squamous cell carcinomas (Tables 3–2 and 3–3). Most homogenous leukoplakic mucosal changes are found on the buccal mucosa, dorsal tongue, and alveolar ridges, anatomic sites in which invasive carcinomas are relatively infrequent. However, it must be stressed that leukoplakic changes in the floor of the mouth, ventral tongue, and soft palate should be clinically viewed with some suspicion because they are occasionally associated with dysplastic changes that signal significant risk for transformation to invasive carcinoma.

Although the association of leukoplakia with invasive carcinoma is relatively uncommon, it has become clear that erythroplakic, or red mucosal, changes are

Table 3–2. **Malignant Transformation of Clinical Oral Leukoplakias**

Reference	No. Patients	No. Subsequent Carcinomas
Pindborg et al., 1963	248	11 (4.4%)*
Silverman, 1968	117	7 (5.9%)†
Einhorn and Wersall, 1967	782	(4%)‡

*3.7 years to development of cancer; seven patients had speckled appearance.
†3.4 years to development of cancer; two patients had speckled appearance.
‡Cumulative frequency for patients observed 20 years.

commonly associated with invasive carcinomas and with a high rate of transformation to malignancy (Mashberg, 1978; Shafer and Waldron, 1975). Erythroplakia is the most common physical finding in early asymptomatic squamous cell carcinoma and therefore must always be viewed with suspicion. The mucosa is thin and consists of altered cells that have matured abnormally. The most common sites of erythroplakia are the floor of the mouth, ventral tongue, soft palate–tonsil complex, pyriform sinus, and hypopharynx. These sites correspond to the common sites of squamous cell carcinomas in the upper aerodigestive tract mucosa. The relatively thin mucosa with submucosal telangiectasis produces the red, velvety appearance of the erythroplakia. Many of the erythroplakias are best categorized as intraepithelial neoplasia, and a sizable percentage of these mucosal alterations are associated with invasive squamous cell carcinomas (Table 3–3).

Although it is agreed that leukoplakic mucosal changes are seldom associated with serious epithelial abnormalities and that erythroplakias have a high association with—or subsequent transformation to—invading carcinoma, the classification of the admixture of these two mucosal changes was for many years erroneously considered a form of leukoplakia.

Table 3–3. **Histopathologic Changes Associated With Mucosal Appearance**

Reference	Histopathologic Changes			
	Leukoplakia			
	Dysplasia		Carcinoma	
Mashberg, 1978	3/43	(7%)	3/43	(7%)
Waldron and Shafer, 1975	153/3256	(5%)	104/3256	(3%)
Silverman, 1968	0/117		12/117	(10%)*
	Speckled			
	Leukoplakia		Erythroplakia	
Mashberg, 1978	6/58	(10%)	33/58	(57%)
	Erythroplakia			
Mashberg, 1978	1/44	(2%)	28/44	(64%)†
Shafer and Waldron, 1975	26/65	(40%)‡	33/65	(51%)

*Ten invasive cancer; two CIS.
†Includes both CIS and invasive cancer.
‡65 biopsies in 58 patients from a series of 65,354 biopsy specimens.

However, it has become evident that this admixture of speckled mucosal changes should be considered a variant of erythroplakia, the most serious of mucosal changes (Mashberg, 1978). It is possible that what was erroneously perceived as a high association of leukoplakia with underlying epithelial abnormalities actually represents leukoplakia with erythroplakia or speckled mucosal change and not pure leukoplakia.

HISTOLOGIC INTERPRETATION OF SQUAMOUS MUCOSAL NEOPLASIA

It is accepted that, in most instances, erythroplakic appearances of squamous mucosa in the aerodigestive tract signify major maturation abnormalities of the mucosa with associated cytologic atypia clearly representing intraepithelial neoplasia. These alterations are analogous to the majority of intraepithelial neoplasia affecting the female genital tract. One major difference is that the upper aerodigestive tract is normally keratinized and often responds to injury by developing surface keratin. This is similar to the keratinizing form of dysplasia affecting the gynecologic tract, a well-recognized subgroup of intraepithelial alterations of the uterine cervix.

In biopsy specimens obtained from relatively thin mucosa with little or no attempts at surface keratinization, the neoplastic nature of the intraepithelial change is usually not a diagnostic problem. This situation is analogous to non-keratinizing dysplasias encountered in the female genital tract, and the observations are similar to those used for the classification or grading of intraepithelial neoplasia. When the mucosa is only partially replaced by a proliferation of immature or morphologically uncommitted cells, a diagnosis of mild or moderate intraepithelial neoplasia or dysplasia is indicated. When there is total or near total replacement of the mucosa by these cytologically uncommitted cells (which resemble basal cells) with little or no evidence of epithelial maturation or organization (differentiation), the intraepithelial changes are advanced and are characteristic of severe dysplasia or CIS. Admittedly, the separation of these four categories is somewhat subjective, but the extent of proliferation of the morphologically uncommitted or undifferentiated cells and the degree of individual cell anaplasia allow application of grading systems similar to those used to evaluate lesions in the uterine cervix.

In my experience, one of the most important criteria for neoplastic transformation in upper aerodigestive tract mucosa is the loss of the organization or polarity indicative of normal maturation within the epithelium. Normally, the squamous mucosa matures in an organized fashion with a well-defined basal layer. The suprabasal cells are small but demonstrate increased cytoplasm as they move toward the surface. The nuclei are generally equidistant from each other, demonstrating an orderly "mosaic" appearance. Near the surface, cytoplasmic keratinization becomes obvious and the cells change their orientation. Loss of this orderly distribution of nuclei and altered cytologic characteristics—including N/C ratio and nuclear pleomorphism—result in the characteristic mucosal alterations of intraepithelial neoplasia or dysplasia (Shafer, 1975).

Individual cell abnormalities are difficult to define, and it must be stressed that assessment of cytologic alterations depends on the location of the cell within the epithelium. Nuclear/cytoplasmic ratios constitute an important parameter in determining cellular atypia because a cell with abundant cytoplasm is normal near the surface of squamous mucosa and distinctly abnormal near the basal portions. Cytoplasmic keratinization is normal near the mucosal surface and markedly abnormal in the depths of the epithelium, indicating disordered intraepithelial maturation. Conversely, the small "uncommitted" cells that normally proliferate near the basal layer are distinctly abnormal when they constitute a substantial portion of the mucosa. The distribution of mitotic figures is commonly useful in the assessment of mucosal maturation. Normally, mitoses are found only in or near the basal layer in the morphologically uncommitted cell populations. Identification of mitoses in the upper layers of the mucosa is another indication of loss of normal maturation. Identification of abnormal mitoses is essentially found only in neoplastic transformed mucosa. Figures 3–3 through 3–7 demonstrate the sequence

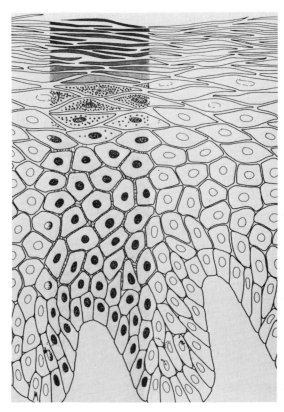

Figure 3–4. This figure represents a thickened mucosa with orderly maturation. There is no evidence of cytologic atypia and it is characteristic of reversible forms of hyperplasia.

of characteristic epithelial alterations affecting upper aerodigestive tract mucosa.

Nuclear alterations also are important parameters in the evaluation of cytologic atypia. It is well established that an increase in nuclear size and nuclear staining are critical factors in the assessment of individual cell atypia. The rationale of this observation is that changes in nuclear size, shape, and staining represent alterations in chromosomal content. Unfortunately, hematoxylin stains a number of nuclear proteins besides DNA. With the Feulgen staining reaction specific for DNA, it has been demonstrated that increased DNA distributions are present in squamous epithelium with the features of intraepithelial neoplasia (Bjelkenkrantz et al., 1983; Giarelli et al., 1977; Grontoft et al., 1978). This abnormal increase in DNA content—hyperdiploid, or aneuploid, chromosomal populations—is associated with neoplastic transformation. The limited studies of this abnormality confirm significant aneuploidy in mucosa with advanced intraepithelial alterations and invasive carcinomas. Unfortunately, sufficient numbers of biopsies with less severe cellular and epithelial alterations have not been obtained, and therefore specific histopathologic criteria for neoplastic transformation have not been conclusively established. However, these studies are important in that they clearly demonstrate that

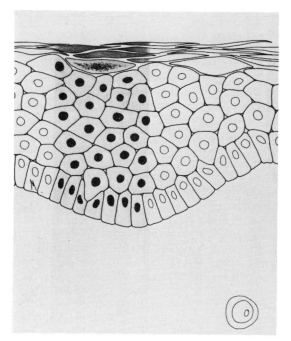

Figure 3–3. Diagrammatic representation of normal squamous mucosa. There is a well-defined basal layer with maturation to the superficial layers of keratinized cells. This is typical of mucosa found on surfaces exposed to mechanical trauma, such as buccal, alveolar ridge, and glottic surfaces.

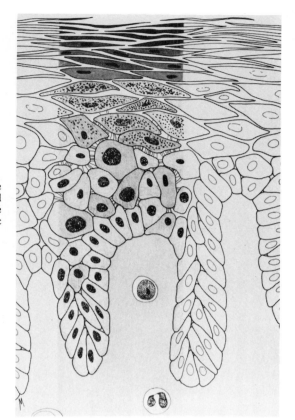

Figure 3–5. This pattern of response to injury demonstrates many of the changes found in Figure 3–4. However, there are some mild maturation and cytologic alterations in the midportion of the mucosa. Although this would be judged as a mild dysplasia, it is highly unlikely to represent a neoplastic process.

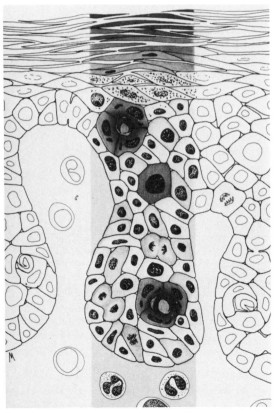

Figure 3–6. The alterations in this diagram are much more severe, with cytologic atypia and an increase in mitotic figures. The most worrisome feature is the "premature" maturation of keratin-forming cells in the lower mucosa. This alteration in maturation often indicates "autonomous expression" of keratinization, a feature of neoplastic transformation The propensity for these mucosal changes to persist or progress is sufficient to justify a diagnosis of intraepithelial neoplasia (Grade II) or moderate dysplasia.

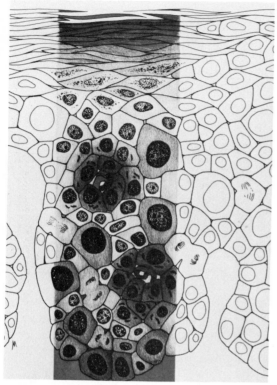

Figure 3–7. This diagram shows severe cytologic and maturation abnormalities. Although there is some evidence of surface maturation, the lacerations are sufficiently severe to be classified as intraepithelial neoplasia (Grade III) or severe dysplasia–carcinoma-in-situ. The differentiation of severe dysplasia and carcinoma-in-situ in the upper aerodigestive tract is extremely difficult and rather arbitrary. It is my preference to reserve the diagnosis of severe dysplasia–carcinoma-in-situ for mucosal alterations that are neoplastic and will continue to persist and often progress to invasive carcinoma. Whether diagnosed as severe dysplasia or carcinoma-in-situ, treatment is needed.

mucosal changes, with the combinations of maturation and cellular abnormalities defined as advanced intraepithelial neoplasia, are unquestionably neoplastic alterations. The critical goal remains the determination of the point at which we can distinguish mild to moderate mucosal alterations that are truly neoplastic from those that occur in response to some other reversible injury. It has been my experience in performing flow cytometry on squamous cell carcinomas that hematoxylin-stained nuclei are very poor indicators of tumor aneuploidy. Even in retrospect, it is extremely difficult to distinguish the diploid and aneuploid cancers histologically by pattern and intensity of nuclear staining. Nuclear size may be a more reliable indicator of chromosomal aneuploidy.

How can we best apply the extensive experience derived in grading of uterine cervical intraepithelial neoplasias to the intraepithelial changes in the upper aerodigestive tract mucosa? In the thin, usually erythroplakic mucosal changes, the criteria applied in the gynecologic tract for grading the majority of dysplasias and diagnosing CIS may be closely applied to upper aerodigestive tract squamous mucosa. Many of the intraepithelial neoplasias of the upper aerodigestive tract are keratinizing, and the criteria for evaluation of these forms of dysplasia/CIS are less clearly established. As a result, the criteria for a diagnosis of severe intraepithelial neoplasia in the head and neck region are controversial. It is my experience that the "classic," "or "non-keratinizing," form of intraepithelial neoplasia is uncommon in upper aerodigestive tract mucosa. The majority of pathologic epithelial proliferations are characterized by the formation of surface keratin. In most instances, the atypical cellular proliferations are found in the depths of the epithelium and are manifested by "premature" expression of keratin (dyskeratosis) or proliferation of morphologically "un-

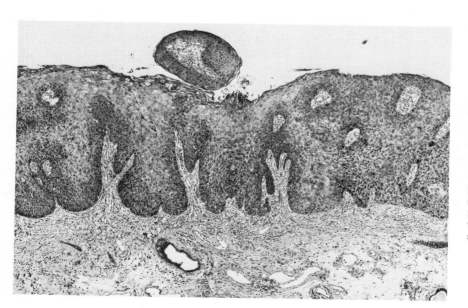

Figure 3–8. Intraepithelial neoplasia of the larynx. This patient had extensive changes similar to those that occur with a thickened mucosa—cellular atypia and maturation abnormalities in the form of premature cellular keratinization. This lesion is representative of intraepithelial neoplasia, Grade III, or severe dysplasia–carcinoma-in-situ. In my opinion, the changes are sufficient to merit a diagnosis of carcinoma-in-situ.

committed," or "undifferentiated," cells. In many instances, both features will be present (Figs. 3–3 to 3–7). "Nuclear pleomorphism," defined as variation in size, shape, and staining, is invariably present, usually accompanied by increased mitoses.

An anatomic site that is characteristic of this form of intraepithelial neoplasia is the laryngeal glottis. The glottis represents a special type of squamous mucosa that possesses a high propensity for development of surface keratin. Injuries to the glottic mucosa usually cause marked proliferation of the epithelium, resulting in acanthosis and some accumulation of surface keratin, appearing leukoplakic on clinical examination (Fig. 3–8). Erythroplakic changes are seldom encountered in the glottis, but they do occur in other sites in the laryngeal mucosa. Although the majority of mucosal insults to the laryngeal glottis are mechanical, carcinogenic influences must always be considered. In several series of carefully studied laryngeal dysplasias and keratoses, between 3.26 and 4.31 percent of patients developed subsequent invasive carcinomas (Table 3–4) (Crissman, 1979; McGavran et al., 1960; Norris and Peale, 1963). The well-differentiated nature of most epithelial proliferations of the laryngeal glottis usually does not demonstrate appreciable cytologic atypia, as reflected by the low frequency of progression to invasive cancers in these series of mucosal hyperplasias with extensive surface keratin formation. It should be noted that a select subgroup of these patients do not demonstrate severe maturation or cytologic abnormalities but do demonstrate intraepithelial neoplastic transformation as the mucosal alterations persist or recur after vocal cord stripping (Crissman, 1982). This is an extremely important point, and recurrence of an intermediate form of intraepithelial neoplasia or moderate dysplasia is a good indicator of neoplastic transformation.

GRADING OF INTRAEPITHELIAL NEOPLASIA

It is my conclusion that the diagnosis of severe, or high-grade, intraepithelial neoplasia should not pose a difficult problem. When sufficient proliferation of small, morphologically uncommitted cells constitute the majority of the mucosal thickness, or when marked maturation and cytologic abnormalities are found (Fig. 3–9), severe intraepithelial neoplasia is an acceptable diagnosis. It is generally agreed, but not adequately

Table 3–4. Frequency of Subsequent Carcinoma in Laryngeal Keratoses/Dysplasia

Reference	No. SCC/No. Patients	Percentage
McGavran et al., 1960	3/84	3.57
Norris and Peale, 1963	5/116	4.31
Crissman, 1979	3/92	3.26

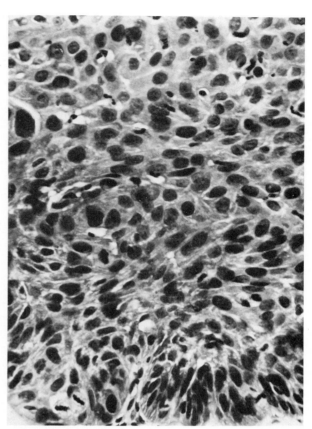

Figure 3–9. The mucosa in this biopsy demonstrates little evidence of differentiation. There is a proliferation of small uncommitted cells without appreciable evidence of intracellular keratinization. There is considerable variation in nuclear and cytoplasmic size and shape, with loss of intercellular organization or mosaic pattern. The nuclei are often crowded, and many appear to exhibit increased staining.

quantified, that these types of mucosal alterations very frequently persist or transform to invasive carcinomas. The separation of these severe alterations into diagnoses of severe dysplasia or CIS is not only difficult but also highly subjective. Both changes are defined as representing degrees in the spectrum of intraepithelial neoplasia that approach invasive carcinoma. Their differentiation represents an estimation of the frequency of progression to invasive cancer, an estimation that is often difficult to derive morphologically. An alternative approach, similar to the scheme proposed for the gynecologic tract, is classification of severe dysplasia and CIS as severe (Grade III) squamous intraepithelial neoplasms (SIN III). This suggestion may provoke controversy, as does any change in terminology. It must be emphasized that the goal of any diagnostic terminology is optimal communication with the surgeon. It is important that the surgeon understand what the pathologist is attempting to define, regardless of the diagnostic terminology used. The pathologist should be cognizant of the surgeon's findings in the interpretation of mucosal biopsies, and the surgeon must understand the nature of the pathologist's definition of diagnostic terms used in the grading of intraepithelial neoplasia.

The major difficulties in classifying and diagnosing intraepithelial neoplasia exist in the moderate, or intermediate group. Lesions in this group display clear epithelial maturation disturbances and cytologic abnormalities (Fig. 3–10), but these atypical findings are not sufficient to permit a comfortable diagnosis of a more severe form of intraepithelial neoplasia (Figs. 3–11 and 3–12). We know that many of these intermediate forms represent reversible hyperplasias, whereas others are early expressions of neoplastic transformation. It is not always possible to differentiate these two important subgroups. For this reason, I suggest that they also be classified in an intermediate group, such as moderate dysplasia or SIN II. It behooves both the pathologist and surgeon to understand that the epithelial changes are worrisome and need to be carefully monitored but that their biologic capacity is not clear.

The final and least disturbing subgroup consists of those epithelial changes that exhibit only minor mat-

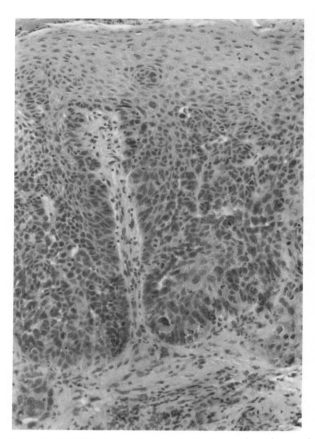

Figure 3–11. This figure also demonstrates good evidence of surface maturation in the form of intracellular and surface keratin formation. However, there are sufficient cytologic alterations with marked variation in nuclear size and staining, often with nuclear crowding, to clearly indicate intraepithelial neoplasia. This biopsy represents a severe dysplasia or squamous intraepithelial neoplasia, Grade III.

uration and cytologic abnormalities (Fig. 3–13). These mucosal injuries are highly unlikely to represent carcinogenic influences and invariably represent reversible hyperplasias that respond to conservative therapy. Because they are unlikely to represent intraepithelial neoplasia, terminology is inconsistent. A term that is descriptive of a reversible process, such as "reactive hyperplasia" or "slight dysplasia," would best inform the surgeon of the pathologist's assessment of the biologic nature of the excised mucosa. These epithelial proliferations will appear abnormal to the surgeon, and their histologic assessment is reassuring to all concerned.

VERRUCOUS CARCINOMA

In 1948, Ackerman described his observations of verrucous carcinoma as follows: "a variety of squamous cell carcinoma whose behavior was unique and had a typical clinical course with characteristic histopathologic growth findings." He reported a lesion that was clinically papillary, or verrucous, in nature with a

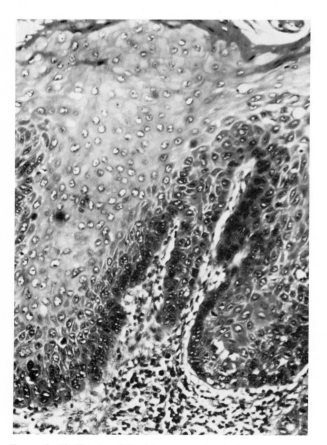

Figure 3–10. This is a difficult biopsy to classify. In my opinion, it is a moderate or intermediate change and may represent a neoplastic alteration. There is clearly significant cytologic atypia (as judged by nuclear pleomorphism, crowding, loss of defined basal layer), but the majority of the epithelium demonstrates more orderly maturation.

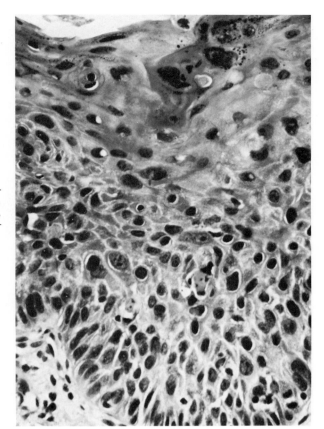

Figure 3–12. This biopsy shows changes similar to those in Figure 3–11, but with less demonstration of superficial mucosal maturation. There is considerable nuclear pleomorphism, with loss of maturation, polarity, and so on. This is another example of severe dysplasia–squamous intraepithelial neoplasia, Grade III.

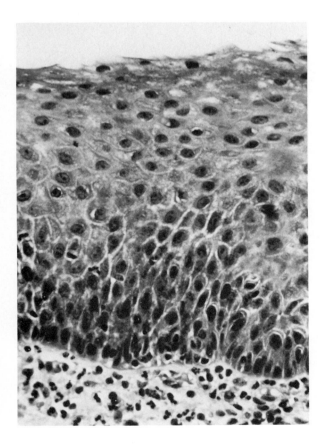

Figure 3–13. This is an example of a hyperplastic mucosa with minor cytologic abnormalities in its deep portions. There is evidence of orderly maturation and no evidence of the abnormalities associated with neoplastic change. This is a form of reactive hyperplasia.

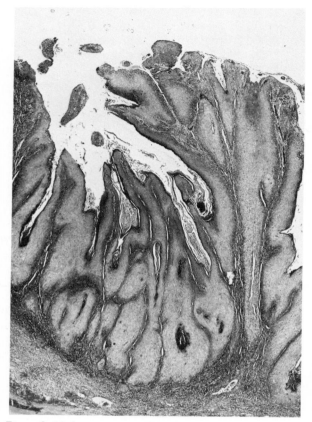

Figure 3–14. Low-power magnification of a verrucous carcinoma of the larynx. The neoplasm is characterized by mature-appearing epithelium with abundant surface keratin. The neoplasm infiltrates the underlying submucosal tissue as demonstrated by the tumor's proximity to the cartilage.

characteristic, somewhat pebbly, mammillated surface. Microscopically, there was an accumulation of keratin on the surface with a downward growth of club-shaped "fingers" of hyperplastic epithelium that gradually pushed into, rather than infiltrated, the deeper tissues (Fig. 3–14). Ackerman emphasized that the epithelium was well differentiated and that the basement membrane appeared intact. The later finding may or may not be true, but the well-organized "pushing border" gives the illusion of epithelial organization that is sufficient for one to assume that it is producing a basement membrane. With further growth, keratin clefts were noted to project deeply into the well-differentiated "fingers" of epithelium, with cystic degeneration sometimes being noted. A submucosal infiltrate of inflammatory cells was commonly present. Many of these features are demonstrated in Figure 3–15. Ackerman went on to state that "the local invasive qualities" are prominent and that all contiguous structures—such as the cheek, soft tissues in the submaxillary area, mandible, and antrum—can be invaded. He referred to this neoplasm as "verrucous carcinoma" and believed that it should be differentiated from other epidermoid carcinomas

on the basis of its excellent prognosis following treatment.

The problems in diagnosing verrucous carcinoma are discussed in many publications and I have no intention of duplicating what has been well described in the literature. In many instances, the initial biopsies, especially small, superficial ones, are often interpreted as benign hyperplasias or as hyperkeratotic, acanthotic squamous proliferations because of the characteristic surface maturation of these neoplasms. This interpretation usually results from the pathologist's failure to appreciate the clinical appearance of the tumor and the corresponding failure of the surgeon to submit an adequate (preferably full-thickness) biopsy. The histopathologic criteria for a diagnosis of verrucous carcinoma are well described in other publications and include demonstration of invasion of the submucosal tissue by the neoplasm (Prioleau et al., 1980). It is interesting that the tumor–host interface of invading tumor was shown to be devoid of basement membrane in some foci and produced abundant basement membrane in other areas. Demonstration of such a

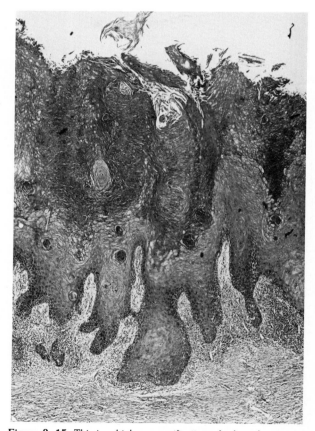

Figure 3–15. This is a higher magnification of a less-characteristic verrucous carcinoma from the buccal mucosa. The surface is covered by extensive accumulations of keratin without the papillary appearance demonstrated in Figure 3–14. This biopsy demonstrates the difficulty in deriving a diagnosis of malignancy with a superficial biopsy. This neoplasm does not have the classic pushing border of invasion, but the organization and broad pegs of invading cancer still qualify it as verrucous carcinoma.

change may require an excisional biopsy, which is not always possible to obtain. An experienced pathologist, working in concert with the head and neck surgeon, may use the biopsy (ideally a full-thickness one) and the gross appearance of the tumor in order to derive a clinicopathologic diagnosis. This approach may require inspection of the tumor-in-situ during endoscopy by both pathologist and surgeon. In my experience, this is the optimal alternative, permitting confident diagnosis of verrucous carcinoma when an excisional biopsy is not feasible.

An epithelial proliferation described as "verrucous hyperplasia" has been described in the literature (Shear and Pindborg, 1980). This entity represents a marked thickening of the squamous mucosa similar to that seen in verrucous carcinoma. The differentiating feature is that verrucous hyperplasia remains superficial to the adjacent mucosa without evidence of submucosal invasion. Because of the high frequency of association with verrucous carcinoma and a histopathologic difference that can be identified only on optimally examined excisional biopsies, I discourage the use of the term "verrucous hyperplasia." It is my impression that the observations described as such represent an early form of the spectrum of verrucous cancers, and the introduction of the term "verrucous hyperplasia" only adds confusion to this difficult area of pathology. Obviously, the best way to diagnose this controversial lesion, while excluding submucosal invasion characteristic of a verrucous carcinoma, is complete excision with histologic examination of multiple sections.

Once a diagnosis of verrucous carcinoma has been rendered, the controversy does not end. However, most experienced head and neck oncologists feel that surgical excision of verrucous carcinoma is the treatment of choice. This is certainly my opinion, and complete excision of the neoplastic mucosa is recommended by others (McDonald et al., 1982). In the larynx, partial or total laryngectomy is indicated. Incomplete excision invariably leads to recurrence, often with an invasive carcinoma. The controversy in therapy concerns anaplastic transformation of verrucous carcinoma. In an exhaustive review of the literature, my colleagues and I determined that the incidence of the development of invasive carcinoma post radiation therapy is increased but that invasive carcinomas are also observed in untreated and surgically treated patients. It is common for clinicians to associate anaplastic carcinomas with "radiation transformation" of verrucous carcinomas, but the literature describes the development of all morphologic grades. These various grades of squamous cell carcinomas have been noted regardless of the type of therapy (or lack of therapy). In a recent clinicopathologic study of 104 patients with verrucous carcinomas, 21 (20 percent) were noted to have a coexisting infiltrating squamous cell carcinoma (Medina et al., 1984). Our conclusions are that surgery remains the treatment of choice but that

radiation therapy was probably as effective a treatment, especially in earlier stage tumors. Transformation to invasive carcinomas occurs with all forms of treatment at roughly similar frequencies and is not a property restricted to patients treated with radiation therapy.

INVERTING PAPILLOMAS

Papillomatosis, or inverting papilloma, is an unusual and perplexing epithelial proliferation occurring primarily in the nasal cavity and paranasal sinuses, although involvement of other sites has been described. The growth pattern and histologic appearance of these inverting papillomas are quite characteristic, and they commonly recur if the tumor is inadequately excised. It must be stressed that resections of these tumors mandate careful pathologic examination of the surgical margins similar to pathologic studies of malignant neoplasms. There are divergent views as to whether these epithelial proliferations represent hyperplasias, extending by metaplasia, or are true neoplasms. Because of the progressive local destructive nature of these inverting epithelial proliferations, I continue to view them as true neoplasms. These tumors are characterized by an inverting proliferation

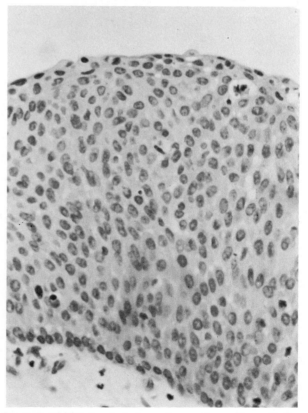

Figure 3–16. This is a typical inverting papilloma. The epithelium is composed of rather monotonous small cells with good intraepithelial organization. The basal layer is present, and squamous change and mucin droplets are not.

of epithelium into the underlying stroma. The epithelium is similar to schneiderian epithelium, often consisting of a monotonous proliferation of small "transitional-appearing" cells (Fig. 3–16). The epithelium may contain mucus droplets or may have prominent squamous differentiation with extensive surface keratin. These histologic variants occasionally cause diagnostic problems, but with the removal of adequate tissues the characteristic inverting growth pattern is obvious. The majority of these neoplasms arise on the lateral wall of the nasal cavity, often near the junction of the atrum and ethmoid sinus. Extension into the maxillary and ethmoid sinuses is common, often with accompanying destruction of adjacent underlying bone.

Associated or subsequent development of squamous cell carcinoma in inverting papillomas is unusual. Fechner and Alford (1968), following an extensive review of the literature, proposed that invasive carcinoma was a rare complication of these tumors. Hyams (1971), in the most definitive study, reported a recurrence rate as high as 66 percent and associated squamous cell carcinoma in 19 (13 percent) of the

inverted papillomas. Difficulty in interpreting inverting papillomas is due to foci of epithelial atypia. These changes have been confused by pathologists as representative of carcinomas (Fig. 3–17). It is my experience that epithelial alterations are relatively uncommon and are best classified as the appropriate grade of intraepithelial neoplasia. Rendering a diagnosis of CIS in an inverting papilloma only further confuses an ill-defined area. There are no data available regarding whether the presence of epithelial atypia increases the already high risk of recurrence. The major effort of the surgical pathologist should be directed toward evaluation of the margins of resection and identification of invasive carcinoma in the papilloma.

PAPILLOMAS AND PAPILLARY CARCINOMAS

The typical benign solitary papilloma occurs in numerous sites in the upper aerodigestive tract of adults and usually does not represent a diagnostic problem (Fig. 3–18). These rare neoplasms need to be clearly differentiated from the juvenile papillomatosis, which is usually viral in origin. However, significant epithelial

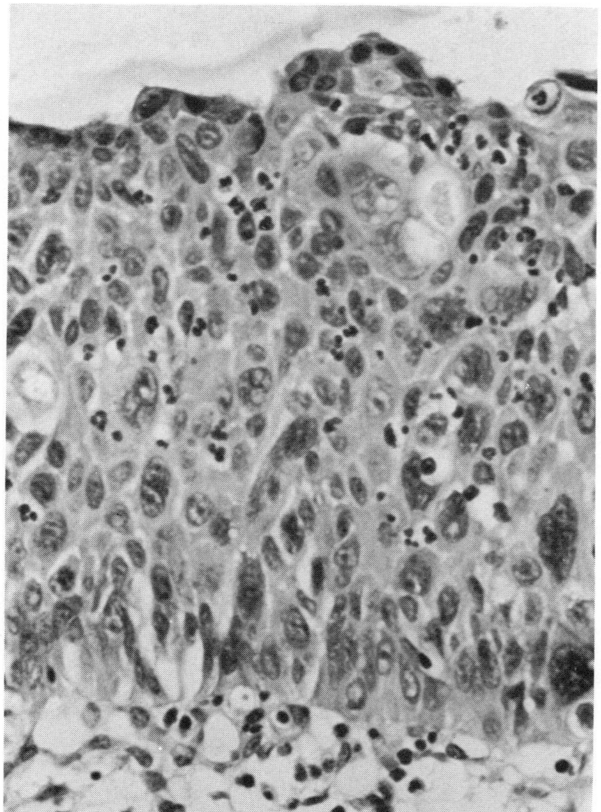

Figure 3–17. This is from the same specimen as Figure 3–16 and demonstrates extreme epithelial atypia consistent with intraepithelial neoplasia (Grade III) or carcinoma-in-situ. The latter diagnosis could possibly cause confusion for a surgeon or clinician not familiar with the high recurrence rates of these neoplasms without epithelial atypia.

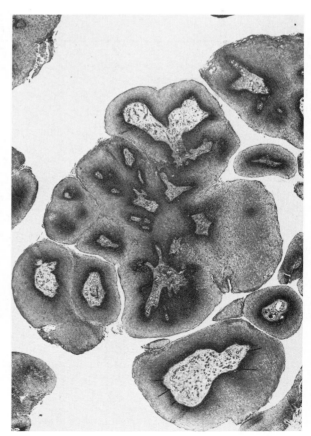

Figure 3–18. This is a typical squamous papilloma without any evidence of epithelial alterations.

maturation and cytologic alterations may be found in isolated exophytic proliferations occurring in adults. The guidelines for interpretation, diagnosis, and treatment of intraepithelial alterations in exophytic papillomas are no different from those used with inverting papillomas. If abnormal foci are identified, excision of the papilloma and the worrisome foci is usually adequate. If epithelial alterations extend to the lines of excision, a more serious situation exists and should be included in the pathology report. In many locations, the entire papilloma may be easily excised. Difficulties develop, however, when papillary outgrowths with epithelial abnormalities arise in the larynx. Partial laryngectomy may be required. When complete excision is not possible and the worrisome areas involve the base of the papilloma, or when a previously excised papilloma recurs with similar histologic changes, the problem becomes more complex. In these situations, the surgeon (and patient) must understand that the substantial risk for subsequent development of invasive carcinoma necessitates a more radical excision. Intraepithelial neoplastic changes do occur in isolated papillomas. The surgical pathologist must determine whether these alterations are confined to the epithelium. If an invasive carcinoma is identified, management of the patient must be appropriately modified.

Papillary carcinomas also are rare and often are difficult to diagnose on small forceps biopsy samples. However, they are not significantly different from papillary carcinomas arising in other anatomic sites. They generally demonstrate a fibrovascular core covered by epithelium with severe maturation and cytologic atypia. This mucosa usually demonstrates the changes of intraepithelial carcinoma but proliferates in an exophytic manner, usually maintaining a well-demarcated delineation between the neoplastic mucosa and fibrovascular stroma (Fig. 3–19). It must be emphasized that these neoplasms, like any non-invasive cancers, are capable of transforming into an invasive carcinoma and must be carefully evaluated so that such foci of transformation can be identified.

DIAGNOSIS OF "EARLY," OR "MICROINVASIVE," CARCINOMA

Differentiation of benign papillary ingrowth of hyperplastic mucosa from early neoplastic invasion of submucosal tissue is often difficult. In many situations, the presence of irregular, poorly organized projections of squamous cells originating from an overlying neoplastic epithelium is easily diagnosed as early, or microscopic, invasion. When the mucosa is hyperplastic, without significant atypia or evidence of SIN, and projections extending into the submucosa are well organized, the correct interpretation is pseudoepitheliomatous growth. The key issues involved in this critical differential diagnosis are the status of the

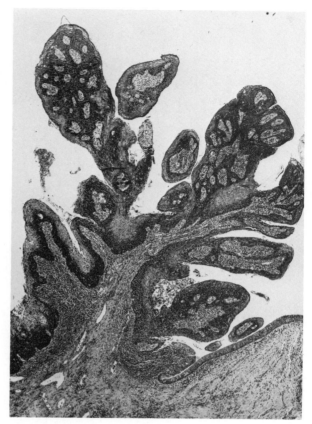

Figure 3–19. For comparison with Figure 3–18, this represents a well-differentiated papillary squamous cell carcinoma. This tumor is from the buccal mucosa and consists of an exophytic proliferation of keratinizing epithelium with the appearance of intraepithelial neoplasia. Multiple sections are necessary to exclude areas of invasive carcinoma. Excision is the treatment of choice.

overlying epithelium (reactive versus neoplastic) and the organization of the suspect areas of squamous epithelium. When a well-defined basal layer with evidence of maturation is present and the epithelium is sufficiently organized to appear capable of producing basement membrane at the epithelial–stromal interface, a diagnosis of papillary ingrowth, or pseudoepitheliomatous change, is indicated. When the suspected focus of invasion is poorly organized with appreciable cellular pleomorphism and irregular intercellular relationships, it is less likely a reactive process, and a diagnosis of invasion is indicated. Figure 3–20 demonstrates a papillary ingrowth in a laryngeal biopsy 6 months post radiation therapy. The biopsies obtained from this ingrowth demonstrated extensive surface hyperplasia with some cellular atypia. These cellular changes (Fig. 3–20), although disturbing, were not judged sufficient for a diagnosis of carcinoma. There is good epithelial–stromal demarcation, and the epithelium appears to be organized sufficiently to suggest the formation of a basement membrane. The extreme cellular atypia in the stroma secondary to radiation effect also should be noted. Figure 3–21

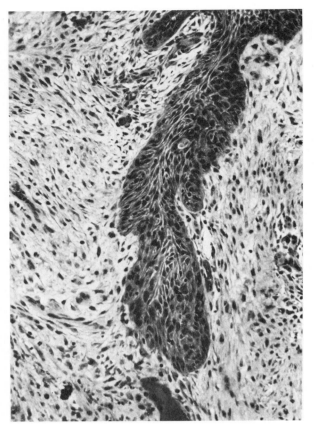

Figure 3–20. This is from a biopsy taken approximately 6 months after radiation treatment for carcinoma of the larynx. The patient developed extensive laryngeal keratosis, and all of the biopsies demonstrated some epithelial atypia but insufficient for a diagnosis of carcinoma-in-situ. The papillary ingrowth has some cytologic and maturation abnormalities, which can be partially explained by the previous radiation. The stroma has a number of abnormal cells which are also consistent with irradiation effect. The epithelial structure is worrisome but has a well-defined border with the host stroma, and the atypia is insufficient for a definite diagnosis of invasive carcinoma.

demonstrates two foci of microinvasive carcinoma. One foci is sufficiently atypical to be unequivocally malignant. It consists of an irregular aggregate of malignant cells with large amounts of keratin-containing cytoplasm. The adjacent focus of infiltrating cancer demonstrates a much better demarcation of the neoplastic cells and host stroma. However, the infiltrating cord of squamous carcinoma has such a degree of cytologic pleomorphism and lack of intraepithelial organization or maturation that it must also be interpreted as invasive carcinoma.

Although the morphologic criteria for the diagnosis of micro-invasion are often difficult, I continue to apply the criteria outlined in the legends of Figures 3–20 and 3–21. If the epithelial ingrowth arises in a focus of intraepithelial carcinoma and has a poorly demarcated border with the host stroma, it is invasive cancer. If the infiltration consists of single groups or cords of cells, it is invasive. When a broad band of epithelium extends into the submucosa, the differen-

tial between reactive and invasive neoplasm becomes more difficult. If there is sufficient cytologic atypia and lack of organization or orderly maturation, the tumor is most likely invasive carcinoma. If there is a well-demarcated epithelial stroma interface and attempts at organization or maturation, I generally take a conservative posture and do not call the lesion invasive. It is hoped that the use of immunohistochemistry to demonstrate the presence or absence of basement membrane (laminin, or type IV collagen) will be helpful in this critical differential. Failure to produce immunologically detectable basement membrane appears to represent a potentially major step in the differentiation of malignant invasion from reactive ingrowths (Barsky et al., 1983). This technique holds great promise and may represent a diagnostic observation in this critical differential diagnosis.

The clinical significance of early invasion, or microinvasion, is not clear, but in circumstances in which the pathologist is confident that the focus of early invasion is the most severe change present—that is, in excisional biopsies or biopsies of small erythroplakic

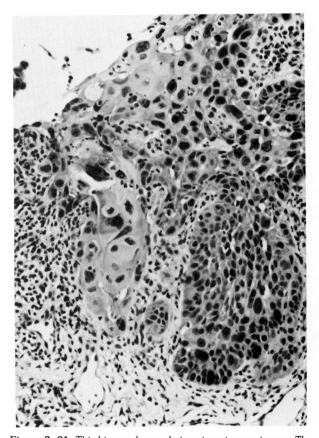

Figure 3–21. This biopsy shows obvious invasive carcinoma. The epithelial structure on the left has a poor demarcation with the host stroma and is clearly composed of malignant-appearing cells. The papillary ingrowth on the right is more difficult to interpret. However, it is (1) arising from overlying cancer, (2) has significant cytologic variation, and (3) is without evidence of maturation, even though the host stromal interface is well defined. These criteria are more than sufficient to merit a diagnosis of invasive cancer.

mucosal changes—a diagnosis of early or microinvasive carcinoma is indicated. It appears that these foci of early invasion have a lower incidence of vascular invasion, as evidenced by the rarity of regional lymph node metastases (Crissman et al., 1980). This will allow the surgeon to modify the choice of treatment and possibly permit a less radical procedure. Selected squamous cell carcinomas have relatively large patches of intraepithelial neoplasm with one or more foci of microinvasion, and it is extremely important for the surgeon to biopsy areas of induration. These foci are most likely to demonstrate the sites of maximal tumor invasion.

In summary, multifocal squamous intraepithelial and invasive carcinomas are being recognized with greater frequency. This growing recognition will undoubtedly be translated into increased biopsies with epithelial precursors to cancer. Although there is not a generally accepted set of criteria for grading intraepithelial alterations of the upper aerodigestive tract, many of the criteria used in other anatomic sites appear applicable. One of the problems inherent in translation is that the majority of upper aerodigestive tract mucosal changes demonstrate appreciable surface keratin production, an uncommon finding in other sites, such as the gynecologic tract.

Histologic clues to grading intraepithelial neoplasia are based on structural intraepithelial maturation and cytologic alteration. The characteristic feature of neoplastic transformation is the development of chromosomal aneuploidy, apparently reflected by both cytologic and intraepithelial maturation alterations. A grading system is described that recognizes unequivocal neoplastic epithelium (severe or Grade III intraepithelial neoplasia, SIN III, or severe dysplasia/CIS) that will usually persist and commonly progress to invasive cancer. Differentiation of severe epithelial changes from questionable categories (intermediate intraepithelial neoplasia, SIN II, moderate dysplasia) also is described.

My criteria for the histology of early or microinvasive carcinomas are presented. The most valuable criteria include origin from overlying carcinoma-in-situ; irregular growth patterns into the underlying host stroma; loss of tumor-stroma interface, characteristic of potential basement membrane formation; and loss of epithelial maturation with cellular abnormalities.

References

Ackerman, L. V.: Verrucous carcinoma of the oral cavity. Surgery 23:670–678, 1948.

Barsky, S. H., Siegal, G. P., Jannotta, F., Liotta, L. A.: Loss of basement membrane components by invasive tumors but not by their benign counterparts. Lab. Invest. 49:140–147, 1983.

Bauer, W. C., and McGavran, M. H.: Carcinoma in situ and evaluation of epithelial changes in laryngopharyngeal biopsies. J. Am. Med. Assoc. 221:72–75, 1972.

Bjelkenkrantz, K., Lundgren, J., Olofsson, J.: Single-cell DNA measurements in hyperplastic, dysplastic and carcinomatous laryngeal epithelium, with special reference to the occurrence of hypertetraploid cell nuclei. Analyt. Quant. Cytol. 5:184–188, 1983.

Cohn, A. M., and Peppard, S. B.: Multiple primary malignant tumors of the head and neck. Am. J. Otolaryngol. 1:411–417, 1980.

Crissman, J. D.: Laryngeal keratosis and subsequent carcinoma. Head Neck Surg. 1:386–391, 1979.

Crissman, J. D.: Laryngeal keratosis preceding laryngeal carcinoma. Arch. Otolaryngol. 108:445–448, 1982.

Crissman, J. D., Gluckman, J. L., Whiteley, J., Quenelle, D.: Squamous cell carcinoma of the floor of the mouth. Head Neck Surg. 3:2–7, 1980.

Einhorn, J., and Wersall, J.: Incidence of oral carcinoma in patients with leukoplakia of the oral mucosa. Cancer 20:2189–2193, 1967.

Fechner, R. E., and Alford, D. O.: Inverted papilloma and squamous carcinoma. Arch. Otolaryngol. 88:73–78, 1968.

Giarelli, L., Silvestri, F., Antonutto, G., Stanta, G.: Observations of the pathologist on precancerous lesions of the larynx. Integrated with histologic data and quantitative analysis of nuclear DNA content. Acta Otolaryngol. 84 (suppl. 344):7–18, 1977.

Gluckman, J. L., and Crissman, J. D.: Survival rates in 548 patients with multiple neoplasms of the upper aerodigestive tract. Laryngoscope 93:71–74, 1983.

Gluckman, J. L., Crissman, J. D., Donegan, J. O.: Multicentric squamous cell carcinoma of the upper aerodigestive tract. Head Neck Surg. 3:90–96, 1980.

Grontoft, O., Hellquist, H., Olofsson, J., Nordstrom, G.: The DNA content and nuclear size in normal, dysplastic and carcinomatous laryngeal epithelium. A spectrophotometric study. Acta Otolaryngol. 86:473–479, 1978.

Hyams, V. J.: Papillomas of the nasal cavity and paranasal sinuses. Ann. Otol. Rhinol. Laryngol. 80:192–206, 1971.

Mashberg, A.: Erythroplasia: The earliest sign of asymptomatic oral cancer. J. Am. Dent. Assoc. 96:615–620, 1978.

McDonald, J. S., Crissman, J. D., Gluckman, J. L.: Verrucous carcinoma of the oral cavity. Head Neck Surg. 5:22–28, 1982.

McGavran, M. H., Bauer, W. C., Ogura, J. H.: Isolated laryngeal keratosis: Its relation to carcinoma of the larynx based on a clinicopathologic study of 87 consecutive cases with long-term follow-up. Laryngoscope 70:932–950, 1960.

Medina, J. E., Dichtel, W., Luna, M. A.: Verrucous-squamous carcinomas of the oral cavity. Arch. Otolaryngol 110:437–440, 1984.

Norris, C. M. and Peale, A. R.: Keratosis of the larynx. J. Laryngol. Otol. 77:635–647, 1963.

Pindborg, J. J., Renstrup, G., Poulsen, H. E., Silverman, S.: Studies in oral leukoplakias: V. Clinical and histological signs of malignancy. Acta Odontol. Scand. 21:404–414, 1963.

Prioleau, P. G., Santa Cruz, D. J., Meyer, J. S., Bauer, W. C.: Verrucous carcinoma. A light and electron microscopic autoradiographic and immunofluorescence study. Cancer 45:2849–2857, 1980.

Shafer, W. G.: Oral carcinoma in situ. Oral Surg. 39:227–238, 1975.

Shafer, W. G., and Waldron, C. A.: Erythroplakia of the oral cavity. Cancer 36:1021–1028, 1975.

Shear, M., and Pindborg, J. J.: Verrucous hyperplasia of the oral mucosa. Cancer 46:1855–1862, 1980.

Silverman, S., Jr.: Observations of the clinical characteristics and natural history of oral leukoplakia. J. Am. Dent. Assoc. 76:772–777, 1968.

Waldron, C. A., and Shafer, W. G.: Leukoplakia revisited. A clinicopathologic study of 3256 oral leukoplakias. Cancer 36:1386–1392, 1975.

Weaver, A., Fleming, S. M., Knecktges, T. C., Smith, D.: Triple endoscopy: A neglected essential in head and neck cancer. Surgery 86:493–496, 1979.

LEWIS B. WOOLNER

4 Lung

The early stages of lung cancer, including possible precursor changes, are rarely encountered by the surgical pathologist studying routine pathologic specimens. Surgically resected lung cancer that is symptomatic or clinically evident usually is advanced lung cancer. Thus, the pathologic findings in the very early, or incipient, stages of bronchogenic carcinoma have been difficult to document. Since the 1970s, documentation of these early stages has been improving owing to a program of screening for early lung cancer (Fontana et al. 1972; Melamed et al., 1977a).

Two screening techniques are available for the detection of early (Stage I) lung cancer: the chest radiograph and the sputum cytology test. These two tests are complementary. The chest radiograph is best for detection of early peripheral parenchymal cancers, whereas the sputum cytology test is the best detector of early, centrally located squamous cancer.

Early lung cancer detected radiographically generally takes the form of a parenchymal rounded nodule and may be of any cell type. The smallest peripheral tumor that can be detected on a chest roentgenogram is approximately 1 cm in diameter. Although small, such peripheral cancers are invasive, and histologically they resemble larger neoplasms in all respects. Little is known of the incipient stages of such parenchymal cancers because they are undetectable either by chest roentgenogram or by sputum cytology.

Radiographically negative lung cancer detected by sputum cytology is known as "occult" lung cancer. Such lesions are intrabronchial in character; involve the subsegmental, or larger, bronchi; and are almost always squamous (Carter et al., 1976; Eggleston et al., 1982; Melamed et al., 1977b; Nasiell et al., 1977; Woolner et al., 1970). Bronchoscopic localization, followed by conservative surgical resection, enables the pathologist to study bronchial cancer of this type at its earliest stages. Special pathologic techniques for processing the surgical specimens are necessary for optimal results.

This chapter on early lung cancer and its possible precursors is based in part on data derived from the author's participation in the Mayo Lung Project, a screening program for the detection of early lung cancer. Some data on the cytologic, pathologic, and roentgenographic aspects of the Mayo Lung Project have been published (Fontana et al., 1975; Fontana et al., 1984; Woolner et al., 1981). In this presentation, the emphasis is directed toward the very earliest stages of the neoplastic process—namely, in-situ and minimally invasive bronchogenic carcinoma—along with available data on possible precancerous, dysplastic changes in the bronchial tree.

PATHOLOGIC CONSIDERATIONS

Special expertise and special techniques on the part of the pathologist may be necessary in the management of early lung cancer cases. Early lung cancer detected by radiography presents few problems. Localization of the tumor is provided by the chest film, on which the carcinoma generally is seen as a rounded, parenchymal nodule that may be as small as 1 cm in diameter. At operation, the line of resection is checked by the pathologist, and the status of peribronchial or other lymph nodes is determined. The pathologic report should include such data as size and cell type of the carcinoma and its relationship to overlying pleura. For this, one complete block through a small tumor or two blocks from a somewhat larger lesion should suffice.

By contrast, radiographically occult lung cancer requires special procedures and expertise at all levels of management. An occult cancer of the lung is suspected in a patient whose sputum contains carcinoma cells or highly atypical squamous cells on repeated examination and in whom an upper airway carcinoma has been excluded. The tumor is localized with the flexible fiberoptic bronchoscope, which facilitates inspection and examination of all parts of the bronchial tree (Sanderson et al., 1974). These occult lung cancers frequently are not visible or are just barely visible to the bronchoscopist. Thus, special

57

procedures, including systematic segmental brushing with multiple spur biopsies of the bronchial tree, are necessary. Conservative surgery is performed after a positive biopsy or positive bronchial brushing confirmed by a second positive examination.

Processing of Surgical Specimen

Because a radiographically occult cancer may not be visible on gross pathologic examination or, if visible, is likely to have poorly defined margins, special care is necessary in processing the surgical specimen. The line of resection is checked by examination of frozen sections during the operation, and the specimen is opened for examination of lobar, segmental, and subsegmental bronchi. After removal of intrabronchial mucus and before the specimen is photographed, it is useful to identify the segmental bronchi with small, typed labels (Fig. 4–1). After formalin fixation, a drawing is made of the opened bronchi, and serial block sectioning is performed. The number of blocks required for an adequate pathologic examination varies according to the specimen. If a gross carcinoma is visible, the entire tumor is sectioned along with a generous margin (at least 1 cm) of adjacent mucosa on either border. If the site of the tumor is identified only by the biopsy site or if resection has been performed on the basis of repeated positive bronchial brushings, the entire segmental bronchus in question or even the bronchi of a resected lobe must be sectioned.

Many occult carcinomas are located in the upper lobe bronchi and may involve the distal lobar bronchus, the trifurcation area, or the orifices of various segmental bronchi. A systematic approach to the

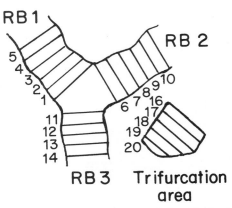

Figure 4–2. Serial block sectioning as carried out for the specimen shown in Figure 4–1.

sectioning of these areas is shown in Figure 4–2. Initial transverse cuts near the orifice of each segmental bronchus leave a triangular trifurcation area that can be carefully sectioned, as shown in the diagram. One margin may be marked with India ink for later reconstruction of the original configuration.

Each section is examined histologically, and any abnormalities found are plotted according to the original diagram. In this way, the exact origin of an occult carcinoma can be indicated, and the extent of in-situ changes as well as the extent and depth of any invasive foci can be determined precisely.

Bronchial Mucosal Abnormalities

The pathologist dealing with early lung cancer should be familiar with the various histologic changes that occur in bronchial epithelium under irritative, inflammatory, or neoplastic conditions. These may be encountered in either biopsy or surgical specimens. The changes include basal cell or goblet cell hyperplasia, squamous cell metaplasia, various squamous cell atypias, and in-situ carcinoma, with or without early microinvasion. These changes are defined and illustrated as follows.

Hyperplasia. The normal bronchial epithelium is composed of five types of cells: basal (reserve) cells, intermediate cells, goblet cells, ciliated columnar cells, and nonciliated columnar cells (Fig. 4–3A). Under inflammatory or irritative stimuli, hyperplasia of bronchial epithelium may occur. This generally takes the form of basal cell, or reserve cell, proliferation and results in a highly cellular epithelium composed largely of nuclei that resemble those of basal cells (Fig. 4–3B). Occasionally, the hyperplastic cells may be somewhat larger and intermediate in size (Fig. 4–3C). Basal cell hyperplasia is frequently associated with, or merges into, squamous cell metaplasia (Fig. 4–3D). Mucus-producing columnar cells (goblet cells), normally present in the bronchial epithelium, also may undergo

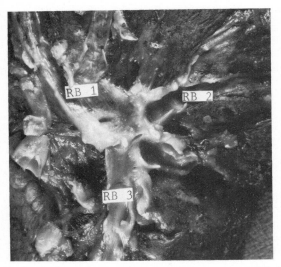

Figure 4–1. In-situ-carcinoma. Processing of specimen. Labeling of opened segmental bronchi as indicated prior to photography aids in subsequent orientation and sectioning of specimen.

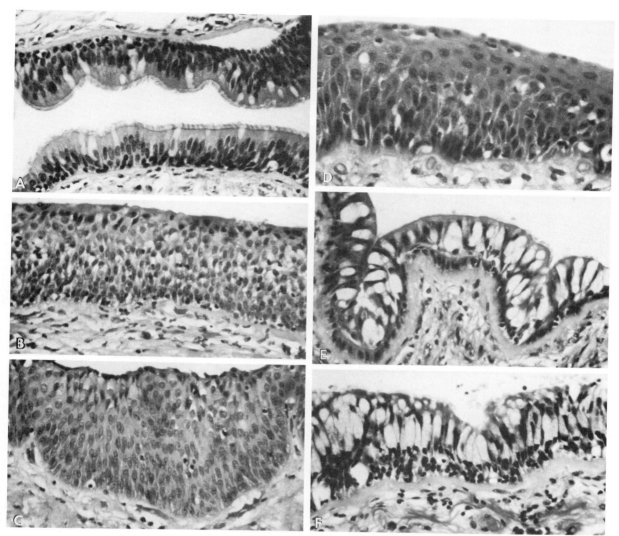

Figure 4–3. Normal and hyperplastic bronchial mucosa. *A*, Essentially normal epithelium lining a small bronchus, including a row of small pyknotic basal cells, slightly larger intermediate cells, tall columnar ciliated cells with somewhat vesicular nuclei, and a few goblet cells. *B* Basal cell hyperplasia. The greatly increased cellularity of bronchial epithelium shown here results largely from a proliferation of basal cells. *C*, Hyperplastic epithelium, showing predominance of larger intermediate cells. The cells appear columnar with regular orientation to basement membrane. *D*, Early squamous metaplasia. The cells above the basal layer show a gradual squamoid transformation. They contain abundant cytoplasm and assume a rounded or polygonal shape with beginning flattening of superficial layers. *E*, Prominent goblet cells. Numerous goblet cells are seen within the superficial layer of columnar cells. There is a suggestion of separation of this epithelium from the underlying prominent basal cell layer. *F*, Goblet cell hyperplasia with some associated basal cell proliferation.

hyperplasia or, in extreme cases, appear to crowd out other constituents of the bronchial epithelium (Fig. 4–3*E* and *F*). Serial block sectioning of the bronchial tree in specimens of lung removed for occult carcinoma may demonstrate areas of desquamation of bronchial epithelium with "slit-formation," often associated with some degree of basal cell or goblet cell hyperplasia (Nasiell et al., 1982). Examples of this phenomenon are shown in Figure 4–4*A* to *C*. Occasionally, this change is noted at the margin of an in-situ carcinoma (Fig. 4–4*D*).

Squamous Metaplasia. This is commonly seen in bronchial mucosa. Early squamoid change is fre-

quently associated with varying degrees of basal cell hyperplasia, but, as the metaplastic change becomes more pronounced, the columnar cells become enlarged and rounded or polygonal with prominent intracellular bridges (prickle cells) (Fig. 4–5*A*). The final stage of advanced squamous change shows a thick layer of fully developed squamous epithelium (Fig. 4–5*B*).

Squamous Cell Atypia. A histologic diagnosis of frank in-situ carcinoma is based on rather marked qualitative changes in surface epithelial cells, including increase in size of cells and nuclei, variation in size and shape of nuclei, abnormal nuclear-cytoplasmic

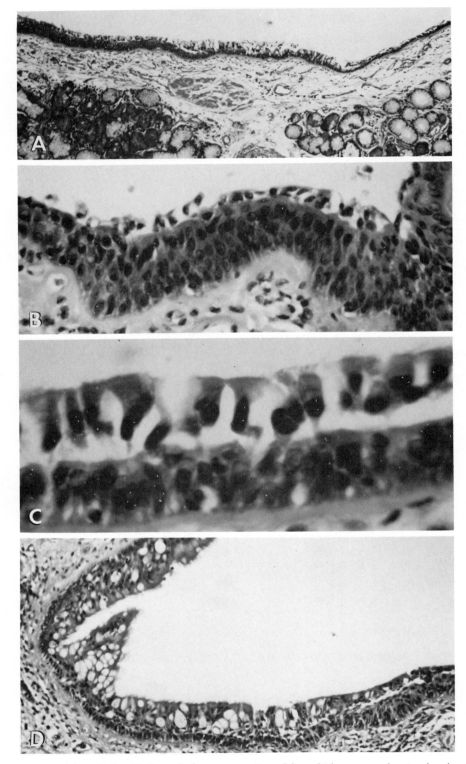

Figure 4–4. Desquamation of bronchial epithelium. *A,* Low-power view of bronchial mucosa, showing basal cell hyperplasia with desquamation of superficial columnar epithelium. *B,* Similar findings from another case. Here the basal layer shows progressive regeneration toward normal. *C,* Same phenomenon as *B* at higher magnification. The desquamating layer of columnar cells is held in place by string-like protoplasmic processes. *D,* Atypical basal cell hyperplasia and "slit-formation" occurring at the advancing margin of an in-situ-carcinoma.

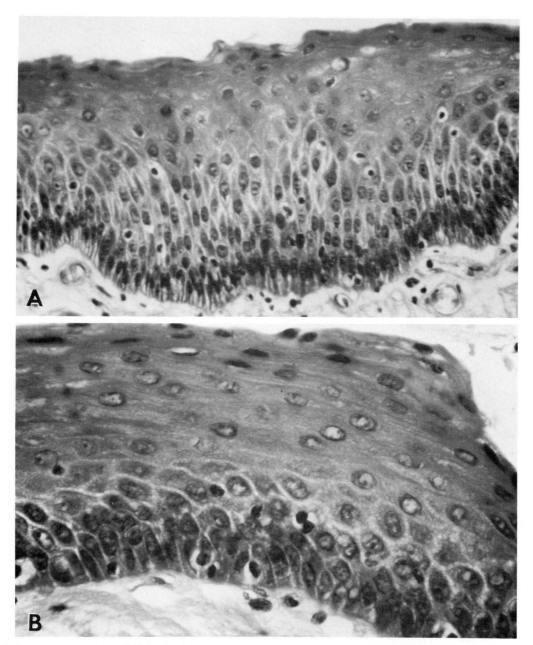

Figure 4–5. Squamous metaplasia. *A,* Fully developed squamous metaplasia of bronchus is shown here with a prominent zone of prickle cells over which the superficial cells become progressively flattened and keratinized. There is no evidence of epithelial atypia. *B,* Advanced stage of the same process. The majority of the cells are flattened and keratinized with pyknotic nuclei in the superficial layers.

ratio, and increased nuclear hyperchromasia, reflecting an increased DNA content of nuclei. More precise details of cellular change indicative of carcinoma can be seen in well-made cytologic preparations from cancerous epithelium.

Degrees of cellular alteration in bronchial epithelium less marked than those of in-situ carcinoma are occasionally encountered. These are commonly referred to as "squamous cell atypias" and correspond in a general way to dysplasia of the uterine cervix. Such changes sometimes may be seen adjacent to, or within, a fully developed area of carcinoma-in-situ of the bronchus, apparently forming a transition between normal and fully cancerous epithelium. Alternatively, atypical foci occasionally may be encountered in a bronchus widely separated from a bronchial carcinoma.

Mild (slight), moderate, or marked degrees of squamous cell atypia may be arbitrarily defined. In mild (slight) atypia, the cellular alteration is minimal. At the other extreme, marked atypia indicates a degree of alteration that is severe but that, in the judgment of the pathologist, falls short of frank carcinoma-in-situ. Moderate atypia is midway between these two extremes. Various grades of cellular atypia are shown in Figure 4–6. (Further discussion of the problem, with illustrations, appears in individual case reports of early carcinoma further on in this chapter.)

Carcinoma-In-Situ. As in other locations, a carcinoma-in-situ of the bronchus is one in which the carcinomatous process is confined to the surface epithelium with no demonstrable invasion of underlying stroma. The ducts of mucous glands are commonly involved by direct extension; less frequently, acinar structures are involved as well. Such ductal or acinar extension should not be mistaken for stromal invasion.

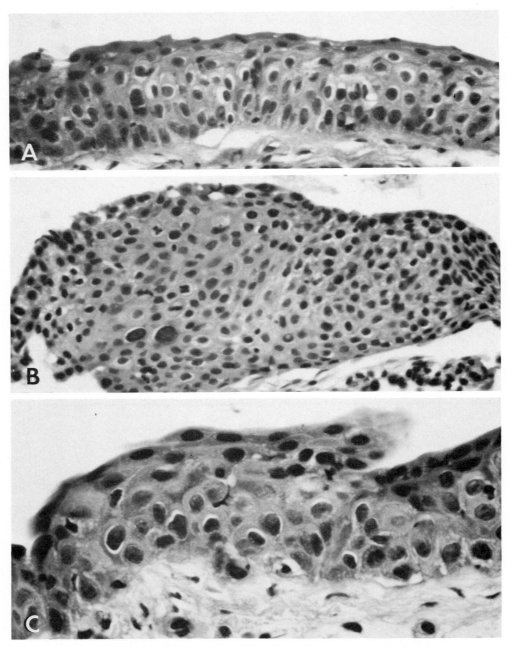

Figure 4–6. Atypical squamous metaplasia. *A,* Squamous metaplasia shown here is associated with slight variation in nuclear size and staining qualities ("slight atypia"). *B,* This metaplastic epithelium shows a more disorderly arrangement of cells along with considerable nuclear variation ("moderate atypia"). *C,* This area of squamous metaplasia shows striking cellular alteration. The metaplastic cells are large and have abundant cytoplasm, and the nuclei vary greatly in size, shape, and staining reaction ("marked atypia"). The changes approach those of carcinoma-in-situ.

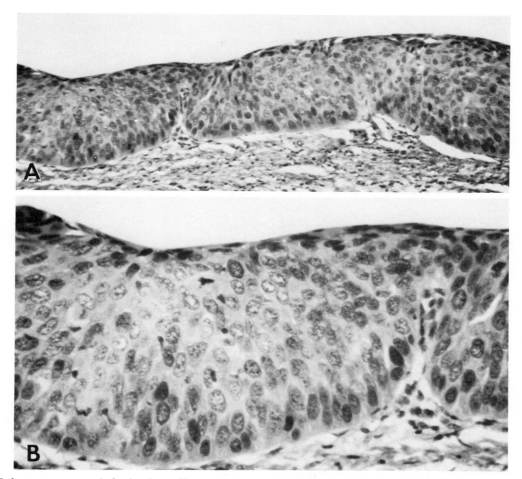

Figure 4–7. In-situ-carcinoma. *A,* In this "typical" example (*see* variants further on), the morphologic changes are convincing for a diagnosis of carcinoma. There is marked cellular proliferation with mitotic figures, and the cells show nuclear hyperchromasia with an alteration in the nuclear-cytoplasmic ratio in favor of the nucleus. *B,* Higher magnification of the same area.

A classic example of in-situ carcinoma is shown in Figure 4–7. Variations in histologic structure of in-situ cancer, from well-differentiated to more anaplastic examples, are discussed in the cases presented further on in this chapter.

Early or Minimal Stromal Invasion. The natural history of in-situ carcinoma presumes an in-situ stage of variable duration followed by invasion of stroma at one or more points, resulting in a "minimally invasive cancer." This initial stage of infiltration is followed by progressively deeper invasion of the bronchial wall or surrounding tissues, with eventual development of lymphatic or blood-borne metastasis.

The earliest evidence of invasion by an in-situ carcinoma is often difficult to diagnose precisely. In general, at the initial stage, small cancerous buds project into the stroma from the overlying cancerous epithelium either on the surface or within ducts or acini (Fig. 4–8*A* to *D*). In turn, these buds elongate or increase in size, and, as a result of further budding and strand formation, a minute "tumor" is formed (Fig. 4–8*E* and *F*). The penetrating tongues of tissue may be sharp and tentacular or more broad-based and expansile in character. Host reaction to invasion by tumor at first is cellular, with lymphocytic or plasma cell infiltration followed by varying degrees of fibrosis. Actual cases illustrating very early and somewhat more advanced microinvasion are presented further on.

CARCINOMA-IN-SITU

Clinicopathologic study of cases derived from a screened population of patients (Woolner et al., 1984) undergoing prompt surgical resection leads to the following conclusions regarding the in-situ stage of bronchogenic carcinoma:

1. In-situ carcinoma may arise in any portion of the bronchial tree, but there is a distinct predilection for the bronchi of the upper lobes at the segmental or subsegmental levels of division.

2. Resected specimens are small (mean diameter, 0.9 cm; range, 0.2 to 1.7 cm), and most are inconspicuous or not visible on gross examination.

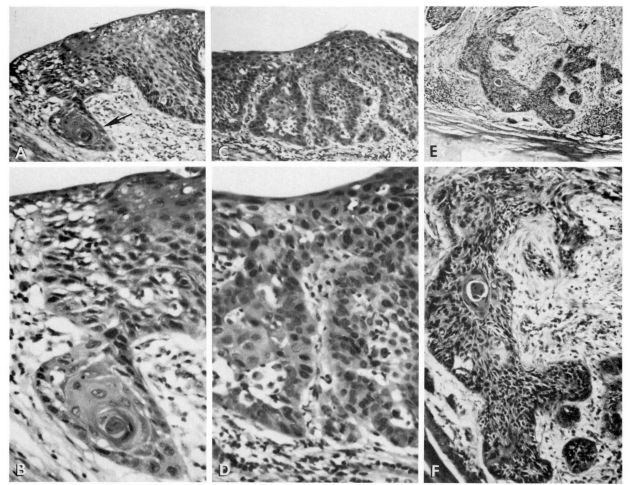

Figure 4–8. In-situ-carcinoma with microinvasion. *A,* Very early evidence of stromal invasion. A cancerous bud *(arrow)* projects downward from the altered surface epithelium. *B,* Higher magnification of focal invasion. *C,* Early but more obvious stromal invasion. The depth of penetration from the surface in this area (measured by micrometer) is 0.25 mm. *D,* Higher magnification of focal invasion. *E,* Advanced stromal invasion. By the process of budding and strand formation, the tumor penetrates almost to bronchial cartilage. *F,* Higher magnification of same area.

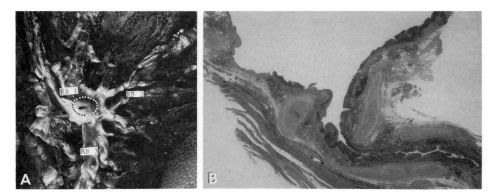

Figure 4–9. Case 1, in-situ-carcinoma. *A,* The carcinoma *(outlined by dots)* involves proximal RB 1, including the orifice of a small unopened branch bronchus. Note the mucosal granularity in the area of carcinoma. *B,* Cross section of RB 1 and small unopened branch bronchus, both lined with carcinoma.

Illustration continued on opposite page

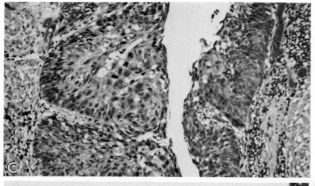

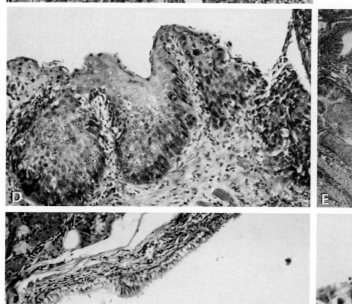

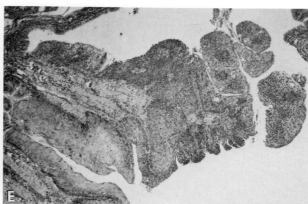

Figure 4–9. *Continued. C,* In-situ-carcinoma involving both walls of small bronchus. Prickle cells predominate. *D,* In this area of adjacent RB 1 there is surface keratinization of tumor cells. *E,* A small papillary component near margin of tumor. *F,* Junction of tumor and adjacent ciliated epithelium in the same area shown at higher magnification. The rather bland appearance of the growing margin suggests a "transitional" stage. *G,* Another tumor margin sharply delineated.

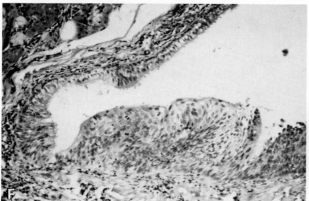

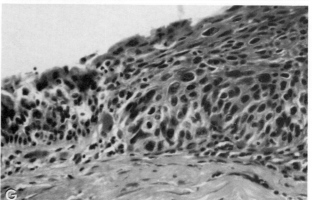

3. Histologically, there is carcinomatous transformation of surface epithelium with frequent direct extension to involve ducts of mucous glands or acini.

4. Some range of histologic variation is observed in a series of in-situ carcinomas, including average, well-differentiated, and more anaplastic examples.

5. The margins of the tumor may be sharp or show a gradual transformation to normal epithelium.

6. The bronchial epithelium adjacent to an in-situ carcinoma may be normal, hyperplastic, metaplastic, or "atypical" in appearance.

7. Distinguishing between an in-situ carcinoma and one in which there is very early minimal stromal invasion may present a difficult diagnostic problem.

A number of variables observed in cases of resected in-situ carcinoma—including size, degree of differentiation, findings at tumor margins, and status of adjacent epithelium— are illustrated in the following seven cases:

Case 1. In-situ carcinoma (1 × 0.9 cm) was visible grossly in RB 1 (right bronchus 1) as mucosal roughening. Histologically, the tumor exhibited an average degree of differentiation, with prickle cells predominating (Fig. 4–9).

Case 2. A very small in-situ carcinoma, not visible grossly, involved the RB 1–2 spur. Histologically, the tumor was rather poorly differentiated and limited to one tissue block (estimated size of tumor, including positive biopsy specimen, less than 0.5 cm). The adjacent mucosa showed some atypical squamous

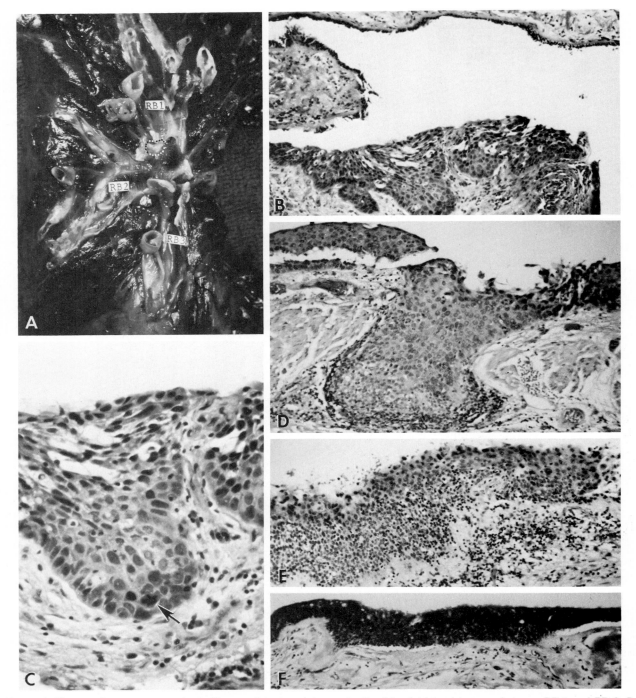

Figure 4–10. Case 2, in-situ-carcinoma. *A,* Very small in-situ-carcinoma *(outlined by dots)* involving spur between RB 1 and RB 2. *B,* Histologic section of the spur shows almost the entire carcinoma. *C,* Higher magnification of tumor, showing pathologic mitotic figure *(arrow). D,* Area on same spur adjacent to tumor shows atypical squamoid change at orifice of mucous gland duct. *E,* Focus of basal cell hyperplasia apart from immediate tumor area, showing surface metaplasia with slight atypia. *F,* Second localized focus of basal cell hyperplasia apart from the tumor area.

metaplasia and focal basal cell hyperplasia (Fig. 4–10).

Case 3. An in-situ carcinoma (1.4 × 0.6 cm) involved RB 1 proximally and was visible grossly as an area of mucosal redness and edema. Histologically,

the tumor was poorly differentiated, with heavy stromal lymphocytic infiltration. The tumor margins were sharp, and the adjacent epithelium was ciliated columnar (Fig. 4–11).

Case 4. In-situ carcinoma (1.5 × 1 cm) involved

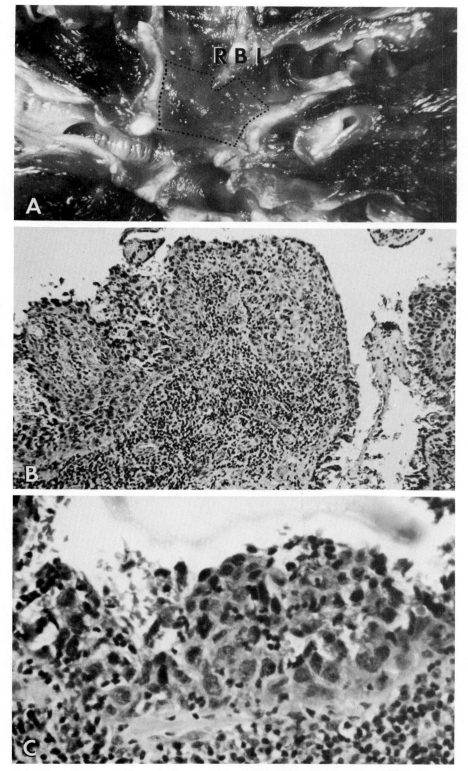

Figure 4–11. Case 3, in-situ-carcinoma. *A,* Mucosal edema involving orifice and proximal portion of RB 1; tumor *(outlined by dots)* was 1.4 × 0.6 cm. *B,* Low-power view of margin of carcinoma shows heavy lymphocytic infiltration of bronchial wall. *C,* Higher magnification of same area shows poorly differentiated carcinoma with no evidence of keratinization.

RB 6 proximally. Histologically, the tumor was fairly active, with deep extension into ducts of mucous glands and acini (Fig. 4–12).

Case 5. An in-situ carcinoma, approximately 1 cm in diameter, was situated on a spur between medial and lateral basal segmental bronchi. Grossly, the tumor was visible as a slightly polypoid projection. Histologically, the carcinoma showed an extreme de-

gree of maturation with keratinization. Adjacent to the tumor were areas of squamous metaplasia and squamous cell atypia (Fig. 4–13).

Case 6. A small carcinoma-in-situ (0.5 cm in diameter) involved the RB 6 spur. A biopsy specimen obtained from this area in the course of localizing bronchoscopy, in which multiple bilateral biopsy and brushing specimens were taken, was positive. Histo-

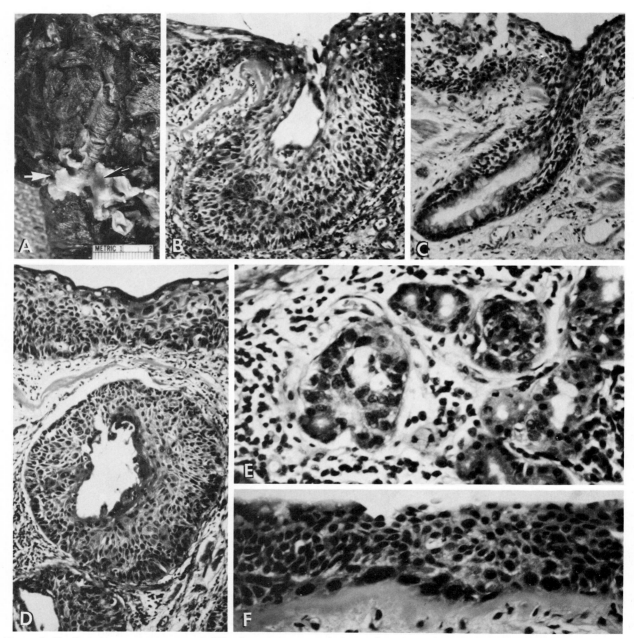

Figure 4–12. Case 4, in-situ-carcinoma. *A,* Whitish, opaque mucosal abnormality at site of carcinoma involving orifice and proximal portion of RB 6 *(arrows).* *B,* Histologic section shows carcinoma-in-situ involving surface epithelium and orifice of duct of mucous gland. The tumor cells are large, and there is surface keratinization. *C,* Early stage of downward extension of surface carcinoma into duct of mucous gland. *D,* Another area shows deeper extension of carcinoma into ducts. Note surface keratinization. *E,* In this area the carcinoma extends into mucous gland acini. *F,* Epithelium at tumor margin shows extension of carcinoma along basal layer of overlying benign epithelium.

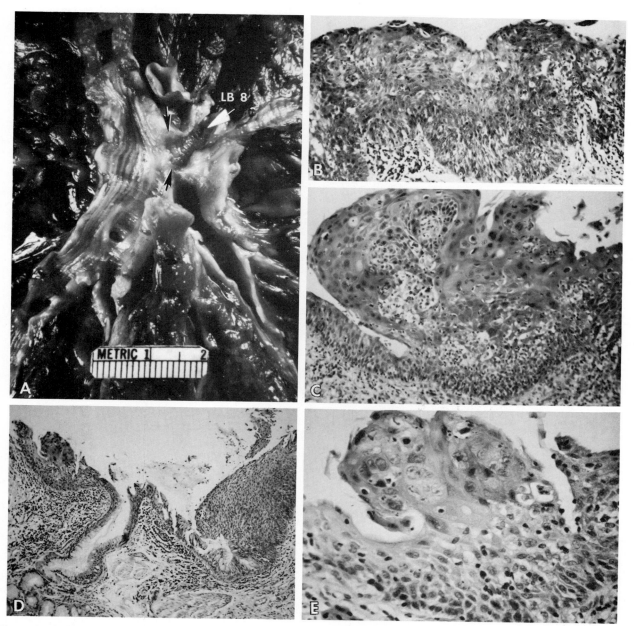

Figure 4–13. Case 5. In-situ-carcinoma. *A,* Slight polypoid thickening of spur represents area of carcinoma *(arrows). B,* Histologic section through center shows a highly differentiated squamous carcinoma. *C,* Section through sharply delineated margin shows polypoid tumor with extreme keratinization. *D,* Adjacent foci of abnormality on same spur—carcinoma at left and marked atypia at right. *E,* High-power view of carcinomatous focus shown in *D.* Basal area appears hyperplastic.

Illustration continued on following page

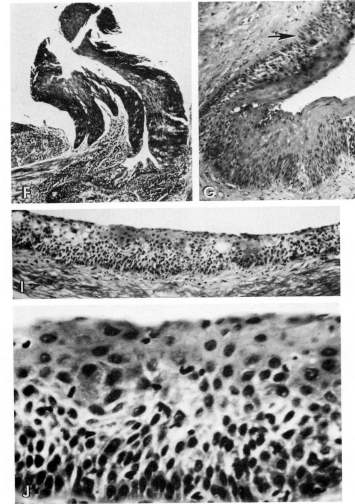

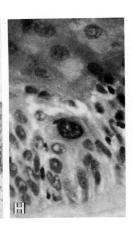

Figure 4–13. *Continued. F,* Another focus of marked atypia adjacent to carcinoma. Note resemblance to cutaneous horn. *G,* Marked squamous metaplasia in region of tumor. One highly abnormal cell is present *(arrow). H,* Higher magnification of the single abnormal cell. *I,* Another area of squamous metaplasia with slight atypia in the vicinity of the tumor. *J,* Higher magnification of same atypical focus.

logically, the cytologic changes are much less impressive than those usually seen in carcinoma-in-situ, and, although this diagnosis is made, the lesion is considered "borderline" (Fig. 4–14). No gross changes were seen in the surgical specimen.

Case 7. A very small carcinoma in LB 6 was detected by serial block sectioning of the entire bronchial specimen. Histologically, the cytologic changes were considered minimal for a diagnosis of carcinoma-in-situ (borderline lesion) (Fig. 4–15).

CARCINOMA-IN-SITU WITH MICROINVASION

The term "microinvasive bronchogenic carcinoma" may be used to describe cases in which beginning stromal invasion has been superimposed on an earlier in-situ stage of the disease. Clinicopathologic study of a series of cases prompts the following conclusions:

1. The time required for the development of mi-croinvasion is unknown. The in-situ stage may be of long duration.

2. Clinical and cytologic findings in microinvasive cancers are similar to those in cases still in situ.

3. Microinvasive cancers tend to be larger than in-situ cancers and are more readily visualized on bronchoscopic or gross pathologic examination.

4. Histologically, the earliest evidence of invasion may be difficult to diagnose precisely; as invasion progresses, the diagnosis becomes more obvious.

5. Classification of radiographically occult bronchogenic carcinoma based on depths of invasion is useful (Woolner and Farrow, 1982). Arbitrary levels include (a) no invasion (in situ); (b) intramucosal invasion (invasion into mucosa 1 mm or less); (c) invasion to inner level of cartilages; (d) deeper invasion to include entire thickness of bronchial wall; and (e) extrabronchial extension.

The following three cases illustrate very early and more obvious examples of microinvasion:

Case 8. A fairly extensive carcinoma-in-situ in-

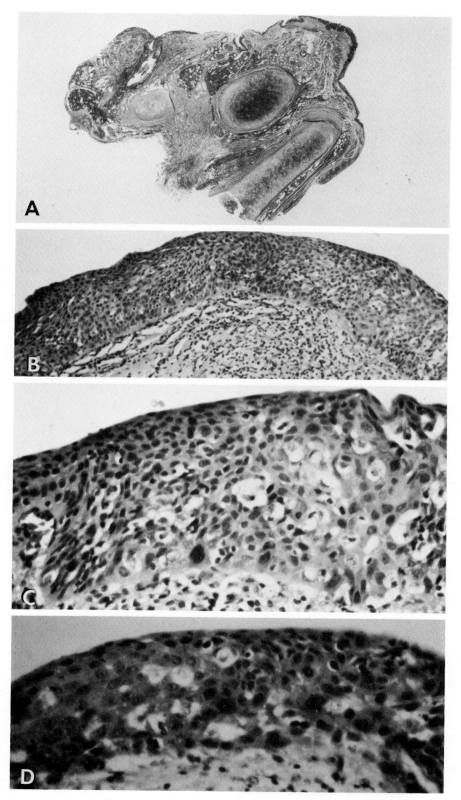

Figure 4–14. Case 6. Carcinoma-in-situ (borderline lesion). *A,* Section through RB 6 spur shows epithelial alteration at the summit. *B,* Histologic section of same spur shows increased cellularity and atypical epithelial changes. *C,* High-power view of a typical area to show the degree of nuclear alteration. Although borderline, the cellular changes are considered sufficient for a diagnosis of carcinoma-in-situ. *D,* Margin of lesion shows gradual transition to normal squamous metaplasia.

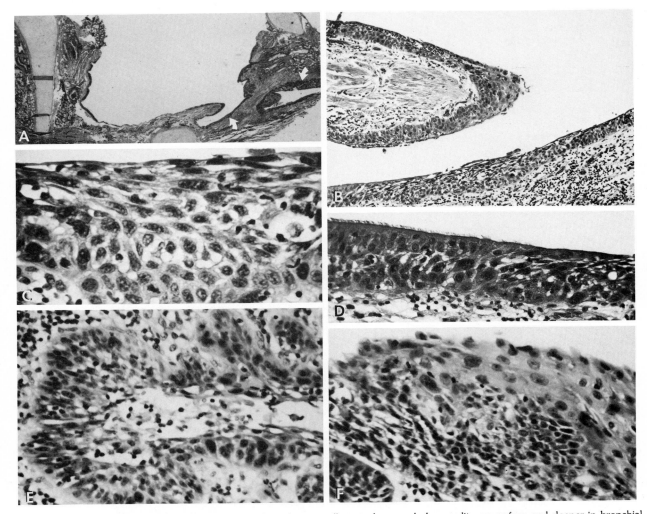

Figure 4–15. Case 7. *A,* Cross section of LB 6 bronchus shows small area of mucosal abnormality on surface and deeper in bronchial wall *(arrows). B,* Higher magnification of surface area shown in *A. C,* High-power view of the same area, representing the most severe cytologic alteration in this case. A diagnosis of carcinoma-in-situ is made, but as in the preceding case, changes are considered borderline. *D,* Margin of the lesion. Atypical cells are undermining the columnar ciliated cells, forming an acute-angle opening from right to left. *E,* High-power view of portion of deep mucosal lesion in *A,* showing extreme hyperplasia and epithelial atypia. *F,* Squamous metaplasia and moderate atypia in surface epithelium adjacent to the carcinoma.

volved a basal segmental bronchus and its two subsegmental branches. Histologically, there was multifocal early microinvasion varying from equivocal, barely detectable foci to definite shallow infiltration of underlying stroma. The margins of the carcinoma varied from a sharply defined junction to one in which a gradual transformation of proliferating atypical basal cells appeared to be occurring (Fig. 4–16).

Case 9. An extensive carcinoma-in-situ with focal microinvasion involved LB 1–2 distally and extended along all three segmental bronchi. The carcinomatous change was visible grossly. Histologically, there was widespread in-situ carcinoma with several foci of shallow microinvasion, all less than 0.1 cm in depth (Fig. 4–17).

Case 10. An extensive carcinoma involved the mucosa of the right upper lobe and extended peripherally along its three subdivisions. Grossly, the mucosa was thrown into folds and greatly thickened. Histologically, there was diffuse in-situ carcinoma with massive extension into ducts of mucous glands and focal invasion to the inner aspect of bronchial cartilages (Fig. 4–18).

MULTICENTRICITY

Multiple primary lung cancers may occur either simultaneously or sequentially (subsequent tumors), in which case a second primary carcinoma develops after "curative" resection of the first one. The frequency of multicentricity of clinically apparent lung

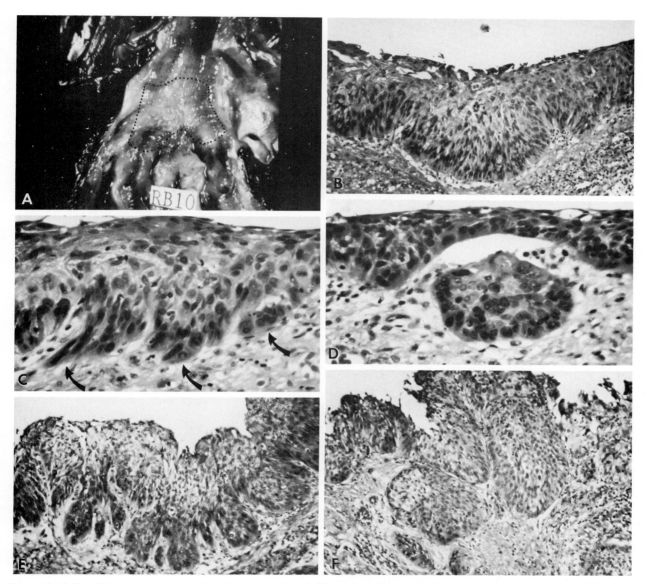

Figure 4–16. Case 8. In-situ-carcinoma with early microinvasion. *A,* Mucosal opacity representing an area of carcinoma-in-situ with minimal invasion. The tumor involves 1 cm of distal RB 10 and 0.6 and 0.2 cm of its subsegmental divisions *(outlined by dots).* *B,* Carcinoma-in-situ with no evidence of invasion. *C,* An adjacent area with equivocal early stromal invasion at junctional zone *(arrows).* *D,* Island of questionable invasion just below the surface in in-situ cancer. *E,* Unequivocal, but shallow, invasion over a wide area. *F,* In-situ change of papillary surface with suggestive minimal invasion beneath.

Illustration continued on following page

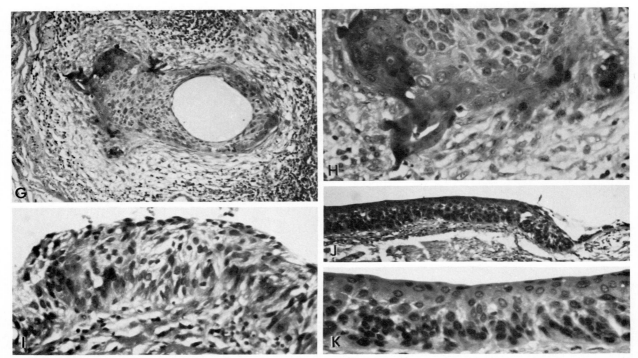

Figure 4–16. *Continued. G,* Carcinoma-in-situ lining duct of mucous gland with associated multifocal early stromal invasion. *H,* Higher magnification of same area, showing details of early stromal penetration. *I,* One margin at which there is abrupt change from abnormal to normal epithelium. *J,* In another marginal area, there is marked basal proliferation underlying benign, but slightly squamoid, cells. *K,* The abnormal basal proliferation at higher magnification.

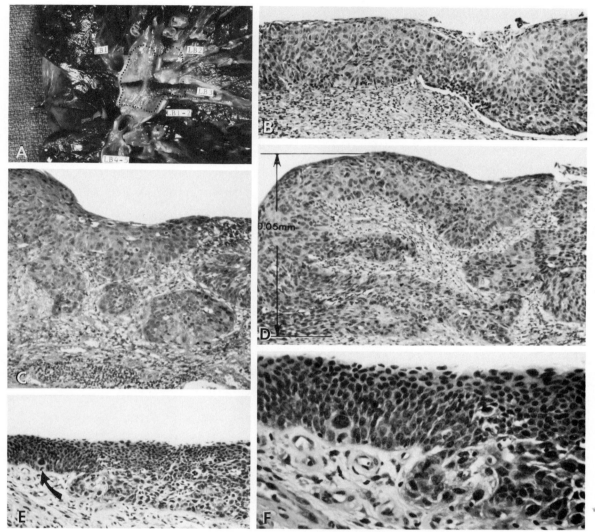

Figure 4–17. Case 9. In-situ-carcinoma with microinvasion. *A,* Granular mucosal changes representing carcinoma-in-situ involving 1.5 cm of distal LB 1–2, 1.4 cm of proximal LB 3, and 0.7 and 0.3 cm of LB 1 and LB 2, respectively (tumor area outlined by dots). *B,* In-situ component of tumor. *C,* One focus of early invasion in which cancerous buds project downward from surface epithelium. *D,* Another invasive focus in which elongating buds and strands of tumor extend less than 0.1 cm into stroma. *E,* One margin of the carcinoma in which lateral extension replaces normal epithelium and appears to be extending into superficial stroma as well. Note single carcinomatous cells in normal epithelium *(arrow)*. *F,* Higher magnification of margin and single cancerous cell shown in *E*.

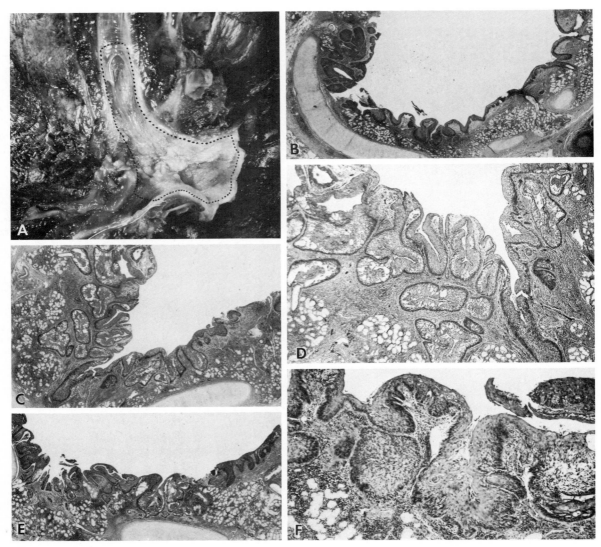

Figure 4–18. Case 10. Carcinoma-in-situ with superficial microinvasion to level of bronchial cartilages. *A,* Thickened mucosa with great accentuation of mucosal folds involving almost entire right upper lobe bronchus and extending 2.5 cm along RB 1 and 1 cm along both RB 2 and RB 3 *(carcinoma outlined by dots). B,* Cross section of right upper lobe bronchus, showing extensive in-situ change and a focus of invasion on left to inner level of cartilages. *C,* Cross section at trifurcation area, showing surface carcinoma and extensive mucous gland duct involvement. *D,* Higher magnification demonstrates peculiar acantholytic change within cancer cells lining the ducts. *E,* Cross section of another area with focal infiltration to inner levels of cartilages. *F,* Higher magnification of infiltrative focus, which is forming a minute ''tumor.''

Illustration continued on opposite page

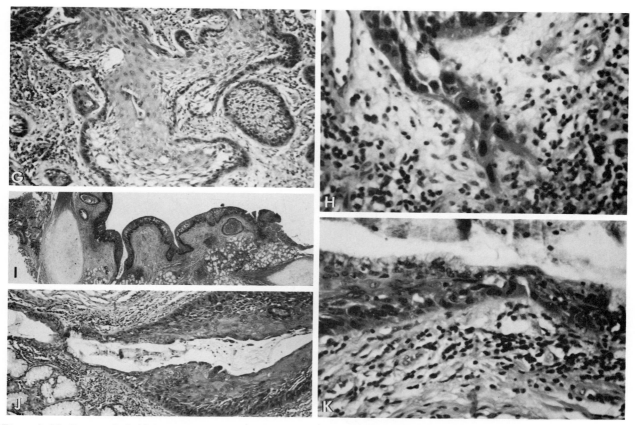

Figure 4–18. *Continued. G,* High-power view, showing details of tumor formation by progressive budding and elongation of strands of carcinoma. *H,* Stromal infiltration at a cellular level. *I,* Cross section of segmental bronchus showing in-situ change extending peripherally. *J,* Higher magnification of same area to show extension into mucous-gland ducts. *K,* High magnification of same duct shows tip of advancing carcinomatous process.

cancer has long posed a difficult problem. Some data have been provided by autopsy studies (Auerbach et al., 1967) and by clinical studies of patients undergoing resective lung surgery (Williams et al., 1981). Information on the multiplicity of in-situ or radiographically occult lung cancer in living patients is difficult to obtain, but some has become available since the introduction of formal screening studies for early cancer detection. The following conclusions are drawn from two such studies (Cortese et al., 1983; Woolner et al., 1984).

1. Initial multicentricity among patients who are surgically treated for occult bronchogenic carcinoma is relatively low. Among 62 patients who had "curative" resection of occult cancers, there were four with simultaneous multicentric tumors. In addition, there were three patients with multifocal or minimally invasive cancer confined to a small area. In these three patients, the separate foci were too closely approximated to be considered multicentric.

2. The risk of a second primary cancer developing after "curative" resection of an initial occult carcinoma is high.

3. The second or third primary cancer is frequently radiographically apparent, invasive, and inoperable.

Problems in diagnosis of multicentricity in occult or in-situ cancer are illustrated by the following case:

Case 11. In this case of bilateral multicentric occult bronchogenic carcinoma, the patient underwent bronchoscopy for localization of occult carcinoma. No abnormality was seen, but mucosa of the lingular bronchus of the left upper lobe (LB 4–5) bled easily on instrumentation. Multiple brush and biopsy specimens were obtained bilaterally. The sites and abnormal biopsy findings from this examination are shown in Figure 4–19A to E. Definite squamous carcinoma was diagnosed in a biopsy specimen from LB 4–5; marked atypia was found, and a biopsy procedure on RB 6 was recommended. The biopsy specimen from LB 2–3 showed metaplasia with slight to moderate atypia; that from LB 6 showed benign squamous metaplasia. A lingulectomy was performed, and a small keratotic squamous carcinoma was found near the orifice of LB 4–5 (Fig. 4–19F to H).

Postoperatively, the sputum continued to show markedly atypical cells, but the thoracic radiograph remained negative. The patient had limited pulmonary reserve, and further bronchoscopic studies were deferred. Two years after lingulectomy, bronchoscopic examination revealed RB 6 to be completely ob-

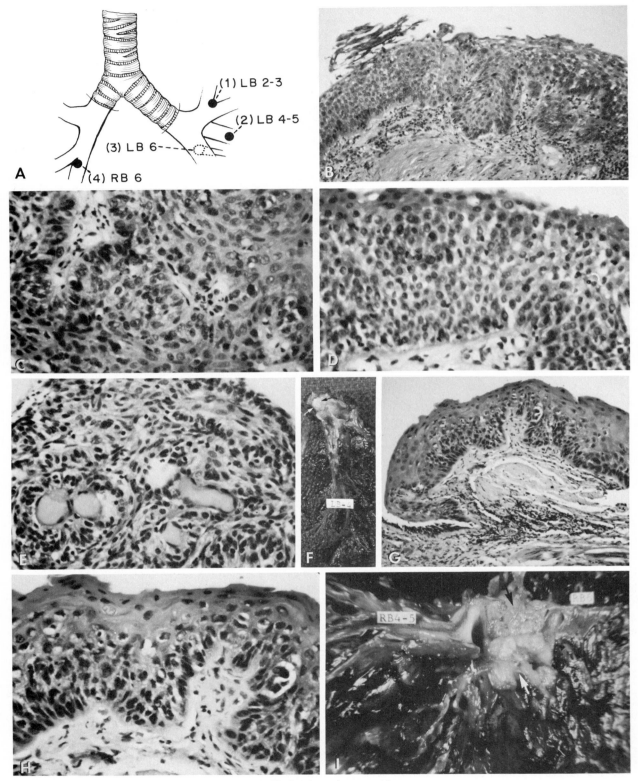

Figure 4–19. *See legend on opposite page.*

structed by tumor. Surgical resection of the right lower lobe was performed, revealing an infiltrative carcinoma involving proximal RB 6 (Fig. 4–19*I*). Sputum cytologic studies were negative postoperatively. The patient died of obstructive lung disease 4 years later, with no evidence of cancer.

INCIPIENT CHANGES

It is widely accepted that, after a variable time period, in-situ carcinoma becomes first a minimally invasive and then a progressively more infiltrative cancer. However, the initial recognizable epithelial changes or possible progressive steps in the evolution of the in-situ stage of bronchial carcinoma are extremely difficult to determine and document. Clues regarding the possible evolution of the in-situ neoplastic process might be provided by study of the smallest (and presumably earliest) resected cancers, by examination of the growing margins and the status of epithelium adjacent to small tumors, and by detection of "atypical" and therefore possibly precancerous foci in bronchial mucosa apart from the cancer. None of these approaches, however, provides conclusive evidence about the evolution of the in-situ cancer into its fully developed form. It is possible that a number of mechanisms may be involved.

In Case 1, the epithelium adjacent to the tumor appeared normal, and there was no clue about the nature of any prior or earlier stage of the in-situ process. In Case 2, a tiny, well-developed in-situ carcinoma showed some adjacent epithelial changes, including focal basal cell hyperplasia and atypical squamous metaplasia. No adjacent epithelial abnormalities were detectable in Cases 3 and 4, both involving fully developed in-situ cancers. In Case 5, the carcinomatous focus was extremely mature and keratotic. Adjacent epithelium showed squamous metaplasia and some basal cell hyperplasia, with foci of atypical squamous metaplasia as well. Thus, there is some evidence in favor of an evolution to in-situ carcinoma through progressive stages of squamous cell atypia. In Cases 6 and 7, there was a tiny area of

in-situ carcinoma with rather borderline cellular alteration. One cannot exclude the possibility that the changes represented a very early stage of development of an "ongoing" in-situ process that was interrupted by the operation.

The time factor in the evolution of an in-situ carcinoma likewise is difficult to determine. Certain cases observed in a screening study suggest that the time for transition from normal to carcinomatous may be rather short, as illustrated by the following case:

Case 12. The patient, a participant in a screening program for early lung cancer, underwent localization with subsequent resection of the right upper lobe for an in-situ carcinoma (0.7 × 0.5 cm) involving the proximal RB 2. Sputum cytology tests at 4-month intervals had been negative for 4⅓ years; they then became positive for carcinoma cells 2½ months prior to resection. A representative area from the center of this small tumor is shown in Figure 4–20*A*, and the margin and adjacent mucosa are shown in Figure 4–20*B* and *C*.

Prior histologic changes in this case are only speculative. The tumor was undergoing keratinization, but the margins did not suggest an origin in a pre-existing area of bronchial squamous metaplasia. The relatively short period of abnormal sputum cytologic findings, beginning abruptly with a diagnosis of cancer cells after 4⅓ years of negative findings, suggested an abrupt change and provided evidence against a prolonged period of transition through stages of mild, moderate, and marked atypia.

By contrast, a slower progression with a possible transition stage is suggested by the following case:

Case 13. The patient, a participant in a screening program, had undergone right upper lobectomy for in-situ carcinoma that was multifocal in the region of the right upper lobe bronchus, the trifurcation area, and orifices of RB 2 and RB 3. Although closely approximated, the in-situ foci were considered separate on serial block sectioning. Prior to the resection, sputum cytologic studies showed marked atypia over a 5-month period, and one specimen was diagnosed as moderately atypical 2 years prior to operation. This finding had been preceded by 3½ years of negative

Figure 4–19. Case 11. *A,* Diagram of bronchial tree, showing sites of origin of abnormal biopsy specimens. *B,* Site 1 (LB 2–3 spur): squamous metaplasia with some surface keratinization. Slight to moderate atypia is apparent in the midportion of the specimen, as indicated by variations in nuclear size and staining. There is some proliferative activity as well, as shown by occasional mitotic figures. *C,* Site 2 (LB 4–5): frank squamous carcinoma of average degree of malignancy. The specimen is cut on the flat—that is, parallel to the surface of the carcinoma—and therefore is not indicative of invasive cancer (see description of resected specimen further on). *D,* Site 3 (LB 6): squamous metaplasia with essentially no evidence of atypia. *E,* Site 4 (RB 6): atypical cytologic change of severe degree (also cut on the flat). A diagnosis of marked squamous cell atypia was made with a recommendation for repeat biopsy procedure at this site. *F,* Resected lingula of left upper lobe. A small keratotic in-situ-carcinoma is visible near the orifice of LB 4–5 *(arrows)*. *G,* Histologic section through in-situ-carcinoma measuring 0.4 cm in diameter. Almost the entire tumor is shown here. *H,* Higher magnification of the central portion of tumor, showing marked surface keratinization. *I,* Resected right lower lobe shows invasive squamous carcinoma involving orifice of RB 6 *(arrows)*. The carcinoma is invasive over 2.5 cm of the proximal broncus and extends 1.2 cm into lung parenchyma.

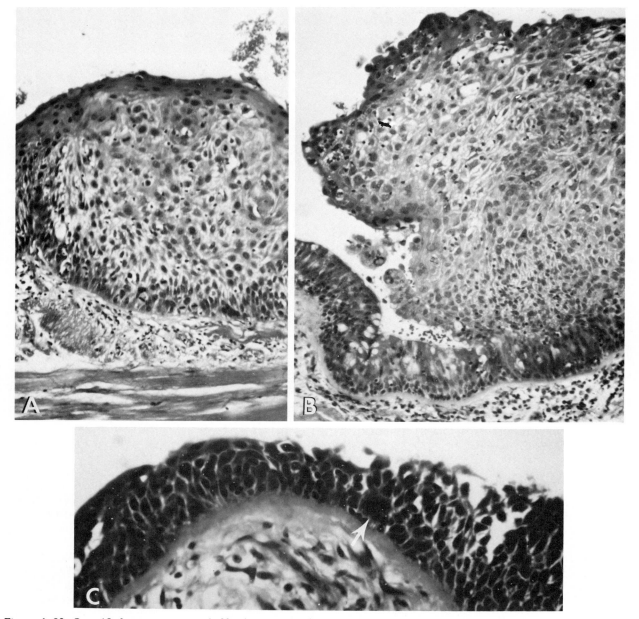

Figure 4–20. Case 12. In-situ-carcinoma. *A,* Histologic section through the center of tumor shows mitotic activity in both deep and superficial levels. There is superficial keratinization present. *B,* Margin of same tumor is sharp, and adjacent normal ciliated epithelium shows only slight basal proliferation. *C,* Mucosa in the vicinity of tumor shows an isolated abnormal cell *(arrow).*

test results. Various histologic changes, including foci of carcinoma-in-situ as well as atypical findings in adjacent mucosa, are shown in Figure 4–21.

The histologic findings in the carcinomatous foci and adjacent epithelium were compatible with the concept of a cancerous change evolving through a series of stages of atypical squamous metaplasia. The longer period of abnormal sputum cytology, including one "moderate" report 2 years preoperatively, also supported a more gradual evolution of the process.

A number of histologic variations at the junction of

carcinoma and adjacent epithelium have been presented in the preceding cases. The transition is usually abrupt, but it may be gradual. A special problem in interpretation of epithelial changes in the vicinity of the tumor is presented in the next case:

Case 14. A sharply circumscribed carcinoma-in-situ with microinvasion (0.6 × 0.4 cm) showed focal cellular changes in adjacent epithelium apparently separate from the main tumor (Fig. 4–22). The question of multifocal carcinoma at a very early stage of development is raised by this case.

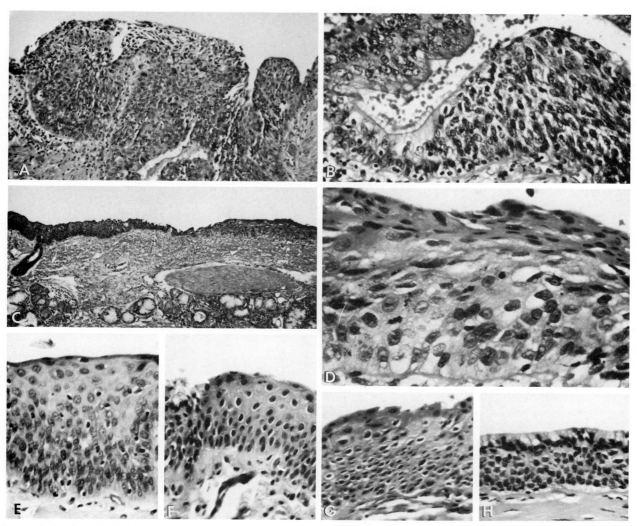

Figure 4–21. Case 13. Multifocal in-situ-carcinoma. *A*, One focus of in-situ-carcinoma with little or no evidence of keratinization. *B*, High-power view of margin of same tumor, showing proliferation of small basaloid cells. *C*, Second focus of in-situ-carcinoma and adjacent squamous metaplasia. *D*, High magnification of in-situ component that shows surface keratinizaiton. *E*, Squamous metaplasia in trifurcation area adjacent to tumor. *F*, Slight squamous cell atypia in same region. *G*, Moderate squamous cell atypia near tumor. *H*, Marked basal cell proliferation in the same area.

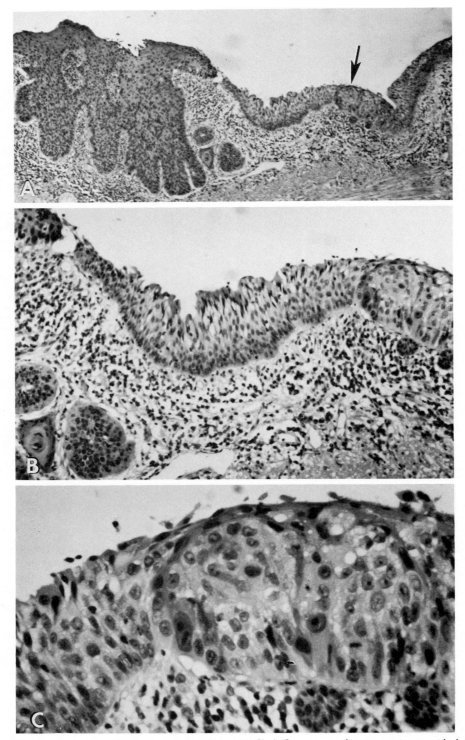

Figure 4–22. Case 14. In-situ-carcinoma with microinvasion (multicentricity?). *A,* One margin of in-situ-carcinoma with shallow microinvasion *(left side).* On right side, focal cellular changes are seen *(arrow). B,* Higher magnification of same margin shows atypical focus separated from main tumor by zone of normal columnar epithelium. *C,* High-power view of same area shows questionable early carcinomatous focus.

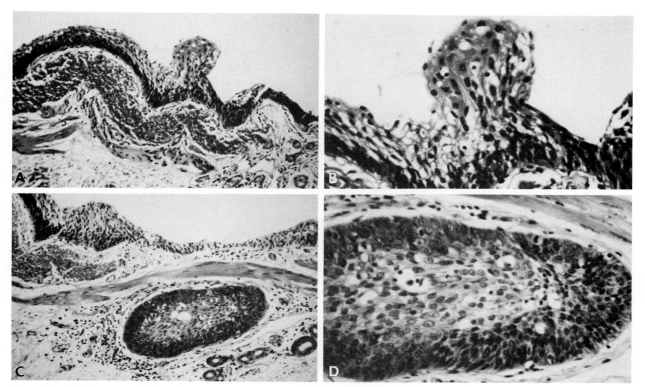

Figure 4–23. Moderate squamous cell atypia. *A,* Focus of atypia, a few millimeters in diameter, in a case of resected in-situ-carcinoma. *B,* Higher magnification of central portion of same area, showing cytologic atypia of moderate degree. *C,* Underlying duct shows changes similar to those seen on the surface. *D,* Higher magnification of the same duct, showing epithelial proliferation with mitotic figures and cellular changes comparable to those on the surface.

Examples of focal atypia, either in the vicinity of the carcinoma-in-situ (Cases 2, 5, and 13) or in widely separated biopsy specimens (Case 11), have been cited. Rare instances of focal atypia in a resected specimen quite separate from the tumor itself have been encountered. One example is shown in Figure 4–23. The carcinoma-in-situ in this case was small (less than 0.5 cm in diameter) and located within a different segmental bronchus.

Atypical changes judged to be moderate also have been encountered in biopsy specimens and present problems in management. One such case, involving a participant in a screening program, is represented in Figure 4–24. The patient had normal cytologic results through 6 years of testing, followed by several atypical specimens over a 1-year period. Localizing bronchoscopy provided a single abnormal biopsy from RB 6. The changes were considered moderate, and surgical resection was not recommended. Sputum cytologic results were negative after bronchoscopy and remained so for 2 years of further screening (to termination of the screening project).

A number of possible pathways of carcinogenesis are suggested by the previous cases, but no firm conclusions can be drawn about the most likely morphologic changes prior to the fully developed in-situ stage of carcinoma. Both a gradual evolution through a series of atypical changes and an abrupt change in previously normal or hyperplastic epithelium seem possible from the evidence at hand.

In summary, the preceding pages depict the variations in histologic and gross findings that the pathologist may encounter in dealing with the earliest stages of intrabronchial carcinoma. Limited data on possible precursor, or "incipient," changes in bronchial epithelium prior to the fully developed in-situ stage have been provided as well. Such information should help one deal with the special problems in diagnosis and management of radiographically occult carcinoma that have been outlined at the beginning of this chapter.

The interpretation of biopsy specimens in cases of radiographically occult carcinoma also presents special problems in diagnosis and management, as indicated in the previous 14 cases. It should be noted that it generally is not possible to diagnose in-situ as opposed to minimally invasive cancer on biopsy evidence. The presence or absence of early microinvasion and its depth of penetration can be determined accurately only after serial block sectioning of the resected specimen. A positive diagnosis of cancer on biopsy calls for prompt conservative resective surgery. Lesser changes require careful management. Squamous metaplasia, a common finding, is not believed to have

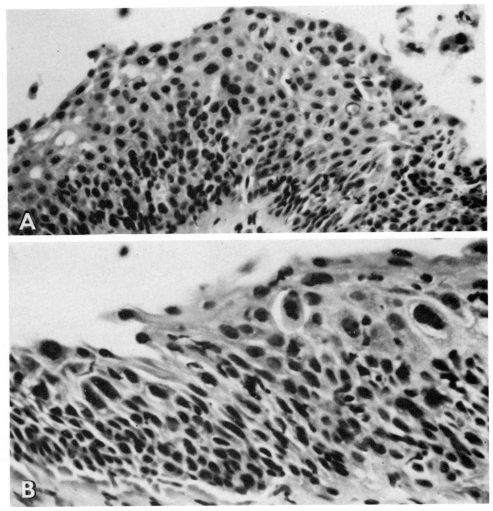

Figure 4–24. Moderate squamous cell atypia. *A*, From subject with abnormal cytologic findings. Metaplastic squamous change is associated with cellular and nuclear atypia considered moderate in degree. *B*, Portion of same biopsy specimen at slightly higher magnification. Nuclear abnormalities within neoplastic cells are obvious.

diagnostic or prognostic significance. Slight squamous cell atypia likewise is not considered a significant change. Marked atypia of any type in a biopsy specimen generally calls for a repeat bronchoscopic examination and repeat biopsy of the suspect area. When there is atypia regarded as moderate (see earlier in this chapter), surgical intervention is not indicated, but careful follow-up is necessary.

The prognosis for patients undergoing surgical resection of in-situ bronchogenic carcinoma, including those with minimal microinvasion, theoretically should be excellent. In a series of such cases subjected to careful pathologic study (Woolner and Farrow, 1982), no examples of lymph node metastasis were observed at the in-situ stage or in those cases involving invasion to the inner levels of bronchial cartilages. By contrast, those cancers with deeper invasion—that is, those extending to the full thickness of the bronchial wall and those infiltrating extrabronchial tissues—one or more peribronchial lymph nodes were found metastatically involved in 20 percent and 69 percent of the cases, respectively.

Survival data for surgically resected, radiographically negative occult lung cancers in the Mayo Lung Project over a 10-year period of observation were reported by Cortese and coworkers in 1983. Of the patients on whom curative resective surgery was performed, 54 were followed for periods ranging from 13 months to 9½ years. Specimens were serially blocked, and the carcinomas were classified according to the classification described earlier. Approximately one third of the occult cancers were entirely in situ, one third showed microinvasion to the inner level of bronchial cartilages, and one third demonstrated deeper invasion up to the extrabronchial level (Woolner et al., 1984). For the 54 cases reported by Cortese and colleagues, the 5-year actuarial survival rate (lung cancer deaths only) was 90 percent.

A major risk factor for patients with occult lung cancer is the development of a second primary carcinoma after curative surgical treatment for the initial lesion. In the series reported by Cortese and colleagues in 1983, approximately 20 percent developed a second primary carcinoma during a period of 8 years of follow-up. The rate of detection of second primaries is approximately 5 percent per year.

References

Auerbach, O., Stout, A.P., Hammond, E.C., Garfinkel, L.: Multiple primary bronchial carcinomas. Cancer 20:699–705, 1967.

Carter, D., Marsh, B.R., Baker, R.R., Erozan, Y.S., Frost, J.K.: Relationships of morphology to clinical presentation in ten cases of early squamous cell carcinoma of the lung. Cancer 37:1389–1396, 1976.

Cortese, D.A., Pairolero, P.C., Bergstralh, E.J., Woolner, L.B., Uhlenhopp, M.A., Piehler, J.M., Sanderson, D.R., Bernatz, P.E., Williams, D.E., Taylor, W.F., Payne, W.S., Fontana, R.S.: Roentgenographically occult lung cancer: a ten-year experience. J. Thorac. Cardiovasc. Surg. 86:373–380, 1983.

Eggleston, J.C., Tockman, M.S., Baker, R.R., Erozan, Y.S., Marsh, B.R., Ball, W.C., Jr., Frost, J.K.: In-situ and microinvasive squamous cell carcinoma of the lung. Clin. Oncol. 1(2):499–512, 1982.

Fontana, R.S., Sanderson, D.R., Miller, W.E., Woolner, L.B., Taylor, W.F., Uhlenhopp, M.A.: The Mayo Lung Project: preliminary report of "early cancer detection" phase. Cancer 30:1373–1382, 1972.

Fontana, R.S., Sanderson, D.R., Taylor, W.F., Woolner, L.B., Miller, W.E., Muhm, J.R., Uhlenhopp, M.A.: Early lung cancer detection: results of the initial (prevalence) radiologic and cytologic screening in the Mayo Clinic study. Am. Rev. Respir. Dis. 130:561–565, 1984.

Fontana, R.S., Sanderson, D.R., Woolner, L.B., Miller, W.E., Bernatz, P.E., Payne, W.S., Taylor, W.F.: The Mayo Lung Project for early detection and localization of bronchogenic carcinoma: a status report. Chest 67:511–522, 1975.

Melamed, M., Flehinger, B., Miller, D., Osborne, R., Zaman, M., McGinnis, C., Martini, N.: Preliminary report of the lung cancer detection program in New York. Cancer 39:369–382, 1977a.

Melamed, M.R., Zaman, M.B., Flehinger, B.J., Martini, N.: Radiologically occult in situ and incipient invasive epidermoid lung cancer: detection by sputum cytology in a survey of asymptomatic cigarette smokers. Am. J. Surg. Pathol. 1:5–16, 1977b.

Nasiell, M., Carlens, E., Auer, G., Hayata, Y., Kato, H., Konaka, C., Roger, V., Nasiell, K., Enstad, I.: Pathogenesis of bronchial carcinoma, with special reference to morphogenesis and the influence on the bronchial mucosa of 20-methylcholanthrene and cigarette smoking. Recent Results Cancer Res. 82:53–68, 1982.

Nasiell, M., Sinner, W., Tornvall, G., Roger, V., Vogel, B., Enstad, I.: Clinically occult lung cancer with positive sputum cytology and primarily negative radiologic findings. Scand. J. Respir. Dis. 58:134–144, 1977.

Sanderson, D.R., Fontana, R.S., Woolner, L.B., Bernatz, P.E., Payne, W.S.: Bronchoscopic localization of radiographically occult lung cancer. Chest 65:608–612, 1974.

Williams, D.E., Pairolero, P.C., Davis, C.S., Bernatz, P.E., Payne, W.S., Taylor, W.F., Uhlenhopp, M.A., Fontana, R.S.: Survival of patients surgically treated for stage I lung cancer. J. Thorac. Cardiovasc. Surg. 82:70–76, 1981.

Woolner, L.B., David, E., Fontana, R.S., Andersen, H.A., Bernatz, P.E.: In situ and early invasive bronchogenic carcinoma: report of 28 cases with postoperative survival data. J. Thorac. Cardiovasc. Surg. 60:275–290, 1970.

Woolner, L.B. and Farrow, G.M.: Mayo Lung Project: pathological findings in occult bronchogenic carcinoma detected through lung cancer screening. Clin. Oncol. 1(2):513–526, 1982.

Woolner, L.B., Fontana, R.S., Cortese, D.A., Sanderson, D.R., Bernatz, P.E., Payne, W.S., Pairolero, P.C., Piehler, J.M., Taylor, W.F.: Mayo Lung Project: pathologic findings and frequency of multicentricity in occult lung cancer. Mayo Clin. Proc., 59:453–466, 1984.

Woolner, L.B., Fontana, R.S., Sanderson, D.R., Miller, W.E., Muhm, J.R., Taylor, W.F., Uhlenhopp, M.A.: Mayo Lung Project: evaluation of lung cancer screening through December 1979. Mayo Clin. Proc. 56:544–555, 1981.

ELAINE S. JAFFE

5 | Lymphoid System

The lymphoid system is distinguished from many other systems by the fact that although polyclonal reactive lymphoid hyperplasias are relatively common, benign tumors of lymphoid cells—namely, benign monoclonal tissue proliferations—have not been recognized. Similarly, the concept of "carcinoma-in-situ" has not been applied to the lymphoid system. One reason for this phenomenon is that in contrast to most cells of the human body, lymphoid cells are normally migratory. Rather than remaining fixed to their tissue environment, they circulate throughout the lymphoid system, following orderly traffic pathways. Thus, benign clonal proliferations of lymphoid cells would likely not remain localized but rather, at their inception, disseminate throughout the lymphoid system following normal traffic patterns (Jaffe, 1983). In contrast, a polypoid adenoma of the colonic mucosa remains confined to the end of its pedunculated stalk. The cells may proliferate and produce mucus, but the lesion remains localized until either one of two events occurs: (1) The lesion may come to clinical attention and be surgically extirpated, or (2) it may undergo malignant transformation and progress to adenocarcinoma. A close relationship between adenocarcinomas of the colon and polypoid adenomas is well recognized. However, in contrast to most benign neoplasms, benign tumors of lymphocytes might disseminate at a time close to their inception and never be identified clinically at a stage at which the entire lesion could be encompassed locally and excised.

Within the lymphoid system, there also are areas that are preferentially populated by B or T lymphocytes. For example, the gut-associated lymphoid tissue, including mesenteric lymph nodes and Waldeyer's ring, contains relatively more B cells than T cells. As one would expect, malignant lymphomas arising in this system are more often of B cell than T cell type. In contrast, T cell lymphomas are more prevalent in lymphoid tissue associated with epithelium, such as the skin and lung. Within individual lymph nodes, B cells are found in the lymphoid follicles and medullary cords, whereas T cells are localized primarily within the paracortex. Compartmentalization of B and T cells is also present in the splenic white pulp and other sites bearing lymphoid tissue. Thus, although the concept of "carcinoma-in-situ" is not normally applied to the lymphoid system, a lymphoma that remains restricted in its normal environment might be considered in situ (Fig. 5–1). For example, follicular lymphomas tend to involve follicular regions of lymph nodes and splenic white pulp.

Although benign tumors of lymphoid cells have not been recognized, with the possible exception of isolated plasmacytoma (discussed further on), reactive lymphoid hyperplasias are relatively common. Moreover, certain atypical reactive hyperplasias and certain atypical immune states have been associated with an increased incidence of malignant lymphoma. These atypical lymphoid hyperplasias could be considered incipient neoplastic events.

On a practical level, the pathologist is called upon regularly to distinguish reactive from neoplastic lesions. If the process shows some features suggestive of a reactive hyperplasia, but the changes are particularly exuberant and lead to partial architectural effacement, the term "atypical lymphoid hyperplasia" may be used. This alerts the clinician that careful clinical follow-up is indicated and that another biopsy may be necessary if symptoms persist. Escalating to the next level of atypia is a process that shows some features suggestive of, but not diagnostic of, malignancy. For such a lymph node, one may use the term "atypical lymphoid proliferation," noting that the process cannot be categorized within the known lymphoid hyperplasias and that it may represent a lymphoma.

One study that examined clinical follow-up in patients with atypical lymphoid hyperplasia demonstrated a 30 percent incidence of malignant lymphoma in subsequent biopsies (Schroer and Franssila, 1979). When the pathologists tried to predict the likelihood of subsequent malignant evolution, they were correct 84 percent of the time. It was noted that a major factor contributing to the inability to arrive at a defin-

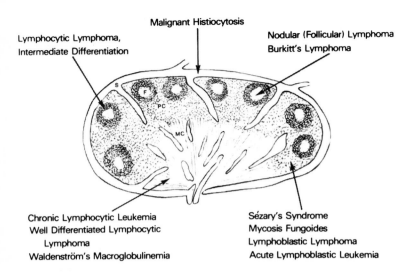

Lymphocytic Lymphoma, Intermediate Differentiation

Malignant Histiocytosis

Nodular (Follicular) Lymphoma
Burkitt's Lymphoma

Chronic Lymphocytic Leukemia
Well Differentiated Lymphocytic
Lymphoma
Waldenström's Macroglobulinemia

Sézary's Syndrome
Mycosis Fungoides
Lymphoblastic Lymphoma
Acute Lymphoblastic Leukemia

Figure 5–1. Schematic diagram of normal lymph node shows relationship of lymphoreticular malignancies to various anatomic and functional compartments of the lymphoid system. Neoplastic diseases tend to involve sites populated by their normal precursors. (Modified after Mann, R. B., Jaffe, E. S., Berard, C. W.: Am. J. Pathol., 94:103–192, 1979.)

itive diagnosis was poor technical quality of the histologic material. The requirement for technically excellent material in evaluating lymph node biopsies cannot be overemphasized.

Immunophenotypic studies may be extremely valuable in distinguishing benign and malignant lesions (Table 5–1). In addition to quantifying the numbers of B and T cells present, one can document the presence of a monoclonal B cell proliferation or demonstrate phenotypic abnormalities of T cells suggestive of malignancy (Jaffe and Cossman, in press).

PROGRESSIVE TRANSFORMATION OF GERMINAL CENTERS

Progressive transformation of germinal centers (PTGC) was described by Lennert and colleagues and by Poppema and coworkers as a lesion resembling

Table 5–1. **Specialized Techniques for the Distinction of Atypical Reactive and Neoplastic Lymphoid Lesions**

Reactive	Neoplastic
Polymorphous: mixture of B and T cells	Monomorphous: predominance of B or T cells
Polyclonality of B or T cells	Monoclonality of B and/or T cells
Normal κ-λ ratio	Restricted light chain expression (B cells)
Absence of clonal band with gene probes	Clonal rearranged band with gene probes for Ig genes (B cells) or T cell antigen receptor (T cells)
Normal diploid karyotypes	Clonal aneuploid karyotypic alterations or chromosomal translocations
Normal antigenic phenotypes with monoclonal antibodies to B and T cell antigens	Aberrant antigenic phenotypes

the nodular form of lymphocyte-predominant Hodgkin's disease (Lennert et al., 1978a; Poppema et al., 1979). Similarly, the lesion is found in an age population commonly affected by this subtype of Hodgkin's disease. It is more prevalent in males than in females and is most common in the fourth and fifth decades of life.

Subsequent studies by Burns and coworkers confirmed the association of PTGC with the nodular form of lymphocyte-predominant Hodgkin's disease in approximately 20 percent of cases (Burns et al., 1984). In some instances, the lesions are seen together in a single lymph node site. In other instances, progressive transformation of germinal centers precedes the development of Hodgkin's disease, and in some patients with a documented diagnosis of lymphocyte-predominant Hodgkin's disease, the diagnosis of progressive transformation of germinal centers may be made in another anatomic site or in recurrent lymphadenopathy following treatment. Thus, the evidence suggests that PTGC may be a preneoplastic lesion that may lead to the development of Hodgkin's disease. Nevertheless, the lesions can be histologically distinguished, and progressive transformation of germinal centers should not be regarded as a malignant neoplasm.

Affected nodes may be involved focally, or the lesion may be extensive, and cause architectural obliteration. In involved lymph nodes, one sees large nodules (Fig. 5–2). Within the center of the nodules are ill-defined structures that resemble germinal centers, but these are often fragmented, with germinal center cells dispersed throughout the nodule. Although cells resembling lymphocyte-predominant variants or L and H cells may be seen, classic Reed-Sternberg cells are not present. Because a lymph node biopsy may show both progressive transformation of germinal centers and lymphocyte-predominant Hodgkin's disease, a lymph node showing the former feature should be extensively sectioned for focal involvement by Hodgkin's disease. If other significant

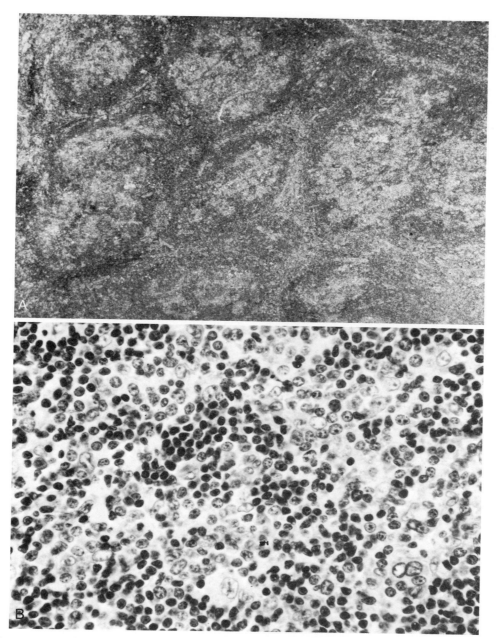

Figure 5–2. Progressive transformation of germinal centers. *A,* Low-power view shows alteration of normal lymph node architecture. Large, ill-defined nodules are seen throughout lymph node. Within nodules are dispersed germinal centers. *B,* High-power view of one of the altered germinal centers. Follicular center cells are mixed with normal lymphocytes and rare cells resembling lymphocyte-predominant variants. Diagnostic Reed-Sternberg cells are not seen.

adenopathy is present in a patient with progressive transformation of germinal centers, a repeat lymph node biopsy is probably indicated to rule out the presence of Hodgkin's disease in other nodal sites.

ANGIOIMMUNOBLASTIC LYMPHADENOPATHY

Angioimmunoblastic lymphadenopathy and a related (if not identical) lesion, immunoblastic lymphadenop-

athy, were described by Frizzera and colleagues (1974) and Lukes and Tindle (1975). At the time of their descriptions, these lesions were considered to represent variants of atypical lymphoid hyperplasia. Affected individuals had generalized lymphadenopathy and systemic symptoms that included fever, polyclonal hypergammaglobulinemia, and often skin rash (Table 5–2). A history of a drug reaction was frequently given, and it was considered that the disease might be related to drug sensitivity and an allergic

Table 5–2. **Clinical Features of Angioimmunoblastic Lymphadenopathy**

Incidence	Males and females
	Adults: median, sixth decade
Presentation	Generalized lymphadenopathy
	Hepatosplenomegaly
	"B" symptoms
	Skin rash/pruritus
	Drug hypersensitivity
Laboratory Data	Polyclonal hypergammaglobulinemia
	Anemia
	Leukocytosis +/−
Clinical Course	Subacute, infectious complications
	Progression to immunoblastic sarcoma (one third of cases)
Therapy	Steroids/cytotoxics

Table 5–3. **Pathology of Angioimmunoblastic Lymphadenopathy**

Complete architectural effacement
Absence of germinal centers or few residual "burned out" germinal centers
Proliferation of small vessels in an arborizing pattern
Polymorphous cellular infiltrate: lymphocytes, immunoblasts, plasma cells, +/− histiocytes, eosinophils
Overall hypocellular appearance with amorphous interstitial material
Open or distended cortical sinus with bridging of capsule by infiltrate.

response. Although treatment with systemic corticosteroids was effective in some individuals, patients remained at risk for infection or organ failure, and the median survival was only approximately 2½ years. It soon became apparent that these patients were at increased risk for the development of malignant lymphomas, and in about 30 percent of patients overt large cell lymphomas of the immunoblastic subtype developed. Moreover, Nathwani and associates (1981) noted that the presence of clusters of immunoblasts within the affected lymph nodes was associated with a more aggressive clinical course and a median survival of only 9 months. Thus, Nathwani's group considered such clusters of immunoblasts to represent evidence of evolution to malignant lymphoma.

Histologically, angioimmunoblastic lymphadenopathy (Table 5–3) is characterized by total architectural effacement (Fig. 5–3). However, peripheral cortical sinuses and trabecular sinuses are often patent and may be dilated. The nodes are replaced by a polymorphous infiltrate of lymphocytes, immunoblasts, and plasma cells, with or without eosinophils, dispersed in an eosinophilic precipitate (Fig. 5–4). Vascular proliferation is conspicuous, and arborizing post capillary venules are seen throughout involved lymph nodes. By definition, reactive or hyperplastic lymphoid follicles are absent, although small atrophic burned-out germinal centers can be seen (Fig. 5–5). The infiltrate characteristically jumps across the lymphoid capsule to infiltrate adipose tissue.

In 1980, Watanabe and coworkers described a variant of peripheral T cell lymphoma associated with polyclonal hypergammaglobulinemia, which histologically bore a striking resemblance to angioimmunoblastic lymphadenopathy. Notably, many of the fea-

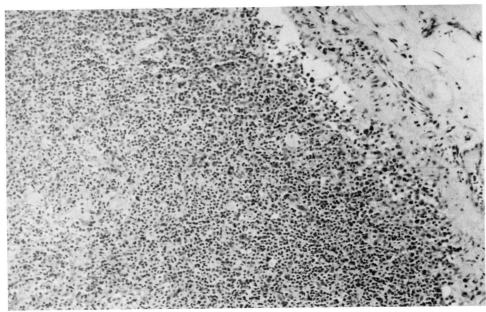

Figure 5–3. Angioimmunoblastic lymphadenopathy. Lymph node architecture is effaced by a diffuse proliferation. However, far cortical sinuses remain open and are often dilated.

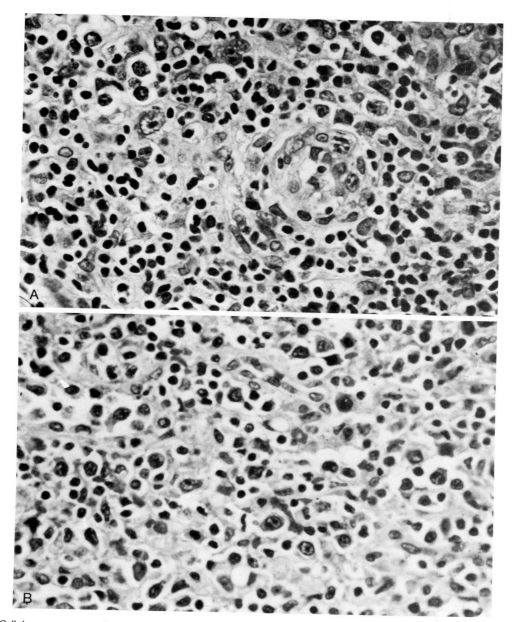

Figure 5–4. Cellular composition of angioimmunoblastic lymphadenopathy. *A,* There is a polymorphous cellular infiltrate composed of lymphocytes, plasma cells, and immunoblasts. Many of the lymphocytes have abundant clear cytoplasm. Note postcapillary venule with numerous lymphocytes in transit through vessel wall. *B,* Abundant amorphous interstitial precipitate is seen in this field.

Illustration continued on following page

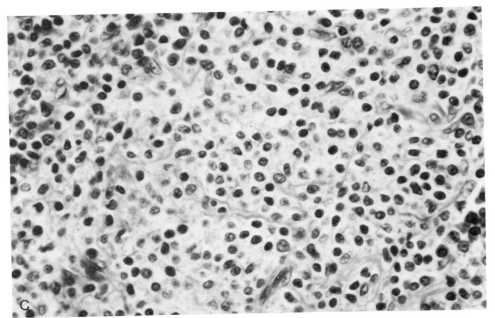

Figure 5–4 *Continued. C,* Plasma cells are particularly numerous in this case.

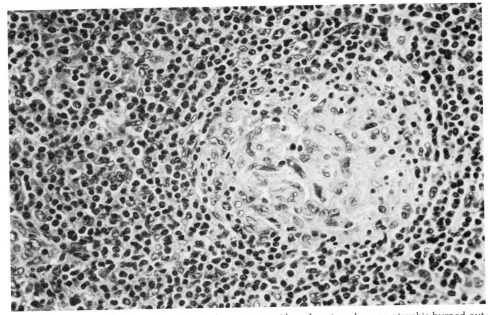

Figure 5–5. Angioimmunoblastic lymphadenopathy. Germinal centers are either absent or show an atrophic burned-out appearance. The diagnosis of angioimmunoblastic lymphadenopathy cannot be made in the presence of florid follicular hyperplasia.

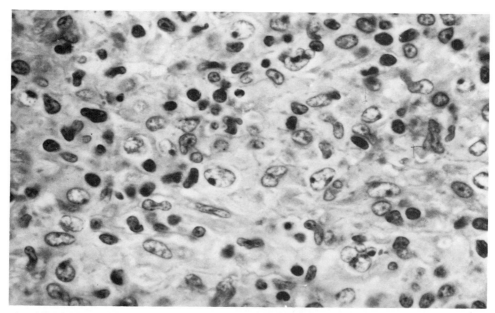

Figure 5–6. Peripheral T cell lymphoma. The polymorphous cellular composition resembles that of angioimmunoblastic lymphadenopathy. Also similar is the presence of immunoblasts with abundant clear cytoplasm. However, in contrast, the background small lymphocytes show significant cytologic atypia in peripheral T cell lymphoma.

tures of peripheral T cell lymphoma are similar to those of angioimmunoblastic lymphadenopathy (Jaffe et al., 1975; Waldron et al., 1977; Jaffe, 1984). Peripheral T cell lymphomas are characterized by a polymorphous infiltrate that effaces lymph node architecture. The atypical large lymphoid cells often have abundant clear cytoplasm (Fig. 5–6). Unlike angioimmunoblastic lymphadenopathy, T cell lymphoma demonstrates atypia in the background small lymphocytes. However, the atypia in the small lymphocytes is often not striking, and thus the distinction between angioimmunoblastic lymphadenopathy and peripheral T cell lymphoma is frequently difficult. Certainly, these observations suggest that angioimmunoblastic lymphadenopathy as initially described may represent a peripheral T cell lymphoma and not an atypical reactive lesion. Future studies for clonality in T cell lesions made possible by the recently described (Hedrick et al., 1984; Siu et al., 1984) T cell receptor probes may permit resolution of this problem and determine whether or not angioimmunoblastic lymphadenopathy is a clonal neoplastic disorder at inception.

DILANTIN HYPERSENSITIVITY

Diphenylhydantoin (Dilantin) and related phenytoin derivatives can produce in certain people a hypersensitivity reaction that may simulate malignant lymphoma (Saltzstein and Ackerman, 1959). The hypersensitivity reaction usually appears within a few weeks to 5 months of the initiation of anticonvulsant therapy. The syndrome appears to be more common in blacks

than in whites (Stanley and Fallon-Pellicci, 1978). It is characterized by skin rash, fever, generalized lymphadenopathy, leukocytosis, and eosinophilia. The acute onset of the lymphadenopathy with white counts that are often markedly elevated may simulate malignant lymphoma. Obtaining appropriate clinical history for treatment with a phenytoin derivative is essential to establishing the diagnosis.

The lymphadenopathy is usually generalized, with conspicuous involvement of cervical lymph nodes. Histologically, the nodes show diffuse infiltration by a mixed population of small and large lymphoid cells (Fig. 5–7). Immunoblasts are numerous, and focal accumulations of immunoblasts may be mistaken for a large cell lymphoma. Eosinophilia is usually conspicuous. Although the lymph node architecture is effaced, one can distinguish the process from lymphoma by the spectrum of lymphoid cells, which represents all stages of lymphocyte transformation. The small lymphoid cells should not show significant cytologic atypia. Histologically, this process belongs within the spectrum of diffuse paracortical hyperplasia. Because of the spectrum of cells present and the associated eosinophilia, a distinction from a peripheral T cell lymphoma is usually the most difficult differential. However, in peripheral T cell lymphomas, cytologic atypia of the small lymphoid cells should be evident.

The skin rash is pruritic, consisting of a generalized macular and papular erythematous eruption. Vesicles can be seen, and there may be desquamation. Histologically, the skin shows a dense superficial atypical lymphoid infiltrate that is primarily perivascular in distribution (Fig. 5–8). However, exocytosis of indi-

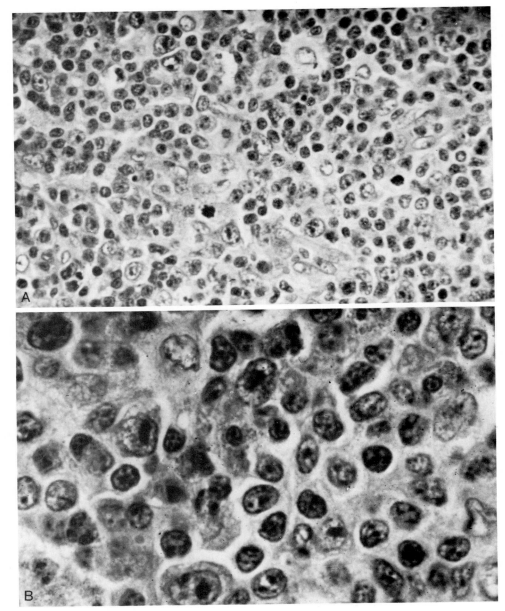

Figure 5–7. Lymph node phenytoin (Dilantin) hypersensitivity reaction. *A,* Lymph node architecture is effaced and is replaced by a mixed population of lymphocytes, immunoblasts, and eosinophils. *B,* Small lymphocytes do not show cytologic atypia, and there is a spectrum in cell size from small to large.

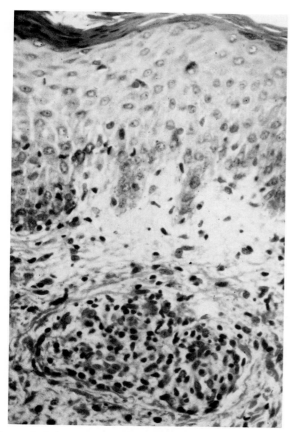

Figure 5–8. Skin phenytoin hypersensitivity reaction. A prominent lymphocytic infiltrate is present in the high dermis and is predominantly perivascular in location. Significant exocytosis by lymphocytes is noted in the epidermis.

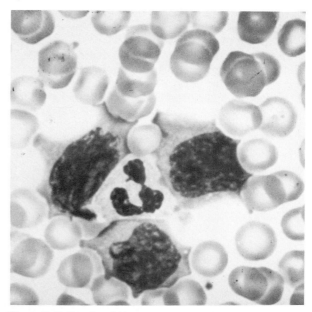

Figure 5–9. Peripheral blood phenytoin hypersensitivity reaction. White blood cell count in this case was 60,000 cells/mm³. The majority of the cells resemble immunoblasts with abundant basophilic cytoplasm. Nuclei contain prominent multiple nucleoli.

vidual cells into the epidermis is usually evident, and the process may be mistaken for Sezary syndrome.

The peripheral blood usually exhibits leukocytosis and eosinophilia. The peripheral white blood cell count can be markedly elevated, as high as 60,000/mm³. Moreover, the atypical cells seen in the peripheral blood resemble immunoblasts and have abundant basophilic cytoplasm and transformed nuclear features. The atypia of the circulating cells may be rather alarming (Fig. 5–9). The atypical immunoblasts in the peripheral blood are T cells (personal observation), and thus again the most difficult differential diagnosis is with the mature T cell malignancies, including adult T cell leukemia/lymphoma, Sezary syndrome, and peripheral T cell lymphoma with peripheral blood involvement.

There have been reports of liver function abnormalities, which can be associated with elevated transaminases and cholestasis. In some cases, the liver function abnormalities may be severe.

It is thought that the pathogenesis of this syndrome is a hypersensitivity reaction to the drug, which is capable of causing significant immune stimulation in laboratory animals. Treatment should, of course, include withdrawal of the anticonvulsant. Systemic corticosteroids may be helpful.

Of a more controversial nature is whether or not phenytoin is associated with an increased incidence of real lymphoma. There exist in the literature a number of case reports of non-Hodgkin's lymphoma and Hodgkin's disease occurring in patients receiving long-term anticonvulsant therapy (Gams et al., 1968). However, whether or not these cases represent an increase over the incidence expected in the general population is not yet established. Patients in whom lymphoma has developed in general have not given a history of phenytoin-induced hypersensitivity reaction, and careful statistical analyses have not shown an incidence higher than that observed in the general population (Matzner and Polliack, 1978).

ANGIOCENTRIC IMMUNOPROLIFERATIVE LESIONS

Angiocentric immunoproliferative lesions are a related group of lymphoproliferative disorders for which several diagnostic terms have been employed: "lymphomatoid granulomatosis," "polymorphic reticulosis," and "atypical lymphocytic vasculitis." All these lesions are angiocentric and angiodestructive proliferations composed of an admixture of lymphocytes and other inflammatory cells (Costa and Martin, 1985; Jaffe, 1984). Despite the polymorphic character of the infiltrate, the lymphocytes may show some cytologic atypia, and approximately 30 percent of patients eventually develop frank malignant lymphoma. Lymphomatoid granulomatosis was initially described by Liebow and associates (1972) as an atypical reactive lesion to be distinguished from Wegener's granulomatosis in the lung. However, recent observations suggest that angiocentric immunoproliferative lesions may be neoplastic at onset, at least in some patients.

The essential feature of all angiocentric immunoproliferative lesions is an angiodestructive and angiocentric lymphoid infiltrate (Fig. 5–10). Small lymphocytes are mixed with plasma cells, histiocytes, and occasional atypical large pleomorphic lymphoid cells. The infiltrate extends through the vascular wall to the endothelium, often resulting in vascular occlusion and extensive tissue necrosis. It has been noted that the proportion of large atypical lymphoid cells correlates inversely with survival, a feature seen in many malignant lymphomas (Katzenstein et al., 1979). For example, in follicular lymphomas, the large lymphoid cells are considered the proliferative element, and when these cells are present in increasing numbers, the disease is associated with a more aggressive clinical course (Mann et al., 1979). The diagnosis of angiocentric lymphoma may be made conclusively when there is striking atypia in the small lymphoid cells or when the large lymphoid cells constitute the major component of the lesion (Fig. 5–11).

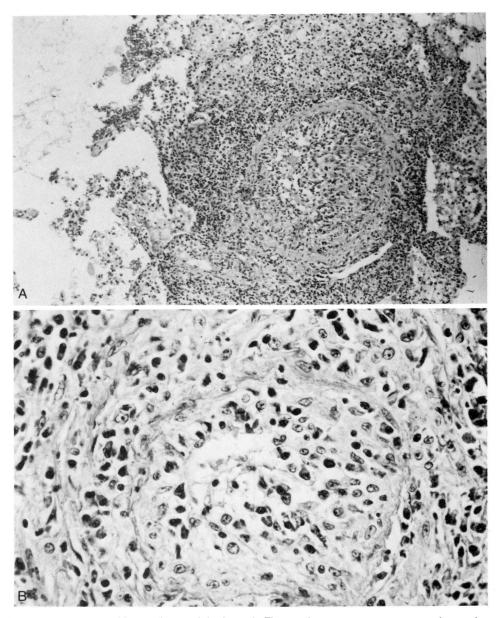

Figure 5–10. Angiocentric immunoproliferative lesion of the lung. A, The unit lesion is an angiocentric and angiodestructive lymphoid infiltrate. B, In many cases the infiltrate is polymorphous with a mixture of lymphocytes, plasma cells, and immunoblasts. Lymphocytes may show minimal cytologic atypia.

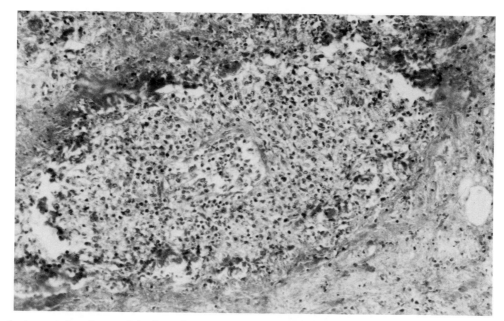

Figure 5–11. Angiocentric lymphoma of the lung. Infiltrate extends through vessel wall, leading to vascular occlusion and extensive necrosis of surrounding lung parenchyma. Infiltrate in this case is monomorphous and composed predominantly of large lymphoid cells.

This author believes that angiocentric immunoproliferative lesions are probably neoplastic at onset. However, when the small cells predominate, the disease is associated with a more indolent clinical course, and combination chemotherapy with regimens such as cyclophosphamide and prednisone have helped achieve complete remissions (Fauci et al., 1982). Frank angiocentric lymphomas pursue an aggressive clinical course and require treatment with aggressive multiagent combination chemotherapeutic regimens commonly used in the treatment of diffuse aggressive non-Hodgkin's lymphomas.

Although lymphomatoid granulomatosis was initially described in the lung, the same lesion can be seen in the nasopharynx and midline nasal sinuses, skin, kidneys, peripheral vessels, and central and peripheral nervous systems. Angiocentric immunoproliferative lesions in the nose and paranasal sinuses are associated with the lethal midline granuloma syndrome and often lead to extensive tissue necrosis and destruction in these sites (De Remee et al., 1978).

Angiocentric immunoproliferative lesions probably represent a variant of peripheral T cell lymphoma. Although only a small number of cases have been studied phenotypically, both in angiocentric immunoproliferative lesions and in frank angiocentric lymphomas, the cells have had mature T cell characteristics. The neoplastic T cells appear to be capable of elaborating a factor that can activate normal macrophages (Simrell et al., 1982; Jaffe et al., 1983). This has led to a hemophagocytic syndrome in patients with AIL.

PAGETOID RETICULOSIS, PARAPSORIASIS EN PLAQUE, AND ALOPECIA MUCINOSA

All the aforementioned lesions represent atypical cutaneous infiltrates, which may precede the development of mycosis fungoides. Mycosis fungoides is a notoriously chronic cutaneous malignancy. Patients in whom mycosis fungoides is ultimately diagnosed frequently give a history of cutaneous eruptions occurring for many years. Multiple skin biopsies occurring over a period of years may be necessary for documentation of the diagnosis of mycosis fungoides. In the early stages, although atypical cerebriform lymphocytes may be seen, diagnostic Pautrier abscesses are absent.

In alopecia mucinosa, the atypical lymphoid cells infiltrate hair follicles, leading to destruction of the follicle and loss of hair. Pagetoid reticulosis is characterized by an atypical infiltrate of cerebriform cells throughout the epidermis (Fig. 5–12) (Braun-Falco et al., 1973). In the Woringer-Kolopp variant, only single isolated keratotic plaques are present, although the lesion histologically resembles mycosis fungoides, and excision of the lesion may result in a sustained clinical remission without recurrence (Burg and Braun-Falco, 1983). However, the disseminated form of pagetoid reticulosis is best considered a morphologic variant of mycosis fungoides and it pursues an aggressive clinical course. It is likely that the isolated form of pagetoid reticulosis represents an isolated mycosis fungoides lesion and that resection of this isolated lesion may result in long-term disease-free survival.

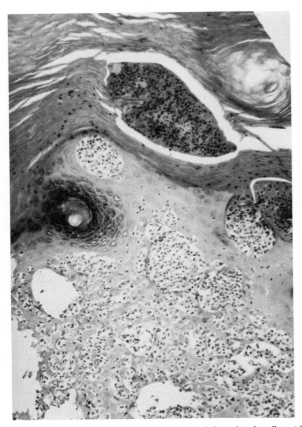

Figure 5–12. Pagetoid reticulosis. Atypical lymphoid cells with cerebriform nuclear features extensively infiltrate the epidermis. The dermal component is minimal. This patient presented with an isolated lesion on the foot and was considered to have the Woringer-Kolopp variant of pagetoid reticulosis. The lesion was resected, but 2 years later the patient developed another similar lesion on the opposite extremity. Most consider this variant of pagetoid reticulosis to represent an early isolated form of mycosis fungoides.

Parapsoriasis en plaque is a disorder characterized by chronic recalcitrant erythematous scaling lesions (Burg and Braun-Falco, 1983). The skin biopsy exhibits a high dermal infiltrate composed of atypical lymphoid cells without demonstrable Pautrier microabscesses. Patients who have large patch lesions or who exhibit the poikiloderma variant frequently progress to mycosis fungoides. However, patients with only small patches may pursue a benign clinical course.

LOW-GRADE B CELL LYMPHOMAS, FOLLICULAR LYMPHOMA, AND SMALL LYMPHOCYTIC LYMPHOMA

These malignant lymphoid proliferations could be considered the "lymphomas-in-situ" of the lymphoid system (Table 5–4). Although these diseases are neoplastic and clonal in nature with proven cytoge-

Table 5–4. **Pathologic and Experimental Characteristics of Low-Grade and High-Grade Malignant Lymphomas**

Low-Grade	High-Grade
Non-destructive growth pattern	Destructive growth pattern
Absence of cellular atypia	Presence of cellular atypia/anaplasia
Respect for privileged sites	Invasion of privileged sites
Response to regulatory influences in vitro and in vivo	Autonomous
Failure to grow in culture	Immortalized in culture
Non-transplantable	Transplantable in immunodeficient host

netic abnormalities (Croce et al., 1984), they are notoriously indolent in their clinical course. Morphologically, the cells of low-grade lymphomas resemble normal cells of the B cell system. The cells of follicular lymphoma resemble the cells of normal lymphoid follicles, and cytologic criteria usually are not useful in distinguishing normal from neoplastic follicular B lymphocytes (Fig. 5–13). Similarly, the cells of chronic lymphocytic leukemia and small lymphocytic lymphoma are morphologically indistinguishable from normal circulating B lymphocytes (Fig. 5–14).

The ability of follicular lymphomas to home to B cell–dependent areas throughout the lymphoid system is well described (Mann et al., 1979). In focally involved lymph nodes, follicular lymphomas often involve cortical follicular zones. Similarly, in spleens involved by this disorder, one sees selective involvement of the B cell–dependent portion of malpighian corpuscle. Although follicular lymphomas are usually disseminated at presentation with involvement of lymph nodes above and below the diaphragm, the disease does not involve privileged sites, and involvement of the central nervous system or testis is virtually never seen in the absence of histologic progression (Jaffe, 1983). Thus, although the disease is disseminated, the cells populate areas normally populated by follicular B lymphocytes.

It had been noted for many years that nodular, or follicular, lymphomas resemble normal lymphoid follicles. To obtain evidence linking follicular lymphomas to the lymphoid follicle, investigators sought an increased incidence of follicular lymphoma in patients with follicular hyperplasia. However, it appears that patients with isolated follicular hyperplasia are not at increased risk to develop follicular lymphoma, and benign follicular hyperplasia probably is not a preneoplastic process. Nevertheless, instances of atypical follicular hyperplasia are not uncommon, and in many instances it may be extremely difficult to distinguish an atypical follicular hyperplasia from follicular lymphoma. Immunologic techniques capable of documenting monoclonality help researchers distinguish benign from malignant follicular proliferations.

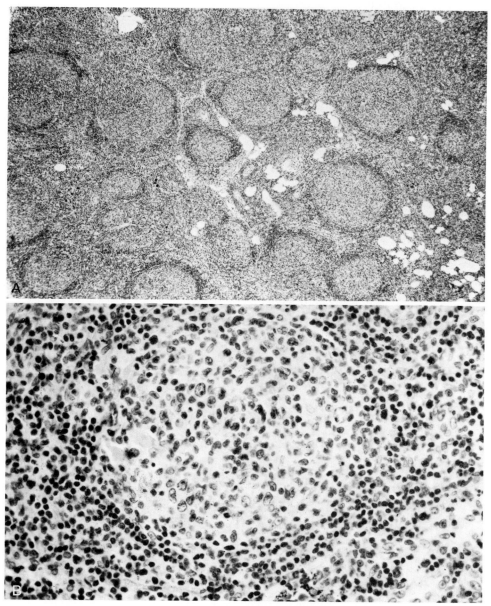

Figure 5–13. Follicular lymphoma. *A,* Follicular proliferation extends throughout lymph node and effaces normal nodal architecture. Follicles generally are of uniform size and shape with little intervening normal lymphoid parenchyma. Cuffs may be present but are ill-defined. *B,* Cytologic composition of follicular lymphoma mimics the cytologic composition of the normal germinal center. A mixture of cleaved and non-cleaved cells is seen.

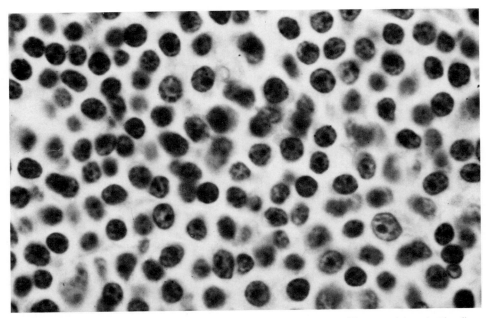

Figure 5–14. Small lymphocytic malignant lymphoma. Cytologically, lymphocytes resemble normal lymphoid cells and do not show cytologic atypia.

PSEUDOLYMPHOMA

The term "pseudolymphoma" has been used to describe atypical lymphoid proliferations of tumor-like proportions. These lesions commonly occur in extranodal sites and have been described in the stomach, orbit, lung, and skin. Pseudolymphomas present as mass lesions clinically, but histologically they are composed of normal lymphoid elements (Table 5–5) (Saltzstein, 1969). Sheets of relatively monotonous small lymphocytes may be seen, sometimes mixed with plasma cells. Interspersed among the small lymphoid elements are cytologically normal germinal centers (Fig. 5–15). Immunoblasts or large transformed lymphoid cells may be present in variable proportions. The more polymorphous the infiltrate and the greater the number of germinal centers, the easier it is to distinguish pseudolymphoma from malignant lymphoma. Because of the preponderance of small lymphocytes in many pseudolymphomas, the principal diagnostic dilemma is usually pseudolymphoma versus a malignant lymphoma of the small lymphocytic subtype.

Definite criteria for the distinction of pseudolymphoma from malignant lymphoma are not universally accepted. The 1983 paper by Koss and colleagues reclassified many pulmonary lesions, formerly diagnosed as pseudolymphomas, as small lymphocytic lymphomas. Nevertheless, many of the patients in this series continued to pursue a benign clinical course, even without systemic therapeutic intervention. Knowles and coworkers (1982) as well as Evans (1982) attempted to use lymphocyte surface markers to distinguish pseudolymphomas from small lympho-

cytic lymphomas in the orbit and skin, respectively. Their studies were not universally successful in that some patients with polyclonal lesions immunologically developed malignant lymphoma. Conversely, some patients with "monoclonal lymphoid proliferations" continued to pursue an indolent course without systemic progression of disease.

It seems apparent that, even if many so-called pseudolymphomas are monoclonal and perhaps neoplastic, these lesions do not undergo rapid dissemination and conservative therapy is indicated. For orbital lesions, localized radiotherapy is probably the treatment of choice. In other anatomic sites, such as the lung, radiotherapy may be more difficult to provide.

In a small number of patients with pseudolymphoma, progression to a high-grade malignant lymphoma, large cell lymphoma, or large cell lymphoma

Table 5–5. **Classic Criteria for the Distinction of Pseudolymphoma from Lymphoma**

Pseudolymphoma	Lymphoma
Presence of skip areas: Normal tissue present between foci of lymphoid proliferation	Absence of skip areas: Continuous lymphoid proliferation throughout tissue
Polymorphous infiltrate	Monomorphous infiltrate
Frequent presence of germinal centers	Absence or rare presence of germinal centers
Absence of cytologic atypia	Cytologic atypia of small and/or large lymphoid cells
Polyclonal B cell population	Monoclonal B cell population

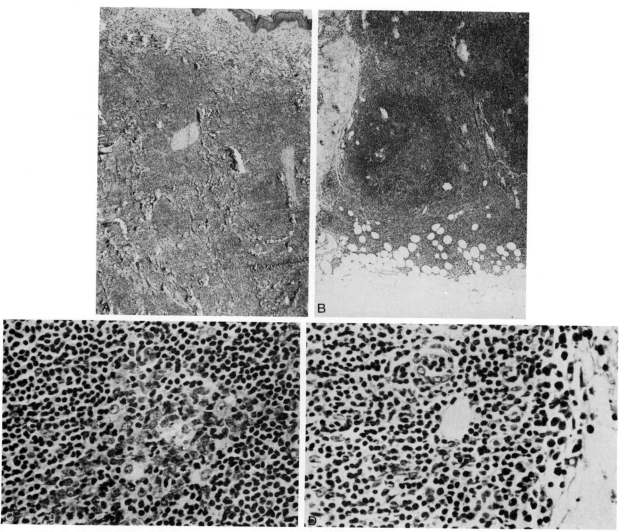

Figure 5–15. Pseudolymphoma of the skin. *A*, Extensive lymphoid infiltrate extends from the dermis to the subcutaneous tissue. *B*, Large hyperplastic germinal centers can be seen adjacent to subcutaneous tissue. *C*, Germinal centers appear normal cytologically and contain starry sky histiocytes. *D*, The interfollicular proliferation consists of lymphocytes, plasma cells, and immunoblasts.

of the immunoblastic subtype has been documented (Wolf and Spjut, 1981). Thus, recurrent disease should always be rebiopsied so that the presence or absence of histologic progression can be documented.

In some sites, identification of the putative stimulus of the atypical lymphoid proliferation may be possible. For example, pseudolymphomas of the stomach are often associated with a chronic gastric ulcer (Brooks and Enterline, 1983). The presence of a chronic ulcer with a granulation tissue or fibrous tissue base is supportive evidence that the lymphoid proliferation associated with it is reactive. In contrast, in lymphomas of the stomach, although the overlying mucosa may be ulcerated, the malignant lymphoid proliferation extends directly to the ulcerated tissue surface. Evidence of chronicity is not an absolute criterion for benignity because, as already noted, pseudolym-

phoma may progress to lymphoma. In such cases, evidence of a chronic ulcer may be seen in the malignant lymphoid proliferation.

ANGIOMATOUS LYMPHOID HAMARTOMA, OR GIANT LYMPH NODE HYPERPLASIA

This lymphoid proliferation has been considered either a hamartomatous or a reactive process (Keller et al., 1972). The lymphoid mass lesion may be seen in the mediastinum, retroperitoneum, or other lymph node–bearing sites. Follicles predominate in this lesion, but T cells are present between the proliferating follicles (Fig. 5–16). The follicles are characterized by prominent central vascular tufts, often creating a hy-

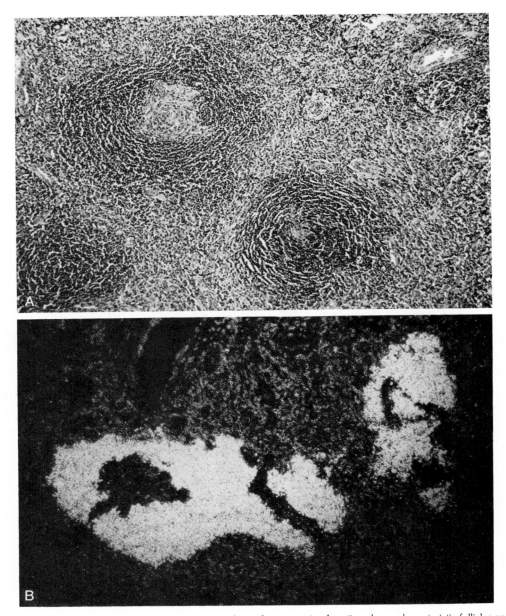

Figure 5–16. Angiomatous lymphoid hamartoma. *A,* Hematoxylin and eosin–stained section shows characteristic follicles containing central vascular tufts surrounded by circumferential rows of normal lymphocytes. The interfollicular stroma contains numerous vessels. *B,* Frozen section of same case rosetted with EAC and viewed with dry dark-field condenser. Reagent red cells adhere to follicles, indicating the presence of complement receptors. The rosetting pattern is similar to that observed with normal follicles.

alinized appearance. Surrounding the follicle are circumferential rows of small normal lymphocytes, so-called onion-skinning.

Between the proliferating follicles the observer sees one of two patterns. In the hyaline vascular type, numerous small blood vessels and hyalinized connective tissue are present in the interfollicular region. In the plasma cell variant, sheets of normal-appearing plasma cells are seen. Patients with the plasma cell variant may have systemic symptoms and a polyclonal hypergammaglobulinemia.

Although patients with angiomatous lymphoid hamartomas are not considered to be at risk for the subsequent development of malignant lymphoma, isolated reports have been described in which the intervening plasma cells are monoclonal (Schlosnagle et al., 1982). At our institution, we have encountered a similar case. Thus, these limited expanded monoclonal proliferations could be considered a preneoplastic event with subsequent risk for malignant evolution. Because malignant lymphomas are not reported in this patient population, either such monoclonal proliferations are extremely rare or secondary malignant transformation is uncommon.

BENIGN MONOCLONAL GAMMOPATHY, ISOLATED EXTRASKELETAL PLASMACYTOMA, AND "BENIGN MONOCLONAL LYMPHADENOPATHY"

Benign monoclonal gammopathy occurs in 1 percent of the general population. The presence of small monoclonal spikes increases with age, and approximately 3 percent of individuals over the age of 60 years will be found to have these spikes. However, this patient population does not appear to be at increased risk for the development of multiple myeloma. If the spike is less than 2 gm percent and if its level remains stable over a period of months to years, development of multiple myeloma is almost never observed. It is likely that such small monoclonal spikes represent exaggerated expanded clones of normal plasma cells or normal immunologic reactions rather than preneoplastic events.

Nevertheless, all cases of multiple myeloma are considered to have their origin in antecedent normal clones of plasma cells. Each individual plasma cell is probably at equivalent risk for neoplastic transformation because the incidence of myeloma subtypes correlates directly with the amount of each immunoglobulin heavy chain class synthesized on a daily basis (Callihan et al., 1983). For example, IgG myeloma is the most frequently observed variant, followed by, in decreasing order of frequency, IgA, IgM, IgD, and IgE myeloma. Moreover, it has been observed that in many patients with multiple myeloma documentation of the antigenic specificity of the abnormal immunoglobulin molecule is possible, and this may correlate with a known antigenic exposure in the affected individual.

Primary extraskeletal plasmacytomas may represent benign clonal plasma cell proliferations. In contrast to B cells, plasma cells do not recirculate but remain sessile once they reach this mature stage (Ford, 1975). Thus, it is not unexpected that localized plasmacytomas do occur. Primarily extraskeletal plasmacytomas may present in lymph nodes as well as other extraskeletal sites (Azar, 1973). Although such lesions frequently are part of a generalized plasma cell dyscrasia, in some instances the tumor is truly isolated, and localized radiotherapy is curative.

Although benign monoclonal lymphadenopathy states theoretically should exist, they have not been documented. In one report, lymph nodes that were histologically benign contained monoclonal B cell proliferation (Levy et al., 1983). However, in many instances the κ-λ ratio was not markedly altered, and in all cases the follow-up period was relatively short. Thus, a definite conclusion cannot be drawn about the clinical evolution of these patients with monoclonal B cell proliferations.

SJÖGREN'S SYNDROME AND RHEUMATOID ARTHRITIS

Individuals affected with the autoimmune complex known as "Sjögren's syndrome" commonly develop an atypical lymphoid hyperplasia (Anderson and Talal, 1972). Involved lymph nodes exhibit reactive follicular hyperplasia, marked plasmacytosis, atypical paracortical hyperplasia, and the presence of monocytoid or plasmacytoid cells in the lymphoid sinuses (Fig. 5–17). Patients with this lymphadenopathy syndrome usually have a polyclonal hypergammaglobulinemia and readily demonstrable rheumatoid factor in the serum.

Individuals with Sjögren's syndrome are also at increased risk for malignant lymphoma. Such lymphomas are usually, but not exclusively, of high-grade B cell types, and in the NZB mouse model for autoimmune disease, B cell lymphomas also are seen (Zulman et al., 1978). The development of a malignant lymphoma in a patient with Sjögren's syndrome is usually accompanied by the disappearance of polyclonal hypergammaglobulinemia and rheumatoid factor from the serum. Thus, it is likely that the reactive lymphoid proliferation disappears and is replaced by a neoplastic lymphoid proliferation no longer producing polyclonal immunoglobulins.

The lymphoid cells isolated from the salivary gland lesions are capable of secreting monoclonal immunoglobulins (Talal et al., 1970), and monoclonal plasma cell proliferations also can be seen in affected minor salivary glands (Lane et al., 1983). It is likely that these small monoclonal proliferations represent a preneoplastic event and that these are the cells at risk for ultimate development of malignant lymphoma. As in multiple myeloma, the ultimate emergence of the malignant disease may represent a "two-hit" phenomenon. The first hit is the creation of an expanded clone of B cells, and the second event is the oncogenic event leading to uncontrolled proliferation of the clone. Nevertheless, salivary gland involvement by lymphoma is not necessarily seen, and the lymphomas are usually both nodal and extranodal in origin.

HASHIMOTO'S THYROIDITIS

Hashimoto's thyroiditis represents another autoimmune syndrome in which affected individuals are at increased risk for the development of malignant lymphoma (Dailey et al., 1955). Hashimoto's thyroiditis occurs more often in females than in males. The thyroid gland is infiltrated by abundant and dense lymphoid tissue containing hyperplastic germinal cen-

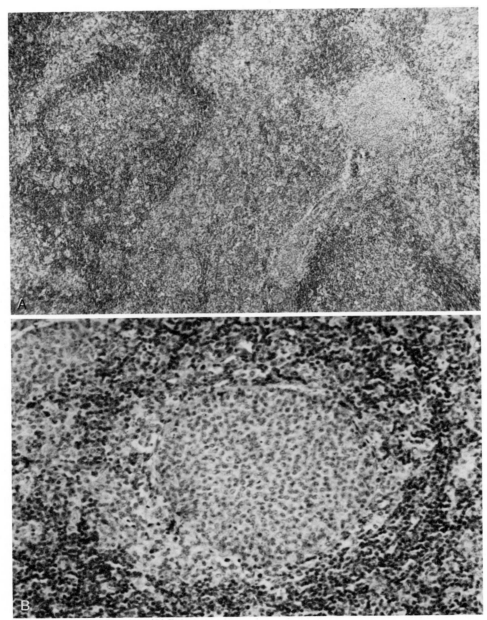

Figure 5–17. Lymph node hyperplasia, Sjogren's syndrome. *A,* Three components to the lymphoid hyperplasia are seen. These include a follicular hyperplasia, a paracortical hyperplasia, and the presence of "monocytoid" cells in the sinuses. *B,* Higher-powered view of one of the sinuses shows accumulation of large lymphoid cells with abundant cytoplasm.

Illustration continued on opposite page

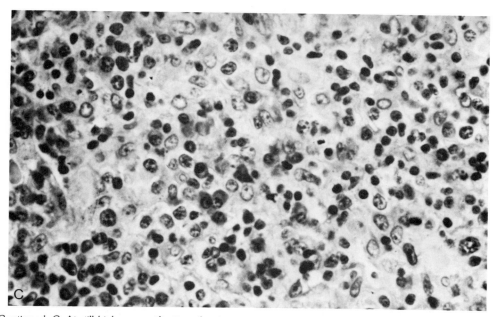

Figure 5–17. *Continued. C,* At still higher magnification, the sinus component is seen to be an admixture of lymphocytes with abundant cytoplasm and plasma cells.

ters. Plasma cells also may be present. The glandular acini are small and atrophic, and the epithelial cells exhibit acidophilic change (so-called Hürthle, or Askanazy, cells).

Both patients with classic Hashimoto's thyroiditis and patients with lymphocytic thyroiditis (without epithelial alterations) are at increased risk for development of malignant lymphoma of the thyroid (Burke et al., 1977). As one might expect, because the reactive proliferations are predominantly of B lymphocytic origin, the malignant lymphomas seen in this population also are predominantly of the B cell type and usually of the aggressive follicular center cell subtypes (large non-cleaved, large cleaved, and small non-cleaved) (Maurer et al., 1979).

GLUTEN-SENSITIVE ENTEROPATHY

Gluten-sensitive enteropathy is a clinicopathologic syndrome associated with villous atrophy, plasmacytosis of the lamina propria, diarrhea, and malabsorption, all of which can be reversed following removal of gluten from the diet. Immunologic abnormalities also have been demonstrated in patients with this syndrome. As with many immune disorders, patients with gluten-sensitive enteropathy or celiac disease have an increased incidence of lymphoma (Otto et al., 1981).

The lymphomas usually occur in the affected small bowel and may be preceded by intestinal ulcerations that are accompanied by an atypical lymphoid infiltrate (Baer et al., 1980). Usually a history of celiac disease has been present for many years, but in some cases the two processes may present simultaneously

(Cooper et al., 1980; Cooper et al., 1982; Swinson et al., 1983).

The ulcerative lesions show at their base a densely cellular infiltrate composed of lymphocytes, immunoblasts, and plasma cells. The infiltrates are usually confined to the submucosa and lamina propria without involvement of the muscularis. All the lymphomas seen in this setting are of the diffuse aggressive subtypes: mixed small and large cell, large cell, and large cell immunoblastic. Although Isaacson and coworkers (1979) have claimed that these lymphomas represent a variant of malignant histiocytosis, other authors have not found evidence for a histiocytic origin of the neoplastic cells (Otto et al., 1981; Saraga et al., 1981). In most studies, monoclonal immunoglobulin has been demonstrated within the neoplastic cells, supporting a B cell origin for these tumors.

IMMUNOPROLIFERATIVE SMALL INTESTINAL DISEASE

Immunoproliferative small intestinal disease, or α-heavy-chain disease, has been described in individuals of lower socioeconomic background from areas of the Mediterranean basin: North Africa, Israel, Iran, and Greece (Nassar et al., 1978; Salem et al., 1977). This disease is clinically characterized by a malabsorption syndrome. Histologic examination of the small bowel reveals villous atrophy and infiltration of the lamina propria by a monomorphous population of cytologically normal plasma cells (Fig. 5–18). A marked plasmacytosis can also be seen in mesenteric lymph nodes. Immunoperoxidase studies show that the plasma cells contain α heavy chain, but light chains

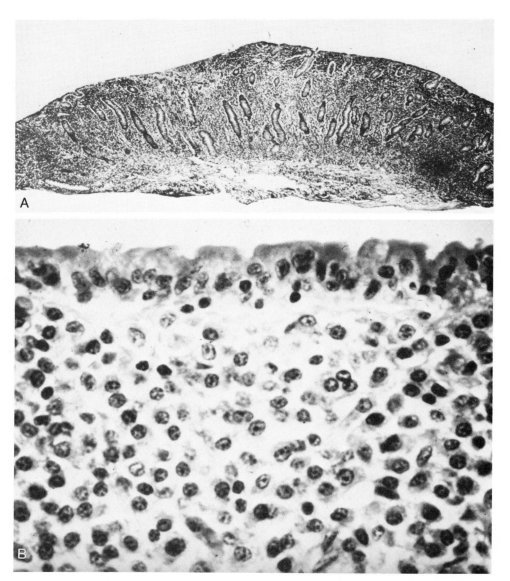

Figure 5–18. Immunoproliferative small-intestinal disease. *A,* Small bowel shows marked villous atrophy. *B,* Lamina propria is infiltrated by normal-appearing plasma cells.

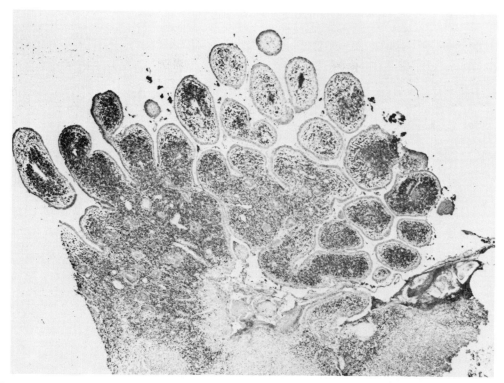

Figure 5–19. Immunoproliferative small-intestinal disease stained for presence of alpha-heavy chain. Virtually all plasma cells demonstrate strong reactivity.

are usually not identifiable (Fig. 5–19) (Isaacson, 1979). The same abnormal α heavy chain is demonstrable in the serum by immunoelectrophoretic techniques.

It has been postulated that α-heavy-chain disease may be related to recurrent and persistent infections of the gastrointestinal tract. In some individuals, treatment with antibiotics alone has produced complete and sustained remissions. However, patients with immunoproliferative small intestinal disease are at a greatly increased risk for the development of high-grade lymphomas of the gastrointestinal tract and mesenteric lymph nodes. Histologically, the lymphomas are classified as large cell immunoblastic in the Working Formulation (Fig. 5–20). Plasmacytoid features may be conspicuous histologically. Immunoperoxidase studies have documented the presence of the same abnormal α heavy chain in the neoplastic lymphoid cells. Thus, immunoproliferative small intestinal disease can be considered a preneoplastic lesion in which the abnormal plasma cells are at increased risk for neoplastic transformation.

IMMUNODEFICIENCY SYNDROMES

Patients with immunodeficiency, either congenital, acquired, or iatrogenic, are at greatly increased risk for the development of malignant lymphoma. Although malignancies are seen with an increased fre-

quency in this patient population, a simple immuno-surveillance mechanism cannot be used to invoke the increased incidence of malignant lymphoma. Malignant lymphomas are by far the most common neoplasm in patients with immunodeficiency, and in some patient populations the incidence may approach 20 percent. The pathogenetic mechanism that leads to development of malignant lymphomas has not been fully explained in this patient population. It is likely that abnormal immunoregulation is the underlying cause.

Immunodeficiency syndromes commonly associated with malignant lymphoma include the Wiskott-Aldrich syndrome, ataxia telangiectasia, and common variable hypogammaglobulinemia. In this clinical setting, virtually all the lymphomas seen are of high-grade histologic types (Fig. 5–21). Disease usually presents in extranodal sites, particularly the brain. Extensive immunologic studies documenting the phenotype of the malignant cells have not been performed.

The recently described epidemic of the acquired immunodeficiency syndrome (AIDS) also has been associated with several significant lesions involving the lymphoid system (Guarda et al., 1983; Ioachim et al., 1983). Early in the course of the disease, patients have generalized lymphadenopathy. Individuals at increased risk for AIDS but lacking criteria for the full-blown syndrome also commonly exhibit generalized lymph node hyperplasia. At this stage, the lymph

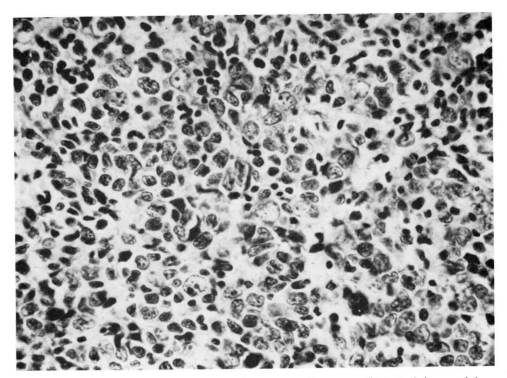

Figure 5–20. Large cell lymphoma supervening in a patient with immunoproliferative small-intestinal disease of the mesenteric lymph node. Large lymphoid cells were shown to contain alpha-heavy chains by immunoperoxidase staining.

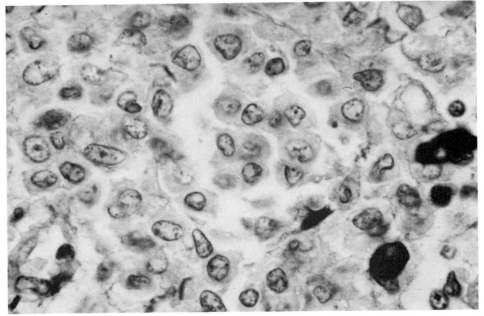

Figure 5–21. Malignant lymphoma, large cell, immunoblastic, arising in a patient with Wiskott-Aldrich syndrome. Although admixed plasma cells contain abundant, intensely stained immunoglobulin, tumor cells were devoid of intracytoplasmic immunoglobulins (immunoperoxidase methodology, ABC technique, hematoxylin counterstain).

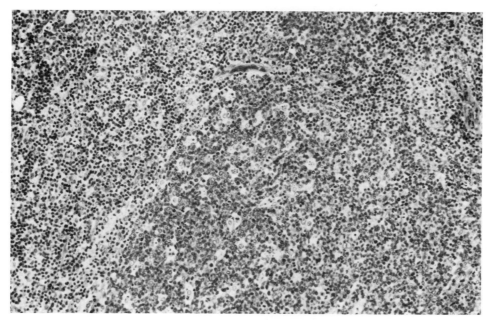

Figure 5–22. Acquired immunodeficiency syndrome, follicular hyperplasia. Hyperplastic germinal centers are prominent but lack well-demarcated lymphoid cuffs. Paracortex does not show significant hyperplasia.

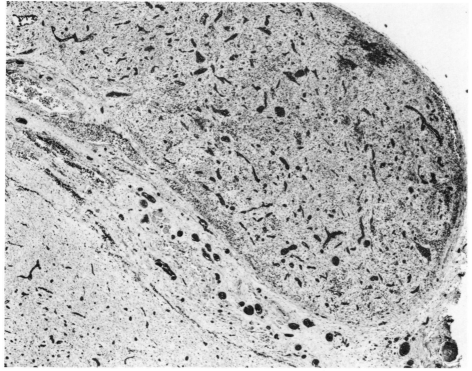

Figure 5–23. End-stage lymph node in acquired immunodeficiency syndrome. There is marked lymphoid atrophy, which affects both B cell–dependent and T cell–dependent areas. Only stromal and reticular elements remain. (Courtesy of Cheryl M. Reichert, M.D., Ph.D., Laboratory of Pathology, National Cancer Institute.)

nodes show marked follicular hyperplasia and plasmacytosis (Fig. 5–22). The paracortex, although not particularly hyperplastic, is not hypocellular. However, with time the paracortex becomes progressively depleted and the hyperplastic follicles stand out against an atrophic, pale paracortical zone. As one might expect, the serum in these patients reflects the B cell activation seen histologically, and polyclonal hypergammaglobulinemia is the rule. Polyclonal B cell activation can also be documented in vitro (Lane et al., 1983). As the disease progresses, progressive lymphoid atrophy, which affects both B cell–dependent and T cell–dependent zones, is seen. Lymphoid cells are lost and are replaced by prominent stromal and reticular elements (Fig. 5–23).

Patients with AIDS are at increased risk for malignancy, in particular Kaposi's sarcoma and malignant lymphoma. Histologically, the lymphomas are primarily of the high-grade B cell types: diffuse small noncleaved, large non-cleaved, and large cleaved (Fig. 5–24). In those cases in which immunologic phenotyping has been performed, B cell markers have been demonstrated. Some cases classified as small noncleaved satisfy criteria for Burkitt's lymphoma. Of interest are the observations that these patients, like patients in Africa with Burkitt's lymphoma, have markedly elevated titers to EBV and that some demonstrate nuclear EBNA positivity (Magrath et al., 1983; Purtilo, 1984).

The pathogenesis of the lymphomas in patients with AIDS and homosexual males without AIDS is not fully elucidated. Simplistically, one could speculate that the polyclonally activated B cells are not properly regulated owing to the T cell deficiency and that continued proliferation results in chromosomal translocations and neoplastic transformation. Although this view fits with existing clinical and laboratory observation, other factors are undoubtedly involved.

EPSTEIN-BARR VIRUS INFECTIONS

The subject of the role of Epstein-Barr virus (EBV) in human lymphoid malignancies—and indeed human neoplasia in general—is extremely complex and beyond the scope of this discussion. However, there are several areas of practical concern to the surgical pathologist. First, it is well established that EBV is the cause of infectious mononucleosis and that this virus can immortalize B lymphocytes in vitro (Klein, 1975). Moreover, most individuals exposed to Epstein-Barr virus carry EBV-infected B cells that can undergo proliferation, both in vivo and in vitro, under appropriate circumstances. However, a direct etiologic role for EBV with any human lymphoid malignancy, including Burkitt's lymphoma, is probably lacking.

Infectious mononucleosis is a subacute illness that occurs in individuals previously unexposed to Epstein-Barr virus. Infants and young children exposed to EBV will not develop any clinical symptoms. However, if exposure to this virus is delayed until adolescence or young adulthood, infectious mononucleosis is seen. This disease is associated with lymphadenopathy, hepatosplenomegaly, and leukocytosis. The lymphadenopathy is usually most conspicuous in the cervical regions. Hepatosplenomegaly can be signifi-

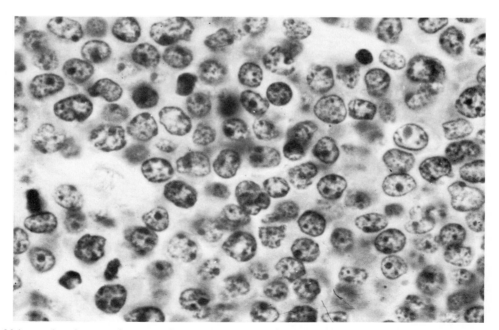

Figure 5–24. Malignant lymphoma in the acquired immunodeficiency syndrome. This tumor was classified as small non-cleaved cell type, which is the most commonly seen histologic subtype in this setting. Other high-grade follicular center cell lymphomas are also seen.

cant and associated with mild liver function abnormalities. The leukocytosis is usually moderate and associated with the presence of atypical lymphocytes called "Downey cells."

Involved lymph nodes may show a spectrum of histologic changes. Characteristically, one sees a follicular hyperplasia, a paracortical hyperplasia, and the presence of monocytoid cells in lymph node sinuses (Fig. 5–25). These monocytoid cells are, in fact, B lymphocytes. As the immunologic reaction to EBV continues, the paracortical hyperplasia may become more pronounced and lead to architectural efface-

ment. Sheets of immunoblasts may be seen, which may be mistaken for a large cell lymphoma by the unwary. However, as with most reactive paracortical hyperplasias, a spectrum of lymphoid cells is evident, ranging from small round lymphocytes to immunoblasts. Necrosis may be conspicuous and is associated with marked nuclear karyorrhexis. However, a neutrophilic response is absent. A similar process may be seen in tonsils and may be associated with ulceration of the overlying mucosa.

The earliest atypical lymphocytes seen in the peripheral blood are EBV-infected cells and have baso-

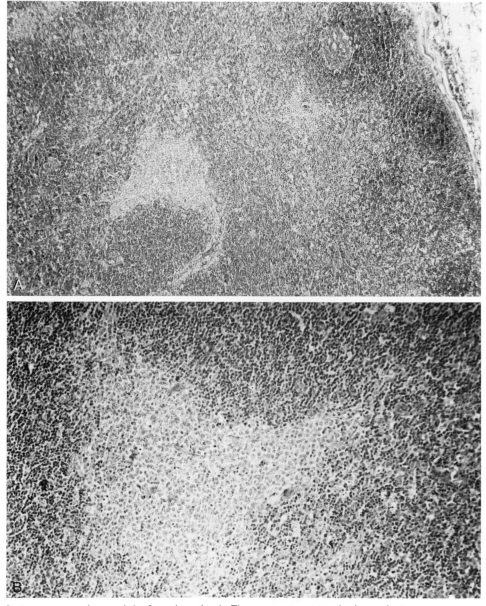

Figure 5–25. Infectious mononucleosis of the Lymph node. *A,* Three components to the hyperplastic process are seen and include a follicular hyperplasia, a paracortical hyperplasia, and the characteristic sinus reaction. *B,* Sinuses are dilated and contain large aggregates of "monocytoid" cells.

Illustration continued on following page

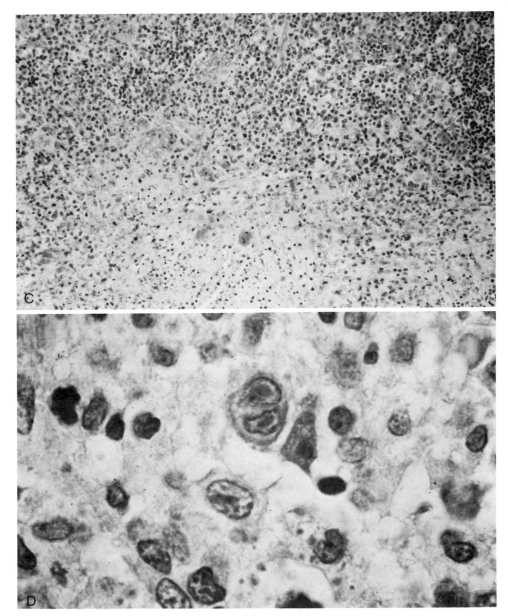

Figure 5–25. *Continued. C,* Necrosis can be conspicuous and is associated with abundant karyorrhectic debris without significant neutrophilic infiltration. *D,* Atypical immunoblasts resembling Reed-Sternberg cells can be identified. Such cells are seen as a component of the paracortical hyperplasia, which may contain numerous immunoblasts.

philic cytoplasm and plasmacytoid features. With time, reactive T cells predominate (Tosato et al., 1979). These have abundant pale cytoplasm with or without azurophilic granules. This T cell response is essential to eradication of the EBV-infected B cell proliferation. In the immunocompromised host, this T cell response is lacking, which may result in an uncontrolled proliferation after EBV infection.

Duncan's disease is an X-linked disorder in which affected males cannot mount an effective immune response to EBV, resulting in a variety of disseminated and progressive lymphoproliferative disorders (Purtilo

et al., 1977). Approximately 75 percent of these individuals develop a fatal form of infectious mononucleosis. More discrete tumor masses also can be seen, most often in the gastrointestinal tract. Morphologically, the cells resemble small non-cleaved, large cell, or immunoblastic lymphomas. However, most immunologic studies have demonstrated the B cell proliferations to be polyclonal.

A similar susceptibility to EBV infection can be seen in individuals receiving immunosuppressive therapy for organ transplantation. The immunosuppressive agent cyclosporin appears to be associated with the highest incidence of these lymphoid proliferations. The subject of post-transplant lymphomas has been a controversial one (Klein and Purtilo, 1981). Lymphoid mass lesions resembling high-grade malignant lymphomas have been reported for many years in patients receiving immunosuppression for organ transplantation (Pinkus et al., 1974; Starzl, 1968). The lymphoid proliferations are usually extranodal, often involving the gastrointestinal tract and central nervous system. Although these lesions have been termed "lymphomas" because of morphologic features, most studies have demonstrated a polyclonal B cell composition (Hanto et al., 1983).

The 1984 report by Starzl and colleagues describes reversibility of these "lymphomas" following withdrawal of cyclosporin and steroids. Thus, these authors postulate that these "lymphomas" are not autonomous lymphoid neoplasms but EBV-immortalized B cell proliferations that can be brought under control by the host if the immunosuppressive therapy is withdrawn. The 1984 report by Cleary and coworkers that these lymphoid proliferations are monoclonal does not necessarily contradict this hypothesis. In fact, when multiple sites were studied by Cleary's group, each individual site represented a different B cell clone. Thus, one could hypothesize that in each site an EBV-infected B cell with a potential growth advantage over other similar cells emerged to form the dominant component at that site. However, the lymphoid cells did not disseminate and remained confined to that site. Subsequent chromosomal translocations may convert such limited B cell clones into autonomous B cell neoplasms (Bird, 1982).

It has been recognized for many years that most patients with African, or endemic, Burkitt's lymphoma have markedly elevated titers to EBV and that EBV viral genome is integrated into the tumor cell DNA (Klein, 1975). However, the identical pathologic and immunologic process, Burkitt's lymphoma in nonendemic regions, is usually not associated with EBV. The common genetic element in all Burkitt's lymphomas is a chromosomal translocation involving the c-myc oncogene and one of the immunoglobulin genes (Croce et al., 1984). It is this translocation that appears to result in neoplastic transformation and autonomous growth. EBV may be a cofactor in that it may promote B cell proliferation, thus increasing the risk for this translocation to occur.

References

Anderson, L.B. and Talal, N.: The spectrum of benign or malignant lymphoproliferation in Sjögren's syndrome. Clin. Exp. Immunol. 10:199–221, 1972.

Azar, H.A.: Pathology of multiple myeloma and related growths. In Azar, H.A., and Potter, M. (eds.): Multiple Myeloma and Related Disorders. Vol. 1, New York, Harper & Row, 1973, pp. 1–85.

Baer, A.N., Bayless, T.M., Yardley, J.H.: Intestinal ulceration and malabsorption syndromes. Gastroenterology 79:754–765, 1980.

Bird, A.G.: Cyclosporin A, lymphomata and Epstein-Barr virus. In White, D.J.G. (ed.): Cyclosporin A. Amsterdam, Elsevier Biomedical, 1982, pp. 307–15.

Braun-Falco, O., Marghescu, S., Wolff, H.H.: Pagetoide reticulose. Hautarzt 24:11–21, 1973.

Brooks, J.J. and Enterline, H.T.: Gastric pseudolymphoma: its three subtypes and relation to lymphoma. Cancer 51:476–486, 1983.

Burg, G. and Braun-Falco, O.: Cutaneous Lymphomas, Pseudolymphomas, and Related Disorders. Berlin, Springer-Verlag, 1983.

Burke, J.S., Butler, J.J., Fuller, L.M.: Malignant lymphomas of the thyroid. A clinical pathologic study of 35 patients including ultrastructural observations. Cancer 39:1587–1602, 1977.

Burns, B.F., Colby, T.V., Dorfman, R.F.: Differential diagnostic features of nodular L&H Hodgkin's disease, including progressive transformation of germinal centers. Am. J. Surg. Pathol. 8:253–261, 1984.

Callihan, T.R., Holbert, J.M., Berard, C.W.: Neoplasms of terminal B-cell differentiation: A morphologic basis of functional diversity. In Malignant Lymphomas: A Pathology Annual Monograph. Norwalk, CT, Appleton-Century-Crofts, 1983, pp. 169–268.

Cleary, M.L., Warnke, R., Sklar, J.: Monoclonality of lymphoproliferative lesions in cardiac-transplant recipients. Clonal analysis based on immunoglobulin-gene rearrangements. N. Engl. J. Med. 310:477–482, 1984.

Cooper, B.T., Holmes, G.K.T., Cooke, W.T.: Lymphoma risk in coeliac disease of later life. Digestion 23:89–92, 1982.

Cooper, B.T., Holmes, G.K.T., Ferguson, R., Cooke, W.T.: Celiac disease and malignancy. Medicine 59:249–261,1980.

Costa, J. and Martin, S.E.: Pulmonary lymphoreticular disorders. In Jaffe, E.S. (ed.): Surgical Pathology of Lymph Nodes and Related Organs. Philadelphia, W.B. Saunders, 1985, pp. 282–297.

Croce, C.M., Tsujimoto, Y., Erikson, J., Nowell, P.: Biology of disease: chromosome translocations and B cell neoplasia. Lab. Invest. 51:258–269, 1984.

Dailey, M.E., Lindsay, S., Skahen, R.: Relation of thyroid neoplasms to Hashimoto's disease of the thyroid gland. Arch. Surg. 70:291–297, 1955.

De Remee, R.A., Weiland, L.H., McDonald, T.J.: Polymorphic reticulosis, lymphomatoid granulomatosis: two diseases or one? Mayo Clin. Proc. 53:634–640, 1978.

Evans, H.L.: Extranodal small lymphocytic proliferation: a clinicopathologic and immunocytochemical study. Cancer 49:84, 1982.

Fauci, A.S., Haynes, B.F., Costa, J., et al.: Lymphomatoid granulomatosis, prospective clinical and therapeutic experience over ten years. N. Engl. J. Med. 306:68–74, 1982.

Ford, W.L.: Lymphocyte migration and immune responses. Prog. Allergy 19:1–59, 1975.

Frizzera, G., Moran, E.M., Rappaport, H.: Angio-immunoblastic lymphadenopathy with dysproteinaemia. Lancet 1:1070–1073, 1974.

Gams, R.A., Neal, J.A., Conrad, F.G.: Hydantoin-induced pseudo-pseudolymphoma. Ann. Int. Med. 69:557–568, 1968.

Guarda, L.A., Butler, J.J., Mansell, P., et al.: Lymphadenopathy in homosexual men. Morbid anatomy with clinical and immunologic correlations. Am. J. Clin. Pathol. 79:559–568, 1983.

Hanto, D.W., Gajl-Peczalska, K.J., Frizzera, G., Arthur, D.C., Balfour, H.H., Jr., McClain, K., Simmons, R.L., Najarian, J.S.: Epstein-Barr virus (EBV) induced polyclonal and monoclonal B-cell lymphoproliferative disease occurring after renal transplantation. Ann. Surg. 198:356–369, 1983.

Hedrick, S.M., Nielsen, E.A., Kavaler, J., Cohen, D.I., Davis, M.M.: Sequence relationships between putative T-cell receptor polypeptides and immunoglobulins. Nature 308:149–153, 1984.

Ioachim, H.L., Lerner, C.W., Tapper, M.I.: The lymphoid lesions associated with the acquired immunodeficiency syndrome. Am. J. Surg. Pathol. 7:543–553, 1983.

Isaacson, P.: Middle East lymphoma and α chain disease. An immunohistochemical study. Am. J. Surg. Pathol. 3:431–441, 1979.

Isaacson, P., Jones, D.B., Sworn, M.J., Wright, D.H.: Malignant histiocytosis of the intestine: report of three cases with immunological and cytochemical analysis. J. Clin. Pathol. 35:510–516, 1982.

Jaffe, E.S.: Follicular lymphomas: possibility that they are benign tumors of the lymphoid system. J. Natl. Cancer Inst. 70:401, 1983.

Jaffe, E.S.: The pathologic and clinical spectrum of post-thymic T-cell malignancies. Cancer Invest., 2:'413–426, 1984.

Jaffe, E.S. and Cossman, J.: Immunodiagnosis of lymphoid and mononuclear phagocytic neoplasms. In Herberman, R. (Ed.) Manual of Clinical Laboratory Immunology, 3rd ed. Washington, DC, American Society of Microbiology, in press.

Jaffe, E.S., Costa, J.C., Fauci, A., et al.: Malignant lymphoma and erythrophagocytosis simulating malignant histiocytosis. Am. J. Med. 75:741–749, 1983.

Jaffe, E.S., Shevach, E.M., Sussman, E.H., Frank, M.M., Green, I., Berard, C.W.: Membrane receptor sites for the identification of lymphoreticular cells in benign and malignant conditions. Br. J. Cancer 31(Suppl. 2):107–120, 1975.

Katzenstein, A., Carrington, C.B., Liebow, A.A.: Lymphomatoid granulomatosis: a clinicopathologic study of 152 cases. Cancer 43:360–373, 1979.

Keller, A.R., Hochholzer, L., Castleman, B.: Hyaline-vascular and plasma-cell types of giant lymph node hyperplasia of the mediastinum and other locations. Cancer 29:670–683, 1972.

Klein, G.: The Epstein-Barr virus and neoplasia. N. Engl. J. Med. 293:1353–1357, 1975.

Klein, G., and Purtilo, D.: Summary: symposium on Epstein-Barr virus induced lymphoproliferative diseases in immunodeficient patients. Cancer Res. 41:4302–4304, 1981.

Knowles, D.M., Halper, J.P., Jakobiec, F.A.: The immunologic characterization of 40 extranodal lymphoid infiltrates. Usefulness in distinguishing between benign pseudolymphoma and malignant lymphoma. Cancer 49:2321–2335, 1982.

Koss, M.N., Hocholzer, L., Nichols, P.W., Wehunt, W.D., Lazarus, A.A.: Primary non-Hodgkin's lymphoma and pseudolymphoma of lung: a study of 161 patients. Hum. Pathol. 14:1024–1038, 1983.

Lane, H.C., Callihan, T.R., Jaffe, E.S., Fauci, A.S., Moutsopoulos, H.M.: Presence of intracytoplasmic IgG in the lymphocytic infiltrates of the minor salivary glands of patients with primary Sjogren's syndrome. Clin. Exp. Rheumatol. 1:237–239, 1983.

Lane, H.C., Masur, H., Edgar, L.C., Whalen, G., Rook, A.H., Fauci, A.S.: Abnormalities of B-cell activation and immunoregulation in patients with the acquired immunodeficiency syndrome. N. Engl. J. Med. 309:453–458, 1983.

Lennert, K., Stein, H., Mohri, N., Kaiserling, E., Muller-Hermelink, H.K.: Malignant lymphomas other than Hodgkin's disease. Berlin, Springer-Verlag, 1978a, p. 38; 1978b, p. 46.

Levy, N., Nelson, J., Meyer, P., Lukes, R.J., Parker, J.W.: Reactive lymphoid hyperplasia with single class (monoclonal) surface immunoglobulin. Am. J. Clin. Pathol. 80:300–308, 1983.

Liebow, A.A., Carrington, C.B. Friedman, R.J.: Lymphomatoid granulomatosis. Hum. Pathol. 3:457–558, 1972.

Lukes, R.J. and Tindle, B.H.: Immunoblastic lymphadenopathy. A hyperimmune entity resembling Hodgkin's disease. N. Engl. J. Med. 292:1–44, 1975.

Magrath, I., Erikson, I., Whang-Peng, J., Sieverts, H., Armstrong, G., Benjamin, D., Triche, T., Alabaster, O., Croce, C.M.: Synthesis of kappa light chains by cell lines containing an 8;22 chromosomal translocation derived from a male homosexual with Burkitt's lymphoma. Science 222:1094, 1983.

Mann, R.B., Jaffe, E.S., Berard, C.W.: Malignant lymphomas: a conceptual understanding of morphologic diversity. Am. J. Pathol. 94:103–192, 1979.

Matzner, Y. and Polliack, A.: Lymphoproliferative disorders in four patients receiving chronic diphenylhydantoin therapy: etiologic correlation or chance association? Israel J. Med. Sci. 14:865–869, 1978.

Maurer, R., Taylor, C.R., Terry, R., Lukes, R.J.: Non-Hodgkin

lymphomas of the thyroid. A clinico-pathological review of 29 cases applying the Lukes-Collins 1-classification and an immunoperoxidase method. Virch. Arch. [A] 383:293–317, 1979.

Nassar, V.H., Salem, P.A., Shahid, M.J. et al.: "Mediterranean abdominal lymphoma" or immunoproliferative small intestinal disease. Part II: Pathological aspects. Cancer 41:1340–1354, 1978.

Nathwani, B.N., Rappaport, H., Moran, E.M., Pangalis, G.A., Kim, H.: Malignant lymphoma arising in angioimmunoblastic lymphadenopathy. Cancer 41:578–606, 1978.

Otto, H.F., Bettmann, I., Weltzien, J.V., Gebbers, J.O.: Primary intestinal lymphomas. Virch. Arch. [A] 391:9–31, 1981.

Pinkus, G.S., Wilson, R.E., Corson, J.M.: Reticulum cell sarcoma of the colon following renal transplantation. Cancer 34:2103–2108, 1974.

Poppema, S., Kaiserling, E., Lennert, K.: Hodgkin's disease with lymphocytic predominance, nodular type (nodular paragranuloma) and progressively transformed germinal centers—a cytohistological study. Histopathology 3:295–308, 1979.

Poppema, S., Kaiserling, E., Lennert, K.: Nodular paragranuloma and progressively transformed germinal centers. Ultrastructural and immunohistologic findings. Virch. Arch. [Cell Pathol.] 31:211–225, 1979.

Purtilo, D.T.: Biology of disease: defective immune surveillance in viral carcinogenesis. Lab Invest. 51:373–385, 1984.

Purtilo, D.T., DeFlorio, D., Hutt, L.M., Bhawan, J., Yang, J.P.S., Otto, R., Edwards, W.: Variable phenotypic expression of an X-linked recessive lymphoproliferative syndrome. N. Engl. J. Med. 297:1077–1081, 1977.

Salem, P.A., Nassar, V.H., Shahid, M.J., et al.: "Mediterranean abdominal lymphoma" or immunoproliferative small intestinal disease. Part I: Clinical aspects. Cancer 40:2941–2947, 1977.

Saltzstein, S.L.: Extranodal malignant lymphomas and pseudolymphomas. Pathol. Ann. 159–185, 1969.

Saltzstein, S.L. and Ackerman, L.V.: Lymphadenopathy induced by anticonvulsant drugs and mimicking clinically and pathologically malignant lymphomas. Cancer 12:164–182, 1959.

Saraga, P., Hurlimann, J., Ozzello, L.: Lymphomas and pseudolymphomas of the alimentary tract. An immunohistochemical study with clinicopathologic correlations. Hum. Pathol. 12:713–723, 1981.

Schlosnagle, D.C.,Chan, W.C., Hargreaves, H.K., Nolting, S.F., Brynes, R.K.: Plasmacytoma arising in giant lymph node hyperplasia. Am. J. Clin. Pathol. 78:541–544, 1982.

Schroer, K.R. and Franssila, K.O.: Atypical hyperplasia of lymph nodes. Cancer 44:1155–1163, 1979.

Simrell, C.R., Crabtree, G.R., Cossman, J., Fauci, A.S., Jaffe, E.S.: Stimulation of phagocytosis by a T cell lymphoma derived lymphokine. In Vitetta, E. and Fox, C.F. (eds.): B and T Cell Tumors: Biological and Clinical Aspects. UCLA Symposia on Molecular and Cellular Biology. Vol. 24. New York, Academic Press, 1982, pp. 247–252.

Siu, G., Clark, S.P., Yoshikai, Y., Malissen, M., Yanagi, Y., Strauss, E., Mak, T.W., Hood, L.: The human T cell antigen receptor is encoded by variable diversity and joining gene segments that rearrange to generate a complete V gene. Cell 37:393–401, 1984.

Stanley, J. and Fallon-Pellicci, V.: Phenytoin hypersensitivity reaction. Arch. Dermatol. 114:1350–1353, 1978.

Starzl, T.E.: Discussion of Murray, J.E., Wilson, R.E., Tilney, N.L., et al.: Five years' experience in renal transplantation with immunosuppression survival, function, complications and the role of lymphocyte depletion by thoracic duct fistula. Ann. Surg. 168:416–35, 1968.

Starzl, T.E., Porter, K.A., Iwatsuki, S., Rosenthal, J.T., Shaw, B.W., Jr., Atchison, R.W., Nalesnik, M.A., Ho, M., Griffith, B.P., Hakala, T.R., Hardesty, R.L., Jaffe, R., Bahnson, H.T.: Reversibility of lymphomas and lymphoproliferative lesions developing under cyclosporin-steroid therapy. Lancet 1:583–587, 1984.

Swinson, C.M., Slavin, G., Coles, E.C., Booth, C.C.: Coeliac disease and malignancy. Lancet 1:111–115, 1983.

Talal, N., Asofsky, R., Lightbody, P.: Immunoglobulin synthesis by salivary gland lymphoid cells in Sjögren's syndrome. J. Clin. Invest. 49:49–59, 1970.

Tosato, G., Magrath, I., Koski, I., Dooley, N., Blaese, M.: N. Engl. J. Med. 301:1133–1137, 1979.

Waldron, J.A., Leech, J.H., Glick, A.D., Flexner, J.M., Collins, R.D.: Malignant lymphoma of peripheral T-lymphocyte origin. Immunologic, pathologic and clinical features in six patients. Cancer 40:1604–1617, 1977.

Wantanabe, S., Shimosato, Y., Shimoyama, M., et al.: Adult T cell lymphoma with hypergammaglobulinemia. Cancer 46:2472–2483, 1980.

Wolf, J.A. and Spjut, H.J.: Focal lymphoid hyperplasia of the stomach preceding gastric lymphoma. Cancer 48:2518–2523, 1981.

Zulman, J., Jaffe, R., Talal, N.: Evidence that the malignant lymphoma of Sjögren's syndrome is a monoclonal B-cell neoplasm. N. Engl. J. Med. 299:1215–1220, 1978.

6 Stomach

Recent technologic developments, especially flexible endoscopy, have made possible the documentation of the initial stages of the gastric neoplastic process in humans. With the new technology it has been shown in some detail what has been known for more than a century: that there are lesions in the gastric mucosa that can be found years before cancer becomes clinically apparent. This was first documented by Kupfer, who described foci of intestinal epithelium in the gastric mucosa more than a century ago (1883), and was discussed extensively afterwards (Jarvi and Lauren, 1951; Masson, 1923; Michalany, 1959; Schmidt, 1896).

It also has been reported that intestinal metaplasia in most cases appears to be a component of a more basic process, chronic atrophic gastritis, which has been characterized on clinical and pathologic grounds (Correa, 1980; Lambert, 1972; Strickland and Mackay, 1973).

Gastric carcinoma is not a homogeneous disease; rather, it appears to involve two independent etiopathogenic entities that have, for convenience, been designated as "intestinal," or "expansive" and "diffuse," or "infiltrative" (Lauren, 1965; Ming, 1977). Our discussion will concentrate on the initial phases of intestinal gastric carcinoma because extensive information is available for this type of carcinoma, unlike the diffuse type, whose initial stages are poorly understood. A few reports describe clusters of poorly organized goblet cells in the gastric epithelium as the initial stage of signet ring cell (diffuse) carcinoma. It has been designated "globoid dysplasia" by Borchard and coworkers (1979). It is not yet clear whether this represents a cancer precursor or foci of carcinoma-in-situ in stomachs that also show invasion of the lamina propria. Further research is needed to characterize the lesion better. Contrary to the "intestinal" type, the great majority of cancers of the diffuse type are not accompanied by precursor lesions in the tumor-free mucosa.

It has been postulated that a continuum of progressive changes precede clinical gastric carcinoma of the intestinal type (Correa, 1983). They all are covered by the term "precursors" but fall into two basic categories: those with mature and those with immature cellular phenotype. Lesions with a mature cellular phenotype are probably remote from the cancer end point, are highly prevalent in populations at high risk, and probably do not deserve any special surveillance or intervention by clinicians because most will never reach the stage of clinical cancer (Correa, 1982). Cells in precursor lesions with immature phenotype have probably reached the stage of irreversibility to normal phenotype, represent a greater threat to the patient, and deserve close clinical surveillance.

The aforementioned changes in the gastric mucosa can be documented with different parameters. We will utilize the morphologic parameters in our presentation. Other parameters will be mentioned only briefly: the histochemistry of mucin and cellular enzymes, the secretion of pepsinogens, and the expression of abnormal antigens.

PRECURSORS WITH MATURE PHENOTYPE

The major lesions in the mature phenotype category are chronic gastritis regenerative hypoplasia, atrophy, and intestinal metaplasia. The immature phenotype category corresponds to the dysplasias.

Chronic Gastritis

Inflammation of the gastric mucosa is probably one of the most frequent clinical syndromes experienced by adults. Ubiquitous irritants such as alcohol, aspirin, and salt are present in most human diets and are frequently abused. Acute gastritis in most instances heals completely, but repeated episodes have the

Work supported by Grant #PO1-CA-28842 of the National Cancer Institute, National Institutes of Health, Bethesda, Maryland.

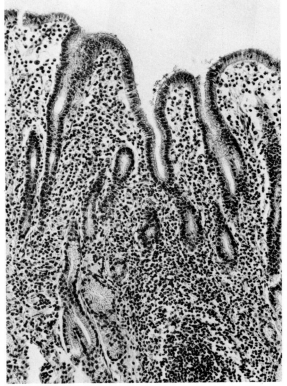

Figure 6–1. Superficial gastritis. Lymphocytic and plasma cell infiltrate in the lamina propria of the upper portion of the mucosa.

potential to induce chronic gastritis. The less advanced form of chronic gastritis is characterized by an infiltrate of mononuclear white blood cells in the superficial layers of the lamina propria (Fig. 6–1). The more advanced forms of chronic gastritis fall into several clinicopathologic entities, which have been discussed elsewhere (Correa, 1980). Some forms, such as hypersecretory gastritis (Fig. 6–2)—which frequently accompanies duodenal peptic ulcer—appear unrelated to gastric cancer. Other forms, such as autoimmune gastritis—which is part of the pernicious anemia syndrome—and environmental gastritis are true precursors of gastric carcinoma. The latter displays the same geographic distribution as epidemic gastric cancer and is probably associated with the same type of diet (Correa, 1982).

Regenerative Hyperplasia

The only cells in the normal gastric mucosa with the capacity to replicate are of the glandular necks. Cell loss in any location triggers cell replication in the neck region, and migration replaces the lost epithelial cells. Migration upward replaces foveolar cells and migration downward replaces glandular cells. Neck cells, therefore, are multipotential and can differentiate either to foveolar or to glandular cells. Gastritis is regularly accompanied by hyperplastic neck cells showing the usual signs of regeneration: large nuclei,

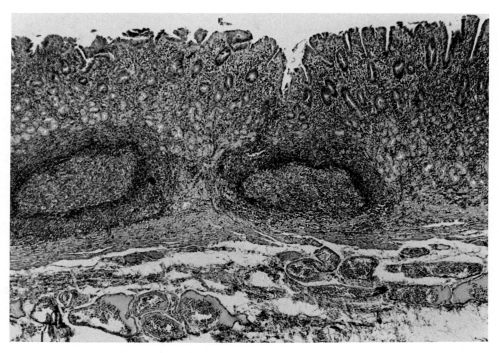

Figure 6–2. Hypersecretory chronic gastritis in patient with duodenal peptic ulcer. Lymphocytic infiltrate involving the full thickness of the mucosa. Prominent lymphoid follicles. Depletion of mucous secretion of the surface epithelium.

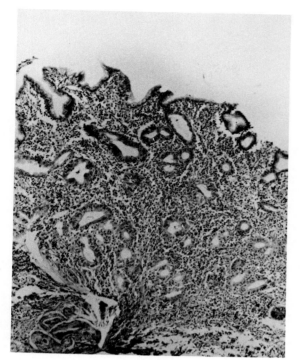

Figure 6–3. Chronic atrophic gastritis with regenerative hyperplasia. Dense inflammatory infiltrate of the lamina propria. The glandular necks are irregular, hyperplastic and of different size and shape. Some nuclei are hyperchromatic.

hyperchromatism, mitosis, and somewhat irregular lumens. Characteristically, those changes are most accentuated in the region of the glandular necks, but migrant hyperchromatic and not yet totally differentiated cells may be seen in other areas, notably the foveolar region. The nuclei of regenerative cells are usually hyperchromatic and round, may overlap, and show frequent mitosis. The background in this situation regularly shows an inflammatory infiltrate and in most cases polynuclear leukocytes participate, indicating acute injury to the mucosa (Figs. 6–3 and 6–4). Occasionally, it is difficult to distinguish regenerative hyperplasia from mild dysplasia. Alcian blue stains should be used to rule out acid mucin, a marker of previous metaplasia that should be absent in true regenerative hyperplasia. If no clear distinction between the two lesions is possible, the pathologist's report should reflect that situation, the patient should be treated for gastritis, and the biopsy should be repeated when the gastritis has subsided.

Atrophy

The loss of gastric glands characterizes all types of gastritis that are epidemiologically linked to gastric cancer (Correa, 1984). It thus appears to be a critical stage in the process of carcinogenesis. Loss of glands is usually accompanied by neck cell hyperplasia, an apparent attempt to regenerate the missing epithelial cells (Fig. 6–5). Atrophic changes are usually observed in a background of chronic gastritis, but the degree of inflammation varies from minimal to prominent. These variable degrees of inflammation have inspired classifications that erroneously suggest that chronic atrophic gastritis and gastric atrophy are different entities. Gastric atrophy consists of atrophic changes and minimal inflammation and is observed in older individuals with extensive lesions, probably representing the advanced stage of the atrophic gastritis process (Fig. 6–6).

INTESTINAL METAPLASIA

Gastric glands lost in the process of atrophic gastritis are frequently replaced by cells with intestinal phenotypes. It is not clear how this process occurs; old explanations referred to "faulty regenerations" that, in modern terminology, called for the expression of some repressed genes in multipotential cells of the glandular necks. Other investigators interpret the change as a true mutation involving structural changes in the DNA molecule (Sugimura et al., 1982). The "faulty regeneration" hypothesis calls for chronic loss

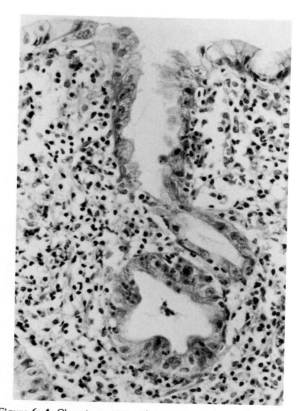

Figure 6–4. Chronic gastritis with regenerative hyperplasia. Large, overlapping nuclei with prominent nucleoli are seen in the glandular neck extending to the foveolar epithelium. Marked mono- and polynuclear infiltrate in the lamina propria.

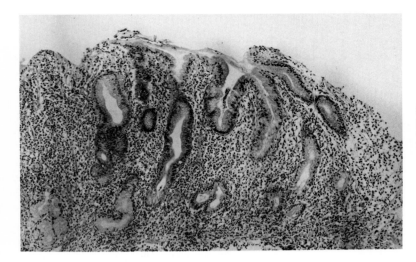

Figure 6–5. Chronic atrophic gastritis. The loss of glands leaves extensive areas of the lamina propria occupied by inflammatory cells only. Glandular neck hyperplasia.

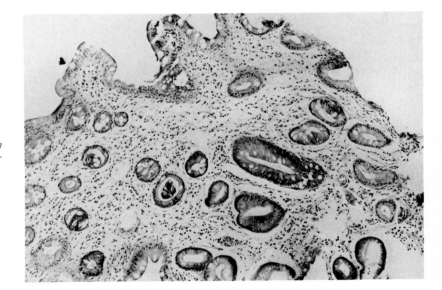

Figure 6–6. Gastric biopsy showing atrophy and mild inflammatory infiltrate. Intestinal metaplasia of glands and surface epithelium.

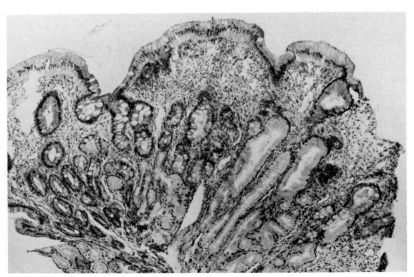

Figure 6–7. Chronic atrophic gastritis with intestinal metaplasia of glands and, to a lesser degree, the surface epithelium. Goblet cells are prominent. The inflammatory infiltrate is mild.

of cells, which could be accomplished by irritants acting alone. The mutation hypothesis postulates the presence of a mutagenic agent in the environment. The fact that some types of chronic gastritis involving cell regeneration, such as hypersecretory gastritis, are not associated with an elevated risk of cancer, favors the mutation hypothesis (Correa, 1980).

Metaplastic glands replace the closely packed tubular glands of the corporal and antral mucosa by crypt-like structures lined by absorptive and goblet cells typical of the intestinal mucosa (Fig. 6–7). Argentaffin and Paneth cells also are present in some intestinalized crypts. Metaplastic glands can also occupy the foveolar region and surface epithelium, especially when this region is thicker than normal, apparently the result of previous foveolar hyperplasia. Structures resembling both small and large intestinal mucosa have been identified in metaplastic lesions of the gastric mucosa. Some observations suggest that in the initial stages of metaplasia the small intestinal type predominates, whereas in advanced lesions colonic type crypts, predominantly populated by goblet cells, are more frequent (Heilmann and Hopker, 1979; Jass and Filipe, 1979; Sipponen et al., 1981; Teglbjaerg and Nielsen, 1978). The two types often coexist, a situation that could be interpreted as a transition from small intestinal to colonic type. Small intestinal metaplasia often produces structures resembling intestinal villi, making its differentiation from true intestinal mucosa difficult in small biopsies (Fig. 6–8). Cells of the small intestinal type of gastric metaplasia secrete the normal small intestinal mucin: It is acid and stains with Alcian blue (pH 2.5), but because it is a sialomucin it does not take the high-iron diamine stain. The same cells usually secrete the complete set of intestinal enzymes: alkaline phosphatase, sucrase, leucine aminopeptidase, trehalase, succinic dehydrogenase, and diaphorase. For this reason, this type has been called "complete metaplasia" (Matsukura et al., 1980).

More advanced stages of the process often show prominent colonic type of metaplasia with straight crypts, lack of villi-like structures, and few, if any, Paneth cells. In this type of metaplastic mucosa, most small intestinal enzymes are absent, although sucrase and leucine aminopeptidase tend to persist. For that reason, this metaplasia has been called "incomplete." The mucin secretion, a mixture of sialomucin and sulfated mucin, is typical of the large bowel; the latter stains positively with high-iron diamine. Several investigators, basing their reports on morphologic observations, have proposed that colonic metaplasia is more closely related to dysplasia and cancer than small intestinal metaplasia is (Heilmann and Hopker, 1979; Jass and Filipe, 1980; Sipponen et al., 1981).

Both small intestinal and colonic types of metaplasia in most cases show signs of "maturity," or good differentiation: Their cells have abundant cytoplasm and basal, round, small, well-spaced nuclei (Figs. 6–7

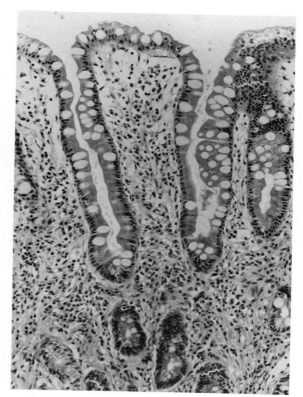

Figure 6–8. Mature intestinal metaplasia, small-intestinal type. Villus-like structures lined by enterocytes and goblet cells. Mild infiltrate of lymphocytes and plasma cells.

and 6–8). In a few cases, this good differentiation is altered, a change that is described as "dysplasia."

DYSPLASIA

Nuclear atypism and partial loss of polarity, the landmarks of dysplasia, have been the subject of several reviews (Grundmann, 1975; Morson et al., 1980; Oehlert et al., 1975; Nagayo, 1981). There is as yet no general agreement on the nomenclature and criteria for the diagnosis of gastric dysplasia (Ming, 1984). It appears that there may be some important interpopulation differences in the type, frequency, and severity of dysplasias. This may reflect the interplay of several etiologic factors because populations at high risk of gastric cancer vary considerably in their diet and therefore may be subject to different intensities of such factors. One etiologic factor prominent in some but not all populations is alcohol. Because alcohol is capable of inducing gastritis it may also modify other lesions. In some patients, dysplasia appears in a background of severe inflammation; in others atrophy, rather than inflammation, is the predominant background. My colleagues and I have identified two main types of dysplasia. They have been designated "adenomatous" and "hyperplastic" in our previous publications (Cuello et al., 1980) and

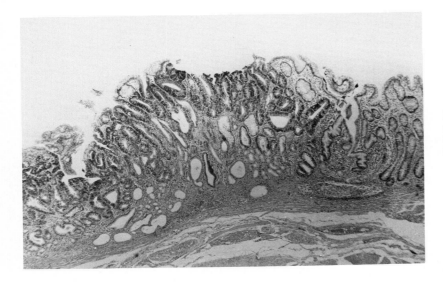

Figure 6–9. Adenomatous dysplasia in flat mucosa, predominantly occupying the glandular neck region. Chronic atrophic gastritis and intestinal metaplasia in the background.

"Type I" and "Type II" by Jass (1983). Although these two types of dysplasia will be described separately the reader should understand that they are not always clearly separable because features of both may coincide or some of the features may not be completely developed.

Adenomatous Dysplasia

Adenomatous dysplasia was described by Sugano and coworkers in 1972 as "atypical epithelium." It usually lies in a background of severe atrophy and consists of a proliferation of closely packed tubular glands lined mostly by cells with eosinophilic cytoplasm that may contain small droplets of acid mucin, requiring Alcian blue stain for their identification. These glands closely resemble those of adenomatous polyps of the large intestine, but they usually occur in flat mucosa (Fig. 6–9). Occasionally, the dysplastic epithelium forms a mass that protrudes into the lumen, an adenomatous polyp (Fig. 6–10). In some preparations, it is possible to determine that the dysplastic

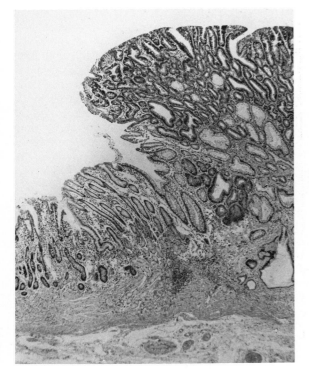

Figure 6–10. Adenomatous polyps. Dysplastic glands proliferate in a background of atrophic gastritis and intestinal metaplasia.

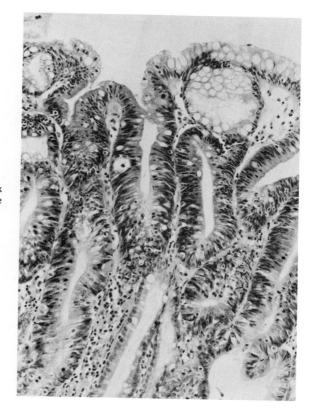

Figure 6–11. Adenomatous dysplasia, prominent in the glandular neck region and extending to the surface epithelium, at which point mature metaplasia predominates.

cells occupy the neck region of the glands, but most frequently cells of this type extend into the foveolar region and cover the surface epithelium (Fig. 6–11). In mild dysplasias, the nuclei are mostly basal and elongated in shape. In moderate degrees of dysplasia, the nuclei are closely packed, elongated, and pseudostratified (Figs. 6–12, 6–13 and 6–14) but retain some degree of polarity. In severe dysplasia, polarity is partially or totally lost, and the nuclei are oval or irregularly shaped, have prominent nucleoli, show frequent mitosis, and often reach the top of the cell (Fig. 6–15). More advanced cases correspond to carcinoma-in-situ and show frankly neoplastic epithelium with total loss of polarity and very irregular nuclei still bound by the original basement membrane of the gland. The transition from mild dysplasia to moderate

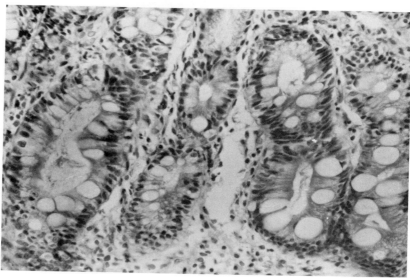

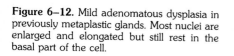

Figure 6–12. Mild adenomatous dysplasia in previously metaplastic glands. Most nuclei are enlarged and elongated but still rest in the basal part of the cell.

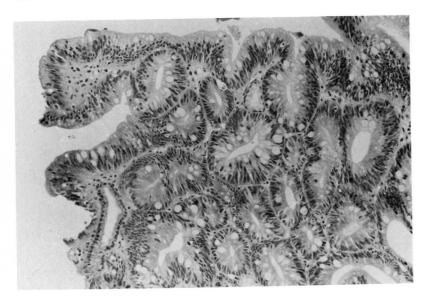

Figure 6–13. Moderate adenomatous dysplasia. Enlarged, elongated nuclei showing pseudostratification.

dysplasia to severe dysplasia to carcinoma-in-situ is difficult to define and rather subjective because there are no clear-cut lines that distinguish one stage from the other.

Carcinomas arising in adenomatous dysplasias usually are of the intestinal, well-differentiated type and appear rather deeply in the mucosa, frequently perforating the muscularis mucosa and invading the submucosa at several independent points (Fig. 6–16).

Hyperplastic Dysplasia

Hyperplastic dysplasia is usually accompanied by severe inflammation and occasionally by foveolar hyperplasia and metaplasia (Figs. 6–17 and 6–18). Glandular atrophy also is usually present but tends to be less severe than in adenomatous dysplasia. Characteristically, the proliferating gland-like structures are irregularly shaped because of branching and forma-

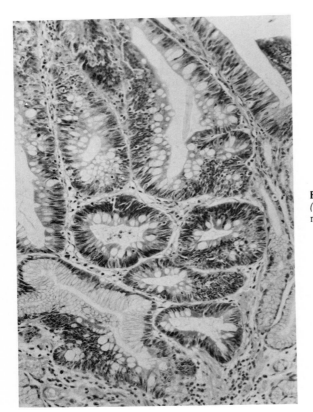

Figure 6–14. Gastric mucosa showing glands with mature metaplasia *(bottom)* and glands with moderate dysplasia. Gradual disappearance of mucous goblets in more advanced dysplastic glands.

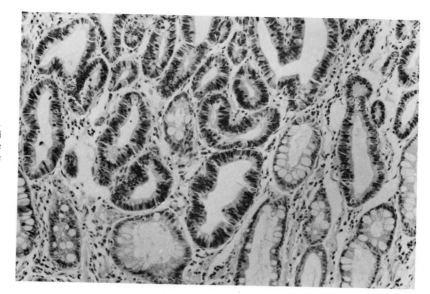

Figure 6–15. Marked adenomatous dysplasia. Large, hyperchromatic, overlapping nuclei reaching the upper part of the cell. Some mature and minimally dysplastic glands are seen at the right side and at the bottom.

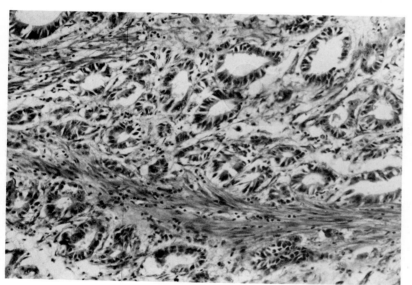

Figure 6–16. Well-differentiated intestinal-type adenocarcinoma infiltrating the submucosa of the stomach. Chronic atrophic gastritis and adenomatous dysplasia were also present.

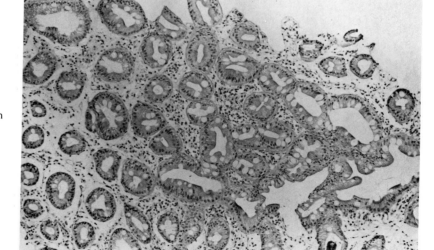

Figure 6–17. Mature intestinal metaplasia in hyperplastic foveolar epithelium.

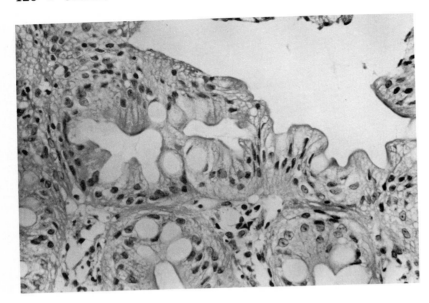

Figure 6–18. Hyperplastic foveolar epithelium with mature intestinal metaplasia.

tion of epithelial folds (Figs. 6–19 and 6–20). In mild forms, some absorptive cells with brush borders and goblet cells are well developed, and the nuclei are elongated but close to the basal side of the cell. In moderate dysplasias, some nuclei reach the upper part of the cell, show partial loss of polarity, and have moderately prominent nucleoli (Figs. 6–20 and 6–21). Severe dysplasias show the original glandular struc-

tures lined by cells with large, irregularly shaped nuclei with frequent mitosis, prominent nucleoli, and total loss of polarity. The transition from severe dysplasia to carcinoma-in-situ is difficult to define, although the former usually shows neoplastic nuclei alternating with nuclei with lesser degrees of atypia (Figs. 6–22 and 6–23).

Carcinomas arising in hyperplastic dysplasias are

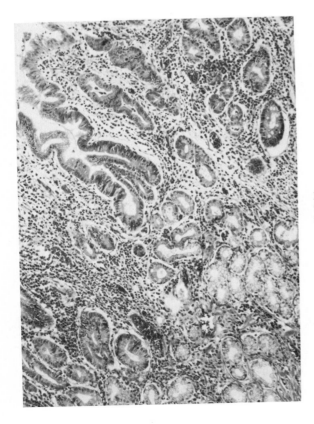

Figure 6–19. Hyperplastic dysplasia in mucosa in a background of intestinal metaplasia. Atrophy is not prominent. Marked inflammatory infiltrate.

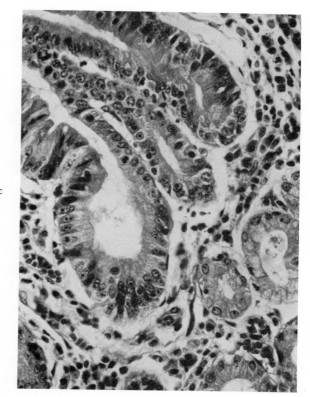

Figure 6–20. Moderate hyperplastic dysplasia. Large, hyperchromatic nuclei and prominent nucleoli. Partial alteration of polarity.

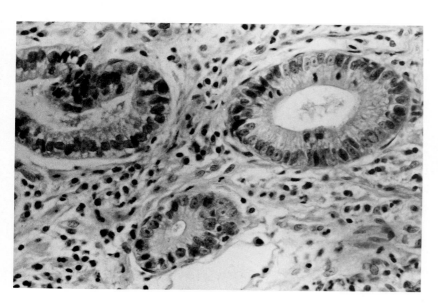

Figure 6–21. Glandular detail in stomach with moderate hyperplastic dysplasia. Hyperchromatic, irregularly-shaped nuclei, partial loss of polarity.

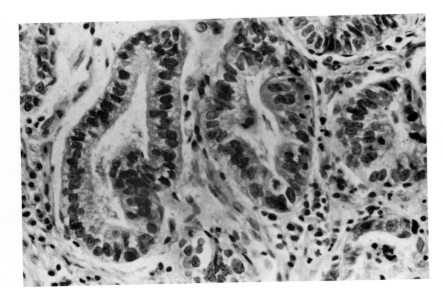

Figure 6–22. Moderate *(left)* and marked *(right)* hyperplastic dysplasia. Irregular shape of nuclei, hyperchromatism, loss of polarity.

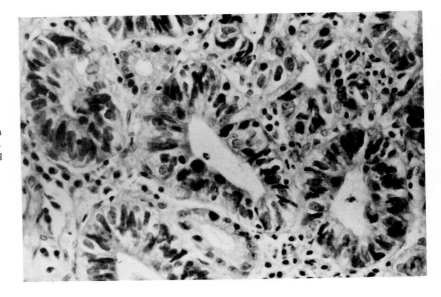

Figure 6–23. Marked hyperplastic dysplasia indistinguishable from carcinoma-in-situ. Marked irregularity of size, shape, and staining of nuclei. Frequent mitosis. Loss of polarity.

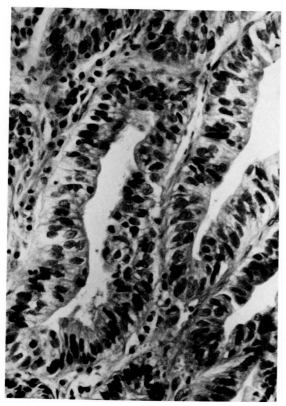

Figure 6–24. Carcinoma-in-situ. All cells show neoplastic phenotype but remain within the bounds of the original glands.

tigens normally found in embryonal and fetal tissue tend to appear in incomplete metaplasia and dysplasia (Higgins et al., 1984). The reappearance of "colonic" antigens in incomplete metaplasia has been interpreted by Nardelli and coworkers (1983) as the expression of fetal duodenal antigens. Invasive carcinoma may express abnormal "adult" and "fetal" antigens.

The level of pepsinogen I in the serum has been associated with metaplasia. It has also been shown that the levels decrease with advanced metaplasia and become lowest in patients who develop gastric carcinoma (Nomura et al., 1980; Stemmermann et al., 1980). This marker probably reflects the gradual loss of parietal cells due to atrophy and metaplasia and can be used to monitor the progress of the disease. When very low levels are present, endoscopy should be performed so that carcinoma can be ruled out.

Another marker of the progress of the precancerous process is the presence of nitrite in the gastric juice. The level of nitrite becomes higher as metaplasia advances and highest in the presence of dysplasia. It probably reflects progressive bacterial colonization of the stomach mucosa by reductase-containing bacteria that transform nitrate into nitrite. Hydrochloric acid secretion also becomes gradually lower but may be

usually of the intestinal type but poorly differentiated and spread laterally, replacing the foveolar epithelium in a considerable extension (Fig. 6–24). This corresponds to the so-called superficially spreading carcinoma (Fig. 6–25). Metastasis of carcinomas originating in hyperplastic dysplasias usually preserves the poorly differentiated intestinal pattern.

OTHER INDICATORS OF PRE-NEOPLASTIC AND INITIAL NEOPLASM

The aforementioned represent increasingly severe lesions that show a progressive loss of differentiation. Classic morphology is but one of the indicators of this progressive loss of differentiation. Histochemical alteration of mucin and of digestive enzymes has already been mentioned. Other noteworthy indicators are the expression of abnormal antigens and the spectrum of pepsinogen secretion.

During fetal development, both gastric and intestinal antigens are present in the gastric epithelium. The intestinal component disappears soon after birth and remains absent in the adult. It reemerges when intestinal metaplasia develops (DeBoer et al., 1969). Antigens found in well-differentiated ("adult") tissues tend to appear in complete metaplasia, whereas an-

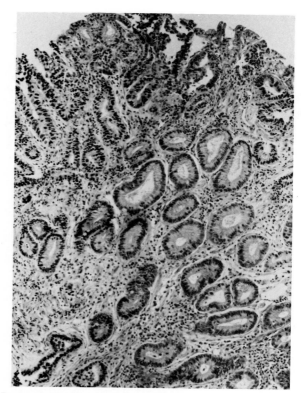

Figure 6–25. Superficially spreading carcinoma occupying an extensive area of the foveolar epithelium and the glandular necks. Moderate hyperplastic dysplasia deeper in the mucosa.

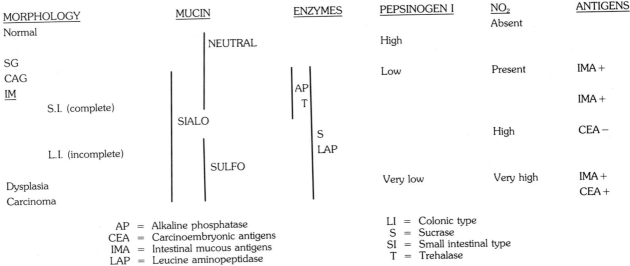

| MORPHOLOGY | MUCIN | ENZYMES | PEPSINOGEN I | NO₂ | ANTIGENS |

Figure 6–26. Diagrammatic representation of the hypothetical model of progression of preneoplastic lesions.

AP = Alkaline phosphatase
CEA = Carcinoembryonic antigens
IMA = Intestinal mucous antigens
LAP = Leucine aminopeptidase

LI = Colonic type
S = Sucrase
SI = Small intestinal type
T = Trehalase

temporarily compensated by gastrin levels that are high as a feedback response to gradual antral atrophy. In patients with advanced atrophy, both gastrin and HCl secretions are expected to drop.

Figure 6–26 represents the model of preneoplastic lesions of the gastric mucosa. A close relationship among morphology, mucin production, digestive enzymes, HCl and pepsinogen secretion, and gastric juice nitrite is postulated.

References

Borchard, F. Mittelstaedt, A., Stux, G.: Dysplasien in Resektionmagen und Klassificationprobleme verschiedener Dysplasieformen. Verh. Dtsch. Ges. Pathol. 63:250–257, 1979.

Correa, P.: The epidemiology and pathogenesis of chronic gastritis: three etiologic entities. Front. Gastroenterol. Res. 6:98–108, 1980.

Correa, P.: Morphology and natural history of precursor lesions. In Schottenfeld, D. and Fraumeni, J. (eds.): Cancer Epidemiology and Prevention. Philadelphia, W. B. Saunders Co., 1982, pp. 90–137.

Correa, P.: Precursor of gastric and esophageal cancer. Cancer 50:2554–2565, 1982.

Correa, P.: The gastric precancerous process. Cancer Surveys, 2:437–450, 1983.

Cuello, C., Correa, P., Zarama, G., Lopez, J., Murray, J., Gordillo, G.: Histopathology of gastric dysplasias: correlations with gastric juice chemistry. Am. J. Surg. Pathol. 3:491–500, 1979.

DeBoer, W. G. R. N., Forsyth, A., Nairn, R. C.: Gastric antigens in health and disease. Behaviour in early development, senescence, metaplasia and cancer. Br. Med. J. 3:93–94, 1969.

Grundmann, E.: Histologic types and possible initial stages in early gastric carcinoma. Beitr. Pathol. 154:256–280, 1975.

Heilmann, K. L. and Hopker, W. W.: Loss of differentiation in intestinal metaplasia in cancerous stomachs. A comprehensive morphologic study. Pathol. Res. Pract. 164:249–258, 1979.

Higgins, P. J., Correa, P., Cuello, C., Lipkin, M.: Fetal antigens in the precursor stages of gastric cancer. Oncology, 41:73–76, 1984.

Jarvi, O. and Lauren, P.: On the role of heterotopias of the intestinal epithelium in the pathogenesis of gastric cancer. Acta Pathol. Microbiol. Scand. 29:26–44, 1951.

Jass, J. R.: A classification of gastric dysplasias. Histopathology 7:181–193, 1983.

Jass, J. R. and Filipe, M. I.: Variants of intestinal metaplasia associated with gastric carcinoma. Histopathology 3:191–199, 1979.

Jass, J. R. and Filipe, M. I.: Sulphomucins of precancerous lesions of the human stomach. Histopathology 4:271–279, 1980.

Kupfer, C.: Fetschrift. Arz. Verein. Munch., p. 7, 1883.

Lambert, R.: Chronic gastritis. Digestion 7:83–126, 1972.

Lauren, P.: The two histological main types of gastric carcinoma: diffuse and so-called intestinal-type carcinoma: An attempt at a histoclinical classification. Acta Pathol. Microbiol. Scand. 64:31–49, 1965.

Masson, P.: Tumeurs Humaines, 1923. Translated by Kobernick, O. Detroit, Wayne University Press, 1970, pp. 643–646.

Matsukura, N., Susuki, K., Kawachi, T., Aoyagi, M., Sugimura, T., Kitaoka, H., Numajiri, H., Shirota, A., Itahashi, M., Hirota, T.: Distribution of marker enzymes and mucin in intestinal metaplasia in human stomachs and relation of complete and incomplete types of intestinal metaplasia to minute gastric carcinomas. J. Natl. Cancer Inst. 65:231–240, 1980.

Michalany, J.: Metaplasia intestinal da mucosa gastrica. Rev. Assoc. Med. Brasil 5:25–36, 1959.

Ming, S. C.: Gastric carcinoma: a pathologic classification. Cancer 39:2475–2485, 1977.

Ming, S.C.: Pathologic features of gastric dysplasias. In Ming, S.C., (ed.): Precancerous conditions and lesions of the stomach. Philadelphia, Praeger, in press.

Morson, B. C., Sobin, L. H., Grundmann, E., Johansen, A., Nagayo, T., Serck-Hassen, A.: Precancerous conditions and epithelial dysplasia in the stomach. J. Clin. Pathol. 33:711–721, 1980.

Nagayo, T.: Dysplasia of the gastric mucosa and its relation to the precancerous process. Gann 72:813–823, 1981.

Nardelli, J., Bara, J., Rosa, B., Burtin, P.: Intestinal metaplasia and carcinomas of the human stomach: an immunohistological study. J. Histochem. Cytochem. 31:366–375, 1983.

Nomura, A. M. Y., Stemmermann, G. N., Samhoff, I. M.: Serum pepsinogen I as a predictor of stomach cancer. Ann. Int. Med. 93:537–540, 1980.

Oehlert, W., Keller, P., Henke, M., Strauch, M.: Die Dysplasien der Magenschleimhaut. Dtsch. Med. Wochenschr. 100:1950–1956, 1975.

Schmidt, A.: Untersuchungen uber des mensliche Magenepithel unter normalen und pathologischen Werhaltnissen. Virch. Arch. [Pathol. Anat.] 143:477–508, 1896.

Sipponen, P., Seppala, K., Varis, K., Hjelt, L., Ihamaki, T., Kekki, M., Siurala, M.: Intestinal metaplasia with colonic type sulfomucins; its association with gastric carcinoma. Acta Pathol. Microbiol. Scand. 88:217–224, 1981.

Stemmermann, G. N., Samhoff, I. M., Nomura, A., Walsh, J. H.: Serum pepsinogen I and gastrin in relation to extent and location of intestinal metaplasia in surgically resected stomach. Dig. Dis. Sci., 25:680–687, 1980.

Strickland, R. C. and Mackay, I. R.: A reappraisal of the nature and significance of chronic atrophic gastritis. Dig. Dis. 18:426–440, 1973.

Sugano, H., Kyoichi, N., Takagi, K.: An atypical epithelium of the stomach. A clinico-pathological entity. Gann Monogr. Cancer Res. 11:257–269, 1972.

Sugimura, T., Matsukura, N., Sato, S.: Intestinal metaplasia of the stomach as precancerous stage. In Armstrong, B. and Bartsch H. (eds.): Host factors in human carcinogenesis. Lyon, France, International Agency for Research on Cancer, Scientific Publication No. 39, 1982, pp. 515–530.

Teglbjaerg, S. and Nielsen, H. O.: Small intestinal type and colonic type intestinal metaplasia of the human stomach. Acta Pathol. Microbiol. Scand. 86:351–355, 1978.

KATHERINE DeSCHRYVER-KECSKEMETI

7 Small Intestine

Fiberoptic endoscopy, which allows visualization of the earliest phases of many lesions in the gastrointestinal tract, has become increasingly available for patients with non-specific or mild symptoms. Consequently, very small lesions, incidental findings, and sequential biopsies now abound in surgical pathology, allowing the pathologist to reconstruct the evolution of many of these lesions. Because clinical data indicate that success in patient management depends to a large extent on early diagnosis, recognition of precancerous lesions has assumed major importance. These precursor lesions, however, as well as the incipient malignant lesions, are often the most difficult ones to evaluate because the pathologist needs to be precise in his diagnosis and yet conservative for the patient's benefit.

In the small intestine, precancerous lesions can be divided into two categories. The first category includes those lesions that are definite precursors of malignancy in that transformation of the cells and subsequent invasion are likely. This information has become available through careful clinicopathologic correlations and follow-up studies. In some of these lesions, histologic examination shows all the cytologic and architectural hallmarks associated with malignancy. However, in the small intestine, as in many other sites, morphologically innocuous-appearing lesions are known to have the capacity for invasiveness in certain clinical settings. Examination of the actual lesion, knowledge about the clinical setting, and familiarity with the precursor changes should allow correct identification by the pathologist in nearly all cases.

The second category of precursor lesions is very different in that some generalized condition predisposes to the malignancy through mechanisms that are as yet unidentified but that possibly include altered immune surveillance or runaway immune response. In such cases, there is no known precursor lesion that develops at the site of the malignancy.

Unfortunately, no attempt can be made within the scope of this chapter to illustrate the full range of precursor lesions found in the small intestine. Instead, we propose to illustrate some lesions that were discovered incidentally on routine radiologic or endoscopic examinations or that were sampled during routine cancer surveillance protocols in our institution, and that represent precursor lesions (incipient or early malignancies). Other cases described in the figure legends presented diagnostic problems because of an incomplete clinical history or unusual appearance of the lesion. We will present criteria for the diagnosis, clinicopathologic correlation, and differentiation of histologic look-alikes for some precancerous lesions occurring in the small intestine. In general, we advocate a conservative approach in providing suggestions to the clinician for treatment and follow-up.

PRECURSORS TO EPITHELIAL LESIONS OF THE SMALL INTESTINE

Adenomas

Adenomas most commonly occur in the large intestine. Recently, however, they have also been reported in the duodenum, probably owing to the increased use of endoscopy (Cooperman, 1978; Dickersin, 1984; Komorowski, 1981; Perzin and Bridge, 1981). Interestingly, adenomas in the small bowel tend to be papillary more often than those in the colon (Perzin and Bridge, 1981), a finding that is attributed to the pre-existing villous architecture used by the proliferating cells. Although villous adenomas may occur in all divisions of the duodenum, they show a predilection for the first and second parts, including the area of the ampulla of Vater (Sobol and Cooperman, 1978). They may be an isolated finding (Fig. 7–1) or may be associated with familial colonic polyposis or Gardner's syndrome. The sporadic form may be solitary or multiple. These neoplasms are in all likelihood premalignant lesions. Of 130 apparently primary small bowel carcinomas in one series, 25 percent histologically demonstrated adenomatous epithelium in the same lesion (Perzin and Bridge, 1981). The benign phase consists of a long period of slow growth without any clinical symptoms. Tumors in this phase

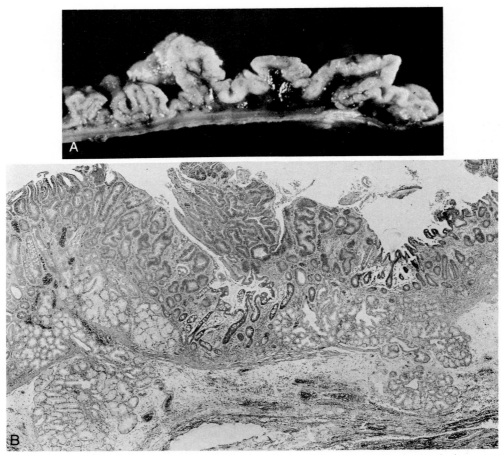

Figure 7–1. This 59-year-old asymptomatic white male was followed for duodenal ulcer disease. The duodenal adenoma was an incidental finding on upper gastrointestinal series. The lesion was not reached on endoscopic examination and was subsequently resected. Grossly (A), the lesion was sessile and polypoid, measuring 5.5 × 3. 5 × 0.5 cm. By microscopy (B), the superficial portions of the mucosa had multifocal villous projections with preservation of the architecture in the basal portions of the mucosa. There was nuclear pseudostratification, epithelial crowding, and cytologic atypia. The tumor had not involved the entire thickness of the mucosa and was completely excised. The patient is well 3½ years later.

are often found incidentally during surgical exploration for some other problem. Their detection is difficult even under these circumstances because they are very soft in consistency and often cannot be felt when the bowel is routinely palpated during abdominal surgery. Not surprisingly, in the clinical series that report small bowel neoplasms in general, malignant tumors predominate because they are symptomatic. This is especially true for the ampullary lesions. The larger the lesion, the more likely that carcinoma will be identified. Carcinomatous changes in villous adenomas tend to be deep and focal, features that often make their recognition by endoscopy or open biopsy unreliable.

Endoscopic biopsies of small bowel that show adenomatous features are labeled simply "villous lesions" in our institution, implying that the nature of the lesion cannot be reliably determined at that time.

Such lesions need to be resected transsubmucosally and blocked in toto to rule out invasive tumor (Perzin and Bridge, 1981). If no invasive carcinoma is present in the specimen, the diagnostic procedure is considered curative. If invasive carcinoma is found, the patient will need to be re-explored and treated with more radical surgical procedures. Frozen-section diagnosis of these tumors is not recommended because the well-known pitfalls of the technique used in this clinical setting may lead to unnecessary surgery.

Cancer surveillance protocols of patients with Gardner's syndrome ordinarily do not include special emphasis on the periampullary region. Villous adenomas in these patients with or without an invasive component do have a predilection for that region, and patients therefore need lifelong surveillance (Fig. 7–2) (Bussey et al., 1978; Iida et al., 1981; Kozuka et al., 1981; Pauli et al., 1980). These patients not uncommonly present with unexplained abnormal liver function tests. They do not necessarily have polyps elsewhere in the small intestine (Scully et al., 1978; Scully et al., 1982); therefore, a high index of suspicion is necessary for early detection.

When dealing with a villous "tumor" of the small intestine, one needs to keep in mind the rare villous hypertrophy that is secondary to a glucagon-producing tumor, which is completely reversible by treatment of the primary condition (Jones et al., 1983). The diagnosis may be suspected on the basis of the more

diffuse involvement seen on barium studies and the identification of the associated dermatologic manifestations, including necrotizing migratory erythema and a persistent maculopapular rash.

Other Polyps

Other epithelial lesions occurring in the small intestine are associated with the Peutz-Jeghers syndrome, which is inherited as an autosomal dominant charac-

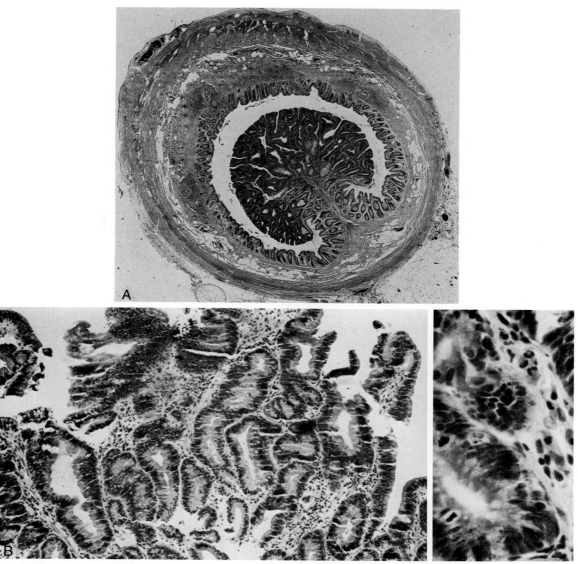

Figure 7–2. The patient is a 37-year-old man who presented one year ago with a family history of colonic polyps and carcinoma. Endoscopy revealed multiple colonic polyps; the possibility of a diagnosis of Gardner's syndrome was entertained. Total colectomy was recommended, and 18 polyps were found in the specimen, one of which had a deeply invasive (Dukes' B) adenocarcinoma. *A*, photomicrograph of a tubular adenoma that was in the appendix. A bulky tumor mass was also resected separately from the mesentery a few months later and was diagnosed as fibromatosis (not shown). As this constellation of lesions is pathognomonic for Gardner's syndrome, the patient has now been under surveillance for the area of the duodenum with special attention to the ampulla. *B*, photomicrograph of the ampullary biopsy with a proliferative epithelial lesion.

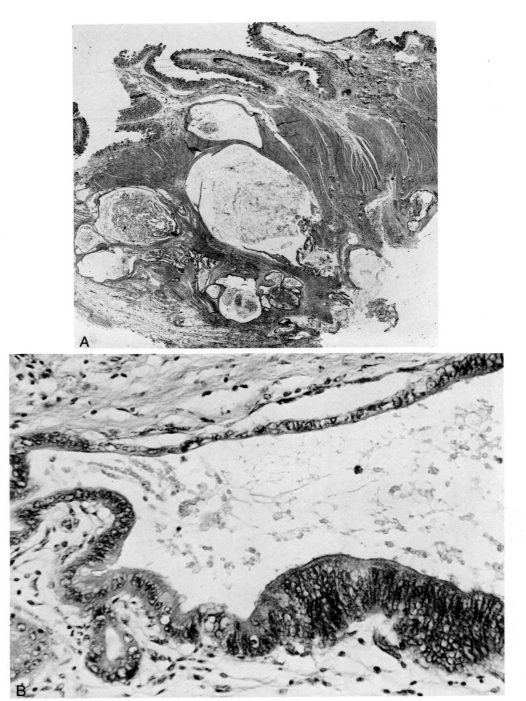

Figure 7–3. A 48-year-old white man had emergency surgery for clinical small-bowel obstruction. He had a recent 40-pound weight loss. At laparotomy, multiple foci of soft gelatinous material were seen on the serosa and adjacent mesentery, and a matted, fibrotic, tumor-like mass was found in the terminal ileum. Multiple frozen sections of the serosal implants showed acellular myxoid material. Although not known at the time of frozen section, the patient had a history of Peutz-Jeghers polyps. A section of the ileum shows benign glands and mucinous cysts throughout the full thickness of the wall, so-called enteritic cystica profunda *(A)*. At higher power *(B)*, some of the glands are lined by a somewhat atypical epithelium. Some cystic spaces are also lined by foamy histiocytes and giant cells. Two-year follow-up on this patient disclosed no malignancy. (Courtesy of Dr. M. Kyriakos, Department of Pathology, Washington University Medical School, St. Louis, MO.)

ter. The hamartomatous polypoid lesions may occur anywhere in the gastrointestinal tract but more often occur in the distal small intestine. The overall incidence of malignancy in this syndrome has been overestimated, according to Kyriakos and Condon (1978), owing to the presence of scattered well-formed glands throughout all layers of bowel wall (Fig. 7–3). Nevertheless, there are documented cases of small bowel malignancy occurring in this syndrome (Bussey et al., 1978). Whether the malignancy arises from normal mucosa, hamartomatous polyp, or associated adenomatous polyps has not been resolved. Epithelial atypia as the precursor to the invasive lesion in the hamartomatous polyp has been suggested (Matuchansky et al., 1979). The status of the precursor lesion in this entity needs further evaluation. Patients with these lesions should be carefully followed.

There is an increase of adenocarcinoma of the small bowel in longstanding gluten-sensitive enteropathy (Swinson et al., 1983). It is not known whether a morphologically recognizable precursor lesion is present in those cases.

Adenocarcinoma of Small Bowel Complicating Crohn's Disease

Patients with longstanding Crohn's disease of the small bowel are also considered at high risk for developing carcinoma (Fresko et al., 1982; Perzin et al., 1984; Radi et al., 1984; Riddell et al., 1983; Shamsuddin and Phillips, 1981; Warren and Barwick, 1983). The mucosa can undergo dysplastic changes that are similar to those described for ulcerative colitis. Surveillance endoscopy in patients with mucosal dysplasia is more difficult and often impossible if strictures or fistulas are present. The latter are areas of predilection for carcinomas (Fig. 7–4). Because of technical factors, terminal ileal biopsies may be obtained at colonoscopy in only a small proportion of patients. Carcinomas arising in patients with regional enteritis

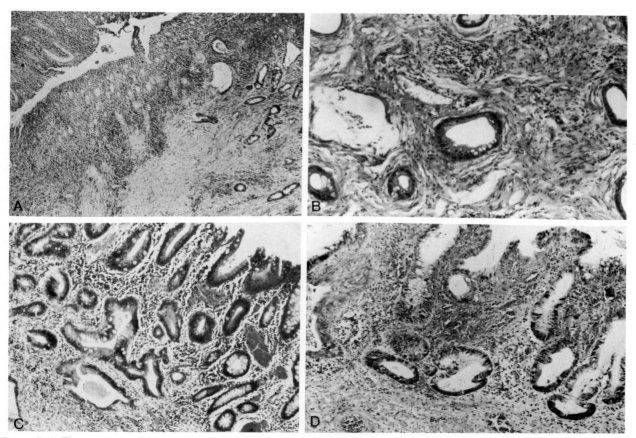

Figure 7–4. The patient is a 36-year-old male with a 13-year history of ulcerative colitis which involved the entire colon and the distal ileum. A recent surveillance biopsy of the sigmoid colon revealed severe dysplasia diagnosed at an outside hospital. Total colectomy was done at our institution. The specimen showed all the gross features typical of long-standing Crohn's disease, including marked thickening of the colon wall and numerous internal fistulas. One of the fistula tracts contained an adenocarcinoma *(A,B)*. The widespread epithelial changes in non-tumoral areas consisted of all degrees of dysplasia, with the same features as described in ulcerative colitis *(C,D)*.

have a predilection for the ileum (76 percent) and occur in the inflamed segments of bowel, with a distribution distinctly different from that of primary small bowel carcinomas in general (Perzin et al., 1984). In many cases, the tumor is not recognizable clinically or even at surgery because it mimics the gross appearance of regional enteritis. Tumors, sometimes multiple, are discovered only when sections are examined microscopically. There are no differences in the incidence of carcinoma in the first, second, and third decades after the onset of symptoms of Crohn's disease. In one third of the patients, the cancer develops in the bypassed segments of bowel (Fresko et al., 1982; Warren and Barwick, 1983). There is a relationship between long-term corticoid therapy and the development of carcinomas in Crohn's disease, the pathogenesis of which is not understood. Immunosuppression has been suggested as a possible mechanism (Valdes-Dapena et al., 1976). Finally, the extent of resection may be difficult to determine, given the multifocal nature of the disease. (See also the discussion of precancerous changes in ulcerative colitis, Chapter 8.)

PRECURSOR LESIONS TO LYMPHOMA

Immunoproliferative Small Intestinal Disease

The term "immunoproliferative small intestinal disease" encompasses a benign phase, followed by a malignant phase (often designated as Mediterranean lymphoma) that includes a spectrum of disorders commonly manifested by diarrhea, weight loss, abdominal pain, and clubbing of the fingers and toes (Khojasteh et al., 1983). Although this disease was initially considered a "Third-World Lesion," recent reports suggest the occurrence of an identical entity in North American children with long-standing immunodeficiency (Neudorf et al., 1983) and in Mexican-American patients (Gray et al., 1982). Because the malignant stage of the disease is believed to be preceded by a long, apparently benign disorder and because a common clonal origin for the lymphoplasmacytic proliferation and the immunoblastic lymphoma has been shown in some cases (Brouet et al., 1977; Ramot et al., 1977), it seems likely that there is an early dysplastic stage in which correct diagnosis is very important, since the disease is potentially curable (Galian et al. 1977). Morphologically, the small intestinal mucosa shows some loss of polarity of the surface enterocytes, transepithelial migration of lymphocytes, and heavy infiltration of the lamina propria with mature plasma cells. The infiltrating cells are thought to be responsible for production of the α-heavy-chain immunoglobulin and formation of a matrix for the evolution of the primary lymphoma (see comment later). Based on a recent study of 22

cases of immunoproliferative small intestinal/α-heavy-chain disease, it was concluded that failure of light chain production is not a constant finding in the disease, that some cases may be associated with secretion of complete IgA molecules, and that other cases represent nonsecretory forms of the disease (Asselah et al., 1983). Moreover, intestinal lymphomas in the Middle East often have a heterogeneous histologic appearance. Although inability to identify a paraprotein in a patient occasionally is due to failure of the techniques that are being used, other causes may be involved (Isaacson, 1979b). Indeed, various studies suggest that this disease is more complex than previously thought and that not all cases of Mediterranean lymphomas are associated with the presence in the serum or duodenal juice of abnormal α heavy chains (Isaacson et al., 1983). The concept of a malignant tumor arising from an abnormal clone of plasma cells that produce α heavy chains or give rise to the "dedifferentiated" immunoblastic type lymphoma has been prevalent. However, another hypothesis suggests that Mediterranean lymphoma should be regarded as a tumor of follicular center cells, which are still receptive to antigenic stimulus. The result is massive plasmacytosis of the intestinal lamina propria in the early stages of disease (Isaacson et al., 1983).

Traditionally, however, a distinction has always been made between the so-called Mediterranean diffuse lymphoma, or malignant stage of immunoproliferative small bowel disease (which is characterized by a proliferation of the small intestine–associated B-lymphoid system and involves the whole length of the small intestine without intervening areas of normal mucosa), and the polypoid, localized Western variety of lymphoma (which has the discrete lesions with intervening non-lymphomatous areas of small bowel) (Gray et al., 1982). In the so-called Mediterranean lymphomas, the atypical plasma cell infiltrates contain an α-chain alone, a light chain alone, or a γ-chain alone, whereas the intervening islands of Ig and J chain–negative lymphoepithelial cells represent tumor. In the Western variety of lymphoma, tumor cells usually contain cytoplasmic Ig of a single light chain class (κ or λ), usually associated with μ and J chains (Isaacson et al., 1983). However, it has been reported that the typical Western variety of intestinal lymphoma can also present with α-heavy-chain disease (Cohen et al., 1978). We have followed two patients who are probably examples of this newly recognized "intermediate type" (Figs. 7–5 and 7–6). In view of these findings and of recent reports of a localized form of colonic lymphoma presenting as α-chain disease (Cho et al., 1982), it is possible that all the foregoing entities represent a group of diseases with the same underlying pathogenic mechanisms, a variable phenotypic expression, and an identifiable precursor stage (Gray et al., 1982; Khojasteh et al., 1983).

In conclusion, careful morphologic and immuno-

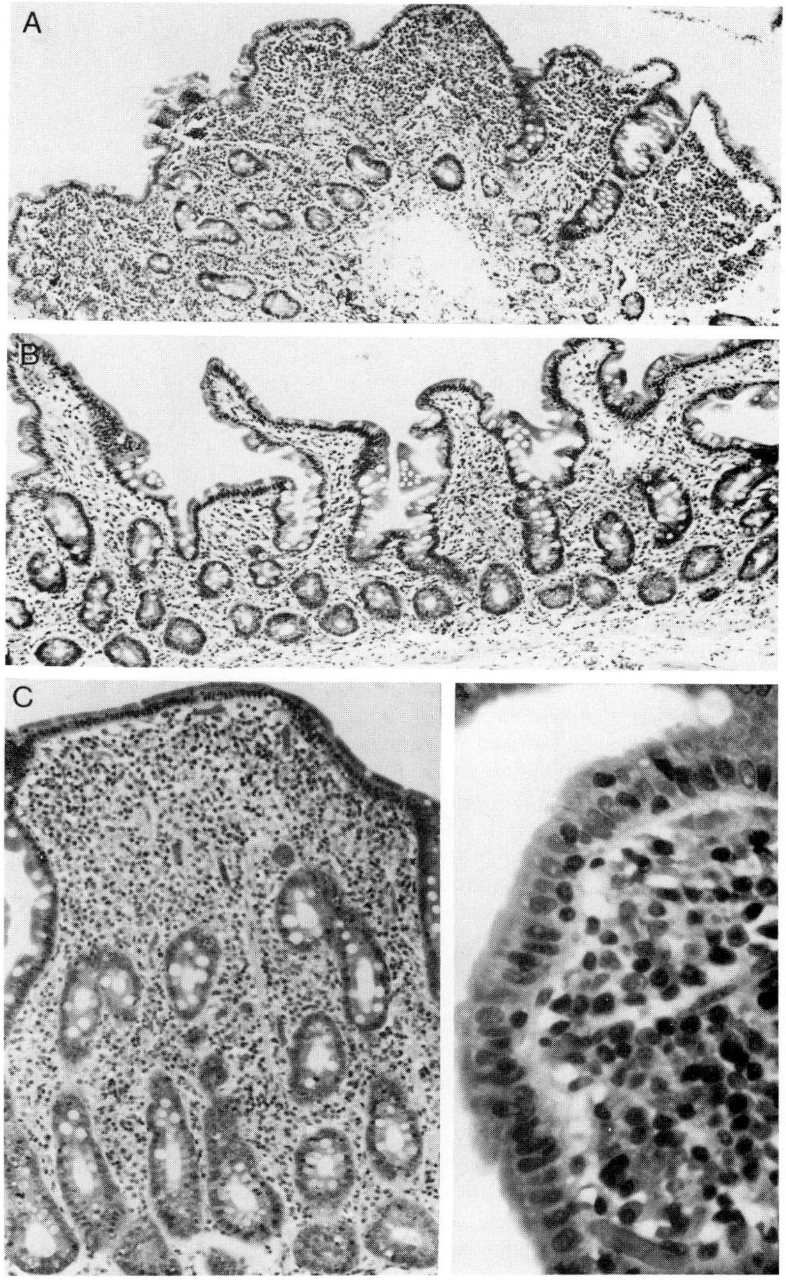

Figure 7–5. The patient is a 75-year-old white female who presented with weight loss, diarrhea, and malabsorption 12 years previously. A small-bowel biopsy at that time *(A)* was read as partial villous atrophy with an atypical plasma cell infiltrate. Following this diagnosis, a hematologic work-up disclosed an IgA paraprotein in the patient's serum. After two courses of melphalan and prednisone, followed by complete clinical improvement, the patient was rebiopsied 4 months later *(B)*. The patient was followed with successive small-bowel biopsies over the years and showed waxing and waning villous atrophy, synchronous atypical plasma cell infiltrates, and clinical symptomatology. The superficial portions of the lamina propria contained only mature plasma cells. The overlying epithelium is lined by columnar and well-differentiated enterocytes. *C,* An episode of relapse 2 years after diagnosis. Six years after the first biopsy, the patient had an exploratory laparotomy for a perforated diverticulum of the sigmoid and had no small-intestinal lesions. She was subsequently lost to follow-up. The patient has not lived or traveled outside the St. Louis area and had no known predisposing condition.

histochemical analyses of cases of Mediterranean lymphoma have demonstrated histologic features that are identical with those of the Western-type follicular center cell lymphomas (Isaacson, personal communication). Thus, an invasive tumor of follicular center cell origin producing the classic lymphoepithelial lesions may evolve from a diffuse, non-invasive, plasmacytic mucosal infiltrate. Although restriction to the small intestine and production of an abnormal α heavy chain may be distinctive, Mediterranean lymphoma appears to be similar in many respects to Western gastrointestinal lymphomas.

Gluten-Sensitive Enteropathy

Gluten-sensitive enteropathy is regularly included with the precancerous conditions of the small intestine (Thompson, 1983). Gluten-sensitive enteropathy, also called non-tropical sprue, mainly involves the proximal small intestine and may have its onset either

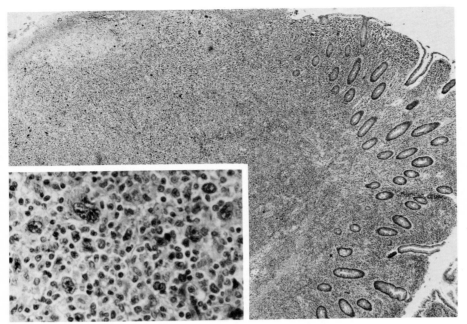

Figure 7–6. A 40-year-old white female with a history of malabsorption, diarrhea, and serum alpha-chains who was followed for 5 years. Small-bowel biopsies at yearly intervals disclosed an atypical lymphoplasmacytic infiltrate with proportional villous changes and preservation of surface enterocytes. The patient then developed splenomegaly and on barium follow-through studies was found to have a jejunal lesion which was ulcerated. It measured 3 cm in length and 7 cm in circumference. The lesion was resected. The histology showed localized lymphomatous involvement of the bowel and one mesenteric lymph node, whereas other nodes, the spleen, and liver were not involved. Pleomorphic, Reed-Sternberg–like cells were numerous, consistent with an immunoblastic lymphoma. The surrounding mucosa showed no atypical lymphoplasmacytic infiltrates.

during early childhood or in later life. Gluten, the protein moiety of wheat, barley, rye, and other cereals, is thought to bind to a receptor on the surface of small bowel epithelial cells and to sensitize the immunocytes located in the mucosa, resulting in damage to the epithelial cells (Trier et al., 1978). This gluten receptor appears to be genetically determined, because 88 percent of patients have the histocompatibility antigen HLA-B8. Histocompatibility genes also code for certain cell surface configurations, which may also function as receptors, capable of serving in these cases as a receptor for gluten. The mechanism of this gluten toxicity is not known, but altered cellular immunity is involved in which the presence of T cells seems to be essential (Katz and Falchuk, 1978). The pathogenesis of the intestinal changes found in dermatitis herpetiformis is not understood either, but both the morphology and the clinical characteristics are similar to those of gluten-sensitive enteropathy (Brow et al., 1971). The incidence of malignant disease, including carcinoma and lymphoma, is greater in adults with unequivocally documented celiac sprue/dermatitis herpetiformis than in the general population (Swinson et al, 1983). The frequency with which lymphoma develops in these patients is not known but appears to be low (Trier et al., 1978). A true histiocytic derivation has been suggested for these lymphomas (Isaacson and Wright, 1978; Isaacson and Wright, 1980) (see also discussion of malignant histiocytosis). A gluten-free diet does not appear to prevent malignancy. Reduced cytotoxicity against tumor cells in vitro may be relevant to the risk of malignancy in these patients in the sense of an altered immune response, with possibly no precursor lesion per se (McClaurin et al., 1971). One must remember that the loss of the normal villous architecture of the mucosa with variable flattening is a characteristic but non-specific response of the small intestine to many forms of mucosal injury, and, consequently, "all that flattens is not sprue" (Katz and Grand, 1979). Many of the clinically and morphologically atypical cases of sprue, which in our experience are quite numerous, may represent early phases of other diseases.

Microscopic Differentiation

The feature most helpful in the differentiation of all the foregoing conditions is the appearance of the surface enterocyte. There is little alteration of the columnar surface cells and only partial villous atrophy in the prelymphoma–lymphoma spectrum of diseases, changes that are proportional to the extent of the lymphoplasmacytic infiltrates in the lamina propria (Fig. 7–7). Conversely, the epithelial and villous changes that occur in sprue/dermatitis herpetiformis are greatly out of proportion with the extent of the plasma cell infiltrate. In addition, biopsies handled routinely (fixed in formalin and imbedded in paraffin) can be stained with monospecific rabbit antiserum to α, γ, μ, κ, and λ chains. The identifiable immunoglobulin component in α-heavy-chain disease has only abnormal α heavy chains; it contains no other heavy chains and no κ or λ light chains. It is found in only 25 to 50 percent of α-chain disease patients in whom serum is examined. Testing serum, urine, and jejunal secretions may improve yield. Testing for its local production may be a more sensitive method (Pangalis and Rappaport, 1977) and would also identify "nonsecretory" forms (Rambaud et al., 1980). Abnormally high-titer anti–α-chain serum is needed to stain the plasma cells of the atypical infiltrate, probably a reflection of molecular abnormality in the elaborated product (Isaacson, 1979b). We recommend serial biopsies in patients with "atypical" lymphoplasmacytic infiltrates—that is, a stromal component out of proportion to the epithelial lesion—with determination of tissue immunologic markers. Use of the J chain as a marker for B cell malignancy will indicate the site at which morphologically atypical cells have actually undergone malignant transformation (Isaacson, 1979a). Karyotyping of the atypical lymphoplasmacytic infiltrate in the mucosa also has been successfully carried out in some cases to ascertain whether the cells were benign or premalignant (Nassar and Khouri, 1974).

Immune-Related Disorders

Primary malignant lymphoma of the small intestine occurs in association with a spectrum of immune-related disorders, such as primary immunodeficiency syndromes and autoimmune disorders, as well as in patients receiving immunosuppressive therapy. We followed a 57-year-old man with hypogammaglobulinemia and diarrhea for 3 years. His initial small bowel biopsy was unremarkable (Fig. 7–8). However, a biopsy obtained 1 year later showed an atypical lymphoid infiltrate. The differential diagnosis, which was between lymphoma and pseudolymphoma, was never resolved. Two years later, the patient demonstrated an unquestionable lymphomatous infiltrate in a biopsy specimen obtained from the small bowel. Cell surface markers identified a B cell neoplasm that elaborated IgM, κ chain only. His acquired immunodeficiency was originally thought to have been a predisposing factor to his malignancy. Rather it is probably an example of a long prelymphomatous stage.

Nodular Lymphoid Hyperplasia

Nodular lymphoid hyperplasia of the small intestine is a condition observed in patients with primary immu-

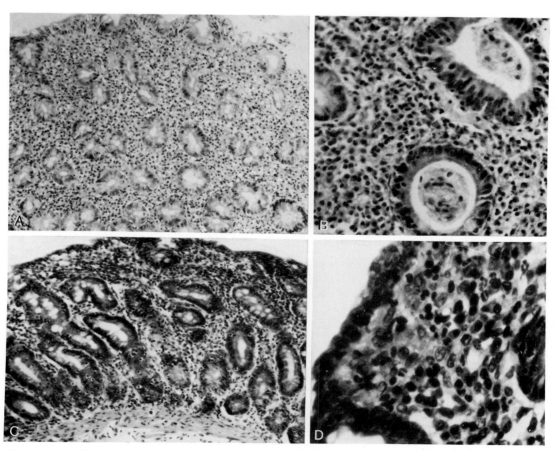

Figure 7–7. A and B, A 53-year-old Jordanian male with symptoms of weight loss and abdominal distention for 6 months. A duodenal biopsy was done in Kuwait on the Arabian Peninsula and was sent for consultation. There is loss of villous architecture but no flattening or loss of polarity of the surface enterocytes. Interepithelial lymphocytes are numerous, and the lamina propria contains a lymphoplasmacytic infiltrate. For comparison, C and D show the small-bowel biopsy in a case of gluten-sensitive enteropathy. The surface enterocyte shows flattening and loss of polarity. The other features of the biopsy are similar to those seen in A and B.

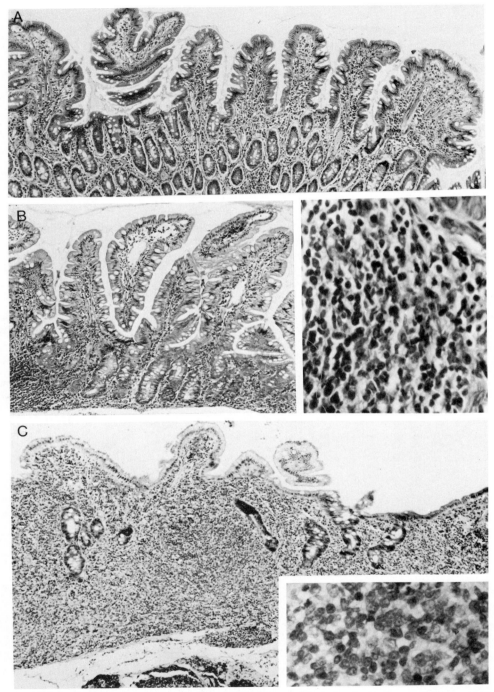

Figure 7–8. At the time of initial work-up the patient, a 57-year-old white man, had chronic diarrhea, weight loss, and hypogammaglobulinemia. A small-bowel biopsy showed minimal non-specific inflammatory changes *(A)*. A year later, a small-bowel series showed abnormal segmentation. A biopsy showed an atypical lymphoid infiltrate in band *(B)*. It was not until 2 years later that a monomorphous frank lymphomatous infiltrate was unequivocally identified *(C)*. Tumor cells expressed IgM kappa.

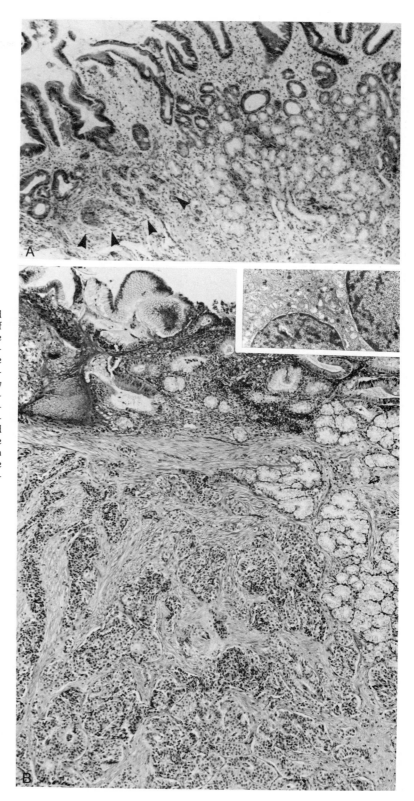

Figure 7–9. A 42-year-old black female who had an upper gastrointestinal barium study because of abdominal pain. A sessile polyp was seen in the duodenal bulb. On endoscopic examination, a 1-cm pinkish-red sessile polyp was visualized in the mid-duodenal bulb, with the intact overlying mucosa having a smooth glistening appearance. *A,* By light microscopy, minute nests of tumor were identified, and the appearance suggested a neuroendocrine neoplasm *(arrows)*. *B,* Subsequent resection of the first portion of the duodenum disclosed extensive transmural involvement by tumor. The patient is alive and well 8 years later. *Inset,* An electron micrograph showing neurosecretory-type cytoplasmic granules in tumor cell cytoplasm (uranyl acetate and lead citrate, × 46,000).

nodeficiency syndromes (Webster et al., 1977). Its histologic features include large lymphoid follicles with well-defined mantles and active germinal centers. The differential diagnosis includes a multicentric nodular malignant lymphoma and the atypical lymphoid hyperplasias often seen in the immediate vicinity of some malignant lymphomas (Matuchansky et al., 1980, 1985). In other cases, it is a variant of immunoproliferative small bowel disease and is associated with a diffuse undifferentiated lymphoma with a "starry-sky" pattern (Nassar et al., 1978). Identification of a monoclonal proliferation of κ or λ chains within the infiltrate will be instrumental in the diagnosis.

Malignant Histiocytosis

Malignant histiocytosis primarily affecting the intestine has been recognized as the malignant condition that most often complicates long-standing gluten-sensitive enteropathy (Isaacson and Wright, 1978; Isaacson and Wright, 1980). The presence of α_1-antitrypsin in the malignant cells is a reliable marker of this condition. The true incidence of malignant histiocytosis of the intestine is not known. According to Isaacson and colleagues, it is far more common than diagnosed cases would lead one to believe owing to the lack of a general awareness of this entity. Tumors of histiocytic nature evolving in association with long-standing immunologic disturbances have long been suspected to occur and have important theoretical implications in tumor biology. According to the same authors, ulcerative jejunoileitis is probably part of the same disease entity. There is often considerable difficulty in establishing a diagnosis of malignancy in this entity. Usually, many sections are needed. The infiltrate not uncommonly has a deceptively benign and polymorphous appearance.

ENDOCRINE TUMORS

Endocrine tumors of the proximal duodenum are usually not incipient neoplasms. They are mentioned because they often present diagnostic difficulties when incidentally sampled on routine endoscopy. Small polypoid or nodular lesions, which are not infrequently found in the first part of the duodenum, usually represent focal epithelial or lymphoid hyperplasia, often related to a long-standing nonspecific inflammatory disease. However, we have seen seven cases in which the polypoid lesion proved at biopsy to be endocrine (carcinoid-like) in nature (Deschryver-Kecskemeti et al., 1984). Such a diagnosis is rarely anticipated by the radiologist or endoscopist. Careful review of endoscopic biopsies and awareness of this entity will help one identify the lesion, despite the small fragments of tumor present in the biopsy (Fig.

7–9). In all our cases in which resection specimens were subsequently available, residual tumor was present in the bowel wall. The prognosis associated with these tumors is good. Complications related to bleeding from the tumor site or to gastrin secretion may cause significant morbidity. The differential diagnosis includes carcinoma and end-stage inflammatory conditions.

References

Asselah, F., Slavin, G., Sowter, G., Asselah, H.: Immunoproliferative small intestinal disease in Algerians. Cancer 52:227, 1983.
Brouet, J. C., Mason, D. Y., Danon, F., Preud'homme, J. L., Seligmann, M., Reyes, F., Navab, F., Galian, A., Rene, E., Rambaud, J. C.: Alpha-chain disease: evidence for common clonal origin of intestinal immunoblastic lymphoma and plasmacytic proliferation. Lancet 1:861, 1977.
Brow, J. R., Parker, F., Weinstein, W. M., et al.: The small intestinal mucosa in dermatitis herpetiformis severity and distribution of the small intestinal lesion and associated malabsorption. Gastroenterology 60:355, 1971.
Bussey, H. J. R., Veale, A. M. O., Morson, B. C.: Genetics of gastrointestinal polyposis. Gastroenterology 74:1325, 1978.
Cho, C., Linscheer, W. G., Bell, R., Smith, R.: Colonic lymphoma producing alpha-chain disease protein. Gastroenterology 83:121, 1982.
Cohen, H. J., Gonzalvo, A., Krook, J., Thompson, T. T., Kremer, W. B.: New presentation of alpha heavy chain disease: North American polypoid gastrointestinal lymphoma. Cancer 41:1161, 1978.
Cooperman, M., Clausen, K. P., Hecht, C., Lucas, J. G., Keith, L. M.: Villous adenomas of the duodenum. Gastroenterology 74:1295, 1978.
DeSchryver-Kecskemeti, K., Clouse, R. E., Kraus, F. T.: Surgical pathology of gastric and duodenal neuroendocrine tumors masquerading clinically as common polyps. Semin. Diag. Pathol. 1:5, 1984.
Dickersin, G. R.: Case Records of the Massachusetts General Hospital (Case 30–1984). N. Engl. J. Med. 311:244, 1984.
Fresko, D., Lazarus, S. S., Dotan, J., Reingold, M.: Early presentation of carcinoma of the small bowel in Crohn's disease (Crohn's carcinoma). Gastroenterology 82:783, 1982.
Galian, A., Lecestre, M.-J., Scotto, J., Bognel, C., Matuchansky, C., Rambaud, J.-C.: Pathological study of alpha-chain disease, with special emphasis on evolution. Cancer 39:2081, 1977.
Gray, G. M., Rosenberg, S. A., Cooper, A. D., Gregory, P. B., Stein, D. T., Herzenberg, H.: Lymphomas involving the gastrointestinal tract. Gastroenterology 82:143, 1982.
Iida, M., Yao, T., Itoh, H., Ohsato, K., Watanabe, H.: Endoscopic features of adenoma of the duodenal papilla in familial polyposis of the colon. Gastrointest. Endosc. 27:6, 1981.
Isaacson, P. Personal communication.
Isaacson, P.: Immunochemical demonstration of J chain: a marker of B-cell malignancy. J. Clin. Pathol. 32:802, 1979a.
Isaacson, P.: Middle East lymphoma and α-chain disease. Am. J. Surg. Pathol. 3:431, 1979b.
Isaacson, P., Al-Dewachi, H. S., Mason, D. Y.: Middle Eastern intestinal lymphoma. J. Clin. Pathol. 36:489, 1983.
Isaacson, P., and Wright, D. H.: Malignant histiocytosis of the intestine. Its relationship to malabsorption and ulcerative jejunitis. Hum. Pathol. 9:661, 1978.
Isaacson, P., and Wright, D. H.: Case 15–1980: celiac disease and intestinal lymphoma. Letter to the editor. N. Engl. J. Med. 303:583, 1980.
Jones, B., Fishman, E. K., Bayless, T. M., Siegelman, S. S.: Villous hypertrophy of the small bowel in a patient with glucagonoma. J. Comput. Assist. Tomogr. 7:334, 1983.

Katz, A. J., and Falchuk, Z. M.: Definitive diagnosis of gluten-sensitive enteropathy. Use of an in vitro organ culture model. Gastroenterology 75:695, 1978.

Katz, A. J., and Grand, R. J.: All that flattens is not "sprue." Gastroenterology 76:375, 1979.

Khojasteh, A., Haghshenass, M., Haghighi, P.: Immunoproliferative small intestinal disease. A "third-world lesion". N. Engl. J. Med. 308:1401, 1983.

Komorowski, R. A., and Cohen, E. B.: Villous tumors of the duodenum. Cancer 47:1377, 1981.

Kozuka, S., Tsubone, M., Yamaguchi, A., Hachisuka, K.: Adenomatous residue in cancerous papilla of Vater. Gut 22:1031, 1981.

Kyriakos, M., and Condon, S. C.: Enteritis cystica profunda. Am. J. Clin. Pathol. 69:77, 1978.

Matuchansky, C., Babin, P., Coutrot, S., Druart, F., Barbier, J., Maire, P.: Peutz-Jeghers syndrome with metastasizing carcinoma arising from a jejunal hamartoma. Gastroenterology 77:1311, 1979.

Matuchansky, C., Morichau-Beauchant, M., Touchard, G., Lenormand, Y., Bloch, P., Tanzer, J., Alcalay, D., Babin, P.: Nodular lymphoid hyperplasia of the small bowel associated with primary jejunal malignant lymphoma. Gastroenterology 78:1587, 1980.

Matuchansky, C., Touchard, G., Lemaire, M., Babin, P., Demeoco, F., Fonck, Y., Meyer, M., Preud'homme, J.-L.: Malignant lymphoma of the small bowel associated with diffuse nodular lymphoid hyperplasia. N. Engl. J. Med. 313:166, 1985.

McClaurin, B. P., Cooke, W. T., Ling, W. R.: Impaired lymphocyte reactivity against tumour cells in patients with coeliac disease. Gut 12:794, 1971.

Nassar, V. H., and Khouri, F. P.: Malignant lymphomas. Tissue karyotyping in doubtful cases. Arch. Pathol. 98:367, 1974.

Nassar, V. H., Salem, P. A., Shahid, M. J., Alami, S. Y., Balikian, J. B., Salem, A. A., Nasrallah, S. M.: "Mediterranean abdominal lymphoma" or immunoproliferative small intestinal disease. Cancer 41:1340, 1978.

Neudorf, S., Snover, D., Filipovich, A.: Immunoproliferative small intestinal disease. N. Engl. J. Med. 309:1126, 1983.

Pangalis, G. A., and Rappaport, H.: Common clonal origin of lymphoplasmacytic proliferation and immunoblastic lymphoma in intestinal α-chain disease. Lancet 2:880, 1977.

Pauli, R. M., Pauli, M. E., Hall, J. G.: Gardner syndrome and periampullary malignancy. Am. J. Med. Genet. 6:205, 1980.

Perzin, K. H., and Bridge, M. F.: Adenomas of the small intestine: A clinicopathologic review of 51 cases and a study of their relationship to carcinoma. Cancer 48:799, 1981.

Perzin, K. H., Peterson, M., Castiglione, C. L., Fenoglio, C. M.,

Wolff, M.: Intramucosal carcinoma of the small intestine arising in regional enteritis (Crohn's disease). Cancer 54:151, 1984.

Radi, M. F., Gray, G. F., Jr., Scott, H. W., Jr.: Carcinosarcoma of ileum in regional enteritis. Hum. Pathol. 15:385, 1984.

Rambaud, J.-C., Modigliani, R., Nguyen Phuoc, B. K., Lejeune, R., LeCarrer, M., Mehaut, M., Valleur, P., Galian, A., Danon, F.: Nonsecretory alpha-chain disease in intestinal lymphoma. N. Engl. J. Med. 303:53, 1980.

Ramot, B., Levanon, M., Hahn, Y., Lahat, N., Moroz, C.: The mutual clonal origin of the lymphoplasmocytic and lymphoma cell in alpha-heavy chain disease. Clin. Exp. Immunol. 27:440, 1977.

Riddell, R. H., Goldman, H., Ransohoff, D. F., Appelman, H. D., Fenoglio, C. M., Haggitt, R. C., Ahren, C., Correa, P., Hamilton, S. R., Morson, B. C., Sommers, S. C., Yardley, J. H.: Dysplasia in inflammatory bowel disease. Standardized classification with provisional clinical applications. Hum. Pathol. 14:931, 1983.

Scully, R. E., Galdabini, J. J., McNeely, B. U.: Gardner's syndrome. Adenomatous polyps of (colon) and small bowel. Adenocarcinomas (two) of small bowel. N. Engl. J. Med. 299:1237, 1978.

Scully, R. E., Mark, E. J., McNeely, B. U.: Villous adenoma with focal carcinoma in situ, periampullary, with extension into common bile duct (Gardner's syndrome), with polyposis of small and large intestine. N. Engl. J. Med. 307:1566, 1982.

Shamsuddin, A. K. M., and Phillips, R. M.: Preneoplastic and neoplastic changes in colonic mucosa in Crohn's disease. Arch. Pathol. Lab. Med. 105:283, 1981.

Sobol, S., and Cooperman, A. M.: Villous adenoma of the ampulla of Vater. Gastroenterology 75:107, 1978.

Swinson, C. M., Slavin, G., Coles, E. C., et al.: Coeliac disease and malignancy. Lancet 1:111, 1983.

Thompson, H.: Precancerous conditions of the small intestine. In Sherlock, P., Morson, B. C., Barbara, L., Veronesi, U. (eds.): Precancerous Lesions of the Gastrointestinal Tract. New York, Raven Press, 1983, p. 205.

Trier, J. S., Falchuk, Z. M., Carey, M. C., Schreiber, D. S.: Celiac sprue and refractory sprue. Gastroenterology 75:307, 1978.

Valdes-Dapena, A., Rudolph, I. Hidayat, A., Roth, J. L. A., Laucks, R. B.: Adenocarcinoma of the small bowel in association with regional enteritis. Cancer 37:2938, 1976.

Warren, R., and Barwick, K. W.: Crohn's colitis with carcinoma and dysplasia. Am. J. Surg. Pathol. 7:151, 1983.

Webster, A. D. B., Kenwright, S., Ballard, J., Shiner, M., Slavin, G., Levi, A. J., Loewi, G., Asherson, G. L.: Nodular lymphoid hyperplasia of the bowel in primary hypogammaglobulinaemia. Gut 18:364, 1977.

KATHERINE DeSCHRYVER-KECSKEMETI

8 Large Intestine

Precursor lesions to colonic neoplasia can be catego-rized according to their gross, endoscopic, and micro-scopic appearances. These subdivisions, however, are arbitrary for didactic purposes and include multiple areas of overlap. In our consideration of these pre-cursor lesions, we will first describe the epithelial changes occurring in polypoid glandular mucosa. This discussion includes the interpretation of surveillance biopsies in polyposis families, of polypoid dysplasia in long-standing ulcerative colitis, and of polyps found on routine lower gastrointestinal endoscopies. Less frequently studied but, equally important are the epithelial changes occurring in nonpolypoid, or flat, glandular mucosa. Some of the neoplasms that de-velop in the colons of patients with chronic ulcerative colitis or following radiation belong to the latter cate-gory, although the lesions are described in the section on polypoid dysplasia. Early neoplasia of the appendix receives special consideration and is followed by a description of rare lesions involving polypoid squa-mous epithelium. A short section will also deal with the possible precursor lesions to lymphomas of the intestine.

Emphasis is placed on the diagnostic criteria for precursor lesions with established biologic behavior. Such interpretative criteria are of immediate impor-tance to the surgical pathologist and to the clinician. Further clinicopathologic correlations are needed to establish the nature of other lesions described in this chapter.

PRECURSOR LESIONS TO CARCINOMAS

Epithelial Atypia in Polypoid Glandular Mucosa

Surveillance Biopsies in Children from Families with Familial Polyposis Syndromes

Gastrointestinal polyposis syndromes in which genetic factors play an essential role represent an area of pathology in which there is considerable confusion

(Bussey et al., 1978; Danes, 1976; Hsu et al., 1983). Colon carcinoma occurring in families with familial polyposis accounts for less than 1 percent of all large intestinal cancers. However, identification of affected family members, in whom the development of carci-noma is certain, allows for true cancer prevention through early surgery. Parameters used in evaluating potential cases of familial polyposis include the num-ber of polyps present, their distribution in the colon and in other parts of the intestine, involvement of sites other than the gastrointestinal tract, and family history. Both familial polyposis coli and Gardner's syndrome are autosomal dominant processes; but as colonic lesions they are essentially the same entity (Gardner, 1983). Once a polyposis patient is identified (>100 polyps), all children in the family who are at risk should be evaluated and registered for indefinite surveillance.

Unfortunately, radiologic and endoscopic studies are usually non-diagnostic in young children or for early lesions. Often, these studies reveal only multiple mucosal nodules (Fig. 8–1) that require biopsy. Ac-curate assessment of the histology of the mucosal nodule then becomes the most important step in determining the nature of the disease (Bussey et al., 1978). The adenomatous change is the earliest man-ifestation of the abnormal tendency for proliferative activity and may involve only a single crypt (Fig. 8–1B). In these polyposis families, adenomatous change is the histologic marker for inheritance of the trait in the young members. Interestingly, even areas of histologically normal mucosa in these patients show cell kinetic abnormalities (Lipkin, 1974; Lipkin, 1975). Moreover, increased tetraploidy has been reported to be a cell-specific feature for the Gardner gene in cultured cells in that it was seen only in those cells taken from sites known to undergo malignant trans-formation and not in all cultured cells from these patients (Danes, 1976).

The policy for treating young patients who show adenomatous change on colonic biopsies varies among institutions. At St. Mark's Hospital in London,

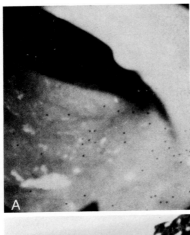

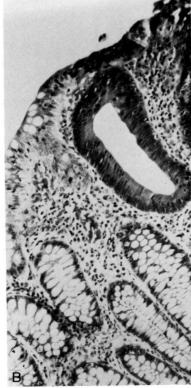

Figure 8–1. The patient is a 9-year-old girl. Gardner's syndrome was recently diagnosed in her mother. *A,* Endoscopic examination showed multiple small (0.2 to 0.3 cm) mucosal protrusions in the right, transverse, lower descending, and sigmoid colons. The differential diagnosis included lymphoid hyperplasia and adenomatous lesions. *B,* By light microscopy, the observed adenomatous change indicated inheritance of the polyposis trait and the need for indefinite surveillance and elective surgery. The patient's 13-year-old sister was screened at the same time and was found to have numerous 0.5-cm polypoid lesions. On the colectomy specimen about 75 adenomatous polyps were found. (*A,* Courtesy of Dr. J. Keating, Division of Pediatric Gastroenterology, Washington University, St. Louis, MO.)

colectomy is usually delayed until the patient is 17 or 18 years old because the risk of cancer before this age is very small, especially when polyps less than 1 cm in diameter are present (Morson, personal com-

munication). Numerous factors, such as social and educational circumstances and psychologic effects, are paramount in deciding the most suitable time for surgery. In our institution, surgery is recommended at an earlier age, even for patients as young as 8 or 9 years, because patient acceptance and adjustment are thought to be better at this age.

Juvenile or "retention," polyps are common lesions affecting young people. Most often they are solitary, sporadic, and of no further clinical significance after removal. Histologically identical lesions, however, may be part of the juvenile polyposis syndrome (Ramaswamy et al., 1984). Initial reports had emphasized the non-neoplastic nature of these retention polyps. More recently, however, several reports have described mixed juvenile and adenomatous features in the same lesion as well as the presence of both kinds of polyps in some patients (Lipper et al., 1981; Mills and Fechner, 1982; Monga et al., 1979). Although no premalignant potential has been assigned to the juvenile polyp itself, several reports have suggested a possible increase in the incidence of gastrointestinal cancer in patients with these polyps and in their families (Bussey et al., 1978; Goodman et al., 1979; Grotsky et al., 1982). These reports justify inclusion of such patients in long-term follow-up studies.

Polypoid Dysplasia in Longstanding Inflammatory Bowel Disease

Carcinoma developing in longstanding inflammatory bowel disease is relatively rare when all cases of colonic carcinoma are considered. However, the comparatively young age of patients at the time of carcinoma presentation (average age, early forties) and the tendency for insidious tumor development heighten our concern about these malignancies. The increased risk of carcinoma has unequivocally been recognized in patients with longstanding inflammatory bowel disease. The actual incidence of carcinoma, however, cannot be accurately estimated because it is difficult to obtain a large cohort of patients. It has been suggested that over 50 percent of this group will ultimately develop carcinoma. Patients with extensive ulcerative colitis for 7 years or more (particularly those in whom onset occurred before 25 years of age) and patients with longstanding Crohn's disease are included in this high-risk population. Prophylactic colectomy in individuals with longstanding colitis has met with little acceptance. Recognition of a prognostically significant epithelial neoplastic but non-invasive change, dysplasia, has brought forth numerous plans for patient management. Surveillance protocols have been established in several institutions, including ours, to follow these patients. Individuals who have had disease for 8 to 10 years are evaluated with a yearly rectal biopsy; for those who have had disease for 10 years or more, proctoscopy or sigmoidoscopy with rectal biopsy is performed every 2 years, and total colonoscopy with biopsies is performed during alternate years. Left-sided or more limited disease may be biopsied at less frequent intervals, approximately every 3 years. Multiple random biopsies from the cecum and the ascending and transverse colon are submitted in one specimen jar. All the biopsy fragments are oriented on Millipore HA filter paper as they are retrieved from the biopsy instrument before fixation, and tissues are processed, cut, and stained on the filter paper. Multiple random biopsies from the left colon (distal transverse, descending, and sigmoid colon) and multiple biopsies from the rectum are submitted separately in a similar manner. Additionally, any visible lesion or suspicious abnormality is biopsied and submitted for evaluation. All specimens are carefully labeled. If numerous lesions are seen, the specimens should be submitted with a drawing that identifies the specific biopsy sites as well as their relationships. Patients who have biopsies that show positive or indefinite dysplasia undergo colonoscopic re-evaluation in 3 months. Biopsies showing severe dysplasia on two separate occasions must be evaluated by a medicosurgical group so that the risk and need for colectomy can be assessed. The final decision is left to the patient and to the attending physician.

Surveillance of patients with longstanding inflammatory bowel disease is difficult. Symptoms of carcinoma may be similar to those resulting from the underlying inflammatory disease, and it is often impossible to make a clinical diagnosis of malignancy. Furthermore, early tumors in longstanding inflammatory bowel disease are finely nodular or plaque-like, making detection difficult by current visualization methods. For these reasons, early "asymptomatic" carcinoma is usually an incidental finding in resected specimens. The infiltrating component is commonly unsuspected on endoscopic biopsy because the superficial portion of the "dysplastic" mucosa closely resembles adenomas occurring in the non-colitic population and the carcinoma may not be recognized. Lesions that are detectable radiologically (Frank et al., 1978) or endoscopically are present in only a small number of patients. These grossly identifiable lesions were originally called "dysplasia-associated lesions" or "dysplasia-associated masses" (Blackstone et al., 1981). Over the years, a spectrum of macroscopic appearances has been recognized, including (1) polyps and polypoid masses; (2) slightly raised nodular and plaque-like areas; (3) villous change with velvety appearance, which is very difficult to detect; and (4) strictures (Fig. 8–2). Typical filiform inflammatory polyps virtually never undergo neoplastic transformation. Inflammatory polyps that appear atypical or adenomatous or that have a distinct head of more than 1 cm in diameter should be excised so that dysplasia can be excluded from the differential diagnosis.

By light microscopy, dysplasia is identified as an unequivocally neoplastic transformation of large bowel epithelium (Riddell et al., 1983). The implica-

tion is that invasive carcinoma may arise directly from this change. "Dysplasia" is synonymous with a variety of other terms, including "premalignant change," "precancerous change," "precancer," "atypia," and "adenomatous change" in ulcerative colitis. Dysplasia includes a spectrum of changes that are now classified according to severity as "high-grade," "low-grade," and "indefinite." The indefinite category may contain "probably negative," "probably positive," and "unknown" subcategories. If atypical "inflammatory" (head > 1 cm) or adenomatous-villous polyps are found, it is necessary to take multiple biopsies around their base because they may be part of a more diffuse dysplastic process. When there is no dysplasia in the surrounding mucosa, the polypoid lesions probably represent "adenomas" of the ordinary variety, particularly in the appropriate age group. Among younger patients, however, adenomatous polyps are unusual and are probably best treated as dysplastic manifestations of a longstanding inflammatory bowel disease. Plaque-like lesions also can harbor dysplasia or an underlying carcinoma. It is stressed that the appearances may be similar, regardless of whether an un-

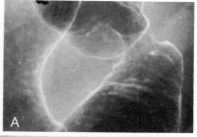

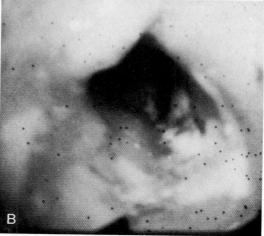

Figure 8–2. The patient is a 36-year-old white male with a 20-year history of ulcerative colitis, which was relatively inactive for the last 10 years. A, Surveillance barium enema showed an area of stricture at the splenic flexure. B, On endoscopy, active disease was seen with multiple ulcers throughout the strictured segment of colon. Because of the stricture, surgery was recommended, but the patient did not agree until a year later. At that time, Dukes' Stage C adenocarcinoma was found in the area of stricture. (Courtesy of Dr. G. Zuckerman, Digestive Disease Center, Washington University Medical School, St. Louis, MO.)

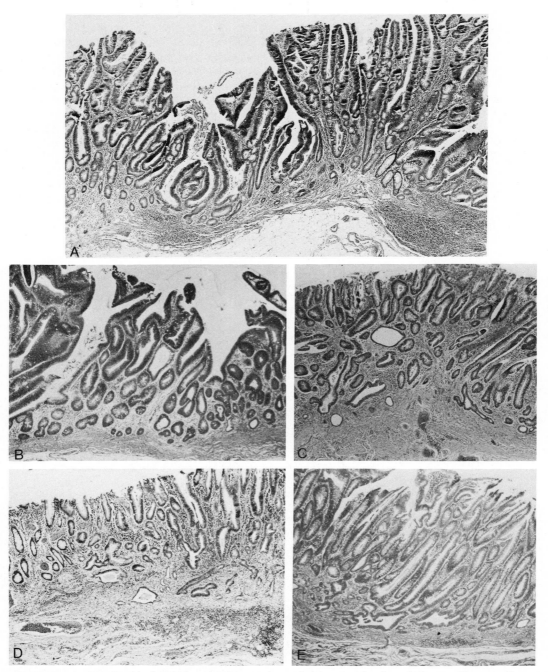

Figure 8–3. The patient is a 74-year-old white male with a history of typical ulcerative colitis for only 3 years. However, the patient had a right hemicolectomy 9 years previously for Dukes' Stage B carcinoma. There is also a history of bloody diarrhea of several weeks' duration 30 years ago, which at the time was thought to have been the result of amebic colitis. Slides from the 1974 partial colectomy were first reviewed with special attention to possible co-existing inflammatory bowel disease which might have been clinically quiescent. Sections from the margins of resection at considerable distance from the tumor showed numerous crypt abscesses. It was concluded that the patient had had inflammatory bowel disease for at least 10 years, and surveillance colonoscopy was performed. The patient had innumerable lesions resembling adenomatous and villous polyps. The biopsy was interpreted as high-grade dysplasia at multiple sites: Examples of lesions from the total colectomy specimen include a villous lesion *(A)*, adenomatous *(B)* and mixed lesions *(C)*, and Dukes' Stage A superficial adenocarcinomas underlying a sessile-villous region *(D,E)*.

derlying carcinoma is present, and that macroscopically—and therefore endoscopically—it is not possible to make this distinction. Further, biopsies of these lesions will reveal dysplasia but rarely the underlying carcinoma if one is present. Many of these lesions do contain invasive carcinoma on resection (Blackstone et al., 1981). For this reason and from a practical point of view, any lesion with a plaque-like appearance is best treated as a carcinoma. In many instances there may be no grossly detectable abnormality, with the diagnosis of carcinoma resulting entirely from the histologic review of random sections. Consequently, resected colons in these cases are thoroughly examined with the "breakfast roll" technique, which allows for almost complete sampling of the specimen.

ᐟ *Positive biopsies* for dysplasia often show architectural changes, such as the presence of a villous or adenomatous configuration. Identification of these changes is important when one is deciding more severe degrees of dysplasia (Fig. 8–3A and B). Dysplasia may also be extensive in non-polypoid, flat mucosa (see also discussion of epithelial atypia in flat mucosa, further on). Dysplasia and cancer in ulcerative colitis may have the same histologic appearance, and lesions thought to be confined to the mucosa, termed "precancer" in a biopsy, not uncommonly

have proved on resection to have come from areas with underlying invasion (Fig. 8–3C).

In low-grade dysplasia, the crypts are enlarged and lined by tall columnar cells, most of which contain mucin. However, there are moderate nuclear pseudostratification and hyperchromatism. Most of the nuclei are confined to the basal half of the cell.

In high-grade dysplasia, the degree of cytologic alteration is greater than in low-grade dysplasia. There are marked nuclear hyperchromatism and pseudostratification that extend into the luminal parts of the cells. Loss of nuclear polarity also may be seen. Often there is lack of mucin production, and the cytoplasm may become intensely eosinophilic (Figs. 8–3 to 8–7). These changes may involve only one part of a crypt or may be widespread.

Negative biopsies for dysplasia include normal mucosa, active disease, and quiescent disease.

Indefinite biopsies do not fit into any of the preceding categories. They can be subdivided into those that are probably negative, those that are probably positive (but in which there is sufficient doubt that the biopsy cannot be included with positive biopsies), and those that are unknown. There is a risk in overinterpreting epithelial changes in mucosal biopsies. If acute inflammation is present, one may have difficulty making a

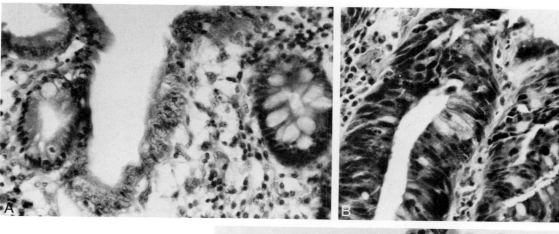

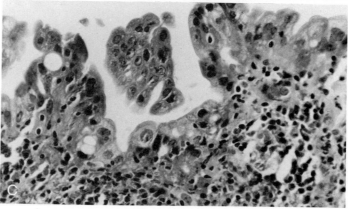

Figure 8–4. In addition to the architectural alterations, varying degrees of cellular changes are present in longstanding ulcerative colitis, ranging from mild and focal nuclear atypia *(A)* to widespread loss of polarity *(B)* and marked pleomorphism *(C)*.

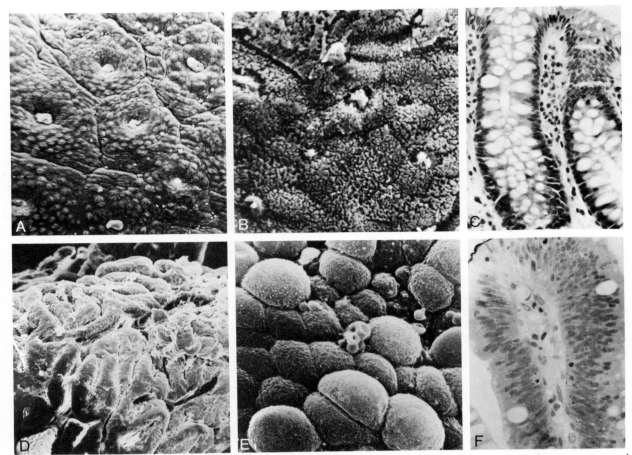

Figure 8–5. The surface changes shown in Figure 8–3 have also been studied by scanning electron microscopy. *A,* Scanning micrographs of normal colon with regular rows of crypts and mucous plugs in crypt orifice. *B,* At higher power polygonal colonic cells are covered with a thick carpet of microvilli. Goblet cells are interspersed and mucus is being extruded. *C,* Same specimen by light microscopy for comparison. *D,* Scanning of colonic biopsy in a patient with longstanding ulcerative colitis. The mucosa has a convoluted appearance, and only rarely are normal crypt orifices seen. *E,* At higher power wide variations are seen in cell size and shape. Microvilli are very sparse. *F,* The corresponding light micrograph. (Courtesy of Dr. H. Shields, Division of Gastroenterology, Beth Israel Hospital, Boston, MA.)

reliable diagnosis of precancer, even when dysplasia is marked. Some degree of epithelial change is commonly seen when there is acute inflammation or regeneration. Those biopsies are best repeated after treatment of active disease is attempted.

In conclusion, a perturbing point needs to be mentioned. Despite regular long-term surveillance, colon cancers continue to develop in optimally followed patients (Lennard-Jones et al., 1983); therefore, some carcinomas arising in patients with longstanding ulcerative colitis must occur in the absence of any significant or morphologically detectable dysplasia. Very rarely, colonic lymphoma develops in patients with longstanding ulcerative colitis.

Alpers and coworkers approached the problem of precancer in ulcerative colitis with thymidine labeling of colonic mucosal explants (Alpers et al., 1980).

These investigators found that regardless of the presence or absence of morphologically identifiable premalignant lesions, the mucosa behaves as if it is resistant to physiologic inhibition to proliferation. Duration of the inflammatory disease was the only important factor in the observed alteration in DNA synthesis, the basis for the uncontrolled proliferative activity. This technique, however, has not found widespread clinical application. Flow cytometry might be a promising alternative approach to this problem.

Lavage cytology has been advocated by Katz and coworkers (1977) as a means for surveillance in patients with longstanding disease. Carcinoembryonic antigen immunostaining is not diagnostically useful because of overlap in staining frequency and intensities among the benign, premalignant, and malignant lesions (Perzin et al., 1984; Rognum et al., 1982).

Surveillance colonoscopy in patients who have Crohn's disease with colon involvement may be in order (Warren and Barwick, 1983) as the pathogenesis of carcinoma arising in longstanding inflammatory disease of the colon may prove to be similar, regardless of the cause, including that associated with schistosomiasis, in which an epithelial precursor has been identified (Ming-Chai et al., 1980).

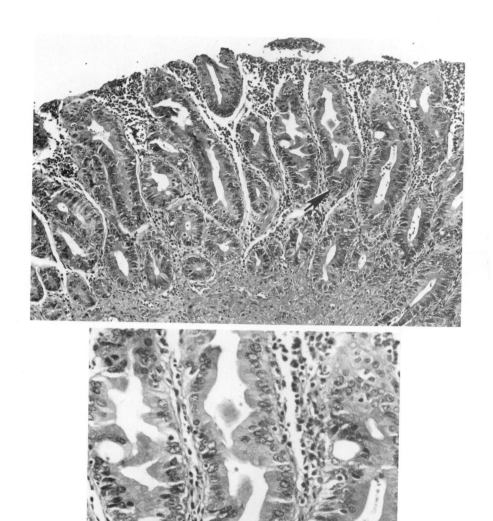

Figure 8–6. Mucosa positive for high grade dysplasia, with serrated crypts. *Top,* Mucin depletion, serrated crypts, and enlarged nuclei. *Bottom,* Detail of area of high grade dysplasia indicated by arrow in top illustration.

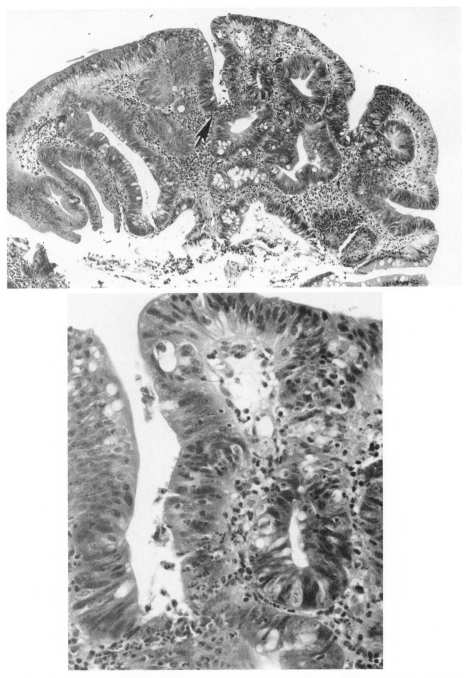

Figure 8–7. Mucosa positive for high grade dysplasia with acute inflammation. *Top*, Typical adenomatous-type glands in a colonoscopic biopsy specimen. *Bottom*, Detail of area (arrow in top illustration) showing an acute inflammatory infiltrate with the formation of crypt abscesses. The dysplastic nature of the epithelium is still apparent, however.

"Polyps" in Routine Surgical Pathology

The possible relationship between colorectal polyps and cancer has been repeatedly addressed and remains controversial. The controversy stems from the impossibility of proving the polyp–cancer sequence in human subjects. In laboratory animals, adenomas and carcinomas of the large intestine behave as distinct entities (Maskens and Dujardin-Loits, 1981). Nonetheless, most authors agree that available evidence does suggest some relationship between adenomatous polyps and carcinomatous change. Epidemiologic data demonstrate that patients with adenomatous polyps are at higher risk for colon cancer (Maskens and Dujardin-Loits, 1981). Moreover, it has been shown that sigmoidoscopic surveillance of large populations with thorough polyp removal not only increases the incidence of detectable curable lesions but also decreases the incidence of rectal cancer (Gilbertsen and Nelms, 1978).

Interestingly, retention type and adenomatous polyps occur following ureterosigmoidostomies (Ali et al., 1984; Moorcraft et al., 1983). The significance and pathogenesis of these polyps have not been established. However, carcinoma at the anastomotic site has been reported after these diversion procedures (Schipper and Decter, 1981), suggesting that a surveillance protocol for these patients may be needed.

Routine colonoscopy in patients with non-specific symptomatology referable to the lower gastrointestinal tract not uncommonly identifies one or several polypoid lesions. These may be subdivided as follows:

Tubular, Tubulovillous, and Villous Adenomas. The risk of adenomas harboring a malignancy depends on the size and type of the adenoma (Qizilbash, 1982). Tubular adenomas (adenomatous polyps) have a low risk of becoming malignant, whereas tubulovillous adenomas (villoglandular polyps) have an intermediate risk. Villous adenomas carry the highest risk of malignancy. Some villous lesions are only a few millimeters in size when detected and might best be designated as "villous hyperplasia" (Fig. 8–8). Villous adenomas were traditionally reported to be uncommon on the right side of the colon, including the cecum and hepatic flexure (Wheat and Ackerman, 1958). Because villous adenomas of the colon do not give rise to the secretory syndrome, they clinically present differently from their rectal counterparts. However, routine colonoscopic examination brings right-sided villous adenomas within reach of the biopsy forceps, and these lesions are rather common findings on routine endoscopic biopsies (Schwob and De-Schryver-Kecskemeti, 1985). Biologic behavior and histologic features are identical with those of their rectal counterpart.

Hyperplastic (metaplastic) polyps, epithelial protrusions that are common in the rectosigmoid area of patients over the age of 40 years, traditionally were considered to have no neoplastic connotation—that

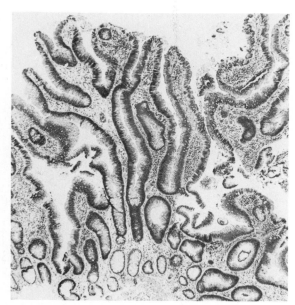

Figure 8–8. Light micrograph of a rectal biopsy in a 68-year-old patient who had a 5-mm polypoid lesion. With routine endoscopy and biopsy, these very small villous or papillary lesions are commonly seen by the surgical pathologist.

is, no role in the adenoma–carcinoma sequence. Not uncommonly, however, hyperplastic polyps contain foci of hyperchromatic and atypical nuclei (Fig. 8–9). In one study, hyperplastic polyps resubmitted to close scrutiny were found to have frank adenomatous foci (Estrada and Spjut, 1980). The clinical significance of these foci remains unknown (Jass, 1983). Carcinoma has been reported in one such lesion (Urbanski et al., 1984). It is our policy to label these lesions "atypical hyperplasias" so that they can be subsequently retrieved and further studied.

Cell kinetic studies of the large intestine and its neoplasms have resulted in an appreciation of differences and histologic appearances and have led to a correlation of histopathology with extent of cellular replicative activity (Fig. 8–10). Thymidine labeling studies have shown that DNA synthesis is restricted to the lower two thirds of the crypts in the normal large intestine (Lipkin, 1974). In contrast, in tubular and villous adenomas, DNA synthesis is not restricted to a particular location. Rather, it occurs more or less randomly on the surface epithelium of tubular adenomas and on the fronds and their bases in villous adenomas (Lipkin, 1974). The same type of cell kinetic disorganization that is seen in adenomas is also found in adenocarcinomas (Lipkin, 1975).

Incidental Carcinoma in Endoscopic Biopsies of "Polyps." Malignant changes in large adenomas may easily be overlooked if only small biopsy fragments from these tumors are examined (Livstone et al., 1977; Qizilbash, 1982). The entire polyp should ideally be removed by cautery snare and properly ori-

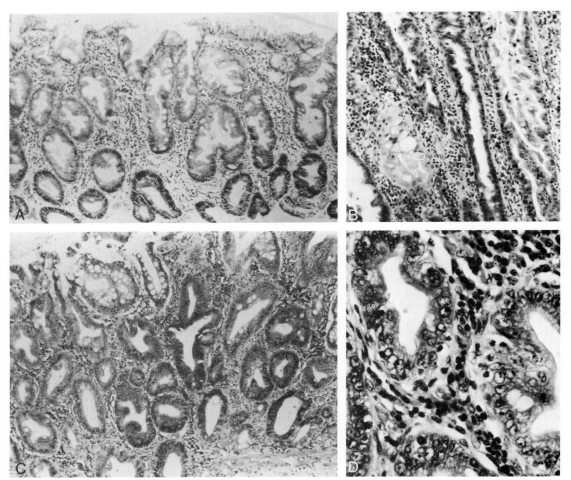

Figure 8–9. *A,* Light micrograph of a polypoid lesion from the sigmoid colon of a 55-year-old patient. In most areas, the features were those of a hyperplastic polyp. *B,* Focally, however, bifurcation of crypts, as evidence of adenomatous proliferation, was present with some nuclear atypia. The patient in *C* and *D* is a 58-year-old male who had a villous adenoma of the cecum 3 years ago. Now the patient has had a right colectomy for a Dukes' Stage C adenocarcinoma of the midtransverse colon. Close to the distal line of resection a polypoid lesion showed a mixed hyperplastic and adenomatous pattern *(C)* with severe epithelial pleomorphism *(D).* For purposes of subsequent identification we label these lesions "atypical hyperplasias."

ented for optimal examination (Lipper, 1983). Multiple sections should be cut in a systematic fashion and include both head and stalk along the long axis. Inking of the base may be helpful in apparently sessile lesions.

Management of patients whose polyps show histologic evidence of malignancy is a matter of controversy. If the carcinoma is superficial and does not extend through the muscularis mucosae, for all practical purposes it will not metastasize (Fenoglio et al., 1973). When invasive beyond the muscularis mucosae, the carcinoma can assume one of three different morphologic appearances: a poorly to moderately differentiated adenocarcinoma or, more rarely, a signet ring cell carcinoma or a small cell undifferentiated (oat cell–like) carcinoma (Mills et al., 1983). Experience indicates that metastases are rare when a pedunculated adenoma contains only superficially inva-

sive well-differentiated carcinoma (Blundell and Earnest, 1980; Blundell and Earnest, 1981). Nevertheless, some authors have concluded that all patients with polyps that contain any invasive type of carcinoma should undergo a standard cancer operation. This assumes that endoscopic polypectomy is inadequate treatment, leaving residual tumor in 15 percent of patients (Colacchio et al., 1981; Wilcox and Colacchio, 1982). Others advocate simple polypectomy unless the tumor is poorly differentiated, has invaded lymphatics, or involves the margin of resection (Cooper, 1983). With this approach, however, 83 percent of patients also had unnecessary surgical resection. More recently, others have found that the most important criterion for residual disease is the presence of cancer at the resection line (Carter et al., 1984; Lipper et al., 1983). There is now a national study aimed at resolving the controversy and provid-

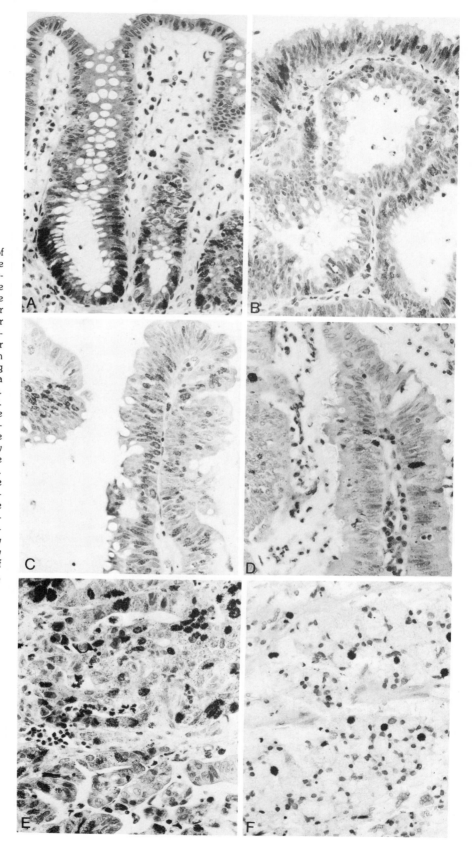

Figure 8–10. *A,* Autoradiographs of various colonic lesions which were pulse-labeled in vitro with tritiated thymidine. Normal large-intestinal surface epithelium and crypts. S-phase cells are marked by dark silver grains over their nuclei and are found only in the lower portions of the crypts. No surface epithelial cells are labeled. *B,* Tubular adenoma. Labeled cells are present in the surface epithelium and underlying neoplastic crypts. *C,* Villous adenoma with low thymidine-labeling index. Only a few labeled cells are present. They are randomly distributed in the villi. *D,* Villous adenoma with high labeling index. Many epithelial cells are labeled in all portions of the villi. They tend to be located adjacent to the stroma rather than toward the surface. *E,* Infiltrating adenocarcinoma of large intestine. Numerous neoplastic epithelial cells and a few stromal cells are labeled. *F,* Poorly differentiated mucinous adenocarcinoma of large intestine. S-phase cells appear to be evenly distributed in the neoplasm. (Courtesy of Dr. J. S. Meyer, Department of Pathology, St. Luke's Medical Center, St. Louis, MO.)

ing uniform guidelines for the appropriate handling of cases of malignancy found during endoscopic removal of a polyp (Cooper, personal communication).

Evaluation of colorectal carcinomas by DNA flow cytometry has shown frequent polyclonality. Multiple stemlines with abnormal DNA content may be present within the same carcinoma (Brattain et al., 1981; Petersen et al., 1980). The presence of hyperdiploid stemlines appears to indicate a high likelihood of relapse after primary surgical therapy and may be applicable to the study of malignant polyps (Wolley et al., 1982). The study of tumor-associated antigens (Strauss and Pascal, 1975) and more recently of monoclonal antibodies (Gilliland et al., 1980; Koprowski et al., 1979; Moldofsky et al., 1984; Sears 1982), may lead to their clinical application in the identification of premalignant lesions and incipient neoplasia.

Epithelial Atypia in Non-Polypoid (Flat) Glandular Mucosa

With thorough colonoscopic examination, small carcinomas are increasingly recognized as only areas of mucosal irregularity (Fig. 8–11). Sometimes, these lesions are no larger than 3 mm in diameter (Haupt and Hamilton, 1983; Shamsuddin et al., 1980; Shamsuddin, 1982; Spjut et al., 1979). The clinical impor-

tance of these small carcinomas, arising presumably in flat mucosa, should be strongly emphasized. Even the smallest mucosal excrescence or focus of discoloration or granularity visible on endoscopy should be subjected to careful scrutiny and biopsy (Crawford and Stromeyer, 1983). Small de novo carcinomas, without a pre-existing visible adenomatous precursor, are important from a theoretical point of view because they indicate that colonic cancers may arise from non-polypoid mucosa. Indeed, non-polypoid mucosa consistently showed epithelial atypia at a distance from the carcinoma in two studies of randomly selected colonic tumors (Saffos and Rhatigen, 1977; Shamsuddin et al., 1981b). Interestingly, most inherited types of large bowel carcinomas are not associated with familial polyposis, yet these types account for 12 to 26 percent of all large bowel cancers. Those that are polyp-associated, however, represent less than 1 percent (Anderson, 1980). The tumors arising in flat mucosa are typically proximal and multiple and occur in younger age groups (Lynch et al., 1977). Adenomatous-polyp precursors have been rarely documented. The nature of the premalignant lesion remains to be determined, although it may correspond to the epithelial dysplasia that occurs in flat mucosa (Fig. 8–12A).

Epithelial dysplasia in flat mucosa as a precursor lesion to invasive carcinomas has been well documented in long-standing inflammatory bowel disease

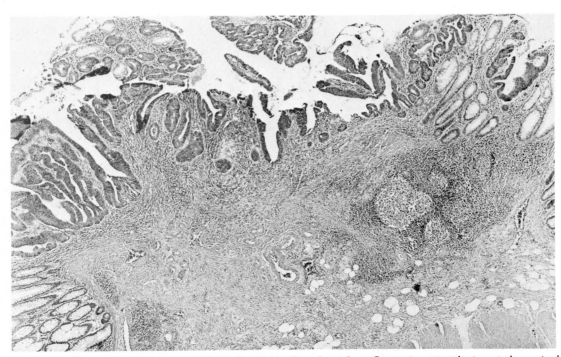

Figure 8–11. The patient is a 69-year-old woman who had clinical work-up for melena. On an air contrast barium study, a raised irregular area was seen at 25 cm into the sigmoid colon. A small (6 mm) intramucosal carcinoma was resected. The patient is well 5 years later.

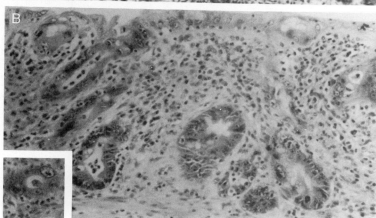

Figure 8–12. *A,* The patient is an 80-year-old male who had a left colectomy for Dukes' Stage C adenocarcinoma. Proximally and at a distance from tumor, epithelial changes were seen on routine sections taken from non-polypoid, flat mucosa. These consist of mild epithelial tufting, and the appearance of large, irregular nuclei and big nucleoli. *B,* Similar but more severe changes seen in colonic mucosa from irradiated areas. The patient had been treated with internal radiation for a gynecologic malignancy. Inset shows nuclear pleomorphism.

(Riddell et al., 1983) (see also previous discussion of polypoid dysplasia in long-standing inflammatory bowel disease).

Radiation-induced malignancy also occurs in flat atrophic mucosa. Atypical, dysplastic changes are not uncommonly seen (Fig. 8–12*B*) (Black et al., 1980; Berthrong and Fajardo, 1981). Because the intestine is unavoidably exposed during radiation treatment of many abdominal and pelvic neoplasms, potential late complications of therapy include the induction of malignant changes (Castro et al., 1973; Greenwald et al., 1978; Shamsuddin and Elias, 1981a). Severe dysplasia in flat mucosa with early stromal invasion has been documented (Shamsuddin and Elias, 1981a), so this condition can now be added to the list of incipient lesions occurring in non-polypoid, or flat, mucosa for which close follow-up of patients at risk is warranted.

Experimental models of colorectal neoplasia also have addressed this question of whether adenocarcinomas originate from adenomas or de novo from the epithelium. The mouse model in which 1, 2-dimethylhydrazine is used as the carcinogen supports the normal mucosa to adenoma to carcinoma sequence (Thurnherr et al., 1973). However, in some strains of rats, the same carcinogen produces adenocarcinomas directly from flat mucosa, without an intervening generation of adenomas (Deschner and Maskens, 1982; Maskens, 1976).

Appendiceal Lesions

Benign, borderline, and malignant neoplasms of the appendix are essentially the same as those occurring in the large intestine but have some special features.

Mucosal Hyperplasia, Mucinous Cystadenoma, and Mucinous Cystadenocarcinoma

The entities of mucosal hyperplasia, mucinous cystadenoma, and mucinous cystadenocarcinoma have been well described previously (Higa et al., 1973). Mucosal hyperplasia is the appendiceal equivalent of the hyperplastic polyp. For differentiating between cystadenoma and cystadenocarcinoma, the only useful histologic feature is the lack of stromal invasion of the former. It is not possible to determine prospectively whether one is dealing with the incipient stage of the malignant process or with a truly benign neo-plasm (Fig. 8–13). This is especially true in view of the epithelial atypia and nuclear crowding present in some cystadenomas. In the appendix, this differential problem is reduced to theoretic grounds because patients with the so-called cystadenomas are cured

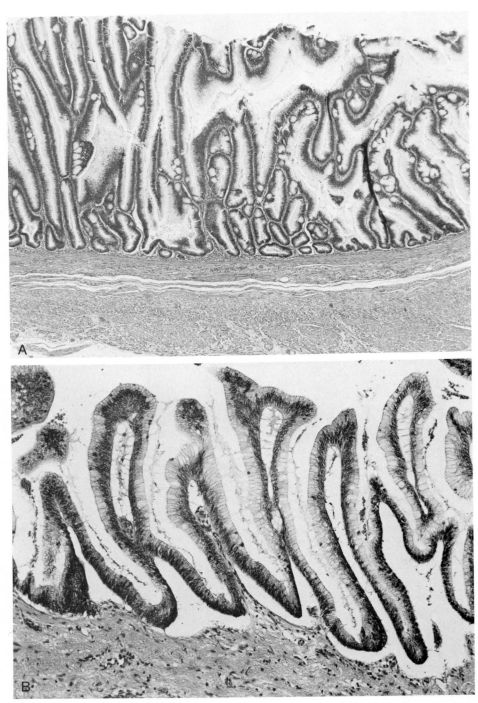

Figure 8–13. Mucinous cystadenoma of the appendix. There was diffuse involvement of the mucosa by a complex papillary pattern of mucin-secreting cells *(A)*. Cellular crowding and pseudostratification is present focally *(B)*. (Courtesy of Dr. J. Rosai, Department of Pathology, Yale University, New Haven, Conn.)

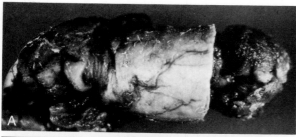

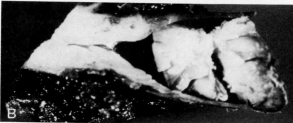

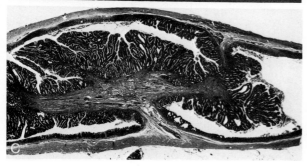

Figure 8–14. *A, B,* Gross appearance of an appendiceal villous adenoma. This presentation is rare in the appendix and resembles villous adenomas in the colon. *C,* Microscopic appearance.

cell carcinoids, adenocarcinoids, the prognosis of patients with these tumors is less favorable than that associated with the usual appendiceal carcinoid. In one series, six of 30 cases were metastatic and behaved clinically as signet ring cell carcinomas (Warkel et al., 1978). Atypical foci, high mitotic rate, and spread beyond the appendix are indicators of aggressive behavior. Right hemicolectomy is advocated for such tumors rather than appendectomy alone. The interesting suggestion has been made by Warkel's group that there may be a spectrum of appendiceal carcinoid tumors: Tubular adenocarcinoid may be associated with intermediate biologic aggressiveness and age of onset and may constitute an evolutionary stage in the development of the goblet cell neoplasm.

We have also seen a case of goblet cell carcinoid of the appendix (Fig. 8–16) that behaved in a highly malignant fashion, despite the absence of mitotic figures, the well-differentiated appearance, and the confinement of the tumor to the wall of the appendix. Electron microscopy disclosed, besides the classic features of the adenocarcinoid (Cooper and Warkel,

by appendectomy. It is, however, an interesting problem in tumor biology. Cystadenomas may be the appendiceal counterpart of adenomatous polyps and villous adenomas. In this sense, the lesions may represent "precursors" to the invasive carcinomas.

Villous adenomas, as we recognize them at other sites, are rarely found in the appendix (Fig. 8–14).

Lesions Containing Both Mucin-secreting and Endocrine Cells

Various tumors in different organs—for example, the stomach, colon, and ovary—often contain endocrine cells mixed with mucinous elements. The question arises whether these tumors are more closely related to carcinoids and thus are associated with a substantially better prognosis than mucinous tumors without the endocrine component. However, the presence of endocrine, argentaffin, or argyrophil cells in a mucinous tumor is not pathognomonic for a carcinoid (Fig. 8–15). Furthermore, contrary to previous opinions regarding the biologic behavior of the so-called goblet

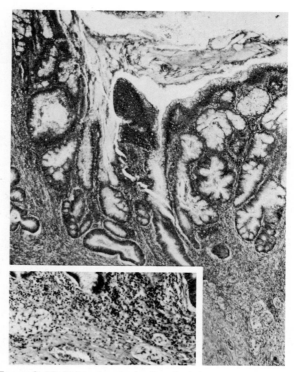

Figure 8–15. Light micrograph of a villous lesion of the appendix found at laparotomy performed for symptoms of acute appendicitis in a 60-year-old patient. Clusters of signet ring cells are present in the submucosa and throughout the wall. On special staining, numerous argyrophil cells were found among the signet ring cells, and the submitting diagnosis was goblet cell carcinoid. However, in spite of the endocrine cells, this lesion represents a villous adenoma with adenocarcinoma in which the invasive portion is of the signet ring variety. The prognosis for this lesion is extremely poor.

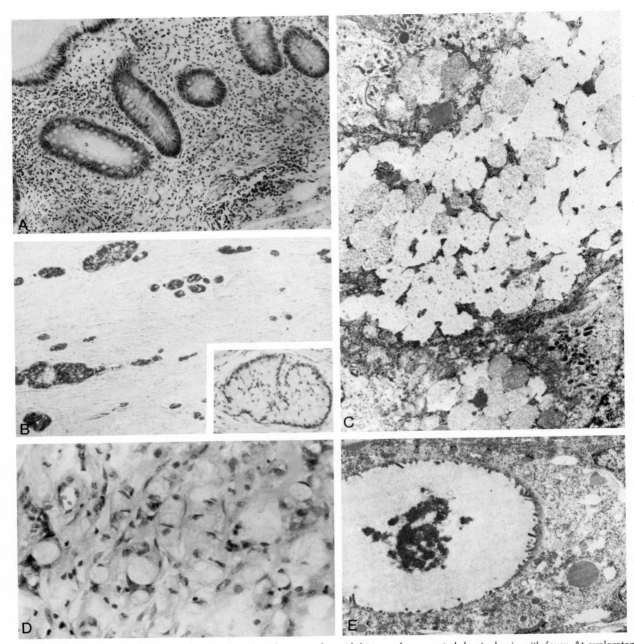

Figure 8–16. The patient is a 59-year-old white female with a several-month history of recurrent abdominal pain with fever. At exploratory laparotomy, the appendix was found to be adherent to the anterior abdominal wall. A frozen section from the point of adherence showed acute and chronic inflammation only. The concluding diagnosis was appendiceal and periappendiceal abscess, and an appendectomy was performed. Sections of the appendix showed infiltration of the wall by regular small smooth-bordered nests of signet ring cells confined to the mucosa and muscularis propria (A,B). On special staining, argyrophil cells were also present in the clusters, supporting the diagnosis of goblet cell carcinoid. No atypia or mitotic figures were present. By electron microscopy, goblet cells and endocrine cells were seen side by side in the clusters (C). Two years later, the patient returned with a hard periumbilical mass, which proved to be recurrent tumor. Signet ring cells diffusely infiltrated the mesentery (D). The patient died of tumor a year later. In retrospect, the tumor behaved more like a mucinous cystadenocarcinoma than a carcinoid. The ultrastructural features were reviewed in the original material and, in addition to the typical goblet and endocrine cell clusters (C), tumor cells forming intracellular lumens were found (E).

1978), occasional tumor cells with intracellular lumens. Similar features were reported in a case of pseudomyxoma peritonei, which was associated with an unexpectedly poor prognosis (Elesha et al., 1981). The presence of intracellular lumens may prove to be a marker for aggressive tumor behavior.

Atypia and Dysplasia

Atypia and dysplasia can also be present in the flat, non-polypoid mucosa in the appendix (Fig. 8–17).

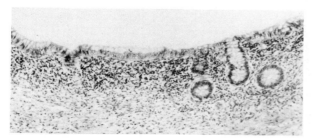
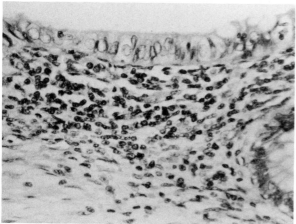
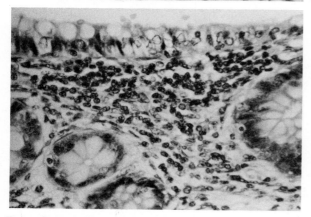

Figure 8–17. A 62-year-old patient had a right hemicolectomy for a large villous adenoma at the hepatic flexure. The patient also had several adenomatous lesions in the specimen. A routine section of the appendix showed considerable epithelial atypia in flat, non-polypoid mucosa.

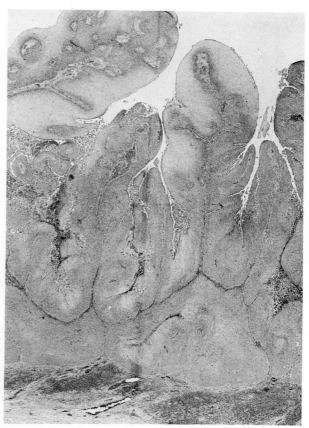

Figure 8–18. The patient is a 47-year-old black female with a 5-year history of intermittent bright red blood from the rectum. The clinical and postendoscopy diagnosis was villous adenoma at the anorectal junction. The lesion involved the entire circumference of the bowel. Multiple biopsies of the villous lesion were interpreted as a well-differentiated squamous cell carcinoma. The patient has had a "squamous papilloma" and a "condyloma acuminatum" removed 4 and 5 years, previously respectively, from the same site. Upon review, the previous biopsies were interpreted as verrucous carcinoma. The resection specimen showed extensive tumor which was well differentiated and only focally and superficially invasive.

Polypoid Squamous Epithelium

Squamous cell carcinomas of the colon are rare (Burgess et al., 1979). Interestingly, however, a high proportion of carcinomas developing in long-standing ulcerative colitis show squamous cell differentiation. Indeterminate basal cell hyperplasia and anaplasia are thought to be related to repeated lesion/repair sequences (Crissman, 1978), although a precursor lesion has not been identified in these tumors. Squamous metaplasia in polyps is occasionally observed and probably does not have clinical significance (Bansal et al., 1984).

Polypoid squamous lesions in colonic mucosa, although rare and mostly benign, cannot be automatically dismissed as squamous papillomas or squamous metaplasias. *Verrucous carcinoma* of the anorectum

(Fig. 8–18) is a rare, low-grade malignancy for which early diagnosis is difficult. Such difficulty is often related to a poor awareness of this lesion. The typical tumor consists of deceptively benign cytologic features, whose presence often causes a considerable delay in establishment of the diagnosis. Papillary fronds, pushing borders, and an underlying inflammatory response are always seen. The differential diagnosis between verrucous carcinoma and squamous papilloma/squamous metaplasia in biopsy specimens often depends more on clinical features, such as the size of the lesion, than on histologic findings. Verrucous carcinoma is large and single (Prioleau et al., 1980). Viral particles are not found by electron microscopy. Perianal and other sites for the lesion are not uncommon (Kraus and Perez-Mesa, 1966), but only two cases have been reported in the rectum (Knoblich and Failing, 1967; Prioleau et al., 1980).

Interestingly, *cloacogenic carcinoma* of the anorectum has recently been described in a report of four anoreceptive homosexual men (Cooper, 1979). No conclusions can be drawn yet about possible precursor lesions or about whether long-term surveillance is warranted in such patients.

PRECURSOR LESIONS TO LYMPHOMAS

There is little available information about the precursors of lymphoma in the colon. It is a rare entity. Some cases of histiocytic lymphoma seem to be associated with longstanding ulcerative colitis (Fig. 8–19). (For a review of the literature on this subject, see Bashiti and Kraus, 1980.)

Clinically significant involvement of the colon in lymphomatoid granulomatosis is rare (Rattinger et al.,

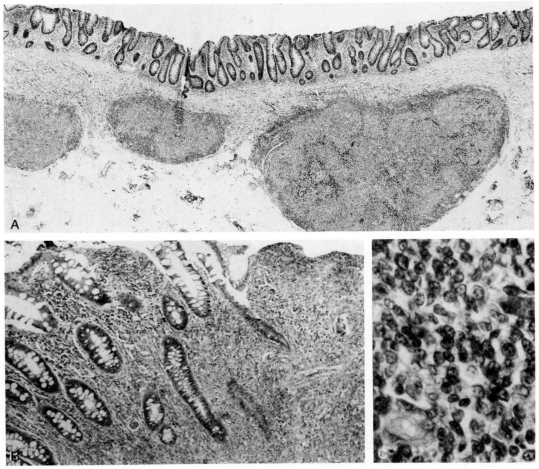

Figure 8–19. The patient is a 42-year-old male who had an 18-year history of ulcerative colitis. He presented at this time with exacerbation of symptoms. On endoscopic examination, multiple masses were found in the descending colon. Advanced ulcerative colitis was also seen. In the proctocolectomy specimen, several lesions were found in the mid-descending colon. *A,* Light micrograph of colonic mucosa between polypoid tumor masses. *B,* Ulcerated colonic mucosa from a "polypoid mass" replaced by a monomorphous tumor, consistent with histiocytic lymphoma. *C,* Higher magnification of the lymphoma cells. (Courtesy of Dr. H. O. Bashiti, Washington University, St. Louis, MO.)

1983; Singh and Hellstrom, 1978) and is due to an ischemic phenomenon secondary to vasculitis. No cases have been described in which lymphoma of the large intestine arose in association with lymphomatoid granulomatosis, a complication that has been reported in the lungs and central nervous system.

Whether there are morphologically recognizable precursor conditions to lymphomatous polyposis, a unique mantle zone lymphoma of the colon, is uncertain (Isaacson, personal communication). The rectal lymphoid polyp, the so-called anal tonsil, is a benign lesion and is not a precursor to lymphoma (Cornes et al., 1961). There is no evidence to implicate benign lymphoid polyp or polyposis of the large intestine in general as a precursor of malignancy except for the indirect relationship of those polyps associated with dysproteinemias that are restricted to the small intestine (see Chapter 7).

Radiation-induced sarcomas and early lesions of Kaposi's sarcoma will be described in detail in Chapter 21.

References

Ali, M. H., Satti, M. B., Al-Nafussi, A.: Multiple benign colonic polypi at the site of ureterosigmoidostomy. Cancer 53:1006, 1984.

Alpers, D. H., Philpott, G., Grimme, N. L., Margolis, D. M.: Control of thymidine incorporation in mucosal explants from patients with chronic ulcerative colitis. Gastroenterology 78:470, 1980.

Anderson, D. E.: An inherited form of large bowel cancer. Muir's syndrome. Cancer 45:1103, 1980.

Bansal, M., Fenoglio, C. M., Robboy, S. J., King, D. W.: Are metaplasias in colorectal adenomas truly metaplasias? Am. J. Pathol. 115:253, 1984.

Bashiti, H. O., and Kraus, F. T.: Histiocytic lymphoma in chronic ulcerative colitis. Cancer 46:1695, 1980.

Berthrong, M. and Fajardo, L. F.: Radiation injury in surgical pathology. Part II. Alimentary tract. Am. J. Surg. Pathol. 5:153, 1981.

Black, W. C., Gomez, L. S., Yuhas, J. M., Kligerman, M. M.: Quantitation of the late effects of X-radiation on the large intestine. Cancer 45:444, 1980.

Blackstone, M. O., Riddell, R. H., Gerald Rogers, B. H., Levin, B.: Dysplasia-associated lesion or mass (DALM) detected by colonoscopy in long-standing ulcerative colitis: an indication for colectomy. Gastroenterology 80:366, 1981.

Blundell, C. R. and Earnest, D. L.: A caution concerning conservative management of colonic polyps containing invasive carcinoma. Gastrointest. Endosc. 26:54, 1980.

Blundell, C. R. and Earnest, D. L.: Cancer in a colonic polyp, or malignant colonic adenomas—is polypectomy sufficient? Gastroenterology 81:625, 1981.

Brattain, M. G., Fine, W. D., Khaled, F. M., et al.: Heterogeneity of malignant cells from a human colonic carcinoma. Cancer Res. 41:1751, 1981.

Burgess, P. A., Lupton, E. W., Talbot, I. C.: Squamous-cell carcinoma of the proximal colon. Dis. Colon Rectum 22:241, 1979.

Bussey, H. J. R., Veale, A. M. O., Morson, B. C.: Genetics of gastrointestinal polyposis. Gastroenterology 74:1325, 1978.

Carter, M., Bak, M., Mitsudo, S., Boley, S. J.: Endoscopically removed malignant colonic polyps—subsequent resection or not? Gastroenterology 86:1041, 1984.

Castro, E. B., Rosen, P. P., Quan, S. H. Q.: Carcinoma of large intestine in patients irradiated for carcinoma of cervix and uterus. Cancer 31:45, 1973.

Colacchio, T. A., Forde, K. A., Scantlebury, V. P.: Endoscopic polypectomy. Inadequate treatment for invasive colorectal carcinoma. Ann. Surg. 194:704, 1981.

Cooper, H. S.: Surgical pathology of endoscopically removed malignant polyps of the colon and rectum. Am. J. Surg. Pathol. 7:613, 1983.

Cooper, H. S., Patchefsky, A. S., Marks, G.: Cloacogenic carcinoma of the anorectum in homosexual men. Dis. Colon Rectum 22:557, 1979.

Cooper, P. H.: Personal communication.

Cooper, P. H. and Warkel, R. L.: Ultrastructure of the goblet cell type of adenocarcinoid of the appendix. Cancer 42:2687, 1978.

Cornes, J. S., Wallace, M. H., Morson, B. C.: Benign lymphomas of the rectum and anal canal. J. Pathol. Bact. 82:371, 1961.

Crawford, B. E. and Stromeyer, F. W.: Small nonpolypoid carcinomas of the large intestine. Cancer 51:1760, 1983.

Crissman, J. D.: Adenosquamous and squamous cell carcinoma of the colon. Am. J. Surg. Pathol. 2:47, 1978.

Danes, B. S.: Increased tetraploidy: Cell-specific for the Gardner gene in the cultured cell. Cancer 38:1983, 1976.

Deschner, E. E. and Maskens, A. P.: Significance of the labeling index and labeling distribution as kinetic parameters in colorectal mucosa of cancer patients and DMH treated animals. Cancer 50:1136, 1982.

Elesha, S. O., Medline, A., Taylor, B. R.: Mucocele of the appendix: pseudomyxoma peritonei and intracytoplasmic canaliculus-like structures. Hum. Pathol. 12:280, 1981.

Estrada, R. G. and Spjut, H. J.: Hyperplastic polyps of the large bowel. Am. J. Surg. Pathol. 4:127, 1981.

Fenoglio, C. M., Kaye, G. I., Lane, N.: Distribution of human colonic lymphatics in normal, hyperplastic, and adenomatous tissue. Gastroenterology 64:51, 1973.

Frank, P. H., Riddell, R. H., Feczko, P. J., Levin, B.: The radiological detection of colonic dysplasia (precarcinoma) in chronic ulcerative colitis. Gastrointest. Radiol. 3:209, 1978.

Gardner, E. J.: Familial polyposis coli and Gardner syndrome—is there a difference? In Ingall, J. R. F., and Mastromarino, A. J. (eds.): Prevention of Hereditary Large Bowel Cancer. Progress in Clinical and Biological Research. Vol. 115. New York, Alan R. Liss, 1983.

Gilbertsen, V. A. and Nelms, J. M.: The prevention of invasive cancer of the rectum. Cancer 41:1137, 1978.

Gilliland, D. G., Steplewski, Z., Collier, R. J., Mitchell, K. F., Chang, T. H., Koprowski, H.: Antibody-directed cytotoxic agents: use of monoclonal antibody to direct the action of toxin A chains to colorectal carcinoma cells. Proc. Natl. Acad. Sci. U.S.A., 77:4539, 1980.

Goodman, Z. D., Yardley, J. H., Milligan, F. D.: Pathogenesis of colonic polyps in multiple juvenile polyposis. Report of a case associated with gastric polyps and carcinoma of the rectum. Cancer 43:1906, 1979.

Greenwald, R., Barkin, J. S., Hensley, G. T.: Cancer of the colon as a late sequel of pelvic irradiation. Am. J. Gastroenterol. 69:196, 1978.

Grotsky, H. W., Rickert, R. R., Smith, W. D., Newsome, J. F.: Familial juvenile polyposis coli. Gastroenterology 82:494, 1982.

Haupt, H. M. and Hamilton, S. R.: Small carcinomas of the colon and rectum. Lab. Invest. 48:35A, 1983.

Higa, E., Rosai, J., Pizzimbono, C. A., Wise, L.: Mucosal hyperplasia, mucinous cystadenoma, and mucinous cystadenocarcinoma of the appendix. A re-evaluation of appendiceal "mucocele." Cancer 32:1525, 1973.

Hsu, S. H., Luk, G. D., Krush, A. J., Hamilton, S. R., Hoover, H. H., Jr.: Multiclonal origin of polyps in Gardner syndrome. Science 221:951, 1983.

Isaacson, P.: Personal communication.

Jass, J. R.: Relation between metaplastic polyp and carcinoma of the colorectum. Lancet 1(8):28, 1983.

Katz, S., Katzka, I., Platt, N., Hajdu, E. O., Bassett, E.: Cancer in chronic ulcerative colitis. Diagnostic role of segmental colonic lavage. Dig. Dis. 22:355, 1977.

Knoblich, R. and Failing, J. F., Jr.: Giant condyloma acuminatum (Buschke-Loewenstein tumor) of the rectum. Am. J. Clin. Pathol. 48:389, 1967.

Koprowski, H., Steplewski, Z., Mitchell, K., Herlyn, M., Herlyn, D., Fuhrer, P.: Colorectal carcinoma antigens detected by hybridoma antibodies. Somatic Cell Genet. 5:957, 1979.

Kraus, F. T. and Perez-Mesa, C.: Verrucous carcinoma: clinical and pathologic study of 105 cases involving oral cavity, larynx and genitalia. Cancer 19:26, 1966.

Lennard-Jones, J. E., Morson, B. C., Ritchie, J. K., Williams, C. B.: Cancer surveillance in ulcerative colitis. Lancet 2:149, 1983.

Lipkin, M.: Phase 1 and phase 2 proliferative lesion of colonic epithelial cells in diseases leading to colonic cancer. Cancer 34:878, 1974.

Lipkin, M.: Biology of large bowel cancer. Cancer 36:2319, 1975.

Lipper, S., Kahn, L. B., Ackerman, L. V.: The significance of microscopic invasive cancer in endoscopically removed polyps of the large bowel. Cancer 52:1691, 1983.

Lipper, S., Kahn, L. B., Sandler, R. S., Varma, V.: Multiple juvenile polyposis. A study of the pathogenesis of juvenile polyps and their relationship to colonic adenomas. Hum. Pathol. 12:804, 1981.

Livstone, E. M., Troncale, F. J., Sheahan, D. G.: Value of a single forceps biopsy of colonic polyps. Gastroenterology 73:1296, 1977.

Lynch, P. M., Lynch, H. T., Harris, R. E.: Hereditary proximal colonic cancer. Dis. Colon Rectum 20:661, 1977.

Maskens, A. P.: Histogenesis and growth pattern of 1,2-dimethyl-hydrazine–induced rat colon adenocarcinoma. Cancer Res 36:1585, 1976.

Maskens, A. P. and Dujardin-Loits, R.-M.: Experimental adenomas and carcinomas of the large intestine behave as distinct entities. Cancer 47:81, 1981.

Mills, S. E., Allen, M. S., Jr., Cohen, A. R.: Small-cell undifferentiated carcinoma of the colon. Am. J. Surg. Pathol. 7:643, 1983.

Mills, S. E. and Fechner, R. E.: Unusual adenomatous polyps in juvenile polyposis coli. Am. J. Surg. Pathol. 6:177, 1982.

Ming-Chai, C., Chi-Yuan, C., Pei-Yu, C., Jen-Chun, H.: Evolution of colorectal cancer in schistosomiasis. Cancer 46:1661, 1980.

Moldofsky, P. J., Sears, H. F., Mulhern, C. B., Jr., Hammond, N. D., Powe, J., Gatenby, R. A., Steplewski, Z., Koprowski, H.: Detection of metastatic tumor in normal-sized retroperitoneal lymph nodes by monoclonal-antibody imaging. N. Engl. J. Med. 311:106, 1984.

Monga, G., Mazzucco, G., Rossini, F. P., Presti, F.: Colorectal polyposis with mixed juvenile and adenomatous patterns. Virch. Arch. [A] 382:355, 1979.

Moorcraft, J., DuBoulay, C. E. H., Isaacson, P., Atwell, J. D.: Changes in the mucosa of colon conduits with particular reference to the risk of malignant change. Br. J. Urol. 55:185, 1983.

Morson, B.: Personal communication.

Perzin, K. H., Peterson, M., Castiglione, C. L., Fenoglio, C. M., Wolff, M.: Intramucosal carcinoma of the small intestine arising in regional enteritis (Crohn's disease). Cancer 54:151, 1984.

Petersen, S. E., Lorentzen, M., Bichel, P.: A mosaic subpopulation structure of human colorectal carcinomas demonstrated by flow cytometry. In Laerum, O. D., Lindmo, T., Thorud, E. (eds.): Flow Cytometry IV. Acta. Pathol. Microbiol. Scand. [A] (Suppl. 274), 1980, pp. 412–416.

Prioleau, P. G., Santa Cruz, D. J., Meyer, J. S., Bauer, W. C.: Verrucous carcinoma. Cancer 45:2849, 1980.

Qizilbash, A. H.: Pathologic studies in colorectal cancer. In Somers, S. C. and Rosen, P. P. (eds.): Pathology Annual, Part I. Vol. 17. New York, Appleton-Century-Crofts, 1982, p. 1.

Ramaswamy, G., Elhossliny, A. A., Tchenthoff, J.: Juvenile polyposis of the colon with atypical adenomatous changes and carcinoma in situ. Dis. Colon Rectum 27:393, 1984.

Rattinger, M. D., Dunn, T. L., Christian, C. D., Jr., Donnell, R. M., Collins, R. D., O'Leary, J. P., Flexner, J. M.: Gastrointestinal involvement in lymphomatoid granulomatosis. Cancer 51:694, 1983.

Riddell, R. H., Goldman, H., Ransohoff, D. F., et al.: Dysplasia in inflammatory bowel disease. Standardized classification with provisional clinical applications. Hum. Pathol. 14:931, 1983.

Rognum, T. O., Elgjo, K., Fausa, O., Brandtzaeg, P.: Immunohistochemical evaluation of carcino-embryonic antigen, secretory component, and epithelial IgA in ulcerative colitis with dysplasia. Gut 23:123, 1982.

Saffos, R. O. and Rhatigen, R. M.: Benign (nonpolypoid) mucosal changes adjacent to carcinomas of the colon. Hum. Pathol. 8:441, 1977.

Schipper, H. and Decter, A.: Carcinoma of the colon arising at ureteral implant sites despite early external diversion. Cancer 47:2062, 1981.

Sears, H. F., Herlyn, M., Del Villano, B., Steplewski, Z., Koprowski, H.: Monoclonal antibody detection of a circulating tumor-associated antigen. J. Clin. Immunol. 2:141, 1982.

Shamsuddin, A. K. M., Bell, H. G., Petrucci, J. V., Trump, B. F.: Carcinoma in-situ and "micro invasive" adenocarcinoma of colon. Pathol. Res. Pract. 167:374, 1980.

Shamsuddin, A. K. M. and Elias, E. G.: Rectal mucossa. Malignant and premalignant changes after radiation therapy. Arch. Pathol. Lab. Med. 105:150, 1981a.

Shamsuddin, A. K. M., Weiss, L., Phelps, P. C., Trump, B. F.: Colon epithelium. IV. Human colon carcinogenesis. Changes in human colon mucosa adjacent to and remote from carcinomas of the colon. J. Natl. Cancer Inst. 66:413, 1981b.

Shamsuddin, A. M.: Microscopic intraepithelial neoplasia in large bowel mucosa. Hum. Pathol. 13:510, 1982.

Singh, G. and Hellstrom, H. R.: Lymphomatoid graulomatosis. Hum. Pathol. 9:364, 1978.

Spjut, H. J., Frankel, N. B., Appel, M. F.: The small carcinoma of the large bowel. Am. J. Surg. Pathol. 3:39, 1979.

Strauss, R. A. and Pascal, R. R.: Invasive and metastasizing carcinoma in a small adenomatous polyp of the colon. Hum. Pathol. 6:256, 1975.

Thurnherr, N., Deschner, E. E., Stonehill, E. H., Lipkin, M.: Induction of adenocarcinoma of the colon in mice by weekly injection of 1,2-dimethylhydrazine. Cancer Res. 33:940, 1973.

Urbanski, S. J., Kossakowska, A. E., Marcon, N., Bruce, W. R.: Mixed hyperplastic adenomatous polyps—an underdiagnosed entity. Am. J. Surg. Pathol. 8:551, 1984.

Warkel, R. L., Cooper, P. H., Helwig, E. B.: Adenocarcinoid, a mucin-producing carcinoid tumor of the appendix. Cancer 42:2781, 1978.

Warren, R. and Barwick, K. W.: Crohn's colitis with carcinoma and dysplasia. Am. J. Surg. Pathol. 7:151, 1983.

Wheat, M. W., Jr. and Ackerman, L. V.: Villous adenomas of the large intestine. Ann. Surg. 147:476, 1958.

Wilcox, G. M. and Colacchio, T. A.: Is polypectomy alone adequate for carcinoma in situ? Gastroenterology 83:716, 1982.

Wolley, R. C., Schreiber, K., Koss, L. G., et al.: DNA distribution in human colon carcinomas and its relationship to clinical behavior. J. Natl. Cancer Inst. 69:15, 1982.

ZSUZSA SCHAFF
KAROLY LAPIS
DONALD EARL HENSON

9 Liver

PRIMARY HEPATOCELLULAR CARCINOMA

Epidemiology

Primary hepatocellular carcinoma is one of the ten most common cancers in the world (Lancet editorial, 1983) and one of the most fatal of all malignancies (Popper, 1979; Szmuness, 1978). It is relatively rare among the white population of the United States (London, 1981; Sandler et al., 1983) and in Europe (Axelsson, 1982; London 1981).

Compared with mortality rates associated with primary hepatocellular carcinoma in low-incidence countries, the death rates are 10 to 20 times greater in high-incidence areas, such as sub-Saharan Africa (Anthony et al., 1973; Kew, 1978; Szmuness, 1978) and Southeast Asia (China, Japan, Korea, Thailand) (Beasly et al., 1981; Gibson et al., 1980; Lai et al., 1981; Nakashima et al., 1983; Okuda, 1980).

According to the World Health Organization, over 250,000 new cases of liver cancer occur each year in the world. In fact, the incidence seems to be increasing. Selected cancer registries covering 37 populations in 18 countries have noted a significant increase in 17 of the populations for males and in 10 for females (Saracci and Repetto, 1980).

All epidemiologic studies have shown a higher incidence of primary hepatocellular carcinoma among males than among females (Saracci and Repetto, 1980).

The age distribution of hepatocellular carcinoma varies with the incidence (Szmuness, 1978). Patients in high-incidence areas are younger; for example, in Mozambique, where the highest rates have been recorded, most cases occur in the third and fourth decades (Kew, 1978). In lower-incidence areas, the

peak age is higher: the mean age was found to be 59.4 years in an Italian study (Pagliaro et al., 1983), 53 years in American blacks, and 61 years in American whites (Steiner, 1960). Primary hepatocellular carcinoma among children is rare, even in high-incidence areas (Landing, 1976).

Etiology

Etiologic factors associated with the majority of cases of primary hepatocellular carcinoma are hepatitis B virus infection, chronic alcohol abuse, and mycotoxins, especially aflatoxin (Popper, 1979). In addition, sex hormones (Williams, 1982), occupational risk factors, medication (Stemhagen et al., 1983), and metabolic alterations (Bannasch et al., 1980) are rare etiologic factors.

It is generally accepted that in humans tumor development takes many years and resembles the multistep process of chemically induced neoplasms in animals (Farber and Cameron, 1980). Studies of chemical carcinogenesis in animals have focused on the early events of neoplastic transformation, in contrast to humans in whom only the late stages of tumor formation can be studied (Farber, 1982).

Prognosis and Diagnosis

Hepatocellular carcinoma is associated with a poor prognosis. Conventional modalities of therapy have not been satisfactory. The median survival is less than 3 months for debilitated patients and less than 6 months for those who are more fit. A particularly fulminant course has been observed in blacks in South Africa. Patients usually die within 4 months after onset of symptoms (Kew, 1978). The poor prognosis is related in part to the advanced stage at the time of

This chapter was prepared under the Bilateral Hungarian–U.S. Cancer Agreement.

167

diagnosis as well as to the large tumor size, multiple sites of origin, and coexistence of cirrhosis.

The treatment of hepatic carcinoma has improved (Kishi et al., 1983; Okuda et al., 1977b). The observation that some primary lesions, especially the minute ones, have a distinct fibrous capsule suggests that at least initially the tumor grows slowly in an expansive, non-infiltrating fashion (Okuda et al., 1977a and b). The most significant factor influencing survival is the size of the tumor at the time of diagnosis. For this reason, research has turned to early detection and diagnosis.

The various diagnostic methods for the detection of primary hepatocellular carcinoma have different values. Alpha-fetoprotein (AFP), the most effective screening marker for advanced disease (Lehmann, 1978), may be a useful indicator of small hepatocellular carcinomas in some cases. Takashima and co-workers (1982), studying 29 small (under 5 cm) carcinomas in 18 patients, showed that lesions less than 1 cm in diameter can be detected only by angiography. Technetium 99m–sulfur colloid liver scans, ultrasonography with gray-scale real time, and computed tomography do not easily demonstrate lesions smaller than 2 cm but can detect those larger than 3 cm (Takashima et al., 1982).

Two important procedures for the diagnosis of primary hepatocellular carcinoma are laparoscopy and liver biopsy. Liver biopsy is desirable in all suspected cases. However, the type of biopsy—"blind," peritoneoscopic, surgical, or fine-needle aspiration—should be carefully considered because of the possibility of postbiopsy bleeding (Reynolds, 1976). Although fine-needle aspiration biopsy is safe and reliable (Lundquist, 1970), coarse-needle biopsy is more widely used (Jacobsen et al., 1983), especially with ultrasonographic guidance (Nosher and Plafker, 1980). Laparoscopy is useful in the diagnosis of early malignant tumors that involve the liver in a focal fashion (Lightdale, 1982). This method has several advantages. It allows one to choose a biopsy site away from surface vessels, to obtain samples by brush cytology, and to collect staging information.

Obviously, the preceding data concerning the epidemiology and prognosis of primary hepatocellular carcinoma only increase the importance for early diagnosis. In the case of "small," or "minute" types, a poor prognosis is also possible (Okuda et al., 1977a), and for this reason increased efforts should be made for an even earlier diagnosis, when the tumor is small and surgical resection is easier to achieve (Chen et al., 1982).

BENIGN TUMORS AND TUMOR-LIKE LESIONS OF THE LIVER

Experimental studies have shown that neoplastic transformation in the liver is a multistep process (Farber, 1982). Similarly, a study of liver tumors in humans suggests that precursor lesions, including most forms of chronic liver disease, especially cirrhosis, also play a role in cancer development (Anthony, 1976; Becker, 1981; Pitot and Sirica, 1980). The role of liver cell dysplasia as a premalignant change seems to be important (Anthony et al., 1973; Cohen et al., 1979). Hepatocellar adenomas and neoplastic nodules experimentally induced in animals share several common morphologic and functional features with liver tumors in humans, including loss or increase of certain enzyme activities and potential regression or progression (Farber, 1982; Thung and Gerber, 1981).

The association of contraceptive steroids with benign liver tumors has attracted considerable attention. Studies have also suggested a connection between adenomas and carcinomas (Tesluk and Lawrie, 1981). The characteristics of premalignant lesions and benign tumors are summarized in Table 9–1.

Liver Cell Adenoma

Liver cell adenomas are usually solitary, well-circumscribed, benign neoplasms (Ishak, 1981). These tumors occur in normal livers, are sharply demarcated from surrounding liver tissue, and are occasionally encapsulated (Fig. 9–1). They vary from less than 1 cm to more than 20 cm in size. The cut surface is usually softer than surrounding liver and has a light yellowish-brown color. Larger tumors often show

Table 9–1. Characteristics of Different Premalignant Lesions and Benign Tumors of the Liver

Lesion	Distribution	Size	Fibrosis	Dysplasia
Cirrhosis	Diffuse	Small or large	Present	Might be present
Focal nodular hyperplasia	Single	Large	Present	Absent
Nodular transformation (NT)	Diffuse	Small	Absent	Might be present
Partial NT	Partially diffuse	Small to large	Absent	
Adenoma	Single	Large	Absent	Might be present

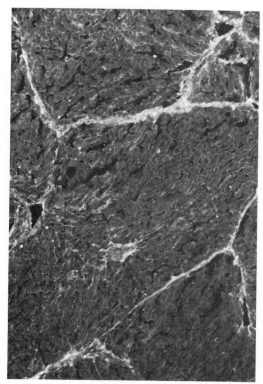

Figure 9–19. Frozen section of cirrhotic human liver stained with fluorescein-isothiocyanate–conjugated antifibronectin. Fibronectin can be seen in septa and along the sinusoids.

entiated tumors, laminin staining was not seen by immunohistochemical methods.

Cholangiocellular carcinomas do not contain fibronectin; only laminin is seen around the tumor cells that formed tubules (Fig. 9–23).

Enzyme Activity Changes

Changes in the activity of certain enzymes as phenotypic markers for malignant cells are becoming important in the diagnosis of early lesions. Enzyme changes have been studied in detail in some animal models. In all these models, there is a brief exposure to an initiating carcinogen followed by exposure to a promoting agent, the effect of which can be simulated in the proliferating liver of a young animal (Peraino et al., 1973) or in the liver of an adult animal after partial hepatectomy (Pitot and Sirica, 1980; Scherer and Emmelot, 1976), or after the proliferation that follows cell necrosis (Ogawa et al., 1980). As a result of different combinations of treatment schedules, foci (clear cell, eosinophilic, basophilic, and mixed), hyperplastic nodules, or neoplastic nodules appear (Figs. 9–24 and 25).

A number of morphologic and functional properties distinguish the altered foci and hyperplastic nodules from the surrounding hepatocytes. The loss of glycose-6-phosphatase (G6P-ase) (Fig. 9–26A), membrane-bound canalicular adenosine triphosphatase (ATP-ase) (Fig. 9–26B), beta-glucoronidase, serine hydratase, acid phosphatase, and glycogen phosphatase activity and the increase in gamma-glutamyltranspeptidase (GGT-ase) activity, expression of preneoplastic antigen, and deficiency to stored iron can be demonstrated histochemically in the hyperplastic nodules and altered foci (Bannasch et al., 1980; Farber, 1982; Ogawa et al., 1980; Pitot and Sirica, 1980).

Less information is available in human cases, although studies suggest a similar pattern of enzymatic changes during neoplastic transformation (Thung and Gerber, 1981; Uchida et al., 1981).

Primary hepatocellular carcinomas show an increase in GGT-ase activity, whereas the activities of G6P-ase and ATP-ase are lost in most cases (Gerber and Thung, 1980; Uchida et al., 1981).

In contrast to carcinomas, liver cell adenomas show ATP-ase and G6P-ase activities but no GGT-ase activity (Gerber and Thung, 1980). Increase in GGT-ase and loss of G6P-ase and ATP-ase were demonstrated in a case of nodular transformation of the liver (Thung and Gerber, 1981).

Text continued on page 187

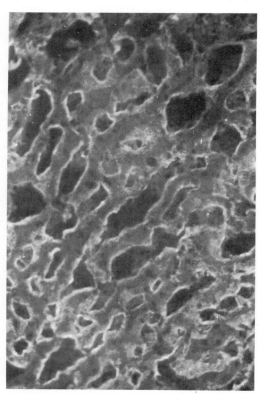

Figure 9–20. Frozen section of focal nodular hyperplasia of the liver stained with fluorescein-isothiocyanate–conjugated antifibronectin. The fibronectin is localized along the distorted sinusoids in a linear form.

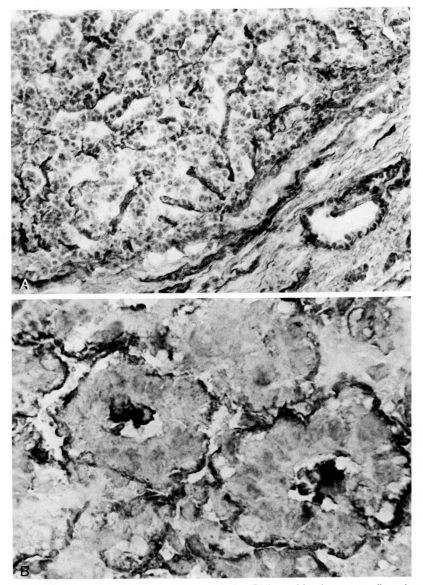

Figure 9–21. Fibronectin is localized around the trabeculae *(A)* and tubules *(B)* formed by the tumor cells and occasionally in the lumen of the tubules *(B)*, in cases of well-differentiated hepatocellular carcinoma (immunoperoxidase).

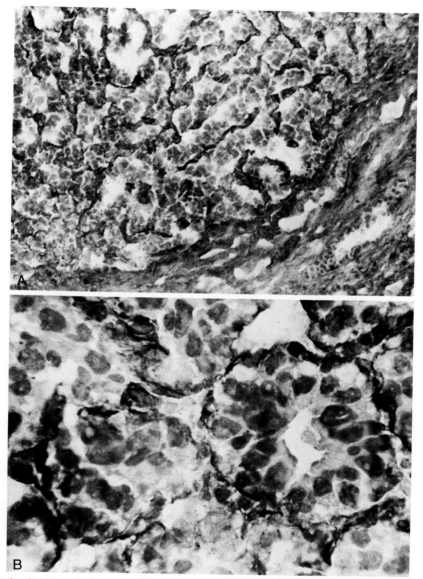

Figure 9–22. Laminin is localized in a similar way to fibronectin around the trabeculae *(A)* and tubules *(B)* formed by the tumor cells in the same cases of primary hepatocellular carcinomas (immunoperoxidase).

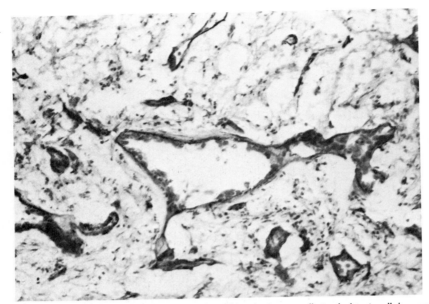

Figure 9–23. Laminin can be demonstrated around the tubules formed by the tumor cells in cholangiocellular carcinoma (immunoperoxidase).

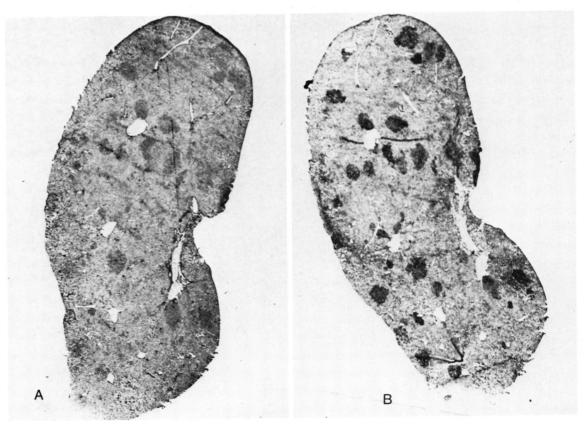

Figure 9–24. Histologic section of rat liver after 3 months of carcinogen (diaminobenzidine) treatment and partial hepatectomy. Neoplastic nodules can be seen on hematoxylin and eosin–stained section (A). Glycogen storage of the nodules can be demonstrated after periodic acid-Schiff reaction (B).

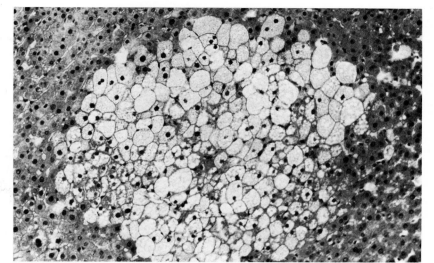

Figure 9–25. Focus composed of clear cells in carcinogen (diaminobenzidine)–treated rat liver.

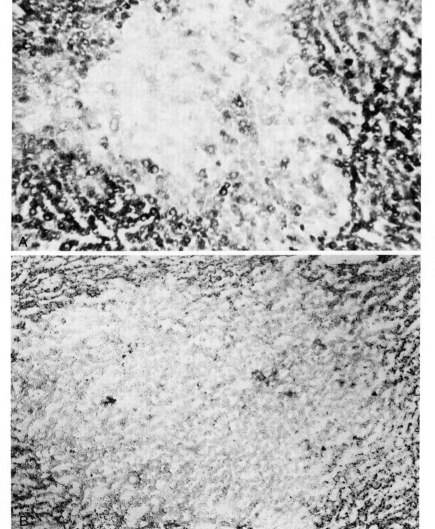

Figure 9–26. Activity of glucose-6-phosphatase *(A)* and adenosine-triphosphatase *(B)* disappears in the foci, in contrast to the surrounding liver in rats treated as in Figure 9–24.

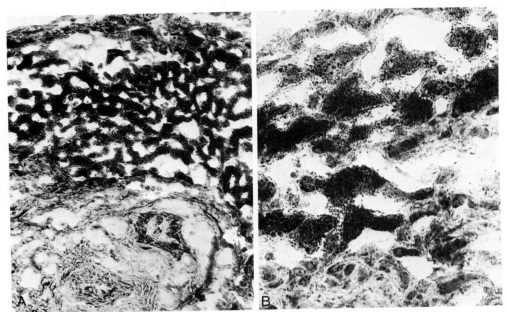

Figure 9–27. A strong positive reaction to gamma-glutamyl-transpeptidase is present in a case of focal nodular hyperplasia of the liver in a 28-year-old woman who has taken oral contraceptives for 2 years.

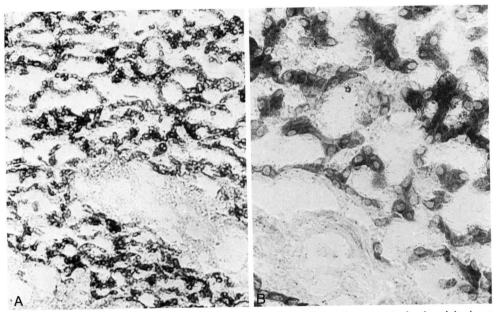

Figure 9–28. *A,B,* A positive (normal) reaction of the activity of glucose-6-phosphatase is present in focal nodular hyperplasia from the same case as in Figure 9–27.

An increased positivity of the GGT-ase (Fig. 9–27) and a normal (positive) reaction of G6P-ase (Fig. 9–28) and loss of ATP-ase activity were detected in focal nodular hyperplasia of the liver (Schaff et al., 1984).

Because there are only a small number of cases studied by histochemical methods, it is not yet possible to draw a conclusion about the phenotypic characteristics of different tumors and tumor-like lesions of the human liver. However, the sporadic cases studied suggest a similar pattern of enzymatic changes during tumor development in humans. These patterns may also be used to define these lesions.

Hepatitis B Virus (HBV) Antigens

Evidence suggesting a causal relationship between HBV infection and primary hepatocellular carcinoma was initially based on epidemiologic observations (Gerin, 1983; Lancet editorial, 1983):

□ Primary hepatocellular carcinoma occurs most commonly in regions where chronic carriers of HBV are found (London, 1982; Popper et al., 1982; Szmuness, 1978)—sub-Saharan Africa, Southeast Asia, and China.

□ Patients with primary hepatocellular carcinoma (in both high-incidence and low-incidence areas) show significantly higher frequencies of serologic markers (HBsAg and anti-HBc) of persistent HBV infection than controls (Blumberg and London, 1981; Szmuness, 1978; Tabor et al., 1977).

□ HBV proteins (HBsAg, less frequently HBcAg) are present in the livers of most patients with primary hepatocellular carcinoma from endemic areas and in many patients from low-incidence areas (London, 1981; Popper et al., 1982).

□ Some cell lines established from primary hepatocellular carcinoma produce HBsAg. Viral antigen production continues even after injection of the tumor into nude mice (Shouval et al., 1982).

□ In high-risk areas of the world, perinatal infection and infection in early life—particularly infection transmitted from chronic carrier mothers to their children—are very important in the development of the carrier state (Blumberg and London, 1981; Tabor et al., 1983).

□ HBV DNA is present in primary hepatocellular carcinoma tissue (Summers and Mason, 1982).

□ Integration of HBV DNA into the host cell genome in HBsAg-producing cell lines and tissues of primary hepatocellular carcinoma has been demonstrated (Brechot et al., 1980; Charkraborty et al., 1980; Edman et al., 1980).

□ Persistent infection with a virus similar to HBV is associated with spontaneous liver cancers of woodchucks (Summers et al., 1978), Chinese domestic ducks, domestic Peking ducks in the United States, and ground squirrels (Blumberg and London, 1981).

□ Immunotherapy of human hepatoma–bearing nude mice in which monoclonal antibodies were used against HBsAg has prevented or suppressed tumor formation (Shouval et al., 1982).

□ Prospective studies have predicted the risk of primary hepatocellular carcinoma in chronic HBsAg carriers (Beasley et al., 1981).

HBV antigens have been localized in tumor cells by immunohistochemical methods (Hirohashi et al., 1982) and orcein staining (Shikata et al., 1974). The proportion of liver tumors that express both HBsAg and HBcAg is small—less than 5 percent (Hirohashi et al., 1982). HBsAg-positive and HBcAg-negative cases were found in three of 60 hepatocellular carcinomas, and HBsAg-negative and HBcAg-positive hepatoma cases were demonstrated in only two of 60 cases studied (Hirohashi et al., 1982). HBsAg was detected in seven of nine serologically HBsAg-positive primary hepatocellular carcinomas. The surface antigen is expressed as fine granules in the cytoplasm of malignant cells. The cytoplasm did not have a ground glass appearance, and cell membranes were negative (Thung et al., 1979). HBcAg was not present in any primary hepatocellular carcinomas in these series. HBsAg is localized only in the cytoplasm, whereas HBcAg occurs in nuclei (Hirohashi et al., 1982). Tumor cells that contained both HBsAg and HBcAg have been reported in only one case (Hirohashi et al., 1982). These results suggest both the production of complete virus by tumor cells and the presence of complete virus genomes within tumor cells (Hirohashi et al., 1982).

A greater number of HBV antigen–positive hepatocytes are found in the non-tumorous areas of the liver. HBsAg is localized either diffusely or within the inclusion bodies in the cytoplasm or in a submembranous pattern (Fig. 9–29), similar to the distribution of HBsAg in other liver diseases (Camilleri et al., 1977; Gudat et al., 1975; Nayak and Sachdeva, 1975). HBcAg has been localized mainly in the nuclei of liver cells and occasionally in the cytoplasm of hepatocytes (Hirohashi et al., 1982). HBsAg and HBcAg are usually expressed in different cells, but occasionally they are observed in the same cell. HBsAg has been localized in some of the dysplastic liver cells, but HBcAg has been seen rarely (Hirhashi et al., 1982).

A 27-nm core particle of the HBV is located in the nuclei of hepatocytes (Fig. 9–30A). The 22 nm–diameter spherical and filamentous particles known to contain HBsAg determinants (Gerber et al., 1974) might be present in the dilated endoplasmic reticulum cisternae (Fig. 9–30B).

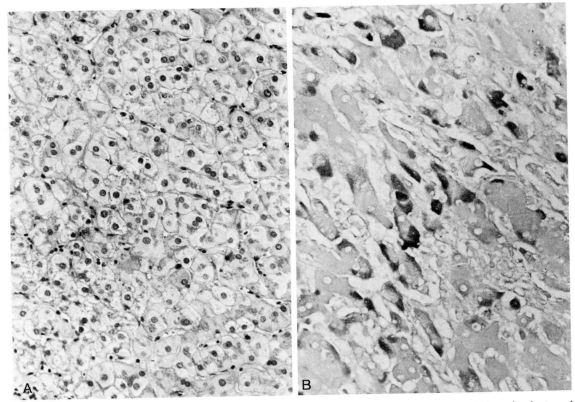

Figure 9–29. *A,* Ground-glass hepatocytes in a chronic carrier of hepatitis B surface antigen (HBsAg). *B,* Different distribution of HBsAg can be seen on section stained with Shikata-orcein in the non-tumorous part of the liver in a case of primary hepatocellular carcinoma.

MORPHOLOGIC CHARACTERISTICS OF PRIMARY HEPATOCELLULAR CARCINOMA

It is not our purpose to furnish a detailed description of the advanced forms of liver cancer. However, to describe the characteristics of early hepatic cancer, we must review the terminology of primary hepatocellular carcinoma.

Gross Anatomy

Several classifications have been used to describe the gross appearance of primary hepatocellular carcinoma. However, none has gained general acceptance because of wide variation in the gross appearance of the tumor.

In general, three types—nodular, massive, and diffuse—are recognized (Edmondson, 1958; Lapis and Johannessen, 1979). In the *nodular* form, the tumor consists of large nodules, clearly delineated from the surrounding non-involved liver tissue. The *massive* type replaces a large area of liver (almost an entire lobe) and infiltrates the surroundings. In the *diffuse* form, the entire liver is usually involved by multiple tumor nodules.

A classification based on the growth pattern of the tumor in relation to the surrounding parenchyma and blood vessels includes the *infiltrative* (spreading), the *expanding* (solitary), the *multinodular* (multiple), and *mixed* types (Nakashima et al., 1983).

Peters (1976) subdivided the gross patterns of primary hepatocellular carcinoma into *diffuse, multicentric, inductive, expanding, megalonodular,* and *sclerosing.* Occasionally, pedunculated forms of primary hepatocellular carcinoma have been observed (Horie et al., 1983). Encapsulated primary hepatocellular carcinoma is considered to be a distinct morphologic entity (Nakashima et al., 1983).

Histologic Patterns

The chief features for characterizing the histologic appearance are cytologic differentiation, the formation of cords, trabeculae or cylindrical structures, and the stromal development of the tumor.

Cytologic Differentiation

One of the most common features of primary hepatocellular carcinoma is the similarity of its tumor cells to non-neoplastic, normal hepatic cord cells. Nonetheless, anaplasia (dedifferentiation) or pleomorphism or both occur to a variable extent. Differentiation is an important criterion for grading liver cell carcinomas. The morphologic appearance of the tumor cells can be characterized by the cytoplasm's staining quality (acidophilic), the cellular form (polyhedral configuration), the nuclear-cytoplasmic ratio, and the cohesiveness of the tumor cells (Jagoe et al., 1982).

Cytoplasmic inclusions such as Mallory bodies, hyalin globules, vacuoles filled with proteinous material, lipid droplets, bile plugs, and fingerprint-like membrane organization (Schaff et al., 1971) often occur in well-differentiated hepatocellular carcinomas (Fig. 9–31). Inability to store hemosiderin is a characteristic of the tumor cells (Edmondson, 1958).

Bile canaliculi can usually be seen by electron microscopy. However, the microvilli surrounding the canaliculi are often decreased in number and usually abnormal (Fig. 9–32) (Schaff et al., 1971). Intracellular lumina lined with numerous microvilli containing pale blue cytoplasmic inclusions are occasionally seen (Fig. 9–32) (An et al., 1983; Lapis, 1979).

An unusual feature of certain types of hepatocellular carcinomas is the presence of clear, oncocytic, giant, and spindle cells. The *clear cells* closely resemble the cells of a renal "clear cell" carcinoma (Fig. 9–33) (Lapis, 1980; Peters, 1976; Wu et al., 1983).

The *oncocytic cell* has a granular eosinophilic cytoplasm packed with mitochondria (Baithun and Pollock, 1983). *Giant cells* are present in some cases (Fig. 9–34), although pure giant cell carcinoma of the liver is rare. Giant cells can contain a single large nucleus, a multilobeted nucleus, or multiple nuclei that number from four to over 100. *Spindle cells* of hepatocellular origin with eosinophilic cytoplasm also can occur in carcinomas of the liver.

Histologic Growth Pattern

The histologic growth pattern of primary hepatocellular carcinoma may be well-developed, moderately developed, or undeveloped.

The *trabecular* arrangement is the most common pattern (Fig. 9–35). In the *acinar* type of growth, a canaliculus is formed by circularly arranged tumor cells. The histologic pattern can appear *tubular* (Fig.

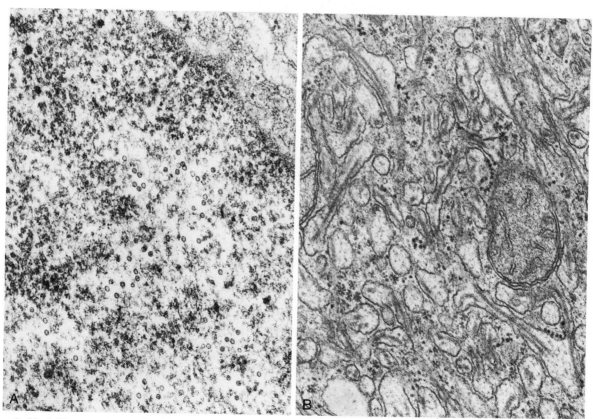

Figure 9–30. *A,* Electron micrograph of 27-nm particles of hepatitis B virus in a chronic carrier. *B,* 22-nm filaments of HbsAg are located in the endoplasmic reticulum of a hepatocyte. (*A,* uranyl acetate and lead citrate.)

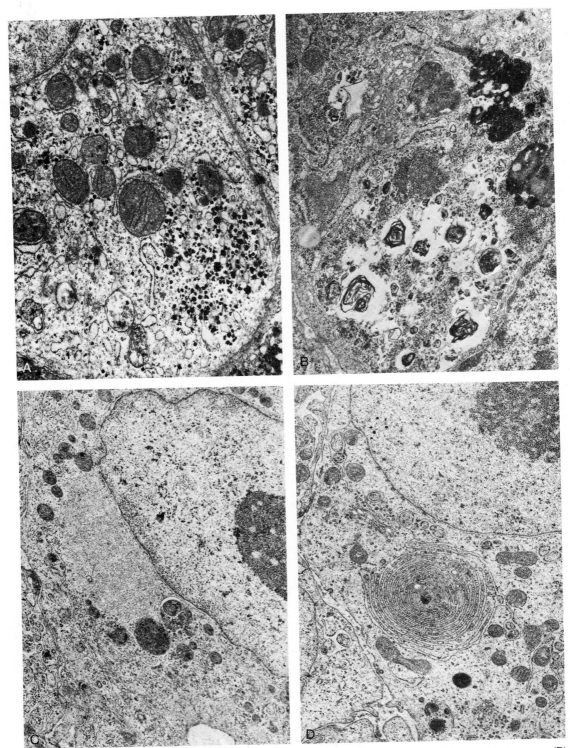

Figure 9–31. Electron micrographs of tumor cells in primary hepatocellular carcinoma. Glycogen particles *(A)*, bile pigments *(B)*, vacuoles filled with proteinaceous material *(C)*, and fingerprint-like organization of the endoplasmic reticulum *(D)* in tumor cells (uranyl acetate and lead citrate).

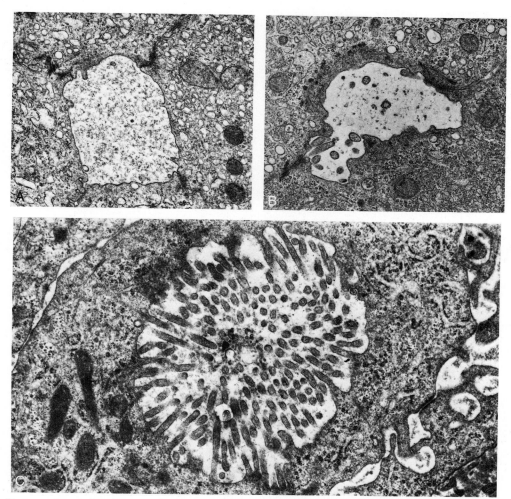

Figure 9–32. Electron micrographs of tumor cells in primary hepatocellular carcinoma. Bile canaliculi are formed by several tumor cells *(A)*. The microvilli are lost or distorted *(A,B)*. Intracytoplasmic lumen lined with numerous microvilli can be seen in a tumor cell *(C)* (uranyl acetate and lead citrate).

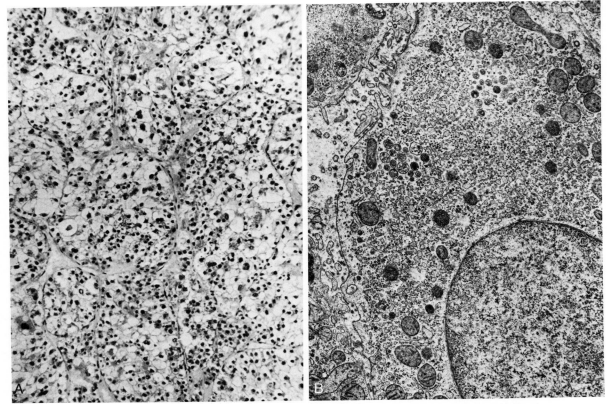

Figure 9–33. Clear cell carcinoma of the liver in a 60-year-old man. The tumor cells are arranged in groups *(A)*. By electron microscopy, an increased number of smooth endoplasmic reticulum vesicles and glycogen particles can be seen *(B)*. *(B,* uranyl acetate and lead citrate).

9–35) or *pseudoglandular* with basally placed nuclei. An increased accumulation of secreted mucinous material can produce an *adenoid* arrangement with flattened cuboidal cells (Fig. 9–36). Tumor cells also can grow in a *solid* pattern without any specific arrangement, creating a "cobblestone" appearance, as described by Peters (1976) (Fig. 9–37).

Histologic growth patterns have also been classified as *sinusoidal, replacing,* and *encapsulated,* designations that indicate the extent of malignancy (Nakashima et al., 1982).

Stromal Development

The amount and arrangement of the fibrous connective tissue and blood vessels seem to affect the histologic growth pattern. Peters (1976) noted that the connective tissue inhibits free development of the trabecular pattern but stimulates a glandular, acinar, or duct-like arrangement of the hepatic tumor cells.

Histologic Grading

The extent of differentiation and the histologic architecture are used to grade hepatocellular carcinomas.

Grade I, or highly differentiated, cancer cells (Fig. 9–38*A)*, which closely simulate normal liver cells, are observed in only a small number (3.3 percent) of liver tumors (Okuda et al., 1980). In *Grade II* (Fig. 9–38*B*), the nuclei are larger and more hyperchromic, and the cytoplasm is granular and more acidophilic. Tubular and acinar growth patterns are frequent. Bile and glycogen are often present. Nuclei are even larger and more hyperchromic in *Grade III* carcinoma. The nuclear-cytoplasmic ratio increases and the cytoplasm is less acidophilic. The trabecular growth pattern is disturbed, and cells can be seen isolated from the cords (Fig. 9–38*C*). Giant cells occur more often. Cells in *Grade IV* carcinomas have large nuclei that often occupy almost the entire cell (Fig. 9–38*D*). The cytoplasm tends to be basophilic. Trabecular or acinar structures are seldom seen. Grade II carcinomas are the most common; Grade IV cancers are the rarest (Nakashima et al., 1983).

Distinct Morphologic Subtypes

Fibrolamellar Carcinoma. This lesion has distinctive clinicopathologic features and represents a special subgroup of hepatocellular carcinomas (Chuong et al., 1982; Craig et al., 1980; Lefkowitch et al., 1983).

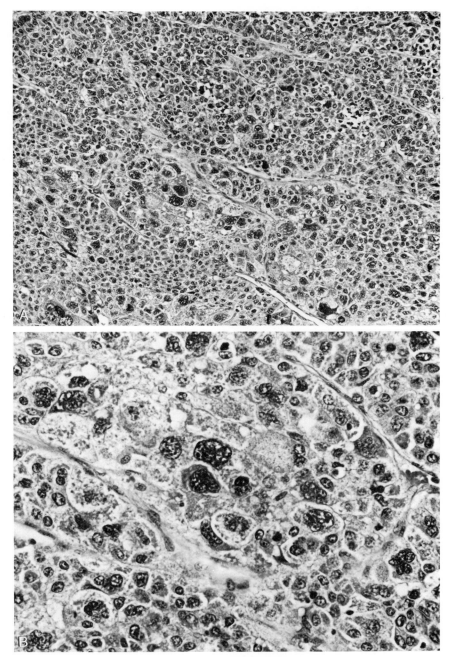

Figure 9–34. *A,B,* Giant cells in a case of primary hepatocellular carcinoma. AFIP Acc. No. 1772607.

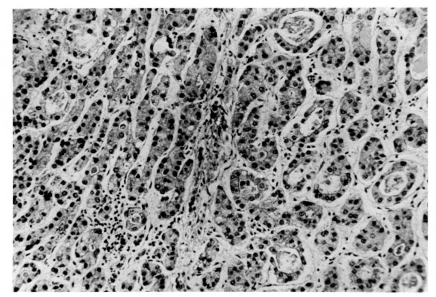

Figure 9–35. Trabecular and tubular arrangement of the tumor cells in primary hepatocellular carcinoma.

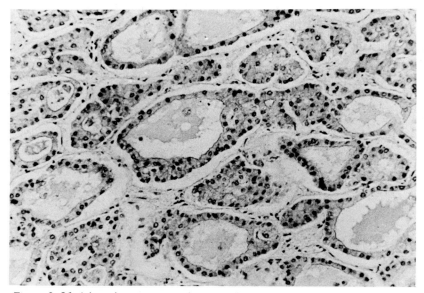

Figure 9–36. Adenoid arrangement of tumor cells in primary hepatocellular carcinoma.

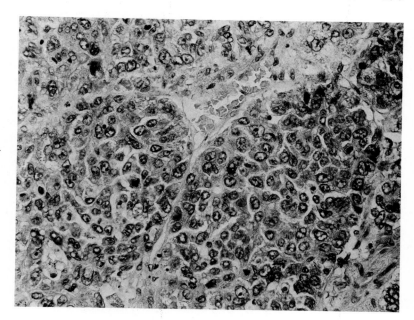

Figure 9–37. Tumor cells in primary hepatocellular carcinoma in a solid pattern.

It characteristically occurs in younger (mean age 23.1 years), non-cirrhotic patients of both sexes.

Macroscopically, the tumor is usually solitary and surrounded by normal liver tissue, although multiple nodules can occur. It can measure from 4 cm to more than 30 cm. It is seldom encapsulated (Farhi et al., 1982). Centrally, an irregular fibrous scar may develop, which causes the tumor to resemble focal nodular hyperplasia of the liver.

Histologically, the most distinct features are the broad collagen bands and fibrocytes arranged in a lamellar, fascicular pattern between groups of deeply eosinophilic polygonal tumor cells (Figs. 9–39 and 9–40). The tumors were generally Grades II to IV (Berman et al., 1980).

By electron microscopy, an increased number of swollen, closely packed mitochondria are found in the tumor cells (Baithun and Pollock, 1983; Craig, et al., 1980; Farhi et al., 1982), a feature that is also characteristic of oncocytes. The term "fibrolamellar oncocytic hepatoma" has been recommended for the tumor (Farhi et al., 1982).

Fibrolamellar carcinoma is characterized clinically by a favorable prognosis. The survival time is longer (68 months) than for other types of primary hepatocellular carcinoma, and the survival at two- and five-year intervals is 82 and 63 percent, respectively (Berman et al., 1980).

The possibility that focal nodular hyperplasia is a precursor to fibrolamellar carcinoma has been suggested but not proved (Berman et al., 1980; Chuong et al., 1982).

Clear Cell Carcinoma. Clear cells are present in focal (about 30 percent of cells) or in diffuse (more than 50 percent of the cells) forms (Lai et al., 1979) (Fig. 9–33). It has been thought that tumors having a large proportion of clear cells are less malignant than other types of hepatocellular carcinomas (Altmann, 1978; Wu et al., 1983). However, in a 1974 study of 13 cases, Buchanan and Huvos were unable to demonstrate any differences in the biologic behavior between clear cell carcinomas and other types of liver cancer. In another study, it was reported that survival is better with the presence of clear cells and that it even improves with increasing proportion of clear cells (Lai et al., 1979).

Clear cells also occur during experimental chemical hepatocarcinogenesis, usually in an intermediate stage of tumor development, before the lipid-and glycogen-poor basophilic malignant cells appear. This raises the possibility that "clear cells" are less malignant than the basophilic malignant hepatocytes in animal systems and that a similar mechanism could exist in humans (Wu et al., 1983).

Background Liver Disorders

As previously noted, the non-cancerous areas of the liver in a high percentage of patients show cirrhosis or extensive fibrosis. Cirrhosis or fibrosis is found in over 80 percent of cases of primary hepatocellular carcinoma (Okuda, 1980; Shikata, 1976). In the majority of cases (63.8 percent), mixed micro- and macronodular cirrhosis is the dominant lesion (Nakashima et al., 1983). Cases in which there are grossly unremarkable parenchymal changes usually show portal inflammation and fibrosis histologically. The weight of the liver with an unremarkable parenchyma

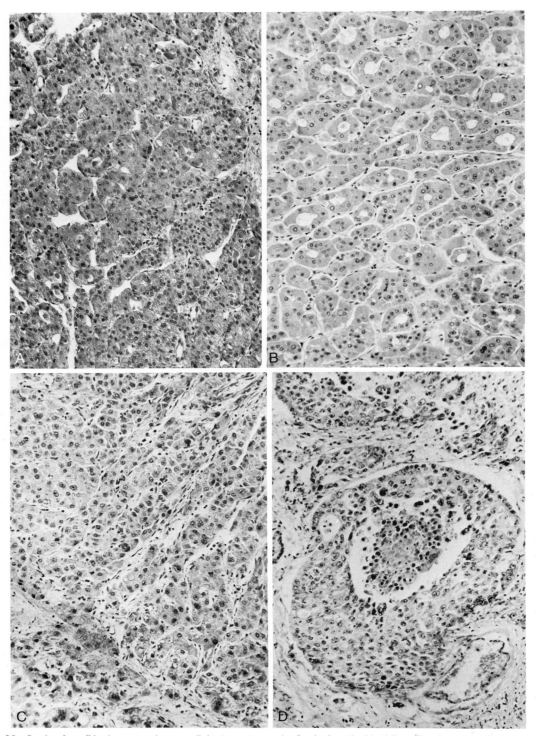

Figure 9–38. Grades I to IV of primary hepatocellular carcinoma. *A*, Grade I or highly-differentiated tumor simulates the normal arrangement of the liver cells. *B*, Grade II shows a tubular arrangement of the tumor cells. *C*, In Grade III the trabecular growth pattern is disturbed; tumor cells are often isolated from the cords of tumor cells. *D*, Grade IV shows anaplastic growth of tumor cells. Large nuclei and necrosis is common.

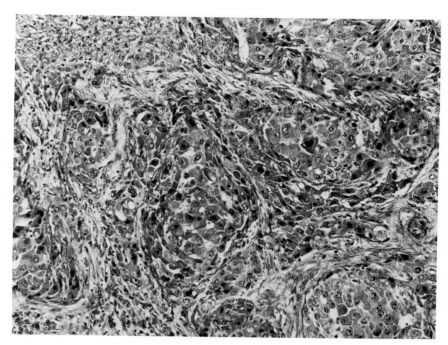

Figure 9–39. Fibrolamellar carcinoma of the liver. Tumor cells, with eosinophilic, polygonal cytoplasm, arranged in groups surrounded by fibrous tissue. AFIP Acc. No. 1720450.

is generally greater than that of a cirrhotic liver in cases of hepatocellular carcinoma. Non-cirrhotic livers can be divided into two groups, based on the extent of fibrosis: those showing a tendency to increasing grade of anaplasia as the degree of fibrosis increases and those demonstrating an inverse correlation between the extent of fibrosis and the anaplasia (Okuda et al., 1982). A history of hepatitis was found in 75 percent of 1556 cases of primary hepatocellular carcinoma in the same series (Okuda, 1980). In another study, it was observed that primary hepatocellular carcinoma developed when cirrhosis was not advanced or in a precirrhotic stage of chronic hepatitis (Lai et al., 1981). A high association (92 percent) between primary hepatocellular carcinoma and postnecrotic cirrhosis has been reported (Lai et al., 1981). Fibrolamellar carcinoma of the liver is not associated with cirrhosis.

Association Between Prognosis and Histology

It was mentioned previously that the fibrolamellar and clear cell types of liver cancer have a better prognosis. However, in a study of 80 cases of primary hepatocellular carcinoma in Hong Kong, no correlation was found between survival and cytologic differentiation, histologic growth pattern, degree of pleomorphism or presence of bile, proteinaceous secretion, giant cells, or hyalin bodies (Lai et al., 1979). The presence of clear cells is the only histologic feature that seems to have prognostic significance.

The histologic growth patterns termed "sinusoidal," "replacing," and "encapsulated" reflect not only the degree of malignancy but also the gross appearance (Nakashima et al., 1982). As a gross anatomic growth pattern, the expanding primary hepatocellular carcinoma is a relatively benign tumor; the infiltrating, or spreading, type is more malignant; and the diffuse type has a rapid fatal course.

The histologic growth pattern of hepatocellular carcinoma seems to depend on the background liver pathology. The negative correlation between fibrosis and anaplasia has already been mentioned. Carcinomas arising in highly cirrhotic livers tend to be more differentiated than those arising in noncirrhotic livers (Okuda et al., 1982).

EARLY CANCER

Diagnosis of liver cancer in its early stage has importance in the treatment. Serum alpha-fetoprotein and celiac angiography seem to be useful in early diagnosis (Okuda et al., 1978).

It has been proposed that liver tumors not exceeding 4.5 cm in diameter or multiple tumors, each one less than 3.5 cm in diameter, be designated "minute hepatocellular carcinoma" (Okuda et al., 1977b). The "small hepatocellular carcinoma" is defined as solitary (less than 5 cm) or multinodular (main tumor less than 4 cm) (Takashima et al., 1982). Fewer than 100 cases of small hepatocellular carcinoma have been published. Almost all the cases have been observed in Japan. No early or minute carcinomas have been

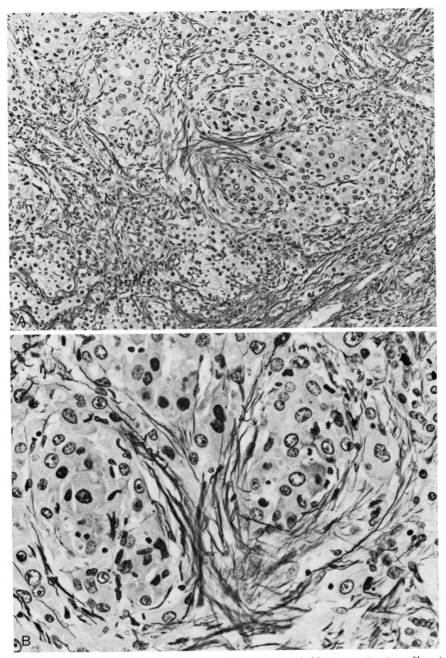

Figure 9–40. Fibrolamellar carcinoma of the liver. Groups of tumor cells are surrounded by connective tissue fibers in a lamellar, fascicular pattern (reticulin stain). AFIP Acc. No. 1720450.

reported from the areas of the world in which primary hepatocellular carcinoma has the highest incidence, such as South Africa.

Small hepatocellular carcinomas are usually found in small livers with advanced cirrhosis (Okuda et al., 1978). They grow slowly and are negative for HBsAg. This suggests that these tumors have a different pathogenesis than those developing rapidly in non-cirrhotic livers. Because data are not available for the early stage of fast-growing cases, only the information accumulated from studies of the "minute" or small forms can be summarized.

Gross Anatomic Findings

The solitary (less than 5 cm) and multiple (less than 4 cm) tumor nodules are usually well circumscribed and round or oval in shape and are frequently located near the capsule, most often in the right lobe (Chen et al., 1982; Kondo et al., 1983). The primary lesion is often surrounded by a fibrous capsule. In one study, 23 cases of minute carcinoma were classified grossly as expanding in 20 cases, spreading in one case, and multinodular in two cases (Nakashima et al., 1983). The diffuse type has not been reported. The tumor has a white or brownish-yellow to green color and a soft consistency (Chen et al., 1982; Kondo et al., 1983; Okuda et al., 1977b). Hemorrhage and necrosis are occasionally seen.

Most of the reported cases of minute carcinoma have been associated with cirrhosis (Kanematsu et al., 1981; Kobayashi et al., 1977; Kondo et al., 1983).

Histology

Well-differentiated carcinomas have been found in most of the cases of minute hepatocellular carcinoma (Kondo et al., 1983; Nakoshima et al., 1983; Yoshida et al., 1982). Trabecular arrangement of the tumor cells is most common (Kondo et al., 1983; Okuda et al., 1977b). The tumor is usually Grade I or II, although Grade III is seen as well. Nuclear atypia is often seen. Mitoses can be observed occasionally.

The cytoplasm of the tumor cells is usually basophilic rather than eosinophilic, and bile congestion can be present. Various degrees of stromal fibrosis, which produces broad anastomosing trabeculae, may occur. Reticulin fibers tightly surround the cords formed by the tumor cells. The tumor nodules are usually separated by a fibrous pseudocapsule from surrounding cirrhotic nodules. Capsular invasion is common, and invasive growth without any encapsulation also has been observed.

Tumor Markers

Alpha-fetoprotein is moderately elevated in 50 percent of cases of early primary hepatocellular carcinoma (Nakashima et al., 1983; Okuda et al., 1977b). As a screening method, AFP seems to be the best, followed by ultrasonography and computed tomography (Takashima et al., 1982). Determination of serum AFP levels and diagnostic ultrasound are recommended for minimization of both cost and radiation exposure. However, no morphologic study of tumor markers in cases of small primary hepatocellular carcinoma has been reported.

Hepatitis B surface antigen was positive in 12 of 13 cases of small hepatocellular carcinoma in Taiwan (Chen et al., 1983) but in only two of 17 similar cases in Japan (Nakashima et al., 1983).

References

Abelev, G. L., Assescritova, I. V., Kraevsky, N. A.: Embryonal serum alpha-globulin in cancer patients. Diagnostic value. Int. J. Cancer 2:551–558, 1967.

Alpert, E.: Human alpha-1-fetoprotein. In Okuda, K., and Peters, R. L. (eds.): Hepatocellular Carcinoma. New York, John Wiley & Sons, 1976, pp. 353–367.

Altmann, H. W.: Pathology of human liver tumors. In Remmer, H., Bolt, H. M., Bannasch, P., Popper, H. W. (eds.): Primary Liver Tumors. Baltimore, University Park Press, 1978, pp. 53–71.

An, T., Ghatak, N., Kastner, R., Kay, S., Lee, H. M.: Hyaline globules and intracellular lumina in a hepatocellular carcinoma. Am. J. Clin. Pathol. 79:392–396, 1983.

Anthony, P. P.: Precursor lesions for liver cancer in humans. Cancer Res. 36:2579–2583, 1976.

Anthony, P. P.: Precancerous changes in the human liver. J. Toxicol. Environ. Health 5:301–313, 1979.

Anthony, P. P., Vogel, C. L., Barker, L. F.: Liver cell dysplasia: a premalignant condition. Am. J. Clin. Pathol. 26:217–223, 1973.

Axelsson, G.: Hepatocellular cancer in Sweden: incidence 1961–62 and 1971–72. J. Chronic Dis. 35:459–466, 1982.

Baithun, S. I. and Pollock, D. J.: Oncocytic hepatocellular tumour. Histopathology 7:107–112, 1983.

Bannasch, P., Mayer, D., Hacker, H. J.: Hepatocellular glycogenosis and hepatocarcinogenesis. Biochem. Biophys. Acta 605:217–245, 1980.

Beasley, R. P., Hwang, L. Y., Lin, C. C., Chien, C. S.: Hepatocellular carcinoma and hepatitis B virus. A prospective study of 22,707 men in Taiwan. Lancet 2:1129–1133, 1981.

Becker, F. F.: Recent concepts of initiation and promotion in carcinogenesis. Am. J. Pathol. 105:3–9, 1981.

Berman, M. M., Libbey, N. P., Foster, J. H.: Hepatocellular carcinoma. Polygonal cell type with fibrous stroma—an atypical variant with a favorable prognosis. Cancer 46:1448–1455, 1980.

Blumberg, B. S. and London, W. T.: Hepatitis B virus and the prevention of primary hepatocellular carcinoma. N. Engl. J. Med. 304:782–784, 1981.

Brechot, Ch., Pourcel, Ch., Louise, A., Rain, B., Tiollais, P.: Presence of integrated hepatitis B virus DNA sequences in cellular DNA of human hepatocellular carcinoma. Nature 286:533–535, 1980.

Buchanan, T. F., Huvos, A. G.: Clear cell carcinoma of the liver. A clinicopathological study of 13 patients. Am. J. Clin. Pathol. 61:529–539, 1974.

Camilleri, J. P., Amat, C., Chousterman, M., Petite, J. P., Duboust,

A., Boddaert, A., Paraf, A.: Immunohistochemical patterns of hepatitis B surface antigen (HBsAg) in patients with hepatitis, renal homograph recipients and normal carriers. Virch. Arch. [A] 376:329–341, 1977.

Chakraborty, P. R., Ruiz-Opazo, N., Shouval, D., Shafritz, D. A.: Identification of integrated hepatitis B virus DNA and expression of viral RNA in an HBsAg-producing human hepatocellular carcinoma cell line. Nature 286:531–533, 1980.

Chen, D. S., Sheu, J. C., Sung, J. L., Lai, M. Y., Lee, C. S., Su, C. T., Tsang, Y. M., How, S. W., Wang, T. H., Yu, J. Y., Yang, T. H., Wang, C. Y., Hsu, C. Y.: Small hepatocellular carcinoma—A clinicopathological study in thirteen patients. Gastroenterology 83:1109–1119, 1982.

Christopherson, W. M., Mays, E. T.: Relation of steroids to liver oncogenesis. J. Toxicol. Environ. Health 5:207–230, 1979.

Christopherson, W. M., Mays, E. T., Barrows, G.: A clinicopathologic study of steroid related liver tumors. Am. J. Surg. Pathol. 1:31–41, 1977.

Chuong, J. J., Livstone, E. M., Barwick, K. W.: The histopathologic and clinical indicators of prognosis in hepatoma. J. Clin. Gastroenterol. 4:547–552, 1982.

Cohen, C., Berson, S. D., Budgeon, L. R.: Alpha-1-antitrypsin deficiency in Southern African hepatocellular carcinoma patients. An immunoperoxidase and histochemical study. Cancer 49:2537–2540, 1982.

Cohen, C., Berson, S. D., Geddes, E. W.: Liver cell dysplasia: association with hepatocellular carcinoma, cirrhosis and hepatitis B antigen carrier status. Cancer 44:1671–1676, 1979.

Craig, J. R., Peters, R. L., Edmondson, H. A., Omata, M.: Fibrolamellar carcinoma of the liver: a tumor of adolescents and young adults with distinctive clinicopathologic features. Cancer 46:372–379, 1980.

Edman, J. C., Gray, P., Valenzuela, P., Rall, L. B., Rutter, W. J.: Integration of hepatitis B virus sequences and their expression in a human hepatoma cell line. Nature 286:536–538, 1980.

Edmondson, H. A.: Tumors of the liver and intrahepatic bile ducts. Armed Forces Institute of Pathology Fascicle 25, 1958.

Edmondson, H. A.: Benign epithelial tumors and tumorlike lesions of the liver. In Okuda, K., Peters, R. L. (eds.): Hepatocellular Carcinoma. New York, John Wiley & Sons, 1976, pp. 309–333.

Farber, E.: Review article: chemical carcinogenesis. A biologic perspective. Am. J. Pathol. 106:271–296, 1982.

Farber, E. and Cameron, R.: The sequential analysis of cancer development. Adv. Cancer Res. 32:125–226, 1980.

Farhi, D. C., Shikes, R. H., Silverberg, S. G.: Ultrastructure of fibrolamellar oncocytic hepatoma. Cancer 50:702–709, 1982.

Foster, J. H.: Benign liver tumors. World J. Surg. 6:25–31, 1982.

Gerber, M. A., Hadziyannis, S., Vissoulis, C., Schaffner, F., Paronetto, F., Popper, H.: Electron microscopy and immunoelectron microscopy of cytoplasmic hepatitis B antigen in hepatocytes. Am. J. Pathol. 75:489–502, 1974.

Gerber, M. A. and Thung, S. N.: Enzyme patterns in human hepatocellular carcinoma. Am. J. Pathol. 98:395–400, 1980.

Gerber, M. A., Thung, S. N., Shen, S., Stromeyer, F. W., Ishak, K. G.: Phenotypic characterization of hepatic proliferation. Am. J. Pathol. 110:70–74, 1983.

Gerin, J. L.: Hepatitis B virus and primary hepatocellular carcinoma. Gastroenterology 84:869–870, 1983.

Gibson, J. B., Wu, P.-C., Ho, J. C. I., Lauder, I. J.: Hepatitis B surface antigen, hepatocellular carcinoma and cirrhosis in Hong Kong. Br. J. Cancer 42:370–377, 1980.

Goldfarb, S.: Sex hormones and hepatic neoplasia. Cancer Res. 36:2584–2588, 1976.

Goodman, Z. D. and Ishak, K.: Hepatocellular carcinoma in women: probable lack of etiologic association with oral contraceptive steroids. Hepatology 2:440–444, 1982.

Gudat, F., Bianchi, L., Sonnabend, W., Thiel, G., Aenishaenslin, W., Stalder, A.: Pattern of core and surface expression in liver tissue reflects state of specific immune response in hepatitis B. Lab. Invest. 32:1–9, 1975.

Hahn, E., Wick, G., Pencev, D., Timpl, R.: Distribution of basement membrane proteins in normal and fibrotic human liver: collagen type IV, laminin and fibronectin. Gut 21:63–71, 1980.

Harada, T., Fukumoto, Y., Kodama, T., Nishimura, H., Nishioka, M., Takemoto, T.: Clinical significance of liver cell dysplasia in chronic liver disease. Bull. Yamaguchi Med. Sch. 26:115–121, 1979.

Hirohashi, S., Shimosato, Y., Ino, Y., Kishi, K.: Distribution of hepatitis B surface and core antigens in human liver cell carcinoma and surrounding nontumorous liver. J. Natl. Cancer Inst. 69:565–568, 1982.

Ho, J. C. I., Wu, P. C., Mak, T. K.: Liver cell dysplasia in association with hepatocellular carcinoma, cirrhosis, and hepatitis B surface antigen in Hong Kong. Int. J. Cancer 28:571–574, 1981.

Horie, Y., Katoh, S., Yoshida, H., Imaoka, T., Suou, T., Hirayama, C.: Pedunculated hepatocellular carcinoma. Report of three cases and review of literature. Cancer 51:746–751, 1983.

Ishak, K. G.: Hepatic lesions caused by anabolic and contraceptive steroids. Semin. Liver Dis. 1:116–128, 1981.

Jacobsen, G. K., Gammelgaard, J., Fuglo, M.: Coarse needle biopsy versus fine needle aspiration biopsy in the diagnosis of focal lesions of the liver. Ultrasonically guided needle biopsy in suspected hepatic malignancy. Acta Cytol. (Baltimore) 27:152–156, 1983.

Jagoe, R., Sowter, C., Dandy, S., Slavin, G.: Morphometric study of liver cell nuclei in hepatomas using an interactive computer technique: nuclear size and shape. J. Clin. Pathol. 35:1057–1062, 1982.

Johnson, P. J. Melia, W. M., Palmer, M. K., Portman, B., Williams, R.: Relationship between serum alpha-foetoprotein, cirrhosis and survival in hepatocellular carcinoma. Br. J. Cancer 44:502–505, 1981.

Kalengayi, M. M. R., and Desmet, V. J.: Liver cell populations and histochemical patterns of adult and fetal type proteins during aflatoxin B1 hepatocarcinogenesis. In Remmer, H., Bolt, H. M., Bannasch, P., Popper, H. (eds.): Primary Liver Tumors. Baltimore, University Park Press, 1978, pp. 467–483.

Kanematsu, T., Sugimachi, K., Kohno, H., Matsumata, T., Kobayashi, M., Inokuchi, K.: Minute liver cancer and concomitant esophageal varices: detection and successful surgical treatment. World J. Surg. 5:707–711, 1981.

Kew, M. C.: Hepatocellular cancer in Southern Africa. In Remmer, H., Bolt, H. M., Bannasch, P., Popper, H. (eds.): Primary Liver Tumors. Baltimore, University Park Press, 1978, pp. 179–183.

Kishi, K., Shikata, T., Hirohashi, S., Hasegawa, H., Yamazaki, S., Makuuchi, M.: Hepatocellular carcinoma. A clinical and pathologic analysis of 57 hepatectomy cases. Cancer 51:542–548, 1983.

Kobayashi, M., Inokuchi, K., Nagasue, N., Saku, M., Iwaki, A.: Successful treatment of early cancer of the liver and portal hypertension in patients presenting with bleeding oesophageal varices. Br. J. Surg. 64:542–544, 1977.

Kojiro, M., Kawano, Y., Isomura, Y., Nakashima, T.: Distribution of albumin- and/or alpha-fetoprotein–positive cells in hepatocellular carcinoma. Lab. Invest. 44:221–226, 1981.

Kolb, A.: Benign liver tumors and oral contraceptives. Acta Chir. Scand. 148:89–91, 1982.

Kondo, Y., Niwa, Y., Akikusa, B., Takazawa, H., Okabayashi, A.: A histopathologic study of early hepatocellular carcinoma. Cancer 52:687–692, 1983.

Lai, C. L., Lam, K. C., Wong, K. P., Wu, P. C., Todd, D.: Clinical features of hepatocellular carcinoma: review of 211 patients in Hong Kong. Cancer 47:2746–2755, 1981.

Lai, C. L., Wu, P. C., Lam, K. C., Todd, D.: Histologic prognostic indicators in hepatocellular carcinoma. Cancer 44:1677–1683, 1979.

Lancet editorial: Prevention of primary liver cancer. Report of a meeting of a W.H.O. Scientific Group. Lancet 1:463–465, 1983.

Landing, B. H.: Tumors of the liver in childhood. In Okuda, K., and Peters, R. L. (eds.): Hepatocellular Carcinoma. New York, John Wiley & Sons, 1976, pp. 205–227.

Lapis, K.: The value of electron microscopy in diagnostic pathology. Case 7. Ultrastr. Pathol. 1:105–109, 1980.

Lapis, K., and Johannessen, J. V.: Pathology of primary liver cancer. In Lapis, K., and Johannessen, J. V. (eds.): Liver Carcinogenesis. Washington, D.C., Hemisphere Publishing Corp., 1979, pp. 145–185.

Lefkowitch, J. H., Muschel, R., Price, J. B., Marboe, C., Braunhut, S.: Copper and copper-binding protein in fibrolamellar liver cell carcinoma. Cancer 51:97–100, 1983.

Lehmann, F. G.: Alpha-1-fetoprotein. In Remmer, H., Bolt, H. M., Bannasch, P., Popper, H. (eds.): Primary Liver Tumors. Baltimore, University Park Press, 1978, pp. 449–463.

Lightdale, C. J.: Laparoscopy and biopsy in malignant liver disease. Cancer 50(Suppl.):2672–2675, 1982.

London, W. T.: Primary hepatocellular carcinoma—etiology, pathogenesis, and prevention. Hum. Pathol. 12:1085–1097, 1981.

Lundquist, A.: Fine-needle aspiration biopsy for cytodiagnosis of malignant tumour in the liver. Acta Med. Scand. 188:465–470, 1970.

Lurie, B., Novis, B., Bank, S., Silber, W., Botha, J. B. C., Marks, I. N.: CRST syndrome and nodular transformation of the liver. Gastroenterology 64:457–461, 1973.

Matsumoto, Y., Suzuki, T., Asada, I., Ozawa, K., Tobe, T., Hohjo, I.: Clinical classification of hepatoma in Japan according to serial changes in serum alpha-fetoprotein levels. Cancer 49:354–360, 1982.

Miyai, K., and Bonin, M. L.: Nodular regenerative hyperplasia of the liver. Am. J. Clin. Pathol. 73:267–271, 1980.

Model, D. G., Fox, J. A., Jones, R. W.: Multiple hepatic adenomas associated with an oral contraceptive. Lancet 1:865, 1975.

Nakashima, T., Kijiro, M., Kawano, Y., Shirai, F., Takemoto, N., Tomimatsu, H., Kawasaki, H., Okuda, K.: Histologic growth pattern of hepatocellular carcinoma: Relationship to orcein (hepatitis B surface antigen)-positive cells in cancer tissue. Hum. Pathol. 13:563–568, 1982.

Nakashima, T., Okuda, K., Kojiro, M., Jimi, A., Yamaguchi, R., Sakamoto, K., Ikari, T.: Pathology of hepatocellular carcinoma in Japan. Cancer 51:863–877, 1983.

Nakopoulou, L., Theodoropoulos, G., Kotsis, L., Papacharalampous, N.: Demonstration of alpha-1-antitrypsin in paraffin sections of hepatoma and cirrhosis. Virch. Arch. [A] 397:163–170, 1982.

Nayak, N. C., and Sachdeva, R.: Localization of hepatitis B surface antigen in conventional paraffin sections of the liver. Am. J. Pathol. 81:479–492, 1975.

Nissen, E. D., Kent, D. R., Nissen, S. E.: Role of oral contraceptive agents in the pathogenesis of liver tumors. In Lapis, K., and Johannessen, J. V. (eds.): Liver Carcinogenesis. Washington, D.C., Hemisphere Publishing Corp., 1979, pp. 61–84.

Nosher, J. L. and Plafker, J.: Fine needle aspiration of the liver with ultrasound guidance. Ultrasound 136:177–180, 1980.

Ogawa, K., Solt, D. B., Farber, E.: Phenotypic diversity as an early property of putative preneoplastic hepatocyte population in liver carcinogenesis. Cancer Res. 40:725–730, 1980.

Okuda, K. and the Liver Cancer Study Group of Japan: Primary liver cancers in Japan. Cancer 45:2663–2669, 1980.

Okuda, K., Misha, H., Nakajima, Y., Kubo, Y., Shimokawa, Y., Nagasaki, Y., Sawa, Y., Jinniouchi, Y., Kaneko, T., Obata, H., Hisamitsu, T., Motoike, Y., Okazaki, N., Kojiro, M., Sakamoto, K., Nakashima, T.: Clinicopathologic features of encapsulated hepatocellular carcinoma. Cancer 40:1240–1245, 1977a.

Okuda, K., Nakashima, T., Obata, H., Kubo, Y.: Clinicopathological studies of minute hepatocellular carcinoma. Gastroenterology 73:109–115, 1977b.

Okuda, K., Nakashima, T., Sakamoto, K., Ikai, T., Hidaka, H., Kibo, Y., Sakuma, K., Motoike, Y., Okuda, H., Obata, H.: Hepatocellular carcinoma arising in noncirrhotic and highly cirrhotic livers: a comparative study of histopathology and frequency of hepatitis B markers. Cancer 49:450–455, 1982.

Okuda, K., Obata, H., Kubo, Y., Nakashima, T.: Early diagnosis and angiographic feature of hepatocellular carcinoma. In Remmer, H., Bolt, H. M., Bannasch, P., Popper, H. (eds.): Primary Liver Tumors. Baltimore, University Park Press, 1978, pp. 149–164.

Pagliaro, L., Simonetti, R. G., Craxi, A., et al.: Alcohol and HBV infection as risk factors for hepatocellular carcinoma in Italy: a multicentric, controlled study. Hepato-gastroenterology 30:48–50, 1983.

Palmer, P. E. and Wolfe, H. J.: Alpha-1-antitrypsin desposition in primary hepatic carcinomas. Arch. Pathol. Lab. Med. 100:232–236, 1976.

Peraino, C., Fry, R. J. M., Staffeldt, E., Kisielski, W. E.: Effects of varying the exposure to phenobarbital on its enhancement of 2-acetylaminofluorene–induced hepatic tumorigenesis in the rat. Cancer Res. 33:2701–2705, 1973.

Peters, R. L.: Pathology of hepatocellular carcinoma. In Okuda, K. and Peters, R. L. (eds.): Hepatocellular Carcinoma. New York, John Wiley & Sons, 1976, pp. 107–169.

Pitot, H. C. and Sirica, A. E.: The stages of initiation and promotion in hepatocarcinogenesis. Biochim. Biophys. Acta 605:191–215, 1980.

Popper, H.: Hepatic cancers in man: quantitative perspectives. Environ. Res. 19:482–494, 1979.

Popper, H., Gerber, M. A., Thung, S. N.: The relation of hepatocellular carcinoma to infection with hepatitis B and related viruses in man and animals. Hepatology 2:1S–9S, 1982.

Qizilbash, A. H. and Castelli, M.: Nodular regenerative hyperplasia of the liver: diagnosis by liver biopsy. Can. Med. Assoc. J. 122:1151–1154, 1980.

Ranstrom, S.: Miliary hepatocellular adenomatosis. Acta Pathol. Microbiol. Scand. 33:225–229, 1953.

Rautenberg, J., Voss, B., Pott, G., Gerlach, V.: Connective tissue components of the normal and fibrotic liver. Klin. Wochenschr. 59:767–779, 1981.

Reintoft, I. and Hagerstrand, I.: Demonstration of alpha-1-antitrypsin in hepatomas. Arch. Pathol. Lab. Med. 103:495–498, 1979.

Reynolds, T. B.: Diagnostic methods for hepatocellular carcinoma. In Okuda, K. and Peters, R. L. (eds.): Hepatocellular Carcinoma. New York, John Wiley & Sons, 1976, pp. 437–448.

Rougier, P., Degott, C., Rueff, B., Benhamou, J.-P.: Nodular regenerative hyperplasia of the liver: report of six cases and review of the literature. Gastroenterolgoy 75:169–172, 1978.

Sakamoto, S., Kawarada, S., Taniuchi, A.: Significance of cirrhotic nodule as a premalignant lesion. Acta Hepat. Jpn. 19:1093, 1978.

Sandler, D. P., Sandler, R. S., Horney, L. F.: Primary liver cancer mortality in the United States. J. Chronic Dis. 36:227–236, 1983.

Saracci, R. and Repetto, F.: Time trends of primary liver cancer: indication of increased incidence in selected cancer registry populations. J. Natl. Cancer Inst. 65:241–247, 1980.

Schaff, Z., Lapis, K., Safrany, L.: The ultrastructure of primary hepato-cellular cancer in man. Virch. Arch. [A] 352:340–358, 1971.

Schaff, Z., Lapis, K., Szecseny, A., Szendroi, M., Faller, J.: Histochemical study of the focal nodular hyperplasia of the liver. Morphol. Igazsagugyi Orv. Sz., 24:64–69, 1984.

Scherer, E. and Emmelot, H. P.: Kinetics of induction and growth of enzyme-deficient islands involved in hepatocarcinogenesis. Cancer Res. 36:2544–2554, 1976.

Sell, S. and Ruoslahti, E.: Expression of fibronectin and laminin in the rat liver after partial hepatectomy, during carcinogenesis, and in transplantable hepatocellular carcinoma. J. Natl. Cancer Inst. 69:1005–1114, 1982.

Shikata, T.: Primary liver carcinoma and liver cirrhosis. In Okuda, K. and Peters, R. L. (eds.): Hepatocellular Carcinoma. New York, John Wiley & Sons, 1976, pp. 53–73.

Shikata, T., Uzawa, T., Yoshiwara, N., Akatsuka, T., Yamazaki, S.: Staining methods of Australia antigen in paraffin sections. Jpn. J. Exp. Med. 44:25–36, 1974.

Shouval, D., Shafritz, D. A., Zurawski, V. R., Isselbacher, K. J., Wands, J. R.: Immunotherapy in nude mice of human hepatoma using monoclonal antibodies against hepatitis B virus. Nature 298:567–569, 1982.

Smith, J. C.: Noncirrhotic nodulation of the liver. Arch. Pathol. Lab. Med. 102:398–401, 1978.

Sogaard, P. E.: Nodular transformation of the liver, alpha-fetoprotein, and hepatocellular carcinoma. Hum. Pathol. 12:1052, 1981.

Steiner, P. E.: Nodular regenerative hyperplasia of the liver. Am. J. Pathol. 35:943–953, 1959.

Steiner, P. E.: Cancer of the liver and cirrhosis in trans-Saharan Africa and the United States of America. Cancer 13:1085–1145, 1960.

Stemhagen, A., Slade, J., Altman, R., Bill, J.: Occupational risk factors and liver cancer. A retrospective case-control study of primary liver cancer in New Jersey. Am. J. Epidemiol. 117:443–454, 1983.

Stocker, J. T., Ishak, K. G.: Focal nodular hyperplasia of the liver: A study of 21 pediatric cases. Cancer 48:336–345, 1981.

Stromeyer, F. W. and Ishak, K. G.: Nodular transformation (nodular "regenerative" hyperplasia) of the liver. Hum. Pathol. 12:60–71, 1981.

Summers, J. and Mason, W. S.: Properties of the hepatitis B–like viruses related to their taxonomic classification. Hepatology 2:61S–66S, 1982.

Summers, J., Smolec, J. M., Snyder, R.: A virus similar to human hepatitis B virus associated with hepatitis and hepatoma in woodchucks. Proc. Natl. Acad. Sci. U.S.A. 75:4533–4537, 1978.

Szmuness, W.: Hepatocellular carcinoma and the hepatitis B virus: Evidence for a causal association. Progr. Med. Virol. 24:40–69, 1978.

Tabor, E., Bayley, A. C., Cairns, J., Pelleu, L., Gerety, R. J.: Horizontal transmission of hepatitis B virus in children and adults in five rural villages in Zambia. Gastroenterology 84(abstr.):1399, 1983.

Tabor, E., Gerety, R. J., Vogel, C. L., Bayley, A. C., Anthony, P. P., Chan, C. H., Barker, L. F.: Hepatitis B virus infection and primary hepatocellular carcinoma. J. Natl. Cancer Inst. 58:1197–1200, 1977.

Takashima, T., Matsui, O., Suzuki, M., Ida, M.: Diagnosis and screening of small hepatocellular carcinomas. Comparison of radionuclide imaging, ultrasound, computed tomography, hepatic angiography, and alpha-1-fetoprotein assay. Radiology 145:635–638, 1982.

Tesluk, H. and Lawrie, J.: Hepatocellular adenoma. Its transformation to carcinoma in a user of oral contraceptives. Arch. Pathol. Lab. Med. 105:296–299, 1981.

Tezuka, F. and Sawai, T.: Hyperplasia of small hepatic cells in the precancerous condition of cirrhotic livers. Tohoku J. Exp. Med. 139:171–177, 1983.

Thung, S. N. and Gerber, M. A.: Enzyme pattern and marker antigens in nodular "regenerative" hyperplasia of the liver. Cancer 47:1796–1799, 1981.

Thung, S. N., Gerber, M. A., Sarno, E., Popper, H.: Distribution of five antigens in hepatocellular carcinoma. Lab. Invest. 41:101–105, 1979.

Uchida, T., Miyata, H., Shikata, T.: Human hepatocellular carcinoma and putative precancerous disorders. Their enzyme histochemical study. Arch. Pathol. Lab. Med. 105:180–186, 1981.

Wanless, I. R., Solt, L. C., Kortan, P., Deck, J. H. N., Gardiner, G. W., Prokipchuk, E. J.: Nodular regenerative hyperplasia of the liver associated with macroglobulinaemia. Am. J. Med. 70:1203–1209, 1981.

Watanabe, S., Okita, K., Harada, T., Kodama, T., Numa, Y., Takemoto, T., Takahashi, T.: Morphologic studies of the liver cell dysplasia. Cancer 51:2197–2205, 1983.

Wessely, Z., Shapiro, S. D., Scherer, J. D.: Focal nodular hyperplasia of the liver: ultrastructural observations. Ann. Clin. Lab. Sci. 12:119–125, 1982.

Wetzel, W. J. and Alexander, R. W.: Focal nodular hyperplasia of the liver with alcoholic hyalin bodies and cytologic atypia. Cancer 44:1322–1326, 1979.

Williams, G. M.: Sex hormones and liver cancer. Lab. Invest. 46:352–353, 1982.

Wu, P. C., Lai, C. L., Lam, K. C., Lok, A. S., Lin, H. J.: Clear cell carcinoma of liver. An ultrastructural study. Cancer 52:504–507, 1983.

Yoshida, T., Okazaki, N., Yoshino, M., Kitaoka, H., Hirohashi, S., Shimozato, Y.: Minute hepatocellular carcinoma without appreciable change in size for seven years: a case report. Cancer 49:1491–1495, 1982.

JORGE ALBORES-SAAVEDRA
DONALD EARL HENSON

10 Gallbladder and Extrahepatic Bile Ducts

For many years, the early changes in the development of invasive carcinomas of the gallbladder were practically unknown. Two reasons can be cited to explain the late recognition of these changes: (1) invasive carcinoma of the gallbladder is an uncommon disease in many countries, and consequently few pathologists have had the opportunity to become familiar with its precursor lesions; and (2) although dysplastic and neoplastic epithelial cells desquamate freely into bile, this fluid is difficult to obtain directly from the gallbladder. Therefore, bile cytology is not a widely used procedure, even in countries in which there is a high prevalence of carcinoma. In recent years, however, a study of multiple random sections of gallbladders excised for cholelithiasis, examination of the mucosa adjacent to invasive carcinomas, and cytologic studies of bile obtained from cholecystectomy specimens have allowed characterization of dysplasia and carcinoma-in-situ (Albores-Saavedra et al., 1980; Alonso de Ruiz et al., 1982; Laitio, 1983a; Laitio, 1983b). Moreover, the histologic criteria for the diagnosis of epithelial atypia secondary to repair, which is often seen in acute and chronic cholecystitis, have been established, and differentiation of this atypia from true dysplasia and carcinoma-in-situ, once thought to be quite difficult, is now possible (Albores-Saavedra et al., 1984).

Carcinoma of the gallbladder is a major cause of death among the populations of some countries (Albores-Saavedra and Henson, 1985). Even in the general population of the United States, in which the mortality rate is considered to be low, this cancer is responsible for 6000 deaths per year (Strauch, 1960; Tanga and Ewing, 1970). Carcinoma of the gallbladder is often associated with the presence of stones, a relationship first observed over 100 years ago. Unfortunately, early diagnosis of gallbladder cancer is difficult. Many cases are not suspected clinically and are first discovered during exploratory laparotomy. Most of the in-situ carcinomas are accidentally found in gallbladders removed for lithiasis. In regard to the early diagnosis, we should emphasize that dysplasia and carcinoma-in-situ can be recognized by cytologic examination of bile collected by gallbladder puncture, a procedure that is not hazardous. Complications are minimal and usually resolve with conservative management (Ropertz and Wagner, 1976). Correct preoperative diagnosis and treatment of these precursor lesions not only will prevent progression but also may reduce the incidence of invasive carcinoma.

DYSPLASIA AND CARCINOMA-IN-SITU OF THE GALLBLADDER

Dysplasia and carcinoma-in-situ are usually not recognized on macroscopic examination because they often occur in association with chronic cholecystitis. Grossly, there are no distinctive features that would alert the pathologist to the presence of these two lesions. The mucosa may appear granular, nodular, plaque-like, or trabeculated. Occasionally, the papillary type of dysplasia or carcinoma-in-situ may exhibit small cauliflower-like excrescences that project into the lumen and that can be recognized on close inspection. However, in most cases of dysplasia and carcinoma-in-situ, the gallbladder shows only a thickened and indurated wall, the result of chronic inflammation and fibrosis.

Histologically, columnar, cuboidal, and elongated cells with variable degrees of nuclear atypia, loss of polarity, and occasional mitotic figures characterize dysplasia. The dysplastic cells are usually arranged in a single layer. However, because of cellular proliferation and nuclear crowding, pseudostratification often occurs (Figs. 10–1 to 10–3). Later, dysplastic cells may extend into the epithelial invaginations and even into the metaplastic antral-type glands (Figs. 10–4 and 10–5) or grow outward and cover small fibrovascular stalks that protrude into the lumen. The large nuclei of dysplastic cells may be round, oval, or fusiform with one or two nucleoli that are more

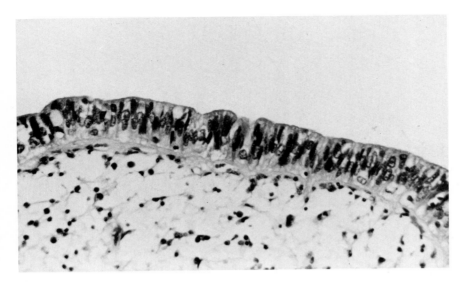

Figure 10–1. Severe dysplasia. There is pseudostratification and hyperchromatism of nuclei. The lamina propria contains foamy histiocytes.

prominent than those of normal cells. The cytoplasm usually stains eosinophilic and contains a variable amount of non-sulphated acid and neutral mucin. Goblet cells are found in one third of the cases (Fig. 10–5). An abrupt transition between normal-appearing columnar cells and dysplastic epithelium is seen in nearly all cases. This transition is an important clue in the differential diagnosis of dysplasia. In general, the cell population of dysplasia is homogeneous, unlike the heterogeneous cell population of the epithelial atypia of repair. In many cases, the dysplastic lesions are continuous with areas of carcinoma-in-situ, although normal-appearing epithelium may separate the two. Because of the widespread involvement of the mucosa by dysplasia and in-situ-carcinoma, we have concluded that some, if not most, invasive carcinomas of the gallbladder arise from a field change within the epithelium (Albores-Saavedra and Henson, 1985).

Cells from carcinoma-in-situ have all the cytologic features of malignancy. Because of the excessive cellular proliferation, mitotic figures are more common and nuclear crowding and pseudostratification are more prominent in cases of carcinoma-in-situ than in cases of dysplasia (Figs. 10–6 and 10–7). Neoplastic cells appear first along the surface epithelium and later extend into the epithelial invaginations and antral-type metaplastic glands. In the late stages of carcinoma-in-situ, the histologic picture is that of back-to-back glands located in the lamina propria but often connected with the surface epithelium (Fig. 10–7). However, not all in-situ carcinomas exhibit this type of growth pattern. Some show distinctive papillary features with small fibrovascular stalks lined by the neoplastic cells. Not infrequently, a combination of these two growth patterns is noted.

An in-situ carcinoma composed of goblet cells, columnar cells, Paneth's cells, and endocrine cells, the last of which were stained with the Grimelius procedure, has been described (Fig. 10–8) (Albores-Saavedra and Henson, 1985). It is assumed that this lesion represents the in-situ phase of the tumor designated "intestinal-type adenocarcinoma" because both the infiltrating and the intraepithelial forms have the same cell population (Albores-Saavedra et al., submitted; Albores-Saavedra and Henson, 1985). Goblet cells may also be a component of the ordinary type of carcinoma-in-situ. Their presence is regarded as an example of intestinal differentiation occurring within the neoplastic epithelium.

Another type of in-situ intestinal carcinoma is composed of cells closely resembling those of colonic carcinomas at the light and electron microscopic levels (Fig. 10–9). The neoplastic columnar cells extend into the epithelial invaginations and the antral-type glands. This tumor also has scattered endocrine cells, most of which contain serotonin. These cells can be demonstrated with the Grimelius and the perioxidase antiperioxidase techniques.

In an effort to learn about the precursor lesions of pure squamous cell carcinomas of the gallbladder, we examined five cases by means of multiple sections that included normal-appearing mucosa. Three of the tumors showed focal areas of squamous dysplasia and carcinoma-in-situ (Fig. 10–10). Such findings suggest that these squamous cell carcinomas, which are unusual in the gallbladder, undergo the same pathologic changes in their development as those arising in other sites (Albores-Saavedra and Henson, 1985).

The wall of the gallbladder with dysplasia or carcinoma-in-situ usually shows inflammatory changes of variable extent. As expected, the most common type of inflammatory response is chronic, with a predominance of lymphocytes and plasma cells, although xanthogranulomatous inflammation or even an acute inflammatory reaction may be present. In some cases,

Text continued on page 209

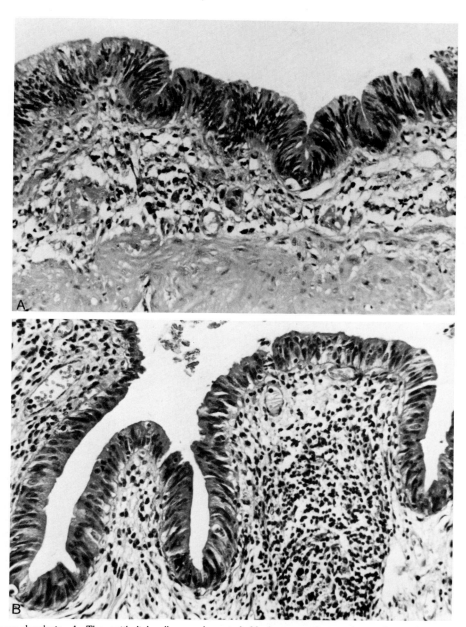

Figure 10–2. Severe dysplasia. *A,* The epithelial cells are elongated. Nuclear crowding and pseudostratification are evident. *B,* The dysplastic cells line folds and extend into epithelial invaginations. An ill-defined lymphoid follicle is present in the lamina propria.

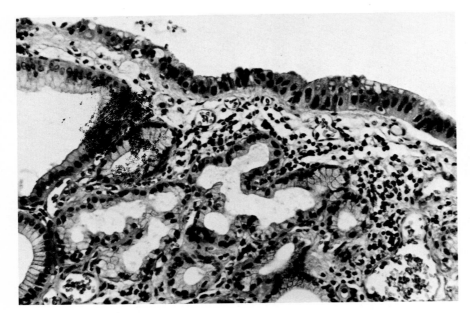

Figure 10–3. The epithelium overlying a group of metaplastic antral-type glands is moderately dysplastic.

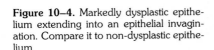

Figure 10–4. Markedly dysplastic epithelium extending into an epithelial invagination. Compare it to non-dysplastic epithelium.

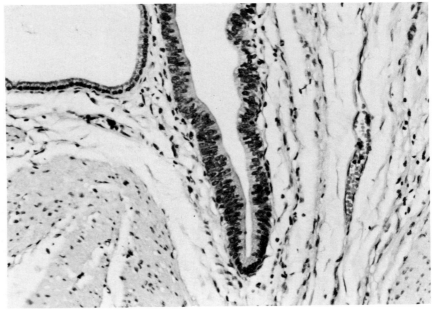

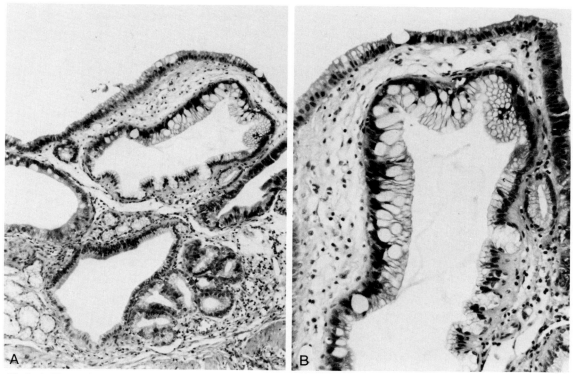

Figure 10–5. *A,* The surface epithelium is only slightly dysplastic and contains few goblet cells, whereas some of the antral-type glands are highly atypical and contain goblet cells. *B,* Higher magnification of *A.* The epithelium of the dilated antral-type gland has been replaced by atypical goblet cells. The surface epithelium shows minimal nuclear atypia.

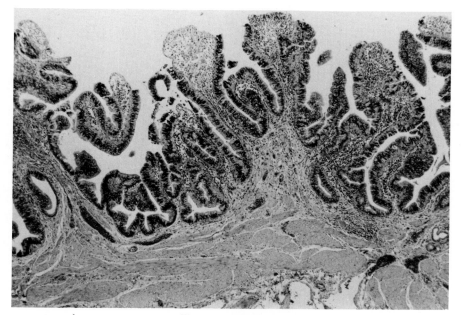

Figure 10–6. Low-power view of an in-situ-carcinoma. The neoplastic epithelium lines mucosal folds and small papillary projections. Gland-like structures are seen in the lamina propria. (Courtesy of Dr. Dale Bennet.)

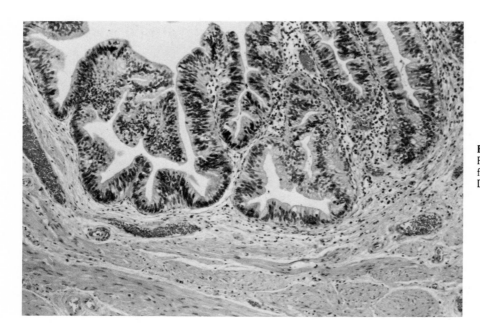

Figure 10–7. Higher magnification of Figure 10–6 showing obvious cytologic features of malignancy. (Courtesy of Dr. Dale Bennet.)

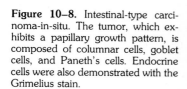

Figure 10–8. Intestinal-type carcinoma-in-situ. The tumor, which exhibits a papillary growth pattern, is composed of columnar cells, goblet cells, and Paneth's cells. Endocrine cells were also demonstrated with the Grimelius stain.

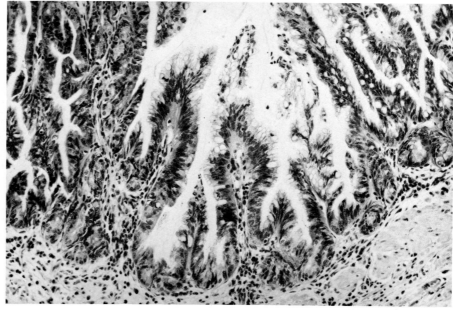

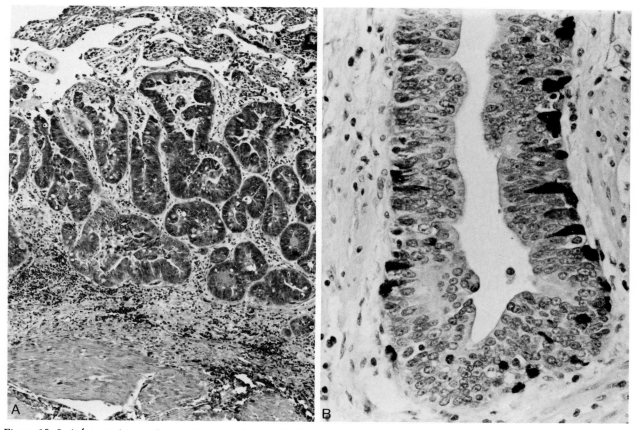

Figure 10–9. *A,* Intestinal-type adenocarcinoma confined to the lamina propria. Tumor cells closely resemble those of a colonic carcinoma. *B,* Numerous serotonin-containing cells are present among columnar cells. Peroxidase-antiperoxidase technique.

lymphoid follicles with germinal centers may even be seen in the lamina propria and muscle layer.

It is recommended that if carcinoma-in-situ is found, multiple sections should be taken to exclude invasion.

Differential Diagnosis

The differential diagnosis between severe dysplasia and carcinoma-in-situ is rather difficult and often impossible in many cases. This is not important because the two lesions, which vary only in degree histologically, may be closely related biologically. However, differentiation of dysplasia or carcinoma-in-situ from the epithelial atypia of repair is of great clinical significance because the last lesion does not progress to carcinoma. The atypia of repair consists of a heterogeneous cell population in which columnar mucus-secreting cells, low cuboidal cells, atrophic-appearing epithelium, and pencil-like cells are present. In addition, there is a gradual transition of the cellular abnormalities, in contrast with the abrupt transition seen in dysplasia and carcinoma-in-situ. Finally, the extent of nuclear atypia is less pronounced in the epithelial atypia of repair than in dysplasia and carcinoma-in-situ.

By immunocytochemical methods it has been shown that carcinoembryonic antigen is present in small quantities in the normal epithelial cells of the gallbladder. Although the reactivity of this oncofetal antigen progressively increases in dysplasia, carcinoma-in-situ, and infiltrating carcinoma (Albores-Saavedra et al., 1983), its cellular localization alone is not useful in distinguishing epithelial atypia of repair from dysplasia or carcinoma-in-situ. In cases of extrahepatic biliary tract cancer, the levels of carcinoembryonic antigen increase in both serum and bile, but an elevated level may be difficult to interpret because extrahepatic duct obstruction from any cause also leads to a rise (Lurie et al., 1975; Tatsuta et al., 1982). This lack of specificity of carcinoembryonic antigen limits its use in the diagnosis of early carcinoma of the gallbladder, but periodic serum determinations are useful in the follow-up of patients with a diagnosis of carcinoma of the gallbladder.

Natural History

Little is known about the natural history of dysplasia and carcinoma-in-situ of the gallbladder. Most of these

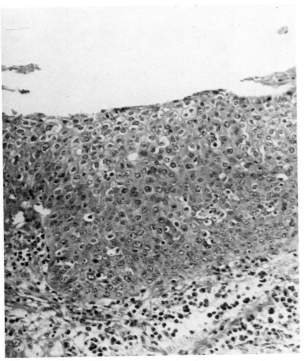

Figure 10–10. Normal columnar epithelium of the gallbladder has been replaced by squamous epithelium with variable atypia at all levels. The lesion can be considered as either severe squamous dysplasia or carcinoma-in-situ.

lesions are diagnosed after cholecystectomy has been performed and the entire lesion removed. This is a limiting factor in the study of their rate of progression. Likewise, the proportion of invasive carcinomas that pass through the sequence of dyplasia and carcinoma-in-situ is unknown. However, there is evidence that progression from in-situ to infiltrating carcinoma does occur. For instance, when in-situ-carcinomas were studied by subserial sections, foci of microinvasion were found in the lamina propria continuous with the overlying carcinoma-in-situ. Dysplasia and carcinoma-in-situ are seen in the areas of intact mucosa that are found adjacent to nearly all invasive carcinomas. These two changes do not represent lateral neoplastic growth because normal or metaplastic epithelium is often seen between the invasive and the in-situ carcinomas. Dysplasia and carcinoma-in-situ are most often found in the fundus and body, the areas of the gallbladder from which most carcinomas arise. Finally, patients with dysplasia and carcinoma-in-situ are 5 years younger than those with invasive carcinoma (Albores-Saavedra et al., 1980).

ADENOMAS AS POSSIBLE CANCER PRECURSORS

In recent years, the role played by adenomas of the gallbladder as possible precursors to invasive cancer has been investigated. Some authors have claimed that the adenoma–carcinoma sequence is the usual route for the development of invasive carcinomas of the gallbladder. Kosuka and associates (1982), for example, based their conclusion on the fact that they were able to demonstrate the remnants of an adenoma in 15 of 79 invasive carcinomas.

We are inclined to believe, however, that what these authors were describing is only the well-differentiated component of some adenocarcinomas. It is

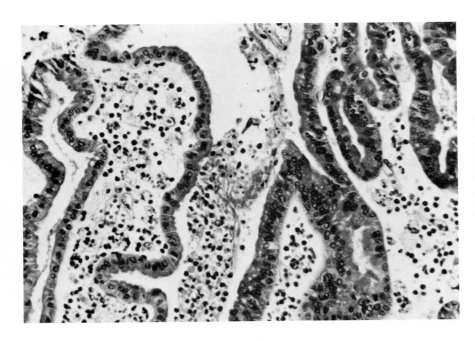

Figure 10–11. Infiltrating carcinoma of the gallbladder. The epithelium on the right shows obvious cytologic features of malignancy, whereas that on the left appears better differentiated and might be interpreted as the remnant of an adenoma. However, the two types of epithilium were also seen in the metastases.

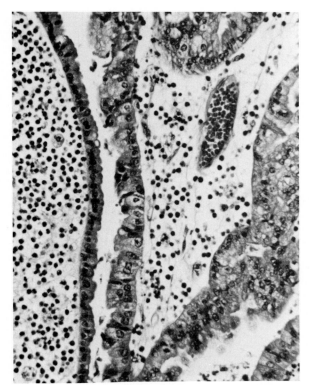

Figure 10–12. Another area of the tumor shown in Figure 10–11. The papillary structures which contain many polymorphonuclear leukocytes are lined by epithelial cells with variable degree of differentiation.

therefore possible that the majority of these adenomas that allegedly gave rise to malignant tumors were carcinomas to begin with. It is generally accepted that well-differentiated adenocarcinomas, including the papillary type, exhibit a broad morphologic spectrum

with areas that may simulate an adenoma or even normal epithelium (Figs. 10–11 and 10–12). Furthermore, hyperplasia of antral-type glands, which often coexists with carcinoma, may easily be confused with the residua of a tubular adenoma. In a study of more than 400 carcinomas of the gallbladder, we were not able to find remnants of tubular or papillary adenomas, even in those carcinomas measuring less than 2 cm. However, adenoma may rarely contain foci ot carcinoma-in-situ. Invasive carcinoma has not been reported from these in-situ lesions.

METAPLASIA AND CARCINOMA OF THE GALLBLADDER

It has long been established that carcinoma of the gallbladder is often associated with cholelithiasis and that chronic irritation caused by the stones can induce a variety of metaplastic changes in the mucosa (Laitio, 1975). Consequently, dysplasia and carcinoma of the gallbladder nearly always arise in an abnormal mucosa (Black, 1980). Antral-type glands, intestinal cells, and superficial gastric-type epithelium are the metaplastic changes most commonly seen (Fig. 10–13) (Laitio, 1975). Other types of metaplastic changes, which are quite rare, include the development of squamous epithelium and fundic-type gastric mucosa. Two or more metaplastic changes may even be seen in the same gallbladder. Because cholelithiasis causes an active cell proliferation of the epithelium (Putz and Willems, 1978), it has been postulated that this stimulates the appearance of endodermal stem cells that can differentiate in several directions, thereby giving rise to cells with intestinal, gastric, or squamous phenotypes (Albores-Saavedra et al., submitted).

These metaplastic changes are first seen on the tips

Figure 10–13. Severe dysplastic epithelium extending into an antral-type gland. Superficial gastric-type epithelium is present between areas of dysplasia.

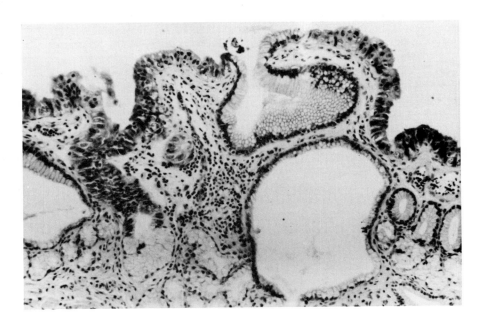

of the mucosal folds, an area that may represent the stem cell zone of the gallbladder epithelium. Furthermore, these metaplastic lesions are found not only in the gallbladder with lithiasis but also in other organs derived from endoderm, such as the esophagus, stomach, small intestine, and colon (Bansal et al., 1984; Symonds, 1974). Moreover, the metaplastic changes are not only associated with inflammation but also have been recognized in benign and malignant epithelial tumors.

Because intestinal-type carcinomas of the gallbladder have the same cell population as intestinal metaplasia and both lesions often coexist in the same specimen, it is possible that these tumors originated from the metaplastic intestinal cells. However, it is possible that the same stem cell that differentiates into cells with mature intestinal phenotypes may become neoplastic, thus eventually giving rise to the intestinal-type carcinomas. Previously, we gave reasons for which we consider squamous cell metaplasia to be the precursor to squamous cell carcinomas. Antral-type glands may show dysplastic and in-situ changes that may be independent of those of the surface epithelium.

PATHOLOGIC STAGE AND PROGNOSIS OF CARCINOMA OF THE GALLBLADDER

As in other sites, a continuum of cellular abnormalities occurs in the gallbladder epithelium during neoplastic transformation. At present, the evidence indicates that the neoplastic change begins along the surface epithelium and later extends into the epithelial invaginations or Rokitansky-Aschoff sinuses and antral-type metaplastic glands located in the lamina propria. In the gallbladder, in-situ carcinoma is designated "pathologic Stage Tis." Cancer that has extended into the lamina propria and muscle layer is designated "pathologic Stage T1." Infiltration of the perimuscular connective tissue or serosa, "pathologic Stage T2," occurs later and is of great clinical significance because these layers contain many lymphatic and blood vessels that facilitate metastasis. In addition, the perimuscular connective tissue is so close to the liver that direct extension is almost unavoidable. As expected, carcinoma-in-situ is cured by cholecystectomy alone. Patients with Stage T1 carcinoma have high survival. However, it is important to recognize that a small proportion of these patients will develop lymph node and liver metastases. Once the tumor has spread beyond the serosa to adjacent organs—"pathologic Stage T3" or "pathologic Stage T4"—the prognosis is very poor. Survival is usually measured in months.

The good correlation that exists between the pathologic stage and survival in gallbladder carcinoma should encourage pathologists to include the information about stage in their reports.

DYSPLASIA AND CARCINOMA-IN-SITU OF THE EXTRAHEPATIC BILE DUCTS

Morphologic studies concerning the precursor lesions of invasive carcinoma of the extrahepatic bile ducts are almost non-existent. A large proportion of these tumors are unresectable at the time of diagnosis. In these cases, a small biopsy is usually taken for histologic confirmation. As a rule, the biopsy specimen does not include adjacent non-involved mucosa. At autopsy, however, these carcinomas, with the possible exception of the papillary type, are quite large and have invaded the adjacent mucosa, obliterating all precursor changes. Another limitation in the study of these lesions is the lack of clinical markers that can be used to identify patients at risk for carcinoma of the extrahepatic bile ducts. These tumors, contrary to those that arise in the gallbladder, are usually not associated with cholelithiasis or choledocholithiasis. In fact, the incidence of cholelithiasis coexisting with carcinoma of the extrahepatic bile ducts is no greater than the expected prevalence of gallstones in the general population. Moreover, there are no known genetic syndromes that increase the risk for cancer of the extrahepatic bile ducts. Occasionally, there are reports of carcinoma of the extrahepatic ductal system occurring in patients with familial polyposis of the colon (Lees and Hermann, 1981). More significant appears to be the association of bile duct carcinoma with ulcerative colitis (Ross and Braasch, 1973). Bile duct carcinoma is also a complication of long-standing primary sclerosing cholangitis (Chapman et al., 1981). However, until the predisposing factors for extrahepatic bile duct carcinoma are further delineated, a systematic search for the precursor lesions is not practical.

With the wider use of cholangiography, computed tomography, and ultrasonography, an increasing number of relatively small carcinomas of the extrahepatic bile ducts have been found and excised along with fragments of normal-appearing mucosa. Histologic examination of the latter has revealed cellular abnormalities that have been interpreted as dysplasia or carcinoma-in-situ and that essentially show the same cell composition and architectural changes as similar lesions occurring in the gallbladder (Laitio, 1983). Our experience with dysplasia and carcinoma-in-situ of the extrahepatic bile ducts is the same as that of Laitio, who has studied these lesions in Finland.

Dysplasia and carcinoma-in-situ usually arise in a background of metaplasia. The most common metaplastic changes encountered in the mucosa consist of antral-type glands and less frequently cells that express intestinal phenotypes such as goblet cells and endocrine cells. The dysplastic and neoplastic cells are first demonstrated on the surface epithelium and subsequently extend downward or project into the lumen as small papillary structures (Figs. 10–14 and 10–15).

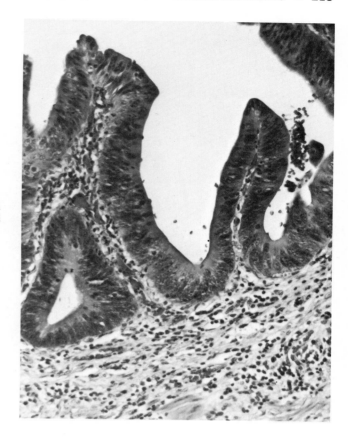

Figure 10–14. Mucosa of the common bile duct adjacent to an infiltrating adenocarcinoma. The epithelium is highly atypical and may be interpreted as either severe dysplasia or carcinoma-in-situ.

In some cases, we have seen carcinoma-in-situ at the margin of resection, which was at a considerable distance from the primary tumor. Residual carcinoma-in-situ at the margins of resection may explain some of the recurrences in the stump of the bile ducts. The mucin and carcinoembryonic antigen contents of these cells are similar to those described for the gallbladder. Independent foci of carcinoma-in-situ are often seen, which again seems to reflect a multicentric origin for cancers arising in the extrahepatic bile ducts.

THE ADENOMA–CARCINOMA SEQUENCE

There is no evidence supporting the concept that patients with solitary adenomas (tubular or papillary) of the extrahepatic bile ducts are at high risk for the development of carcinoma. Certainly, most clinical observations do not support the adenoma–carcinoma sequence. The finding of an "adenomatous residue" by some authors (Kosuka et al., 1984) can be explained, as in the gallbladder, by the broad morphologic spectrum of these tumors, most of which contain a well-differentiated component, as well as by the presence of metaplastic antral-type glands. Further complicating the interpretation is the fact that these glands may even show dysplastic and in-situ changes.

CYSTADENOMA AS A CANCER PRECURSOR

Cystadenoma is a rare but distinctive neoplasm of the biliary tree, more often found within the liver or pancreas than in the bile ducts or gallbladder. Occasional cases, however, have originated in the extrahepatic bile ducts. Malignant epithelial transformation has been seen in cystadenomas arising in the liver (Ishak et al., 1977; Marsh et al., 1974), but the malignant potential of the extrahepatic bile duct tumors is unknown.

PAPILLOMATOSIS OF THE EXTRAHEPATIC BILE DUCTS

Papillomatosis is characterized by multiple and complex papillary lesions that may involve extensive areas of the biliary tree, including the gallbladder and intrahepatic bile ducts. Even extension into the pancreatic ducts has been observed. Although the disease is rare and only a few cases have been reported, progression to invasive carcinoma is well documented (Neumann et al., 1976). For this reason, papillomatosis should be regarded as a precancerous condition.

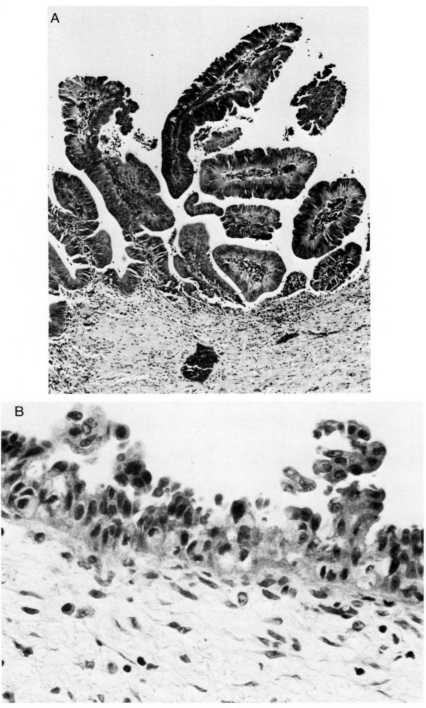

Figure 10–15. *A*, Papillary carcinoma-in-situ of common bile duct. Papillary structures are lined by tall columnar pseudostratified epithelium with features of malignant change. Microinvasion was seen in other areas. *B*, Carcinoma-in-situ is seen in flat mucosa of the common bile duct.

References

Albores-Saavedra, J., Alcantara-Vazquez, A., Curz-Ortis, H., Herrera-Geopfert, H.: The precursor lesions of invasive gallbladder carcinoma. Cancer 45:919–927, 1980.

Albores-Saavedra, J. and Henson, D. E.: Tumors of the Gallbladder and Extrahepatic Bile Ducts, 2nd Series, Fascicle 26. Washington, D.C., Armed Forces Institute of Pathology, 1985.

Albores-Saavedra, J., Manrique, J. J., Angeles-Angeles, A., Henson, D. E.: Carcinoma in situ of the gallbladder. A clinicopathologic study of 18 cases. Am. J. Surg. Pathol. 8:323–333, 1984.

Albores-Saavedra, J., Nadji, M., Henson, D. E., Mones, J., Weissman, J.: Intestinal metaplasia of the gallbladder. Hum Pathol., submitted.

Albores-Saavedra, J., Nadji, M., Morales, A., Henson, D. E.: Carcinoembryonic antigen in normal, preneoplastic and neoplastic gallbladder epithelium. Cancer 52:1069–1072, 1983.

Alonso de Ruiz, P., Albores-Saavedra, J., Henson, D. E., Monroy, M. N.: Cytopathology of precursor lesions of invasive carcinoma of the gallbladder. Acta Cytol. 6:144–152, 1982.

Bansal, M., Fenoglio, M. C., Robboy, S. T., King, D. W.: Are metaplasias in colorectal adenomas truly metaplasias? Am. J. Pathol. 115:253–265, 1984.

Black, W. X.: The morphogenesis of gallbladder carcinoma. *In* Fenoglio, C. M. and Wolff, M. (eds.): Progress in Surgical Pathology. Vol. 2. New York, Masson Publishing Co., 1980, pp. 207–223.

Chapman, R. W. G., Burroughs, A. D., Bass, N. M., Sherlock, S.: Long-standing asymptomatic primary sclerosing cholangitis. Dig. Dis. Sci. 26:778–782, 1981.

Ishak, K. G., Willis, G. W., Cummins, S. D., Bullock, A. A.: Biliary cystadenoma and cystadenocarcinoma. Cancer 39:322–338, 1977.

Kosuka, S., Tsubone, M., Hachisuka, K.: Evolution of carcinoma in the extrahepatic bile ducts. Cancer 54:65–72, 1984.

Kosuka, S., Tsubone, M., Yasui, A., Hachisuka, K.: Relation of adenoma to carcinoma in the gallbladder. Cancer 50:2226–2234, 1982.

Laitio, M.: Goblet cells, enterochromaffin cells, superficial gastric-type epithelium and antral-type glands in the gallbladder. Beitr. Pathol. 156:343–358, 1975.

Laitio, M.: Carcinoma of the extrahepatic bile ducts. A histopathologic study. Pathol. Res. Pract. 178:67–72, 1983.

Laitio, M.: Histogenesis of epithelial neoplasms of human gallbladder. I. Dysplasia. Pathol. Res. Pract. 178:51–56, 1983a.

Laitio, M.: Histogenesis of epithelial neoplasms of human gallbladder. II. Carcinoma. Pathol. Res. Pract. 178:57–66, 1983b.

Lees, C. D. and Hermann, R. E.: Familial polyposis coli associated with bile duct cancer. Am. J. Surg. 141:378–380, 1981.

Lurie, B. B., Loewenstein, M. S., Zamcheck, N. P.: Elevated carcinoembryonic antigen levels and biliary tract obstruction. J.A.M.A. 233:326–330, 1975.

Marsh, J. L., Dahms, B., Longmire, W. G., Jr.: Cystadenoma and cystadenocarcinoma of the biliary system. Arch. Surg. 109:41–43, 1974.

Neumann, R. D., LiVolsi, V. A., Rosenthal, N. S., Burrell, M., Ball, T. J.: Adenocarcinoma in biliary papillomatosis. Gastroenterology 70:779–782, 1976.

Putz, P. and Willems, G.: Proliferative changes in the epithelium of the human lithiasic gallbladder. J. Natl. Cancer Inst. 60:283–287, 1978.

Ropertz, S. and Wagner, K.: Die laparaskopische Gallenblasenpunktiontechnik und diagnostische. Leber Magen Darm 6:19–24, 1976.

Ross, A. P. and Braasch, J. W.: Ulcerative colitis and carcinoma of the proximal bile ducts. Gut 14:94–97, 1973.

Strauch, G. O.: Primary carcinoma of the gallbladder. Surgery 47:368–383, 1960.

Symonds, D. A.: Paneth cell metaplasia in diseases of the colon and rectum. Arch. Pathol. 97:343–347, 1974.

Tanga, M. R. and Ewing, J. B.: Primary malignant tumors of the gallbladder. Surgery 67:418–426, 1970.

Tatsuta, M., Yamamura, H., Yamamoto, R., Morii, T., Okuda, S., Tamura, H.: Carcinoembryonic antigen in the bile in patients with pancreatic and biliary cancer. Cancer 50:2903–2909, 1982.

PATRICK J. FITZGERALD
ANTONIO L. CUBILLA

11 Pancreas

The belief that the first morphologically recognizable form of carcinoma is carcinoma-in-situ appears to be correct for all human cancers arising from epithelium of glands and surfaces. Whether there are precursor lesions, actual or potential, to carcinoma-in-situ appears to depend on the organ that is involved. Even within each organ there may be different precursors for different types of carcinoma. In many circumstances, there may be no recognizable precursor lesions, with the carcinoma-in-situ arising de novo from "normal" epithelium (Rosai and Ackerman, 1978; Stewart, 1960).

Until the advent of recent advances in imaging and endoscopic techniques, the pancreas had been a relatively inaccessible retroperitoneal organ and its tissue had been available for examination only at operation or autopsy. There are no reported studies that have followed the process of pancreatic carcinogenesis in the human from an early to a late stage as, for example, there are with carcinomas of the uterine cervix (Albert, 1981; Barron and Richart, 1968). There is no direct evidence that any one of the many benign lesions suggested as a precursor progresses to in-situ or to invasive carcinoma.

In the pancreas, as in other gastrointestinal organs, there are lesions such as metaplasia, hyperplasia, polyp, papillary hyperplasia, adenoma, papilloma, and villous papilloma that are associated with pancreatic ductal cancer. There are also carcinomas that appear to arise in otherwise normal epithelium (Cubilla and Fitzgerald, 1976; Cubilla and Fitzgerald, 1984a). The pertinent questions are whether the benign lesion is an obligate stage in the transformation process, an ancillary non-malignant manifestation of a neoplastic state, fertile ground for the appearance of an in-situ carcinoma, or an incidental finding unrelated to the carcinogenic process.

In a search for lesions associated with pancreatic cancer that might be considered possible precursors, we examined ductal and ductular epithelium of resected pancreas following surgery and also at autopsy in a group of patients with invasive pancreatic cancer matched with a control group of patients of similar age and sex who died without pancreatic cancer (Table 11–1) (Cubilla and Fitzgerald, 1976).

We have also had an opportunity to examine five cases of in-situ carcinoma, or minimally invasive cancer, of the pancreatic ductal system (Cubilla and Fitzgerald, 1984a).

BENIGN NEOPLASMS AS POSSIBLE PRECURSORS OF PANCREATIC CANCER

Polyp, Papilloma, and Adenoma of the Ampulla of Vater

Polyp, papilloma, and adenoma of the ampulla of Vater have been suggested as possible precursors of cancer in the ampulla (Cattell and Pyrtek, 1950).

A neoplastic polyp or an adenoma may be a precursor of a cancer of the ampulla or of the pancreatic ductal system. Both are rare (Cubilla and Fitzgerald, 1984a). Klöppel states that in 20 percent of cases of ampullary carcinoma a sessile villous adenoma of the duodenal mucosa precedes the carcinoma (Klöppel and Heitz, 1984). Of 31 patients with cancer of the ampulla, 21 had a papillary configuration (Cubilla and Fitzgerald, 1980b), although it is not known how many, if any, had arisen from a papilloma.

Pancreatic ductal papillomatosis has been reported in a small number of patients (Patient 1, Cubilla and Fitzgerald, 1984a; Habán, 1936; Klöppel and Heitz, 1984), and in the first two reports, invasive pancreatic cancer was found. In our Patient 1, foci of papilloma, villous papilloma, papillary carcinoma, and carcinoma-in-situ were found in the pancreatic ductal system. However, papilloma of the pancreatic duct is rare. In most cases of pancreatic cancer, papillomas are not a predominant feature (Table 11–2), and they

Table 11–1. **Duct Epithelial Changes with Pancreas Cancer***

	Surgical (100 cases) (%)	Autopsy (127 cases) (%)	Combined (227 cases) (%)	Control† (100 cases) (%)
Squamous metaplasia	7	6	6	12
Pyloric gland metaplasia	31	18	24	17
Mucous cell hypertrophy	48	24	35	28
Focal epithelial hyperplasia	7	6	6	5
Ductal papillary hyperplasia	50	26	37	12
Marked atypical hyperplasia	27	14	20	0
Carcinoma-in-situ	24	13	18	0

*Comparison of associated lesions present in invasive pancreatic cancer patients and in a control group of patients with non-pancreatic cancer.

†One hundred autopsies of patients with non-pancreatic cancer matched for age and sex with the autopsy pancreas cancer cases. (From Cubilla, A. L. and Fitzgerald, P. J.: Cancer Res. 35:2234–2246, 1975.)

probably are not precursors of any significant percentage of cancers of the pancreatic ductal system.

Carcinoid tumors have been reported in the ampulla region (Cubilla and Fitzgerald, 1984a), but whether they were malignant from the onset or were transformed from a benign carcinoid tumor is not known.

Serous Cystadenoma

Serous cystadenoma is a benign lesion, and carcinoma is not believed to arise from it (Compagno and Oertel, 1978a; Cubilla and Fitzgerald, 1984a; Klöppel and Heitz, 1984). Glenner and Mallory (1956) have divided this group of tumors into those with papillae (presumably having a greater likelihood for transformation into a cystadenocarcinoma) and those without papillae that are benign. We have studied two cases at autopsy of serous cystadenomas with a few foci of papillae of benign-appearing epithelium, but no evidence of invasion or metastases was present (Cubilla and Fitzgerald, 1984c). In none of the 34 cases of Compagno and Oertel (1978a) was there any evidence of spread of this tumor or metastasis. We have

Table 11–2. **Primary Malignant Neoplasms of the Non-endocrine Pancreas***

	Patients Number (%)		Patients Number (%)
Duct (ductule) cell origin	573 (88.8)	*Connective tissue origin*	4 (0.6)
Duct cell carcinoma (494)		Leiomyosarcoma (1)	
Giant cell carcinoma (27)		Malignant fibrous histocytoma (1)	
Giant cell carcinoma (osteoclastoid type) (1)		Malignant hemangiopericytoma (1)	
Adenosquamous carcinoma (20)		Osteogenic sarcoma (1)	
Adenosquamous (spindle cell) carcinoma		Fibrosarcoma	
Microadenocarcinoma (solid microglandular) (16)		Rhabdomyosarcoma	
Mucinous ("colloid") carcinoma (9)		Malignant neurilemoma	
Cystadenocarcinoma (mucinous) (5)		Liposarcoma	
Papillary cystic tumor (1)			
Mucinous-carcinoid carcinoma		*Uncertain histogenesis*	59 (9.2)
Carcinoid		Pancreaticoblastoma (simple type)	
Oncocytic carcinoid		Pancreaticoblastoma (mixed type) (1)	
Oncocytic carcinoma		Unclassified (58)	
Oat-cell carcinoma		Large cell (50)	
Ciliated cell carcinoma (?)		Small cell (7)	
		Clear cell (1)	
Acinar cell origin	8 (1.2)		
Acinar cell carcinoma (7)		*Malignant lymphoma (?)*	
Acinar cell cystadenocarcinoma (1)		Histiocytic	
		Plasmacytoma	
Mixed cell type	1 (0.2)		
Duct-islet cell (1)		*Total*	645
Duct-islet-acinar cell			
Acinar-islet cell			
Carcinoid-islet cell			

*Classification of malignant lesions of the pancreas and the relative frequency of the types at Memorial Hospital, New York, NY. Figures obtained from over 500,000 surgical specimens and 13,882 autopsies. 821 patients were listed as having pancreas (non-islet) cancer; adequate clinical and pathologic material was available for study in 645 patients. Diagnoses without (numbers) indicate that such a cancer did not occur in the Memorial Hospital patients during the years of the review (1949 to 1978) but has been reported in the literature or was seen by us subsequent to 1978.

(From Cubilla, A. L. and Fitzgerald, P. J.: Tumors of the Exocrine Pancreas. Atlas of Tumor Pathology, Second Series, Fascicle 19. The American Registry of Pathology, Armed Forces Institute of Pathology, 1984.)

examined a case of predominantly serous cystadenoma with some foci of columnar cells containing mucin (Cubilla and Fitzgerald, 1984c). Conceivably, these foci of cells with mucin could give rise to a mucinous cystadenocarcinoma, a more likely transformation to carcinoma than that of serous cystadenoma to carcinoma (see following discussion).

Mucinous Cystadenoma

It has been believed for many years that there is a benign cystic lesion of the pancreas, mucinous cystadenoma, in which the cysts contain mucin produced by benign-appearing, mucin-producing epithelium lining the cyst wall. The finding of foci of carcinoma in some of the cysts, recurrences of the cystic tumor after surgery, and metastasis after inadequate surgery have led to the conclusion (Compagno and Oertel, 1978b; Cubilla and Fitzgerald, 1984a; Klöppel and Heitz, 1984) that these tumors should be considered malignant or to have such a high potential for malignant transformation that surgical extirpation should be carried out if possible. One cannot deny the possibility that there exists a mucinous cystadenoma; if it does exist, it should be regarded as a likely precursor for some mucinous cystadenocarcinomas.

Acinar Cell Cystadenoma

We have reported a case of acinar cell cystadenocarcinoma (Cantrell et al., 1981), and the possibility of there being a benign counterpart, acinar cell cystad-

enoma, was discussed. Such a tumor would appear to be very rare, although possibly among the cystic lesions of the pancreas previously encountered or reported there may have been some that were acinar cell in origin.

Acinar Cell Adenoma

Acinar cell carcinoma has been reported to account for from 1 percent (Cubilla and Fitzgerald, 1984a) to 11 percent (Webb, 1977) of human pancreatic cancers. A possible precursor lesion to acinar cell carcinoma, acinar cell adenoma (Fig. 11–1), is said to be rare although a few have been described (Cubilla and Fitzgerald, 1984a; Glenner and Mallory, 1956; Webb, 1977).

Longnecker and coworkers (1980) have described in the human pancreas a 44 percent incidence of what they call "dysplasia" of acinar cells and suggest that this is a lesion that is a precursor of acinar cell carcinoma. Neither Klöppel and Heitz (1984), Pour (1978), nor our group (Cubilla and Fitzgerald, 1984c) were able to confirm this high incidence, which seems to be disproportionately high in view of the relatively low incidence of acinar cell carcinoma.

A few patients with foci of adenomatous hyperplasia have been recorded (Cubilla and Fitzgerald, 1984a; Glenner and Mallory, 1956). Their rarity may be a matter of limited sampling and examination of the pancreas.

The advent of animal models of acinar cell tumors (Hayashi and Hasegawa, 1971; Longnecker and Crawford, 1974; Shinozuka et al., 1980) has provided

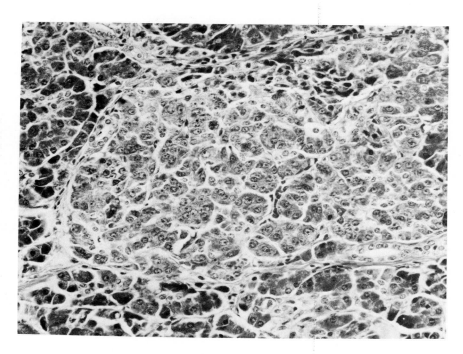

Figure 11–1. Pancreatic nodule of lightly staining cells without ductules or islet cells and with a thin rim of collagen at periphery. Acini are irregular and have decreased basophilia; some contain more nuclei than the normal acinus. Cells have decreased basophilia of the cytoplasm, large nuclei, and more prominent nucleoli than the normal acinar cell. Possible adenoma. Patient had invasive ductal cancer elsewhere.

opportunity to trace the pathogenesis of this rare tumor. In these models, both acinar cell adenomas and acinar cell carcinomas occur. Shinozuka and associates (1980) have reported two patients with an acinar cell nodule in the pancreas; in one patient there was also an insulinoma, suggesting that ductular tissue may be the source of the islet and acinar cell adenomas (Pour, 1978). It should be instructive to determine by more detailed examination of the human pancreas whether similar adenomas are present in humans, and, if so, their relationship to acinar cell carcinoma.

Islet Cell Adenoma

Islet cell neoplasms are the bane of the morphologist. The distinction between islet cell hyperplasia and adenoma and the distinction between adenoma and carcinoma are usually difficult or impossible to make. The problem is complicated by the fact that an islet cell "adenoma" that has behaved as such in the patient for years may suddenly present clinically with metastasis. Heitz, who has had abundant experience with islet cell tumors, states that with the exception of a small number of highly malignant, clearly invasive tumors, the only reliable criterion of the malignant nature of the tumor is massive infiltration of adjacent organs or metastases or both (Klöppel and Heitz, 1984).

Among the possible precursors of islet cell carcinoma are the normal islet cell, islet cell hyperplasia, islet cell adenoma, and the pancreatic ductular cell (Pour, 1978). Heitz believes that the origin of pancreatic endocrine tumors is the pancreatic ductular epithelial cell (Klöppel and Heitz, 1984; Pour, 1978).

Neoplasms of the connective tissue of the pancreas are rare (Cubilla and Fitzgerald, 1975; Cubilla and Fitzgerald, 1984a), and no precursor study of these tumors of the pancreas is known to us.

NON-NEOPLASTIC OR DYSPLASTIC POTENTIAL PRECURSORS OF PANCREATIC CANCER

With many types of cancer, different benign lesions have been postulated as precursors, notably metaplasia, hyperplasia, papillary hyperplasia, and dysplasia.

Squamous Metaplasia

Squamous metaplasia may be the setting in which the uncommon adenosquamous cell cancer of the pancreas (Cubilla and Fitzgerald, 1975; Cubilla and Fitz-

gerald, 1984a) arises, as suggested by the case reported by Hartsock and Fisher (1961). They found carcinoma-in-situ in multiple foci of squamous metaplasia. However, most squamous cancers of the pancreas also have an adenocarcinoma component and are called "adenosquamous carcinomas." In one of our cases of invasive adenosquamous carcinoma, there was an in-situ carcinoma that was primarily adenocarcinoma in configuration (Cubilla and Fitzgerald, 1984c).

The incidence of squamous metaplasia is significant in patients with pancreatic diseases such as chronic pancreatitis and in the elderly (Kozuka et al., 1979), and it is many times greater than the incidence of adenosquamous cell cancer, so that one or more additional factors is needed to explain the transformation of the relatively frequent metaplasia to the relatively rare adenosquamous carcinoma.

Papillary and Adenomatous Hyperplasia

We found a much higher incidence of papillary hyperplasia (Fig. 11–2) in the ductal epithelium of patients with carcinoma of the pancreas than in the duct epithelium of patients who had non-pancreatic cancer (Table 11–1). Others have reported similar results (Sommers et al., 1954b; Klöppel et al., 1980; Kozuka et al., 1979). However, the problem of obstruction was present in all our pancreatic cancer patients. It is known that obstruction, inflammatory changes, or aging can induce papillary hyperplasia in the pancreatic ducts (Klöppel and Heitz, 1984; Kozuka et al., 1979). Rarely, the latter is so marked as to be mistaken grossly for a nodule of carcinoma (Cubilla and Fitzgerald, 1984b). Klöppel believes that papillary hyperplasia is a reactive process that entails no significant risk for the development of pancreatic cancer (Klöppel and Heitz, 1984).

Evaluations of the significance of the formation of a connective tissue stalk in a papillary structure show that the proliferation of epithelium in a rigid tubular structure would cause the increase of cells to expand into the lumen and form mounds, hillocks, or papillae of epithelial cells. Whether a core of connective tissue accompanies the projection of cells is probably related to many factors, including the degree of hyperplasia. In many of the in-situ-carcinomas composed of papillae, no significant stromal reaction is apparent; in others, there is considerable stalk formation. It is important in discussing associated lesions to differentiate papillary hyperplasia (Fig. 11–2) from the papillary growth pattern of an expanding neoplasm. In Patient 1, the neoplastic lesion was predominantly papilliferous, and most papillae had a connective tissue stromal stalk, but some had no connective tissue core.

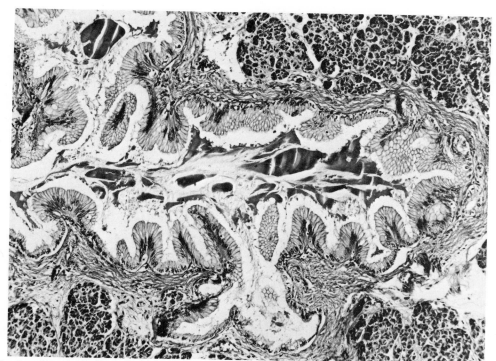

Figure 11–2. Papillary hyperplasia of main duct associated with obstruction caused by carcinoma of the head of the pancreas. Papillae lined with columnar mucinous cells project into the lumen of the duct, which contains inspissated secretion. Some normal epithelium between papillae. No atypia or neoplastic changes present.

One of the features of pancreatic ductal cancer is that in most cases the invasive neoplasm is primarily non-papillary (Table 11–2) (Cubilla and Fitzgerald, 1984a), which implies that the source of the cancer was a non-papillary one, or that if the cancer came from a papillary precursor, it had changed its morphology to a non-papillary invasive carcinoma.

Papillary hyperplasia or adenomatous hyperplasia or both may be a setting conducive to the development of a carcinoma-in-situ while being completely independent of the neoplastic process, or the carcinoma-in-situ may be randomly superimposed upon one or both lesions. More evidence is required for papillary hyperplasia and adenomatous hyperplasia to be considered precursor lesions, an essential step in the transformation process.

Marked Atypia (Dysplasia)

In our studies we found that, as in most cancers, there were debatable lesions, primarily nuclear abnormalities, in the pancreatic ductal cells that were highly suggestive of cancer but that lacked some features and were not sufficiently distinctive for us to label "carcinoma" (Fig. 11–3). Other pathologists might believe that these lesions had crossed the border to carcinoma-in-situ. We have called this group "marked

atypia (dysplasia)" (Cubilla and Fitzgerald, 1976; Cubilla and Fitzgerald, 1984a). In 20 percent of patients with pancreatic cancer there were ductal cells with marked atypia and in the control patients there were none, suggesting that this change was a significant one.

In some of our cases, the atypical epithelium was part of a papillary or hyperplastic lesion, but it also occurred in many flat areas of epithelium or in small papillae of carcinoma-in-situ, particularly in Patients 2 to 5. This lesion has sometimes been viewed as a transition phase between hyperplasia and neoplasia, but such an interpretation is speculative inasmuch as the lesion occurs in the absence of hyperplasia. Some definitive objective finding, such as an immunocytochemical "cancer marker," is needed for tissue sections in these cases in which the subjective factor becomes more prominent in the diagnosis than in the generally accepted criteria for the diagnosis of carcinoma-in-situ.

Other Possible Precursors

Other mentioned precursor possibilities such as focal epithelial hyperplasia, mucinous hypertrophy, and pyloric metaplasia were not significantly increased in our studies of cases of pancreatic cancer compared with

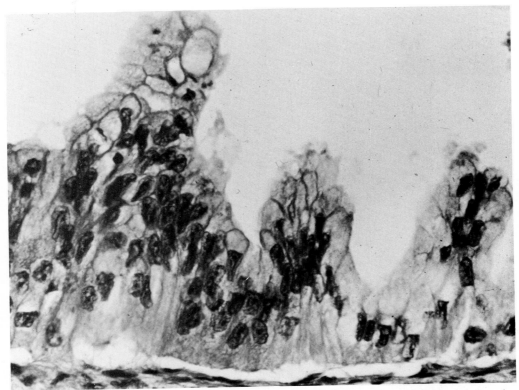

Figure 11–3. Area of marked atypia in Patient No. 2. Papillae of cells with some variation in size and shape of nuclear chromatin as well as prominent nucleoli and some loss of nuclear polarity. Mucin present in most cells. Variation not believed great enough to warrant diagnosis of carcinoma-in-situ, but lesion debatable.

control cases of non-pancreatic carcinomas (Table 11–1) (Cubilla and Fitzgerald, 1976).

CARCINOMA-IN-SITU ASSOCIATED WITH INVASIVE CARCINOMA

Many investigators have found foci of ductal carcinoma-in-situ (Figs. 11–4 to 11–7), associated with but separate from invasive ductal cancer, with the percentage of patients with such lesions varying from 3 percent (Sommers and Meissner, 1954b) to over 30 percent (Edis et al., 1980; Tryka and Brooks, 1979). Our own studies showed 24 percent in surgical specimens and 13 percent in autopsy studies (Table 11–1) (Cubilla and Fitzgerald, 1976). We believe that the difference was caused by the greater amount of tissue sampled by the more numerous histologic sections taken from the surgical specimen than from the pancreas at autopsy, albeit there may have been more overgrowth of in-situ lesions in the cancers in the autopsy tissues.

Many authors have noted that most carcinomas-in-situ are found close to the invasive cancer (example of the field theory) but that a lesser percentage of carcinomas-in-situ are found at a greater distance from the invasive cancer—for example, in the body or the

tail or both when the invasive cancer is in the head of the pancreas (Cubilla and Fitzgerald, 1984a). Possibly, such findings are in part the result of an inadequate sampling of tissue at a distance from the main invasive tumor.

CARCINOMA, IN-SITU OR WITH MINIMALLY INVASIVE CANCER

There have been a small number of cases reported of carcinoma-in-situ of the pancreas in the absence of invasive pancreatic cancer found at autopsy, in a surgically resected pancreas, or in a biopsy of the pancreas. In the few cases reported, the patients have generally been over 40 years. Gray and Scott (1968) described carcinoma-in-situ of the terminal portions of both the pancreatic duct and the common bile duct in a patient with invasive carcinoma of the common bile duct. Hartstook and Fisher (1961) noted multiple foci of carcinoma-in-situ in areas of squamous metaplasia of pancreatic ducts.

Pour and associates (1982), reporting on autopsies in 87 men from 40 to 87 years of age, recorded four patients (5 percent) with in-situ pancreatic cancer. This relatively high incidence of carcinoma-in-situ may be partly explained by the thoroughness of the path-

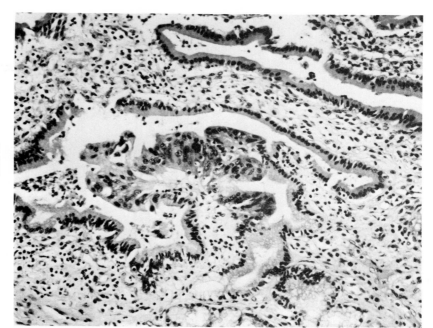

Figure 11–4. Small duct with mostly normal epithelium and a papillary area with foci of carcinoma-in-situ. Patient had invasive ductal cancer elsewhere.

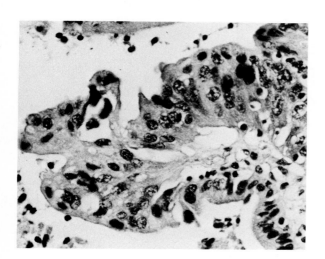

Figure 11–5. Section adjacent to that in Figure 11–4. Marked hyperchromasia of nuclei that vary in size, shape, and polarity. Relatively normal epithelium at lower right.

Figure 11–6. Focus of carcinoma-in-situ in patient who had invasive carcinoma elsewhere in duct. There is piling up of nuclei in a zone of "flat" epithelium. Larger than normal nuclei show great variation in size, shape, and polarity. Large and multiple nucleoli are present, and there is disorganization of epithelial architecture.

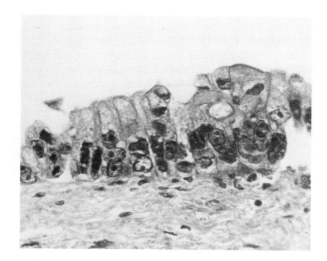

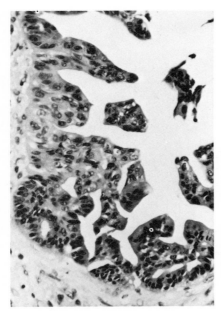

Figure 11–7. Carcinoma-in-situ of dilated duct with piling up of hyperchromatic cells showing bridging and gland formation. Nuclei of cells are varied in size, shape, and polarity. Nucleoli are prominent. Patient had invasive carcinoma elsewhere.

ologic study. The entire organ was fixed and cut into blocks of tissue, and many histologic sections of each block were examined. The figure of 5 percent, however, seems very high in view of the incidence of invasive pancreatic cancer if one believes that most carcinomas-in-situ progress to invasive carcinoma. Mukada and Yamada (1982) discovered five similar cases in 206 autopsies (2.5 percent) of patients from 10 to 88 years of age. Kozuka and colleagues, in an examination of 713 autopsies of patients 40 years of age or older in which there was no invasive pancreatic cancer, described five cases of atypical hyperplasia (stated to be synonymous with carcinoma-in-situ) of pancreatic ductal epithelium (0.7 percent). It is apparent that further studies of extensive and detailed examination of the human pancreas for the presence of carcinoma-in-situ are needed.

We have examined five cases of cancer of the human pancreatic ductal system collected from different hospitals. These lesions were carcinoma-in-situ or carcinoma-in-situ with no gross evidence of invasion or metastasis (Figs. 11–8 to 11–17) (Cubilla and Fitzgerald, 1984a).

Patient 1. An 83-year-old white diabetic woman with painless jaundice was subjected to exploratory surgery. A cholecystectomy and a common bile duct examination were performed, and a tumor was palpated in the second portion of the duodenum. Subsequently, endoscopy revealed "polyps" in the duodenum. At a second operation, two papillomas of the duodenum were found, one at the ampulla of the

major (Wirsung) duct and the other at the ampulla of the minor (Santorini) pancreatic duct. There was a gallstone impacted in the common bile duct just proximal to the ampulla of Vater, and both the common bile duct and the pancreatic duct systems were dilated proximal to it. The surgeon performed a total pancreatectomy.

Grossly, the entire ductal system of the pancreas contained tumor, and there was virtually complete atrophy of acinar tissue with replacement by fibrous connective tissue and collagen. Microscopically, a diffuse papillomatosis (Fig. 11–8) with foci of papillary carcinoma of the duct epithelium (Figs. 11–9 and 11–13) was present from the ampullas throughout the rest of the ductal system of the head, body, and tail of the pancreas. In some places the tumor completely filled the lumen of the duct, and in other foci there were fronds of less well differentiated papillary carcinoma (Fig. 11–13). Some areas of carcinoma-in-situ were present in papillae with stroma (Figs. 11–8 and 11–13). Small foci of in-situ cancer without stroma were often interspersed between papillae (Fig. 11–9).

There was relatively little in-situ-carcinoma present in the small ducts or ductules. Only rarely were acinar cells present, and there was a decrease of islet tissue. The mucosa of both ampullas showed in-situ-carcinoma, and there was carcinoma present in the stroma of the ampulla of Vater and of the wall of the duodenum. The portion of the common bile duct containing the impacted stone showed chronic inflammation but no cancer. Microscopic examination of three peripancreatic lymph nodes revealed no carcinoma. The patient died at home 2 years after the operation of what was described as carcinomatosis; no autopsy was performed.

Habán (1936) has recorded a somewhat similar case of multiple papillomatosis of the pancreatic ductal

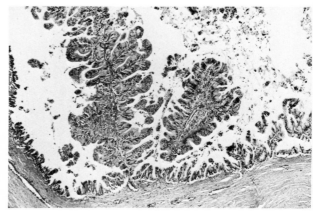

Figure 11–8. Patient No. 1. Papillae in main duct with epithelium ranging from benign to marked atypia and carcinoma-in-situ. Papilliferous epithelium between papillae appears to be abnormal. No evidence of invasion of ductal wall.

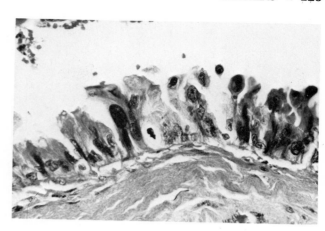

Figure 11–9. Patient No. 1. Papilliferous epithelium of duct wall between large papillae shown in Plate 11–2. Marked variation in size of nuclei, particularly to left of center where abnormal mitotic figure is also present. No invasion of ductal wall.

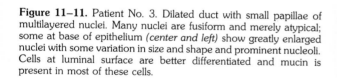

Figure 11–10. Patient No. 2. Piling up of epithelium of a dilated duct with cells showing hyperchromasia of nuclei of varying size and shape. Many nuclei show one or more prominent nuclei, condensation of chromatin at the nuclear membrane, and loss of polarity.

Figure 11–11. Patient No. 3. Dilated duct with small papillae of multilayered nuclei. Many nuclei are fusiform and merely atypical; some at base of epithelium *(center and left)* show greatly enlarged nuclei with some variation in size and shape and prominent nucleoli. Cells at luminal surface are better differentiated and mucin is present in most of these cells.

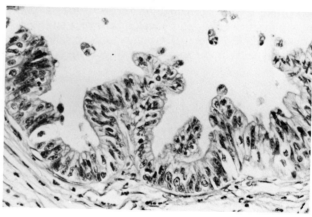

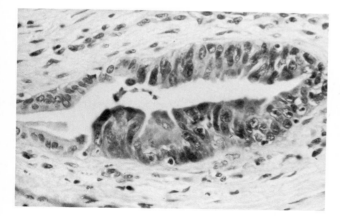

Figure 11–12. Patient No. 4. Small duct showing normal epithelium *(left)* and carcinoma-in-situ, the latter showing piling up of many layers of large cells with large nuclei of varying size and shape, variation in distribution of nuclear chromatin, and lack of polarization. Prominent nucleoli are common. (Courtesy of Dr. M. Huntrakoon.)

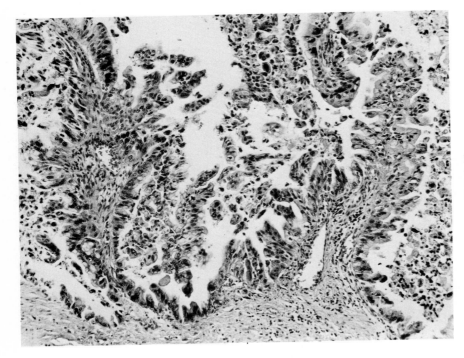

Figure 11–13. Patient No. 1. Papillary carcinoma in main duct. Papillae contain cells ranging from atypia to marked atypia to carcinoma-in-situ.

system in which there were multiple foci of carcinoma-in-situ and one area of invasive carcinoma. Klöppel and Heitz (1984) have reported two cases of ductal papillomatosis.

Patient 2. A 65-year-old white man with anorexia, persistent back pain, and a weight loss of 9 kg (20 lb) showed by abdominal computed tomographic scanning and celiac and superior mesenteric arteriography

abnormal findings suggestive of cancer in the head of the pancreas.

At surgery, a diffusely infiltrative thickening of the pancreas extended from the neck of the pancreas throughout the body and tail. A total pancreatectomy was performed, and the patient died shortly after the operation. No autopsy was performed.

Gross examination of the resected pancreas re-

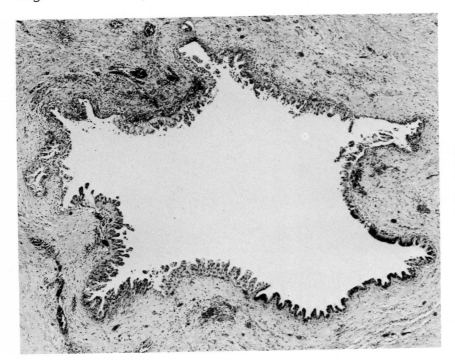

Figure 11–14. Patient No 2. Dilated main duct showing variation of epithelium from normal to hyperplastic to marked atypia to carcinoma-in-situ. Atrophy of acinar and islet tissue and replacement by fibrous connective tissue.

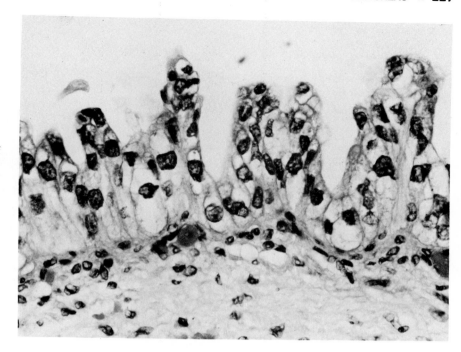

Figure 11–15. Patient No. 2. Focus of carcinoma-in-situ in dilated duct. Papillae of large cells with greatly enlarged nuclei of different size, shape, and polarity. Nucleoli prominent and multiple in some cells. Mucin present in some cells.

vealed that the head of the pancreas was unremarkable, but the neck, body, and tail showed diffuse atrophy with replacement by fibrotic tissue. No gross tumor was identified. The Wirsung duct was patent throughout with considerable variation in diameter in the body and tail (Fig. 11–14).

Throughout the head, body, and tail of the pancreas, the epithelium of the main ducts revealed abnormal findings—papillary hyperplasia, marked atypia, or carcinoma-in-situ (Figs. 11–10, 11–14, and 11–15). The in-situ cancer was mainly in the largest ducts, but there was considerable involvement of the secondary duct system; only rarely was a ductule involved. Carcinoma-in-situ was found in the periphery of one islet.

The carcinoma-in-situ foci were widespread

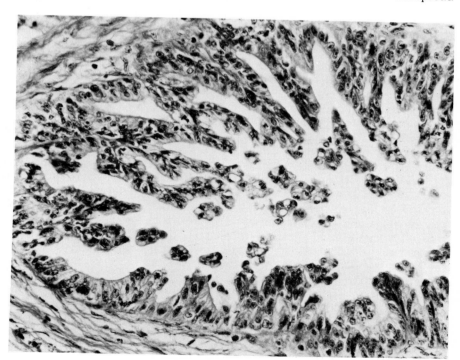

Figure 11–16. Patient No. 3. Duct with papillae of atypical epithelium, marked atypia, and carcinoma-in-situ at 5 to 7 o'clock.

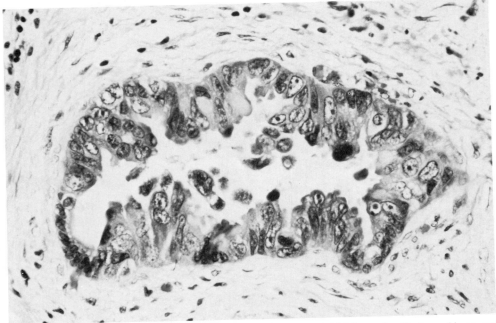

Figure 11–17. Patient No. 4. Small duct with focus of normal epithelium *(lower left)*. Multilayered epithelium of large epithelial cells with variably sized large nuclei and prominent nucleoli piled up into hillocks and papillae. Variation in the amount and distribution of nuclear chromatin. (Courtesy of Dr. M. Huntrakoon.)

throughout the gland with "skip" areas of normal epithelium, hyperplasia, and marked atypia between the foci. The lesions did not occur as those in the florid papillary pattern of Patient 1 but were prominent, arranged in relatively "flat" ductal hillocks of piled-up malignant cells (Fig. 11–14).

In the very small amount of parenchymal acinar and islet tissue remaining in the body and tail of the pancreas, there was no evidence of marked atypia, adenoma, or carcinoma. There was carcinoma present in a perineural space. Three of 58 lymph nodes of the superior body group (Cubilla et al., 1978) examined microscopically were shown to have carcinoma. The biliary tract was negative.

Patient 3.* A 52-year-old white woman with a chronic pancreatitis associated with alcohol abuse had a total pancreatectomy for a cancer of the body of the pancreas. Carcinoma-in-situ was confined to the pancreatic duct system except for a small focus of invasion of the parenchyma in the body. Foci of marked atypia and carcinoma-in-situ were present in many ducts (Figs. 11–11 and 11–16). Ectasia of ducts occurred, and the flattened epithelium of these ducts was in marked contrast to the ducts of normal size, which at low magnification revealed the large columnar cells with pale-staining cytoplasm of carcinoma-in-situ cells. The in-situ cancer was papilliferous in some areas (Figs. 11–11 and 11–16) but occurred in

"flat" epithelium in others. Nuclear abnormalities at the base of the epithelium were diagnostic (Figs. 11–11 and 11–16).

The patient has survived 5 years after the operation, a very rare occurrence in pancreatic cancer of the body or tail of the pancreas.

Patient 4.* A 58-year-old white man who was known to imbibe alcohol excessively became jaundiced, and at operation a pseudocyst was found to obstruct the common bile duct. A Whipple resection revealed chronic pancreatitis and many areas of carcinoma-in-situ of the large and small ducts (Figs. 11–12 and 11–17). Hillocks of large cells with prominent nuclei showed pleomorphism of nuclear chromatin and a lack of nuclear polarity. Often, papillae of similar cells and even an occasional papilla with a stalk of stroma were present. In microscopic fields with carcinoma-in-situ, adjacent relatively normal ductal cells were seen (Fig. 11–12). Carcinoma was present in perineural spaces. There appeared to be invasion of the parenchyma in a few areas. Carcinoma-in-situ was present in the margin of surgical resection (Fig. 11–17). Microscopic examination of lymph nodes revealed no carcinoma.

The patient re-entered the hospital 6 months later, and at operation the abdomen was said to be "full of tumor." He was discharged and died at home; no autopsy was performed.

*Tissue sections kindly furnished by Dr. Joseph Eggleston, Baltimore, Maryland.

*Case kindly furnished by Dr. M. Huntrakoon, Kansas City, Kansas.

Patient 5.† A 60-year-old white man died of massive gastrointestinal bleeding associated with cirrhosis of the liver (alcoholic) and rupture of esophageal varicosities. At autopsy, a chronic pancreatitis was present. There were multiple foci of carcinoma-in-situ of the large and small ducts in the tail of the pancreas, with a few foci of possible invasion of the parenchyma. The nuclei of the cancer cells showed marked variation in the amount and distribution of chromatin, and there was loss of polarity. No carcinoma was found on microscopic examination of peripancreatic lymph nodes. The carcinoma was present in areas of papillary hyperplasia and in non-papillary areas as well.

Discussion. All our five patients with carcinoma-in-situ, or early invasive carcinoma, had chronic pancreatitis.

Patient 1 represents a very rare type of diffuse papillomatosis of the ductal system that either alone or with the obstruction of the ductal system by a stone led to virtually complete absence of the acinar cell parenchyma and fibrosis. The papillomatosis was associated with foci of papillary carcinoma and in-situ carcinoma; the latter occurred in both papillary and non-papillary areas. The origin of the invasive carcinoma must have been the ductal system, but whether it was from one or more papillomas, from a papillary carcinoma, or from a carcinoma-in-situ from non-papillary epithelium cannot be determined. The patient was a known treated diabetic of 15 years' duration, but no history concerning alcohol or smoking was available.

Patient 2 had a focal chronic pancreatitis with marked atrophy of the parenchyma of the body and tail and a relatively normal head of the pancreas. Carcinoma-in-situ occurred throughout the ductal system. No mention of alcohol, cigarette smoking, or biliary symptoms was made in the patient's record, but the focal nature of the chronic pancreatitis (Sarles et al., 1980) would suggest an alcoholic factor. Carcinoma-in-situ was present primarily in non-papillary neoplastic ductal epithelium.

Patient 3 was prone to excessive use of alcohol and had chronic pancreatitis. Only minimal invasion of the parenchyma of the pancreas and no perineural or lymph node involvement were found on microscopic examination. The in-situ carcinoma was present mostly in non-papillary neoplastic ducts and ductules.

Patients 4 and *5* had chronic pancreatitis associated with excessive alcohol use, and their foci of in-situ carcinomas occurred mostly in non-papillary neoplastic ductal epithelium.

Thus, chronic pancreatitis associated with alcoholism occurred in three, possibly four, of our patients. Unfortunately, no cigarette smoking history was available in these patients. In only 1 percent of our 645 patients with pancreatic cancer was there a history of chronic pancreatitis (Cubilla and Fitzgerald, 1978), so chronic pancreatitis would seem to be an unlikely precursor of any large percentage of cases of pancreatic cancer. Chronic alcoholism is generally not considered to be a causative agent in cancer of the pancreas (Buncher, 1980). Our findings in the three, possibly four, patients who were alcoholics might be related to the bias of a small number of cases; they could represent a systematic bias because of the presence of chronic pancreatitis, which led to more frequent operations and/or more extensive histologic study of the pancreas in surgical resections or at autopsy; or they could represent a small subset of patients with pancreatic cancer caused by the combined action of alcohol and cigarette smoking (Cubilla and Fitzgerald, 1978b), as found with esophageal cancer (Day, 1982).

In summary, carcinoma-in-situ is the precursor of invasive cancer of the pancreatic ductal system.

Marked atypia (severe dysplasia) is a likely precursor of carcinoma-in-situ in some cases, although subjective factors play a more prominent role in this diagnosis than in the diagnosis of carcinoma-in-situ.

Mucinous cystadenoma or acinar cell cystadenoma (if either exists as an entity) may be a precursor of the respective cystadenocarcinoma.

The villous adenoma of the ampulla of Vater is said to be a precursor of ampullary carcinomas in about 20 percent of cases.

The very rare papilloma of the pancreatic ductal system is probably not a precursor for any significant number of cancers of the pancreas.

Papillary hyperplasia is present in the majority of cases of ductal pancreatic cancer, but it is also present in a significant percentage of cases of ductal obstruction and inflammation, and it increases with age. Most cancers of the pancreas are not predominantly papillary. Foci of carcinoma-in-situ can occasionally be found in papillary hyperplasia, but they also occur in the absence of the lesion. Convincing evidence for papillary hyperplasia as an essential step in the carcinogenic process is lacking.

Squamous metaplasia may be a precursor of the uncommon adenosquamous carcinoma of the pancreatic ductal system, although there is relatively little evidence available to support such a possibility.

Other lesions, such as focal epithelial hyperplasia, pyloric metaplasia, and mucinous hyperplasia, do not appear to be precursors of pancreatic ductal cancer.

Islet cell cancers are an enigma to the morphologist inasmuch as they are diagnosed by invasion or metastasis or both. They may arise from pre-existing adenoma, islet cells, islet cell hyperplasia, or ductular cells; no conclusive studies are available.

---

†Case kindly furnished by Dr. Douglas MacGregor, U.S. Veterans Hospital, Kansas City, Missouri.

The rare acinar cell carcinoma of the pancreas in humans might arise from ductular epithelium, from an acinar cell adenoma, or de novo from the acinar cell. The advent of animal models with the presence of acinar cell adenoma and acinar cell carcinoma should help one considerably in interpreting acinar cell lesions in humans. More detailed examination of the human pancreas is needed to provide evidence concerning the prevalence of possible precursors of acinar cell carcinoma.

Of the many problems involving possible precursors of pancreatic carcinomas, it is obvious that limited sampling of the pancreas has been a major defect in most studies. In addition, the matter of proper control groups of patients—matched for age, sex, the presence of inflammatory or ductal obstructive changes, and the influence of diabetes, alcohol, cigarette smoking, and other possible carcinogens—has to be met. Only when these two major conditions are satisfied may one determine the significant association of the various lesions with the cancer and whether they occur in the proper time sequence to qualify as a possible precursor state. Then the problem of the relationship of an associated change can be examined more critically.

A small subset of alcoholic patients with chronic pancreatitis who are also excessive cigarette smokers might be at higher risk for pancreatic cancer, similar to the greater risk for these patients for cancer of the esophagus.

It is not known at what age carcinoma-in-situ of the pancreas appears, although most of the small number of reported cases were found in patients over 40 years. The rate of progression of pancreatic cancer from a morphologically recognizable in-situ lesion to invasive cancer is unknown, and the rate of progression of invasive pancreas cancer to metastasis is also unknown. At present, when a carcinoma of the pancreatic ductal system is discovered clinically, there is no evidence as to whether the cancer has been present for months or for years. The natural history in both temporal and morphologic aspects is completely unknown.

References

Albert, A.: Estimated cervical cancer disease state, incidence and transition rates. J. Natl. Cancer Inst. 67:571–576, 1981.

Barron, B.A. and Richart, R.M.: A statistical model of the natural history of cervical carcinoma based on a prospective study of 557 cases. J. Natl. Cancer Inst. 41:1343–1353, 1968.

Buncher, C.R.: Epidemiology of pancreatic cancer. In Moosa, A.R. (ed.): Tumors of the Pancreas. Baltimore, Williams & Wilkins Co., 1980, pp. 415–427.

Cantrell, B.B., Cubilla, A.L., Erlandson, R.A., Fortner, J., Fitzgerald, P.J.: Acinar cell cystadenocarcinoma of human pancreas. Cancer 47:410–416, 1981.

Cattell, R.B. and Pyrtek, L.J.: Premalignant lesions of the ampulla of Vater. Surg. Gynecol. Obstet. 90:21–30, 1950.

Compagno, J. and Oertel, J.E.: Microcystic adenomas of the pancreas (glycogen-rich cystadenomas). Am. J. Clin. Pathol. 69:289–298, 1978a.

Compagno, J. and Oertel, J.E.: Mucinous cystic neoplasms of the pancreas with overt and latent malignancy (cystadenocarcinoma and cystadenoma). Am. J. Clin. Pathol. 69:573–580, 1978b.

Cubilla, A.L. and Fitzgerald, P.J.: Morphological patterns of primary non-endocrine human pancreas carcinoma. Cancer Res. 35:2234–2246, 1975.

Cubilla, A.L. and Fitzgerald, P.J.: Morphological lesions associated with human primary invasive nonendocrine pancreas cancer. Cancer Res. 36:2690–2798, 1976.

Cubilla, A.L. and Fitzgerald, P.J.: Pancreas cancer (nonendocrine): A review. Part I: Clin. Bull. (Memorial Sloan-Kettering Cancer Center) 8:91–99, 1978; Part II: Clin. Bull. 8:143–155, 1978.

Cubilla, A.L. and Fitzgerald, P.J.: Cancer (non-endocrine) of the pancreas. A suggested classification. In Fitzgerald, P.J. and Morrison, A.B. (eds.): The Pancreas. Intl. Acad. Pathol. Monogr. Baltimore, Williams & Williams Co., 1980a, pp. 82–110.

Cubilla, A.L. and Fitzgerald, P.J.: Surgical pathology aspects of cancer of the ampulla–head-of-pancreas region. In Fitzgerald, P.J. and Morrison, A.B. (eds.): The Pancreas. Baltimore, Williams & Wilkins Co., 1980b, pp. 67–81.

Cubilla, A.L. and Fitzgerald, P.J.: Tumors of the Exocrine Pancreas. Atlas of Tumor Pathology, Second Series, Fascicle 19. Bethesda, MD, The American Registry of Pathology, Armed Forces Institute of Pathology, 1984a.

Cubilla, A.L. and Fitzgerald, P.J.: Pancreatitis and the false diagnosis of pancreatic cancer. In Gyr, K.E., Singer, M.V., Sarles, H. (eds.): Pancreatitis. Concepts and Classification. Excerpta Medica, Amsterdam, 1984b, pp. 367–369.

Cubilla, A.L. and Fitzgerald, P.J.: Unpublished data, 1984c.

Cubilla, A.L., Fortner, J., Fitzgerald, P.J.: Lymph node involvement in carcinoma of the head of the pancreas area. Cancer 41:880–887, 1978.

Day, N.E.: Esophagus. In Schottenfeld, D. and Fraumeni, J.F. (eds.): Cancer Epidemiology and Prevention. Philadelphia, W.B. Saunders Co., 1982, pp. 596–623.

Edis, A.J., Kiernan, P.O., Taylor, W.F.: Attempted curative resection of ductal carcinoma of the pancreas. Mayo Clin. Proc. 55:531–536, 1980.

Glenner, G.G. and Mallory, G.K.: The cystadenoma and related nonfunctional tumors of the pancreas. Cancer 9:980–996, 1956.

Gray, B. and Scott, R.: Carcinoma in situ in common bile duct and pancreatic duct. Br. J. Surg. 55:309–311, 1968.

Habán, G.: Papillomatose and Carcinom des Gangsystems der Bauchspeicheldrüse. Virch. Arch. [A] 297:207–220, 1936.

Hartsock, R.J. and Fisher, E.R.: Cancer in situ in pancreatic squamous metaplasia. Arch. Surg. 82:674–678, 1961.

Hayashi, Y. and Hasegawa, T.: Experimental pancreatic tumor in rats after intravenous injection of 4-hydroxyamino-quinoline 1-oxide. Gann 62:329–330, 1971.

Klöppel, G., Bommer, G., Ruckert, K., Seifert, G.: Intraductal proliferation in the pancreas and its relationship to human and experimental carcinogenesis. Virchows Arch. [A] 387:221–233, 1980.

Klöppel, G. and Heitz, P.U.: Pancreatic Pathology. Edinburgh, Churchill Livingstone, 1984.

Kozuka, S., Sassa, R., Taki, T., Masamoto, K., Nayasawa, S., Saga, S., Hasegawa, B., Takeuchi, M.: Relation of pancreatic duct hyperplasia to carcinoma. Cancer 43:1418–1428, 1979.

Longnecker, D.S. and Crawford, B.G.: Hyperplastic nodules and adenomas of exocrine pancreas in azaserine-treated rats. J. Natl. Cancer Inst. 53:573–577, 1974.

Longnecker, D.S., Shinozuka, H., Deker, A.: Focal acinar cell dysplasia in human pancreas. Cancer 45:534–540, 1980.

Mukada, T. and Yamada, S.: Dysplasia and carcinoma in situ of the exocrine pancreas. Tokushima J. Exp. Med. 137:115–124, 1982.

Pour, P.M.: Islet cells as a component of pancreatic ductal neoplasms. I. Experimental study: ductular cells, including islet cell precursors, as primary progenitor cells of tumors. Am. J. Pathol. 90:295–316, 1978.

Pour, P.M., Sayed, S., Sayed, G.: Hyperplastic, preneoplastic and neoplastic lesions found in 83 human pancreases. Am. J. Clin. Pathol. 77:137–152, 1982.

Rosai, J. and Ackerman, L.V.: The pathology of tumors. Part 1: Precancerous and pseudomalignant lesions. CA 28:331–342, 1978.

Sarles, H.C., Figarella, O., Piscornia, E., et al.: Chronic calcifying pancreatitis (CPC). Mechanism of formation of the lesions. New data and critical studies. *In* Fitzgerald, P.J. and Morrison, A.B. (eds.): The Pancreas. Baltimore, Williams & Wilkins Co., 1980, pp. 48–66.

Shinozuka, H., Lee, R.E., Dunn, J. L., Longnecker, D.S.: Multiple atypical acinar cell nodules of the pancreas. Hum. Pathol. 11:389–391, 1980.

Sommers, S.C. and Meissner, W.A.: Unusual carcinomas of the pancreas. Arch. Pathol. 58:101–111, 1954a.

Sommers, S.C., Murphy, S.A., Warren, S.: Pancreatic duct hyperplasia and cancer. Gastroenterology 27:629–640, 1954b.

Stewart, F.W.: The problem of the precursor lesions. Postgrad. Med. 27:317–323, 1960.

Tryka, A.F. and Brooks, J.R.: Histopathology in the evaluation of total pancreatectomy for ductal carcinoma. Ann. Surg. 190:373–381, 1979.

Webb, J.N.: Acinar cell neoplasms of the exocrine pancreas. J. Clin. Pathol. 30:103–112, 1977.

EDWIN W. GOULD
AZORIDES R. MORALES

12 Breast

The subject of incipient neoplasia of the breast has never been more pertinent than it is now. The modern emphasis on the early detection of breast cancer has led to the biopsying of very small lesions that are often of controversial significance. As a result, the pathologist is frequently called upon to interpret and diagnose a variety of epithelial hyperplasias and minimal carcinomas. Therefore, it is relevant that we examine our knowledge of the morphologically recognizable lesions that may precede the development of invasive carcinoma of the breast. It is also essential to review the evidence indicating which histomorphologic patterns represent risk factors without actually being precursors per se.

CARCINOMA-IN-SITU

It is generally accepted that the intraluminal multiplication of neoplastic cells that we identify as ductal or lobular carcinoma-in-situ of the breast precedes the development of invasive carcinoma. However, as in other organs, carcinoma-in-situ in the breast is not a morphologic component of every infiltrating carcinoma because the growing tumor may destroy its point of origin. Furthermore, histologically recognizable in-situ carcinoma is not necessarily an obligatory precursor to invasive carcinoma.

Intraductal carcinoma can express itself in a number of different histomorphologic patterns that often occur together. Of these, comedocarcinoma (Fig. 12–1) is the easiest to identify because it contains all the cytologic hallmarks of malignancy. However, the micropapillary (Fig. 12–2) and cribriform (Fig. 12–3) variants may be difficult to recognize because of the bland appearance of the tumor cells. Transitions from these more subtle forms of intraductal carcinoma to comedocarcinoma led early observers to recognize their significance. It has been demonstrated that an apocrine variant of cribriform intraductal carcinoma is frequently associated with infiltrating tubular carcinoma.

The biology of intraductal carcinoma has never been studied adequately in controlled prospective investigations because a mastectomy is usually performed in such cases. There are, however, a few reports of studies of small numbers of patients with intraductal carcinoma treated by biopsy only. In one series, 15 patients with intraductal carcinoma—all were low-grade micropapillary except one—were followed for an average of 21.6 years (Rosen, 1981). Ten developed carcinoma in the same breast after an average of 9.7 years. Eight of the cancers were infiltrating ductal of no special type, one was a medullary carcinoma, and one became a bulky intraductal lesion. In a similar study, Page and associates (1982) followed 25 women with the micropapillary and cribriform variants of intraductal carcinoma for more than 3 years. Seven of those women (28 percent) developed invasive carcinoma after an average of 6.1 years from the time of biopsy. Six of the tumors were invasive ductal carcinoma of no special type, and one was a mucinous carcinoma.

It is clear from these data that if left untreated, some but not all patients with low-grade intraductal carcinoma will develop invasive ductal carcinomas. One cannot assume that the entire tumor was removed in the initial biopsy because Carter and Smith (1977) showed that 66 percent of mastectomy specimens contain residual intraductal carcinoma following the diagnostic biopsy. Thus, two thirds of patients with biopsy-proven intraductal carcinoma theoretically have residual tumor and may be able to develop invasive carcinoma. This is certainly a more impressive figure than the 28 percent found in Page's study and more in agreement with the 10 of 15 cases (66 percent) reported by Rosen (1981).

Lewis and Geschickter (1938) reported eight cases of comedocarcinoma that were treated by local excision only. Six of these eight patients had a local recurrence within a 4-year period; four of these latter recurrences were within only 1 year. Furthermore, when a radical operation was performed for the recurrences, three of the six had axillary nodal metas-

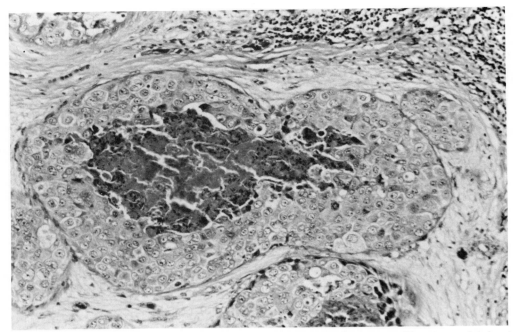

Figure 12–1. Large anaplastic cells distend "duct" with central necrosis in typical comedocarcinoma. There is associated periductal fibrosis and chronic inflammation.

tases. These data suggest that intraductal comedocarcinoma is a more aggressive disease than the low-grade micropapillary/cribriform intraductal carcinoma.

The significance of lobular carcinoma-in-situ was recognized because of its morphologic and temporal relationship to a specific form of invasive carcinoma.

Foote and Stewart (1941) in their classic report followed by the studies of many others reported cases of in-situ lobular carcinoma that were followed by the development of invasive carcinoma over variable periods of time. Clinically, in-situ lobular carcinoma is a disease of premenopausal women. In 60 to 70 percent

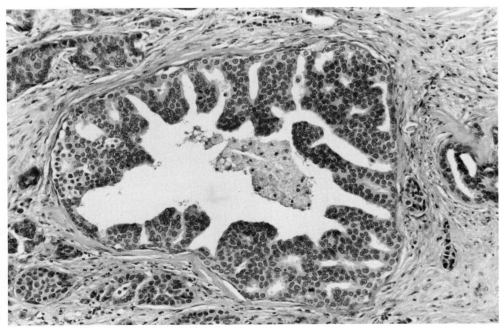

Figure 12–2. The stratification of a uniform cell population forms micropapillary projections in a dilated lumen. Focally there is a cribriform pattern. Invasive carcinoma is also present.

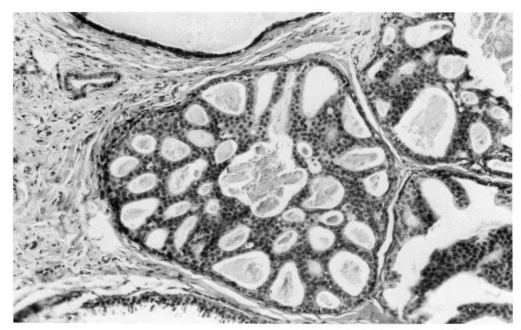

Figure 12–3. Uniform cell population is evenly distributed around well-formed circular lumina in the cribriform pattern of intraductal carcinoma.

of cases, the lesion is multicentric in one breast (Shah et al., 1973; Warner, 1969) and has been reported to be bilateral in approximately 35 percent of cases (Rosen et al., 1981). It is a non-palpable microscopic lesion that is often discovered when the patient is biopsied for some other process, usually fibrocystic disease. In two series, the incidence of this lesion in breast biopsies has been 1.5 percent (Andersen, 1974) and 2.5 percent (Giordano and Klopp, 1973), respectively.

The histologic appearance of the typical lesion (Figs. 12–4 and 12–5) has been well described (Foote and Stewart, 1941; McDivitt et al., 1968; Haagensen, 1971); nevertheless, there is still confusion as to the

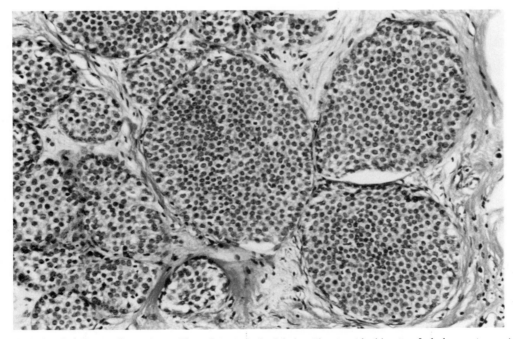

Figure 12–4. Small uniform cell population fills and distends the lobule without residual lumina. Lobular carcinoma-in-situ.

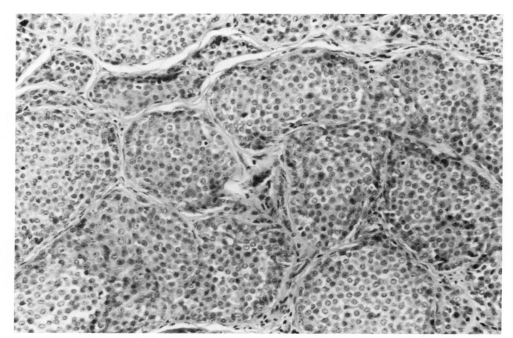

Figure 12–5. Compared with Figure 12–4, a slightly larger, more pleomorphic cell population fills and distends the lobule. The cells are less cohesive and have nucleoli.

minimal qualitative and quantitative criteria needed for the diagnosis of lobular carcinoma-in-situ.

The natural history of in-situ lobular carcinoma is understood better today than it was in the past because of the publication of three detailed studies of patients with untreated tumors of this type (Andersen, 1974; Haagensen et al., 1973; Rosen et al., 1978). These investigators reported that the risk of subsequent invasive carcinoma in patients with lobular carcinoma-in-situ is seven to twelve times greater than it is in an age-corrected population. The majority of their patients, however, remained disease free for 20 years or longer. The carcinomas that did develop in those patients were as likely to occur in the ipsilateral breast as in the contralateral one. Furthermore, less than 50 percent were purely invasive lobular; the majority were ductal or intraductal alone or in combination with the lobular small cell component. Haagensen found that many of the subsequent carcinomas were of a favorable histologic subtype, namely intraductal, tubular, papillary, or medullary. Moreover, it takes many years for invasive carcinoma to develop. In Rosen's study population, the average time required for the development of ductal carcinoma was 16.3 years; that required for infiltrating lobular carcinoma was 24 years.

It is apparent that, in spite of these investigations, the enigma of lobular carcinoma-in-situ remains. Is it truly a preinvasive carcinoma that only occasionally becomes invasive? Why are the cancers that develop often not lobular but ductal histologically? Is there spontaneous regression of this lesion in the majority of patients who remain disease free after simple

biopsy? Does the disease spontaneously regress at menopause? Some hypothetical answers have been proposed for these difficult questions; Rosen found intraductal carcinoma coexisting with lobular carcinoma-in-situ in 11 percent of 75 consecutive biopsy or mastectomy specimens. Therefore, he suggests that many of these patients do develop infiltrating ductal carcinoma. Furthermore, he has found that the average rate of progression from intraductal to invasive ductal carcinoma is 10 years, as opposed to 20.4 years for lobular carcinoma. Therefore, it is to be expected that in many cases only the invasive ductal component will manifest itself. This also explains the presence of residual lobular carcinoma-in-situ in patients who develop ductal carcinoma. The fact, however, that the majority of patients do *not* subsequently develop invasive carcinoma raises the question of the appropriateness of the designation "lobular carcinoma-in-situ." It is for this reason that Haagensen and others opt for the more conservative term "lobular neoplasia," which signifies the uncertainty of the progress of this disease in any given patient. Thus far, no subset of lobular carcinoma-in-situ patients has been delineated that is at increased risk for the development of invasive carcinoma.

PRECURSORS OF CARCINOMA-IN-SITU

Although it is generally agreed that invasive carcinoma of the breast is preceded by the development of carcinoma-in-situ, the morphologic precursors of intraductal and lobular carcinoma-in-situ have not yet been clearly defined. There are, however, an array of benign epithelial proliferations of the breast that have been implicated as predisposing to, or directly resulting in, carcinoma. The possible cause and effect relationships between these lesions and carcinoma are discussed subsequently.

Ductal and Lobular Epithelial Hyperplasia

Morphologic studies suggest that a number of ductal and lobular hyperplastic lesions may be linked over time to the development of carcinoma-in-situ. Following their exhaustive study of cancerous breasts, using a subserial whole-organ sectioning technique, Gallager and Martin (1969) concluded that there is a morphologic continuum from hyperplasia to mammary carcinoma. Black and Chabon (1969) graded the extent of hyperplasia and atypia that may occur within the duct system of the breast. In that and later publications (Black and Kwon, 1980) Black concludes that there is a morphologic continuum from atypia to in-situ carcinoma to invasive carcinoma. However, he also concludes that most patients with epithelial atypia or carcinoma-in-situ do not develop invasive breast carcinoma within 10 to 20 years after local resection.

Wellings and Jensen and their associates performed a series of elegant studies on whole human breasts using a three dimensional "subgross" sampling technique followed by histologic study (Cardiff et al., 1977; Jensen et al., 1976; Wellings, 1980; Wellings and Jensen 1973; Wellings et al., 1975). Their studies show that ductal and lobular carcinoma-in-situ are localized in the terminal ductal lobular unit, which consists of the extralobular terminal duct, the intralobular terminal duct, and the ductules. They described an atypical lobule, a potential precursor lesion, at the subgross level in the terminal ductal lobular unit. This atypical lobule is essentially a large hyperplastic lobule that can be graded from I to V in a morphologic continuum from the normal lobular structure to ductal carcinoma-in-situ (Figs. 12–6 and 12–7). All grades of atypical lobules examined at autopsy were significantly more common in cancerous breasts than in non-cancerous ones. According to these studies, increasing epithelial hyperplasia in the atypical lobule results in progressive unfolding of the terminal ductal lobular unit with eventual formation of large dilated cystic spaces filled with neoplastic cells. Examination of these large spaces, in routine histologic preparations, has led other observers to erroneously conclude that the origin of such resultant hyperplasias and carcinomas is the large duct system.

The evidence that both carcinoma and hyperplasia begin in the terminal ductal lobular unit is compelling and has been corroborated by Squartini and Sarnelli (1981) who used the same "subgross" technique. However, the evidence for a morphologic sequence from Grade I to a higher atypicality and to carcinoma

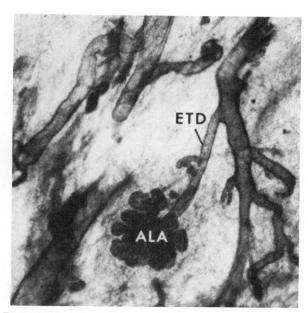

Figure 12–6. Subgross photograph of an atypical lobule of type A (*ALA*). *ETD*, Extralobular terminal duct. (From Wellings, S. R., et al.: J. Natl. Cancer Inst. *55*(2):231, 1975.)

is less convincing. Azzopardi (1979) points out that Grades I and II atypical lobules illustrated by Wellings and coworkers (1975) correspond to adenosis or blunt duct adenosis, a lesion that is not associated with a significant risk for the subsequent development of carcinoma. Other intermediate forms indicated by Wellings as preceding carcinoma-in-situ are lesions with varying degrees of hyperplasia, that most of us

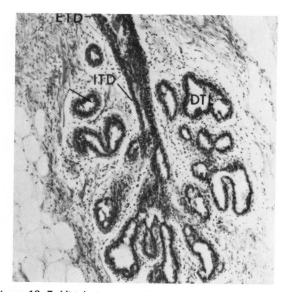

Figure 12–7. Histologic preparation corresponding to Figure 12–6. The extralobular terminal duct (*ETD*), intralobular terminal duct (*ITD*), and ductules (*DTL*) are shown. Arrow points to ductules with cytoplasmic apical blebs protruding into lumen, a Grade I atypical lobule of type A (*ALA*). (From Wellings, S. R., et al.: J. Natl. Cancer Inst. *55*(2):231, 1975.)

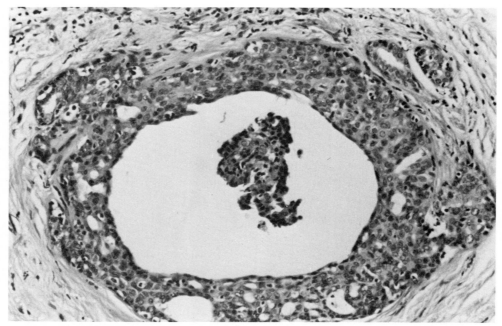

Figure 12–8. Benign epithelial hyperplasia (papillomatosis) in dilated lumen. The bland cellular population has indistinct cell borders with intraepithelial lymphocytes.

would refer to as "benign ductal hyperplasia" or "papillomatosis."

Is "papillomatosis," or "epitheliosis" (interchangeable terms), a precursor to intraductal carcinoma? This is a difficult question because a range of morphologic changes is included under these terms (Figs. 12–8 to 12–10). In fact, the names apply to any benign epithelial proliferation that tends to fill the terminal ducts.

Sandison (1962) in an autopsy study found epitheliosis in 22 percent of normal breasts. Foote and Stewart (1945) originally demonstrated that papillomatosis without atypia is as common in noncancerous breasts as in cancerous ones. Others (Nizze, 1973)

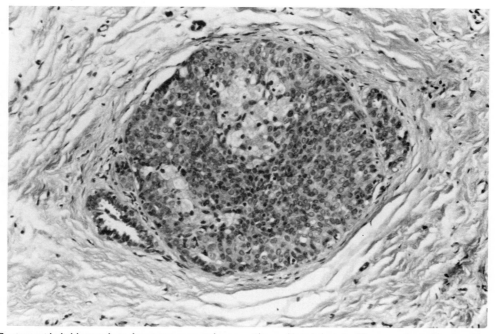

Figure 12–9. Benign epithelial hyperplasia forming a syncytial mass within a dilated ductule. There are typical foam cells centrally located.

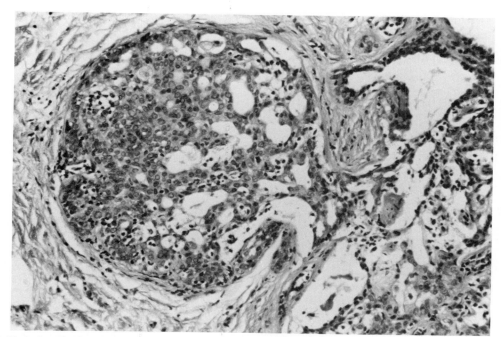

Figure 12–10. Marked epithelial hyperplasia (papillomatosis) flowing into the terminal duct. There are irregular spaces and lymphocyte accumulation within the epithelium.

have demonstrated that the incidence of epitheliosis (papillomatosis) in breasts contralateral to breasts treated for carcinoma is no greater than in normal control specimens.

More recently, Simpson and colleagues (1982) in an investigation of 500 consecutive mastectomy specimens reported that cancerous breasts from patients 26 to 55 years of age contained epitheliosis at 2.6 to 9.5 times the expected frequency. In contrast, after the age of 55 years, the frequency of epitheliosis in cancerous breasts was close to that seen in normal controls. These findings suggest a relationship between epitheliosis and carcinoma in the premenopausal years, implying either a direct transformation of the hyperplastic epithelium into carcinoma or a predisposition that might lead to cancer elsewhere in the breast.

Reasoning that minute cancers might reveal their exact origins before the cancer overgrows and obscures them, Azzopardi studied 15 microcancers, 14 of which measured no more than 3 mm in diameter. He could find no evidence of transition from epitheliosis to cancer, "except perhaps in one case." He concluded that "early carcinoma rarely has its origin in solid areas of epitheliosis or other types of benign epithelial hyperplasia" and that "the earliest changes usually take place de novo in epithelium which is not affected by previous solid benign hyperplasia."

It is certainly more appealing to construct a morphologic continuum between normal hyperplasia and neoplasia. There is well-documented precedence for such a sequential development which is based on the mouse mammary tumor system (DeOme et al., 1959).

Furthermore, such a progression is seen in other epithelial neoplasms in the human body. However, the precursors to what we call "intraductal carcinoma" have not been convincingly identified. If there is a subset of papillomatosis that is truly preneoplastic, it has yet to be identified.

Morphologic precursors to lobular carcinoma-in-situ are not definable because the minimal definition of "lobular carcinoma-in-situ" is not clear. Nevertheless, the term "atypical lobular hyperplasia" has been employed when hyperplasia in the lobule exists but not to the extent that a diagnosis of lobular carcinoma-in-situ is warranted. It is an ill-defined term that is used when only a part of one lobule is involved by the hyperplastic process or when ductal lumina persist in the involved lobule.

Page and coworkers (1978) reported that the risk of subsequent carcinoma in patients with atypical lobular hyperplasia is approximately four times greater than expected, over a 15- to 24-year follow-up; by contrast, the risk is seven to 12 times greater in association with lobular carcinoma-in-situ. Because it often appears that the cytology of the cells in atypical lobular hyperplasia is identical with that in lobular carcinoma-in-situ and only the degree of lobular involvement differs, one wonders whether the number of cells within a given lesion does not relate best to the biologic progression of the disease. However, both Haagensen's and Rosen's studies demonstrate that the degree of acinar distention, presumably related to the number of cells present, does not predict which patients are more likely to develop invasive carcinoma. However, Haagensen (1983) compared the frequency of certain quantitative and qualitative variations in the morphology of lobular neoplasia occurring alone and in conjunction with frank carcinoma. Three of nine microscopic features studied were found to be considerably more common in lobular neoplasia coexisting with overt carcinoma than in lobular neoplasia occurring alone. They are as follows: (1) loss of cohesion among the cells filling the lobules; (2) formation of macroacini; and (3) maximal lobular neoplasia.

If invasive breast cancer evolves through stages of epithelial proliferation to carcinoma-in-situ, as many believe, one would expect that risk factors already established for invasive breast carcinoma might apply as well to these precursor lesions. That concurrence should provide epidemiologic support for a biologic progression. Unfortunately, epidemiologic investigations of benign breast disease have yielded inconsistent and conflicting results with respect to major risk factors known for carcinoma (Brinton et al., 1983; Cole et al., 1978; Ernster, 1981; Sartwell et al., 1978; Soini et al., 1981).

Brinton and associates (1983) in a case-control study for the Breast Cancer Demonstration Detection Project analyzed for the presence of several well-recognized risk factors for breast carcinoma in over 1500 cancer study subjects, patients with benign breast disease, and controls. Patients with in-situ or invasive breast cancer had many of the same epidemiologic factors, except for the following that were only related to invasive cancer: (1) obesity, (2) oophorectomy, and (3) history of a sister with breast cancer. Patients who had benign or malignant breast disease shared no epidemiologic characteristics, with one minor exception—a history of a previous breast biopsy. Their study certainly supports the concept that in-situ and invasive cancer represent different stages of the same disease; however, no conclusion can be drawn with respect to a relationship between benign breast disease and subsequent carcinoma. One case control study (Soini et al., 1981) contained an evaluation of the epidemiologic characteristics of certain subcategories of benign breast disease. The following were considered: (1) ductal epithelial proliferation; (2) other dysplasias including cysts, adenosis, duct ectasia, fibrosclerosis, gynecomastia, and other non-neoplastic proliferative lesions; (3) adenomas and papillomas, and (4) fibroadenomas. They concluded that none of the foregoing groups of benign lesions exhibited risk factors resembling those of breast cancer. It is obvious that further study and more refined pathologic subgroupings are needed.

Papillomatous Lesions

Any discussion of the histologic precursors of invasive carcinoma also must include the papillomatous lesions of the breast, which as a group are one of the most confusing subjects within surgical pathology. Both terminology and criteria for differentiating benign from malignant lesions have contributed to this confusion. Therefore, it would seem advisable to begin by defining the basic lesions involved.

The papilloma is a grossly visible, solitary neoplasm, usually found in a centrally dilated lactiferous duct. Clinically, it presents with a discharge from the nipple. Microscopically (Figs. 12–11 and 12–12), the papilloma is composed of variably sized fibrovascular stalks upon which there sits a double-layered epithelium resembling the epithelium of the major ducts. Mitoses are sparse in large duct papillomas, but in some instances bleeding with organization and fibrosis can cause these lesions to look quite alarming.

Multiple papillomas are visible grossly and appear to arise simultaneously and independently in many ducts. Multiple papillomas are bilateral in 26 percent of the cases (Haagensen, 1971). Histologically, the epithelium within the multiple papillomas ranges from perfectly bland to severely atypical, making it difficult at times for the pathologist to distinguish them from papillary carcinoma. Apocrine metaplasia and adenosis are often associated with the multiple papillomas and should be considered an integral part of the disease (Haagensen, 1971).

Many authors believe that the solitary intraductal papilloma is not premalignant (Haagensen et al., 1951; Hendrick, 1957; Kraus and Neubecker, 1962; Murad et al., 1981); others, however, claim the opposite (Buhl-Jorgensen et al., 1968; Carter, 1977; Pellettiere, 1971). Pellettiere and coworkers do not discriminate adequately between papillomas and epitheliosis (papillomatosis). This failure exemplifies the problems encountered in the evaluation of papillary lesions of the breast; so often microscopic and macroscopic diseases are grouped together under the category of papillomatosis. Although Buhl-Jorgensen and colleagues (1968) presented a compelling study in support of the relationship between the intraductal papilloma and carcinoma of the breast, they did not distinguish those patients who had multiple papillomas, a wholly different entity. Carter (1977), however, in a well-designed study of 64 patients who had a simple excision of a solitary intraductal papilloma, concluded that the solitary papilloma represents a risk factor for developing carcinoma and that the risk increases with concommitant papillomatosis or multiple papillomas. With the possible exception of Carter's study, there is no supporting evidence to suggest that the solitary papilloma bears any significant relationship to carcinoma.

An increasing body of evidence indicates that multiple papillomas, unlike solitary papilloma, do predispose to the development of carcinoma. Thus, Carter (1977) found that one third of all patients with multiple papillomas subsequently developed carcinoma; Murad and colleagues (1981) reported that six of 21 patients (28.6 percent) with multiple papillomas de-

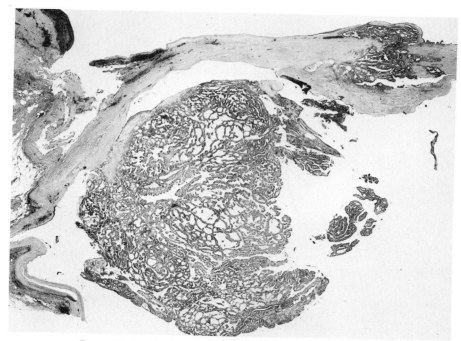

Figure 12–11. Papilloma entirely contained within an ectatic duct.

veloped carcinoma, usually with cribriform, papillary, or cartwheel patterns. Haagensen found that 15 of 39 patients (38%) with multiple papillomas had simultaneously or subsequently developed carcinoma of the intraductal apocrine, papillary, or cribriform types. Other aspects of this entity include a high rate of recurrence and a tendency to affect younger women.

The propensity of these lesions to occur in younger women is particularly interesting in view of a recently described entity, juvenile papillomatosis (Kiaer et al., 1979; Rosen et al., 1982; Rosen et al., 1980). This

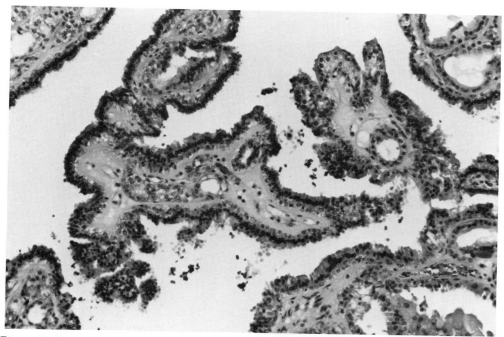

Figure 12–12. Figure 12–11 at higher power, demonstrating broad fibrovascular stalks lined by two cell layers.

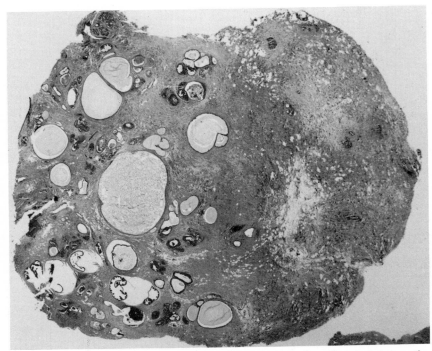

Figure 12–13. Well-circumscribed mass containing prominent ectatic ducts and papillomatosis in juvenile papillomatosis.

lesion affects women 10 to 44 years of age, with a mean age of 21 years, and usually presents as a localized mass (Rosen et al., 1980; Rosen et al., 1982). Grossly, these lesions are nodular with variably sized cysts, usually less than 1 cm in diameter; yellow "flecks" appear in the stroma as do dilated cysts or ducts with papillary lesions. Microscopic features include duct papillomatosis, apocrine and non-apocrine cysts, papillary apocrine hyperplasia, sclerosing adenosis, and duct stasis (Figs. 12–13 and 12–14). Rosen et al. (1982) found that three of 84 patients had concurrent carcinoma; two of the lesions were

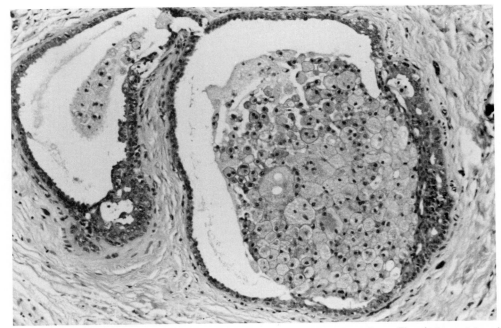

Figure 12–14. Figure 12–13 at higher power, showing ectatic ducts with apocrine metaplasia. The ducts contain minimal epithelial hyperplasia and foam cells.

secretory carcinomas and one was a lobular carcinoma-in-situ. Although the long-term risk for the development of carcinoma in patients with this condition is not known, it is significant that 26 percent of the patients studied by Rosen and colleagues (1982) had female relatives, usually grandmothers or great aunts, with a history of breast cancer. This high incidence suggests that juvenile papillomatosis is a morphologic marker for breast cancer in a family and that the patients themselves may be at increased risk for developing carcinoma of the breast.

Papilloma or adenoma of the nipple is a distinctive although uncommon clinical pathologic entity. This lesion usually presents as a nodule just below the nipple, often with a discharge and/or an erosion of the skin surface mimicking Paget's disease. Histologically, it is characterized by the proliferation of glands and ducts within a fibrous stroma, a pattern that may be difficult to distinguish from infiltrating carcinoma. However, the cellular population in the adenomatous glands tends to be uniform and contains two different cell types resembling the epithelium of the normal milk sinuses. Papillary proliferation is almost invariably present with these lesions and may appear in smaller ducts (papillomatosis) and/or in larger ducts, resembling intraductal papilloma. Some authors (Perzin and Lattes, 1972; Taylor and Robertson, 1965) maintain that papillary adenoma is not a precancerous condition. However, Bhagavan and colleagues (1973) have described two cases in which there was a morphologic transition to ductal carcinoma. The malignant potential of these lesions, however, is probably low because so few cases have been reported (Bhagavan et al., 1973).

FIBROCYSTIC DISEASE

Up to this point, we have considered whether certain benign conditions are precursor lesions. It is now our intent to examine these benign conditions as part of fibrocystic disease and to evaluate the evidence that these lesions represent histologic risk factors.

Traditionally the diagnosis of "fibrocystic disease" is based on the criteria set down by Foote and Stewart (1945) and depends on the presence of one or more of the following lesions: cyst, duct papillomatosis, blunt duct adenosis, sclerosing adenosis, apocrine epithelium, and fibrosis. However, the incidence of these various histologic changes is extremely high. Furthermore, these changes are not always associated with clinical symptoms, such as a palpable lump or mastodynia. The prevalence of these various histologic changes in autopsy studies of "normal" breasts exceeds 40 percent (Frantz et al., 1951; Kramer and Rush, 1973; Sandison, 1962). In fact, in one such investigation (Sloss et al., 1957), the changes were so universal that the authors stated: "The mere qualitative presence of blunt duct adenosis, apocrine epithelium, and intraductal epithelial hyperplasia in the breasts of women is insufficient to warrant that such tissue be considered as diseased."

The ubiquity of these changes in normal and asymptomatic breasts, together with the pathologist's penchant for applying the term "fibrocystic disease" to any surgical pathology specimen not containing overt carcinoma, has rendered the term meaningless and therefore some favor abandoning it entirely (Love et al., 1982; Scanlon, 1981).

Nevertheless, numerous reports have suggested some correlation between fibrocystic disease and carcinoma of the breast. In reviewing these reports, we cannot but wonder as McDivitt did ". . . what, in fact, is being correlated (McDivitt, 1978)!"

In many of these studies, a patient population defined by a biopsy diagnosis of "fibrocystic disease" has been followed for the development of carcinoma. In 1940, Warren reported his study of 1044 patients from Toronto and Massachusetts who had been diagnosed as having fibrocystic disease. After an average of 9 years postbiopsy, he calculated that the risk of carcinoma for this group was 4.5 times greater than that for most of the general female population of Massachusetts. This study is impressive because of the large number of patients; however, it is disconcerting because a disproportionate number of carcinomas developed in the Boston population; furthermore, this study was undertaken prior to the recognition of lobular carcinoma-in-situ. Its inclusion in their data would most certainly have altered their conclusions. In this regard, it is interesting that a follow-up study (Monson et al., 1976) was conducted involving the Massachusetts population only. In that study, 733 women were followed for an average of 30.3 years; among this group, the risk of developing breast cancer was 2.5 times that expected in the general population, as compared with 4.5 times in the original study. In another frequently cited study, Davis and associates (1964) followed 284 women with the biopsy diagnosis of fibrocystic disease for an average of 13 years and found that the risk for carcinoma in those who had epithelial hyperplasia was 2.5 times the expected rate; for non-hyperplastic lesions, the risk was 1.2 times the expected rate. However, the criteria for the histologic diagnosis of fibrocystic disease and hyperplasia in that study are open to question because the authors state that "No matter how much piling up of epithelium, the condition is considered benign cystic disease with epithelial hyperplasia unless there is invasion into the stroma or marked atypism of cells." It is reasonable to assume, therefore, that some forms of intraductal carcinoma that show little cytologic atypia—such as the micropapillary and cribriform variants—were probably designated "fibrocystic disease with epithelial hyperplasia" in that study.

In a more recent study, Donnelly and associates (1975) followed 370 women with a diagnosis of a benign lesion established between 1935 and 1949.

After a median follow-up of 13.5 years, these authors found that the risk of breast carcinoma in patients with chronic cystic mastitis was 2.9 times the expected rate. However, in only 25 percent of the cases was the original material available for histologic review, and it is almost certain that some of the original diagnoses would have been changed if current diagnostic criteria had been used. This contention is supported by Black and coworkers (1972), who found in reviewing 77 previously diagnosed benign biopsies that 16 (21 percent) could be reclassified as carcinoma-in-situ.

Finally, many of these studies did not include an adequate control group. For example, Veronesi and Pizzocaro (1968) studied patients in Italy but based their calculations on a control group from the United States. More importantly, none of the earlier studies (Clagett et al., 1944; Lewison and Lyons, 1953) were controlled with respect to most of the major known risk factors for breast carcinoma other than increasing age. That means that the increased risk may have been related to other factors, such as a family history of breast carcinoma that influenced the physician to be more aggressive in performing biopsies.

It is clear that fibrocystic disease is a histologically heterogeneous group, and one would not expect the risk of carcinoma to be the same for each component. In an attempt to identify those components that might constitute an increased risk for subsequent carcinoma, Page and coworkers (1978) followed 925 women for 15 to 24 years and identified atypical lobular hyperplasia as *the* histologic lesion having the greatest risk for the development of carcinoma, six times the expected rate in women under 45 years and three times the rate in those over 45 years. After the age of 45 years, three ductal epithelial proliferative lesions—ductal hyperplasia, papillary apocrine change, and apocrine-like ductal hyperplasia—were associated with an increased risk of 2.6, 2.7, and 2.1 times the expected rates, respectively (only the first two however, were significant at a P level of 0.02). Ductal hyperplasia was defined as any lesion that had three or more epithelial cell layers without atypia above the basement membrane. Apocrine-like ductal hyperplasia is similar to the previous category, but there is in addition apocrine differentiation of the cell. Papillary apocrine change was characterized by apocrine cells two to three cell layers that thickly projected into a central lumen. The two aforementioned categories of ductal hyperplasia plus the category of atypical ductal hyperplasia include most of the lesions that fall into the spectrum of "papillomatosis," according to the authors. No increased risk of carcinoma was observed with any of the following non-hyperplastic lesions: cysts, duct ectasia, apocrine change (non-papillary), sclerosing adenosis, and fibroadenoma.

Hutchinson and coworkers (1980) studied 1441 women with an average follow-up of 12.9 years and found an increased risk of carcinoma in those women whose fibrocystic disease was characterized by epithelial hyperplasia or papillomatosis. The risk was further increased from 2.7 to 5.2 by the presence of histologic calcification in these lesions. No increased risk was associated with cysts, apocrine metaplasia, sclerosing adenosis, or fibroadenoma.

Neither Page's nor Hutchinson's investigation confirmed the conclusion of Haagensen and others (Harrington and Lesnick, 1981; Jones and Bradbeer, 1980) that there was a two- to threefold increased risk for the subsequent development of carcinoma in women with gross cystic disease of their breasts.

STELLATE SCAR AND TUBULAR CARCINOMA

Evidence presented by several authors (Fisher et al., 1983; Linell et al., 1980) suggests that carcinoma of the breast may evolve from a morphologically distinctive stellate scar. This lesion has been described with a variety of names, including "radial scar" (Hamperl, 1975), "infiltrating epitheliosis" (Azzopardi, 1979), "sclerosing papillary proliferation" (Fenoglio and Lattes, 1974), and "non-encapsulated sclerosing lesion of the breast" (Fisher et al., 1979). The characteristic puckered lesions range from less than 1 mm to about 1 cm in diameter and usually appear as an incidental microscopic finding. Histologically the lesion (Fig. 12–15) is composed of multiple tubules and lobules radially arranged around a sclerotic center that often contains abundant elastic material. At times, it is difficult to distinguish between this entity and tubular carcinoma; in fact, Linell and coworkers (1980) have presented evidence that tubular carcinomas of the breast may arise in these radial scars.

Furthermore, according to the 1980 study of Linell's group, as tubular carcinomas grow larger they progress to less well-differentiated ductal carcinomas; therefore, they hypothesize that radial scars are the first recognizable lesions in the development of more than 50 percent of all breast carcinomas. In 1983, Fisher and coworkers, while assessing pathologic findings in the National Surgical Adjuvant Breast Project, found that 38 percent of carcinomas could be traced to a scar, which in 14 percent of cases resembled a radial scar.

The concept of tubular carcinoma (Figs. 12–16 and 12–17) progressing to a larger, less-differentiated tumor is suggested by several lines of evidence. First, the frequency of pure tubular carcinoma without any ductal component in a large series of breast carcinomas, such as the NSABP, has been reported to be 1.2 percent (Fisher et al., 1975). However, the frequency rises to 9 percent in a study of breast cancers derived from mass screening clinics using mammography (Patchefsky et al., 1977). Clearly, the ability to detect smaller lesions is increasing the yield of tubular

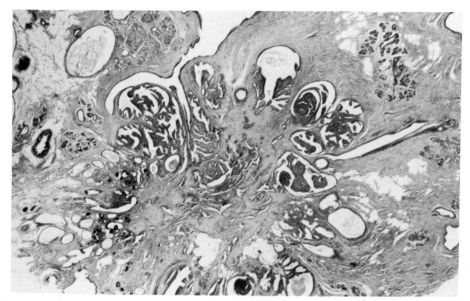

Figure 12–15. Stellate lesion composed of radially arranged tubules containing papillomatosis. There is abundant elastosis centrally.

carcinomas. The difference between these two series is hard to reconcile. One possible explanation is that this tumor is so indolent in its growth that it rarely becomes palpable or perhaps even spontaneously regresses. Another possible explanation is that tubular carcinomas do indeed transform into a less well-differentiated histologic subtype. Cooper and associates (1978) found that pure tubular carcinoma was on the average smaller than the tumor that contained both a tubular and an infiltrating ductal component, although this finding was not statistically significant. In addition, they found that the infiltrating ductal component often lay peripheral to the well-differentiated tubular component. This latter arrangement has also been seen by others (McDivitt et al., 1982). Furthermore, it is well recognized that tubular carcinoma is

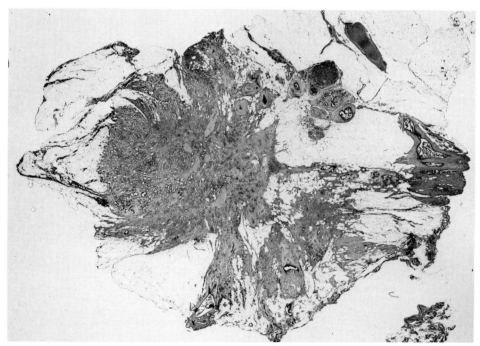

Figure 12–16. Stellate tubular carcinoma. The tubules extend into the fat.

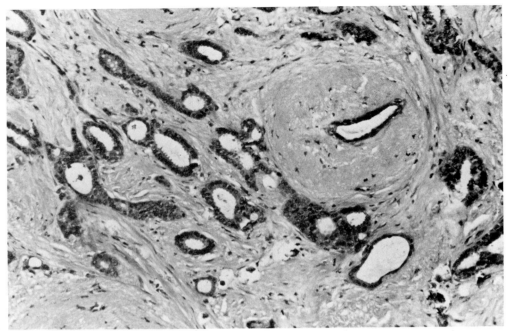

Figure 12–17. Tubular carcinoma at high power. The tubules contain apocrine "snouts" and transverse bridges. There is typical periductal elastosis.

found mixed with another histologic subtype more often than it is found pure. In fact, the varying frequencies of tubular carcinoma reported partly reflect the extent to which another less well-differentiated component might be found in a single lesion and still be designated "tubular carcinoma." It is also worth noting that Peters and coworkers (1981) found that in small carcinomas, the proportion of the tubular component decreased as the diameter of the lesion increased. All these observations suggest that tubular carcinomas may transform into infiltrating ductal carcinomas.

Egger and associates (1982) studied 65 small breast cancers, 60 of which had maximum diameters of less than 10 mm. These authors found that 34 of the 65 cancers had at their centers obliterated ducts with periductal elastosis and that 12 showed a pre-existing stellate scar in the center of the invasive tumor. In addition, 38 of the 65 small tumors exhibited tubular differentiation either alone or in combination with solid invasive cords. These investigators suggest that ductal obliteration and periductal elastosis do not cause the development of cancer but "mark the site of active transformation and hence the "at-risk" zone for cancerogenesis."

It is apparent that a sizeable proportion of small cancers less than 1 cm in diameter have an abundant tubular component and contain elastotic areas. However, it is not clear how these small cancers relate to the radial scar. Also, it is not known whether the elastosis precedes or follows the development of carcinoma. As additional studies, such as mammography, continue to detect increasingly smaller lesions, more data should be obtained about this interesting problem.

The secretarial expertise of Lee Ann Moffett is greatly appreciated.

References

Andersen, J.A.: Lobular carcinoma in situ: a longterm follow-up in 52 cases. Acta Pathol. Microbiol. Immunol. Scand. [A] 82:519, 1974.

Azzopardi, J.G.: Problems in Breast Pathology. Vol. 2. Major Problems in Pathology. Philadelphia, W.B. Saunders Co., 1979.

Bhagavan, B.S., Patchefsky, A., Koss, L.G.: Florid subareolar duct papillomatosis (nipple adenoma) and mammary carcinoma. Report of three cases. Hum. Pathol. 4:289, 1973.

Black, M.M., Barclay, T.H.C., Cutler, S.J., Hankey, B.F., Asire, A.J.: Association of atypical characteristics of benign breast lesions with subsequent risk of breast cancer. Cancer 29:338, 1972.

Black, M.M., and Chabon, A.B.: In situ carcinoma of the breast. Pathol. Ann. 4:185, 1969.

Black, M.M., and Kwon, S.: Precancerous mastopathie: structural and biological considerations. Pathol. Res. Pract. 166:491, 1980.

Brinton, L.A., Hoover, R., Fraumeni, J.F., Jr.: Epidemiology of minimal breast cancer. J.A.M.A. 249:483, 1983.

Buhl-Jorgensen, S.E., Fischermann, K., Johansen, H., Petersen, B.: Cancer risk in intraductal papilloma and papillomatosis. Surg. Gynecol. Obstet. 127:1307, 1968.

Cardiff, R.D., Wellings, S.R., Faulkin, L.J.: Biology of breast neoplasia. Cancer 39:2734, 1977.

Carter, D.: Intraductal papillary tumors of the breast. Cancer 39:1689, 1977.

Carter, D. and Smith, R.R.L.: Carcinoma in situ of the breast. Cancer 40:1189, 1977.

Clagett, O.T., Plimpton, N.C., Root, G.T.: Lesions of the breast: the relationship of benign lesions to carcinoma. Surgery 15:413, 1944.

Cole, P., Elwood, J.M., Kaplan, S.D.: Incidence rates and risk factors of benign breast neoplasms. Am. J. Epidemiol. 108:112, 1978.

Cooper, H.S., Patchefsky, A.S., Krall, R.A.: Tubular carcinoma of the breast. Cancer 42:2334, 1978.

Davis, H.H., Simons, M., Davis, J.B.: Cystic disease of the breast: relationship to carcinoma. Cancer 17:957, 1964.

DeOme, K.B., Faulkin, L. J., Jr., Bern, H.A., Blair, P.B.: Development of mammary tumors from hyperplastic alveolar nodules transplanted into gland-free mammary fat pads of female C3H mice. Cancer Res. 19:515, 1959.

Donnelly, P.K., Baker, K.W., Carney, J.A., O'Fallon, W.M.: Benign breast lesions and subsequent breast carcinoma in Rochester, Minnesota. Mayo Clin. Proc. 50:650, 1975.

Egger, H., Tulusan, A.H., Schneider, M.L.: A contribution to the natural history of breast cancer. II. Precursors and lesions associated with small cancers of the breast. Arch. Gynecol. 231:199, 1982.

Ernster, V.L.: The epidemiology of benign breast disease. Epidemiol. Rev. 3:184, 1981.

Fenoglio, C., and Lattes, R.: Sclerosing papillary proliferations in the female breast. Cancer 33:691, 1974.

Fisher, E.R., Gregorio, R.M., Fisher, B., et al.: The pathology of invasive breast cancer. A syllabus derived from findings of the national surgical adjuvant breast project (Protocol No. 4). Cancer 36:1, 1975.

Fisher, E.R., Palekar, A.S., Kotwal, N. Lipana, N.: A non-encapsulated sclerosing lesion of the breast. Am. J. Clin. Pathol. 71:240, 1979.

Fisher, E.R., Palekar, A.S., Sass, R., Fisher, B.: Pathologic findings from the national surgical adjuvant breast project (Protocol No. 4):IX. Scar cancers. Breast Cancer Res. Treat. 3:39, 1983.

Foote, F.W., and Stewart, F.W.: Lobular carcinoma in situ. A rare form of mammary cancer. Am. J. Pathol. 17:491, 1941.

Foote, F.W., and Stewart F.W.: Comparative studies of cancerous versus non-cancerous breasts. Ann. Surg. 121:6–53; 197–222, 1945.

Frantz, V.K., Pickren, J.W., Melcher, G.W., Auchincloss, H., Jr.: Incidence of chronic cystic disease in so-called "normal breasts." Cancer 4:762, 1951.

Gallager, H.S., and Martin, J.E.: Early phases in the development of breast cancer. Cancer 24:1170, 1969.

Giordano, J.M., and Klopp, C.T.: Lobular carcinoma in situ: incidence and treatment. Cancer 31:105, 1973.

Haagensen, C.D.: Diseases of the Breast, 2nd ed. Philadelphia, W.B. Saunders Co., 1971.

Haagensen, C.D., Lane, N., Bodian, C.: Coexisting lobular neoplasia and carcinoma of the breast. Cancer 51:1468, 1983.

Haagensen, C.D., Lane, N., Lattes, R., Bodian, C.: Lobular neoplasia (so-called lobular carcinoma in situ) of the breast. Cancer 42:737, 1978.

Haagensen, C.D., Stout, A.P., Phillips, J.S.: The papillary neoplasms of the breast—I. Benign intraductal papilloma. Ann. Surg. 133:18, 1951.

Hamperl, H.: Strahlige Narben und obliterierende mastopathie. Virch. Arch. [A] 369:555, 1975.

Harrington, E., and Lesnick, G.: The association between gross cysts of the breast and breast cancer. Breast 7:13, 1981.

Hendrick, J.W.: Intraductal papilloma of the breast. Surg. Gynecol. Obstet. 105:215, 1957.

Hutchinson, W.B., Thomas, D.B., Hamlin, W.B., Roth, G.J., Peterson, A.V., Williams, B.: Risk of breast cancer in women with benign breast disease. J. Natl. Cancer Inst. 65:13, 1980.

Jensen, H.M., Rice, J.R., Wellings, S.R.: Preneoplastic lesions in the human breast. Science 191:295, 1976.

Jones, B.M., and Bradbeer, J.W.: The presentation and progress of macroscopic breast cysts. Br. J. Surg. 67:669, 1980.

Kiaer, H.W., Kiaer, W.W., Linell, F., Jacobsen, S.: Extreme duct papillomatosis of the juvenile breast. Acta Pathol. Microbiol. Immunol. Scand. [A] 87:353, 1979.

Kramer, W.M., and Rush, B.F., Jr.: Mammary duct proliferation in the elderly. A histopathological study. Cancer 31:130, 1973.

Kraus, F.T., and Neubecker, R.D.: The differential diagnosis of papillary tumors of the breast. Cancer 15:444, 1962.

Lewis, D., and Geschickter, C.F.: Comedocarcinoma of the breast. Arch. Surg. 36:225, 1938.

Lewison, E.F., and Lyons, J.G., Jr.: Relationship between benign breast disease and cancer. Arch. Surg. 66:94, 1953.

Linell, F., Ljungberg, O., Anderson, I.: Breast carcinoma aspect of early stages, progression and related problems. Acta Pathol. Microbiol. Scand. [A] 272:1, 1980.

Love, S.M., Gelman, R.S., Silen, W.: Fibrocystic "disease" of the breast—a nondisease? New Engl. J. Med 307:1010, 1982.

McDivitt, R.W.: Breast carcinoma. Hum. Pathol. 9:1, 1978.

McDivitt, R.W., Boyce, W., Gersell, D.: Tubular carcinoma of the breast. Clinical and pathologic observations concerning 135 cases. Am. J. Surg. Pathol. 6:401, 1982.

McDivitt, R.W., Stewart, F.W., Berg, J.W.: Tumors of the breast. Atlas of Tumor Pathology, 2nd Series, Fascicle 2. Bethesda, MD, The American Registry of Pathology, Armed Forces Institute of Pathology, 1968.

Monson, R.R., Yen, S., MacMahon, B., Warren, S.: Chronic cystic mastitis and carcinoma of the breast. Lancet 2 (Part 1):224, 1976.

Murad, T.M., Contesso, G., Mouriesse, H.: Papillary tumors of large lactiferous ducts. Cancer 48:122, 1981.

Nizze, H.: Fibrous cystic mastopathy and epitheliosis in the opposite breast of mammary carcinoma patients. Oncology 28:319, 1973.

Nomura, A., Comstock, G.W., Tonascia, J.A.: Epidemiologic characteristics of benign breast disease. Am. J. Epidemiol. 105:505, 1977.

Page, D.L., Dupont, W.D., Rogers, L.W. Landenberger, M.: Intraductal carcinoma of the breast: follow-up after biopsy only. Cancer 49:751, 1982.

Page, D.L., Vander Zwaag, R., Rogers, L.W., Williams, L.T., Walker, W.E., Hartmann, W.H.: Relation between component parts of fibrocystic disease complex and breast cancer. J. Natl. Cancer Inst. 61:1055, 1978.

Patchefsky, A.S., Shaber, G.S., Schwartz, G.F., Feig, S.A., Nerlinger, R.E.: The pathology of breast cancer detected by mass population screening. Cancer 40:1659, 1977.

Pellettiere, E.V., II: The clinical and pathologic aspects of papillomatous disease of the breast. Am. J. Clin. Pathol. 55:740, 1971.

Perzin, K.H., and Lattes, R.: Papillary adenoma of the nipple. (Florid papillomatosis, adenoma, adenomatosis). A clinicopathologic study. Cancer 29:996, 1972.

Peters, G.N., Wolff, M., Haagensen, C.D.: Tubular carcinoma of the breast. Clinical pathologic correlations based on 100 cases. Ann. Surg. 193:138, 1981.

Rosen, P.P.: Clinical implications of preinvasive and small invasive breast carcinomas. Pathol. Ann. 16(2):337, 1981.

Rosen, P.P., Braun, D.W., Jr., Lyngholm, B., Urban, J.A., Kinne, D.W.: Lobular carcinoma in situ of the breast: preliminary results of treatment by ipsilateral mastectomy and contralateral breast biopsy. Cancer 47:813, 1981.

Rosen, P.P., Cantrell, B., Mullen, D.L., DePalo, A.: Juvenile papillomatosis (Swiss cheese disease) of the breast. Am. J. Surg. Pathol. 4:3, 1980.

Rosen, P.P., Lieberman, P.H., Braun, D.W., Jr., Kosloff, C., Adair, F.: Lobular carcinoma in situ of the breast. Detailed analysis of 99 patients with average follow-up of 24 years. Am. J. Surg. Pathol. 2:225, 1978.

Rosen, P.P., Lyngholm, B., Kinne, D.W., Beattie, E.J.: Juvenile papillomatosis of the breast and family history of breast carcinoma. Cancer 49:2591, 1982.

Sandison, A.T.: An autopsy study of the adult human breast. National Cancer Institute Monograph 8, DHEW PHS, US 6 PO, Washington, D.C., 1962.

Sartwell, P.E., Arthes, F.G., Tonascia, J.A.: Benign and malignant breast tumors; epidemiological similarities. Int. J. Epidemiol. 7:217, 1978.

Scanlon, E.F.: The early diagnosis of breast cancer. Cancer 48:523, 1981.

Shah, J.P., Rosen, P.P., Robbins, G.F.: Pitfalls of local excision in the treatment of carcinoma of the breast. Surg. Gynecol. Obstet. 136:721, 1973.

Simpson, H.W., Mutch, F., Halbert, F., Griffiths, K., Wilson, D.: Bimodal age-frequency distribution of epitheliosis in cancer mastectomies. Cancer 50:2417, 1982.

Sloss, P.T., Bennett, W.A., Clagett, O.T.: Incidence in normal breasts of features associated with chronic cystic mastitis. Am. J. Pathol. 33(No. 6):1181, 1957.

Soini, I., Aine, R., Lauslahti, K., Hakama, M.: Independent risk factors of benign and malignant breast lesions. Am. J. Epidemiol. 114:507, 1981.

Squartini, F., and Sarnelli, R.: Structure, functional changes and proliferative pathology of the human mammary lobule in cancerous breasts. J. Natl. Cancer Inst. 67:33, 1981.

Taylor, H.B., and Robertson, A.G.: Adenomas of the nipple. Cancer 18:995, 1965.

Veronesi, U., and Pizzocaro, G.: Breast cancer in women subsequent to cystic disease of the breast. Surg. Gynecol. Obstet. 126:529, 1968.

Warner, N.E.: Lobular carcinoma of the breast. Cancer 23:840, 1969.

Warren, S.: The relation of "chronic mastitis" to carcinoma of the breast. Surg. Gynecol. Obstet. 71:257, 1940.

Wellings, S.R.: A hypothesis of the origin of human breast cancer from the terminal ductal lobular unit. Pathol. Res. Pract. 166:515, 1980.

Wellings, S.R., and Jensen, H.M.: On the origin and progression of ductal carcinoma of the human breast. J. Natl. Cancer Inst. 50:1111, 1973.

Wellings, S.R., Jensen, H.M., Marcum, R.G.: An atlas of subgross pathology of the human breast with special reference to possible precancerous lesions. J. Natl. Cancer Inst. 55:231, 1975.

A. B. JENSON
W. D. LANCASTER
R. J. KURMAN

13 Uterine Cervix

Invasive squamous cell carcinomas of the uterine cervix are preceded by a heterogeneous group of premalignant lesions designated "dysplasia" and "carcinoma-in-situ." Although the concept of carcinoma-in-situ as a preinvasive cancer was not well accepted until the 1930s, illustrations of this lesion as a cancer invading submucosal glands appeared in Amann's textbook on gynecologic histology in 1897 (cited in Koss, 1979). Recognition of carcinoma-in-situ as a biologic entity was a major step toward clarification of the pathogenesis of cervical cancer and its establishment as a model for human carcinogenesis. Problems persisted, however, in the classification of less severe but related intraepithelial abnormalities arising in cervical squamous epithelium. These difficulties were reconciled, in part, at the First International Congress on Exfoliative Cytology in 1961 (Weid, 1962), when "carcinoma-in-situ" was defined as a lesion in which undifferentiated cells occupied the full thickness of the epithelium; all other disturbances of differentiation were designated "dysplasias." Subsequently, cervical dysplasia was also regarded as a preinvasive lesion, although it was recognized that the majority of dysplasias remained stable or regressed and that only a small fraction progressed to invasive cancer. (Nasiell et al., 1983; Spriggs, 1981). Although uncertainties exist even today about the biologic potential of individual lesions, it is well recognized that women with cervical dysplasias are at a significantly increased risk for developing both carcinoma-in-situ and invasive squamous cell carcinoma (Koss, 1979).

Since the 1960s, epidemiologic studies have linked cervical cancer and its precursors to sexually transmitted diseases with a predilection for metaplastic squamous epithelium of the transformation zone of uterine cervix (Figs. 13–1 and 13–2) (Kessler, 1977; Rotkin, 1973). Immunocytochemical and molecular DNA hybridization studies have revealed human papillomavirus (HPV) structural proteins or DNA sequences or both in the majority of all malignant and premalignant lesions (Gissmann et al., 1984; Lancaster et al., 1985; Pfister, 1983). These studies suggest that these lesions represent a heterogeneous group of HPV-associated hyperplasias, dysplasias, and neoplasias. In this chapter, we will address the problems related to histologic diagnosis, terminology, and management of cervical dysplasias as well as the relationship of cervical dysplasia to HPV infection.

ETIOLOGY

It is generally believed that squamous cell cancer of the cervix and associated precancerous lesions are causally related to sexually transmitted diseases (Alexander, 1973; Kessler, 1977; Rotkin, 1973). Support for this belief includes observations that the most consistent etiologic cofactors are early intercourse and multiple sexual partners. The male is a silent but primary reservoir. Monogamous women have an increased risk of developing cervical cancer if their sexual partners previously had sexual relations with women with cervical carcinoma or if their partners are concurrently sexually active with many people. Most of the evidence since 1970 has implicated herpes simplex virus Type 2 (HSV-2) in the etiology of these diseases. The evidence was based upon seroepidemiologic case control studies showing a higher prevalence of HSV-2 serum antibodies in patients with cervical dysplasia, carcinoma-in-situ, and invasive squamous cell carcinoma (Nahmias et al., 1974; Rawls et al., 1969). Recently, however, a prospective, carefully matched seroepidemiologic study of over 10,000 women followed for up to 8 years showed no difference in the prevalence of HSV-2 antibody among women with cervical dysplasia or neoplasia and matched controls (Vonka et al., 1984a; Vonka et al., 1984b). Furthermore, there is a lack of immunologic and virologic data identifying HSV structural antigens and DNA sequences in cervical dysplasia and cancer.

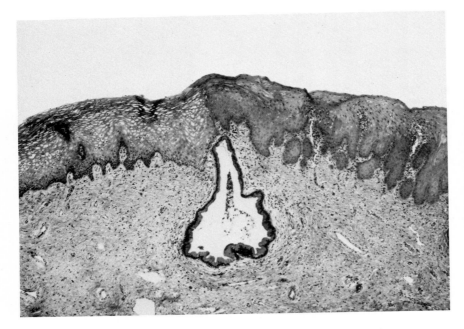

Figure 13–1. Glycogenated squamous epithelium of normal exocervix (*left*) undergoes abrupt transition at transformation zone (depicted by submucosal gland) into metaplastic squamous epithelium on endocervix (*right*). Metaplastic squamous epithelium may be more susceptible to different types of human papillomavirus infection than is mature squamous epithelium. (Courtesy of Armed Forces Institute of Pathology.)

Thus, there is little evidence to support the role of HSV-2 in the etiology of cervical neoplasia.

It was not until the late 1970s that HPV was implicated in the pathogenesis of cervical dysplasia, when Meisels and coworkers (1976) and Purola and Savia (1977) noted the similarity between exfoliated cells from mild cervical dysplasia and those from condyloma acuminata. On the basis of these findings, Meisels and colleagues (1977) subsequently reclassified 90 percent of mild dysplasias as flat condylomas. Since then, it has been estimated that 1 to 2 percent of all young women screened by cytologic examination have evidence of HPV infection (Meisels and Fortin, 1976; Meisels et al., 1977; Syrjanen et al., 1981). Moreover, morphologic evidence of HPV infection is present in the majority of dysplasias and in over 40 percent of in-situ-carcinomas (Kurman et al., 1983). Recently, HPV genus-specific structural antigens (Fig. 13–3) or DNA sequences or both were found in 90 percent of all dysplasias and in-situ-carcinomas (Lancaster et al., 1983; Okagaki et al., 1983). However, seroepidemiologic studies aimed at clarifying the relationship of HPV infection to cervical neoplasia have not yet been performed because a reliable serologic assay for HPV is not available.

NOMENCLATURE

Terms currently in use are "dysplasia/carcinoma-in-situ" (Poulson et al., 1975) and "cervical intraepithelial neoplasia" (Richart, 1968). The former, which is subdivided into mild, moderate, and severe, has been adopted by the World Health Organization. The latter is subclassified into cervical intraepithelial neoplasia Types I, II, and III. Type I is equated with mild dysplasia (Figs. 13–3 to 13–6), Type II with moderate dysplasia (Figs. 13–7, 13–13, and 13–14), and Type III with severe dysplasia (Figs. 13–8 to 13–15) and carcinoma-in-situ. Use of Type III as a category eliminates the morphologic distinction between severe dysplasia (Figs. 13–8 to 13–10) and carcinoma-in-situ (Figs. 13–11 to 13–15). Clinically there is no difference in the management of these lesions.

Recognition of the putative role of HPV in cervical dysplasia and neoplasia has created some confusion regarding the appropriate terminology for the various types of intraepithelial lesions. The term "flat condyloma" was proposed to describe mild dysplasia with histologic evidence of HPV infection, with the implication that this is a benign viral infection that is distinct from "true dysplasia," which is preneoplastic (Meisels and Fortin, 1976; Purola and Savia, 1977). Similarly, the term "atypical condyloma" has been applied to moderate and severe dysplasias that have histologic evidence of HPV infection (Meisels et al., 1981). However, because available evidence suggests that most cervical lesions are associated with HPV infection, it seems prudent to retain the traditional classification and include in the report whether or not there is histologic evidence of HPV infection (Editorial, 1983). It is conceivable that in the future correlation of specific HPV types with various grades of dysplasia will shed further light on their behavior and result in a new classification of intraepithelial neoplasia.

HISTOPATHOLOGY OF DYSPLASIAS

Dysplastic lesions were characterized by Reagen in 1953 as being composed of proliferating cells that did not involve the full thickness of the epithelium. The

Text continued on page 258

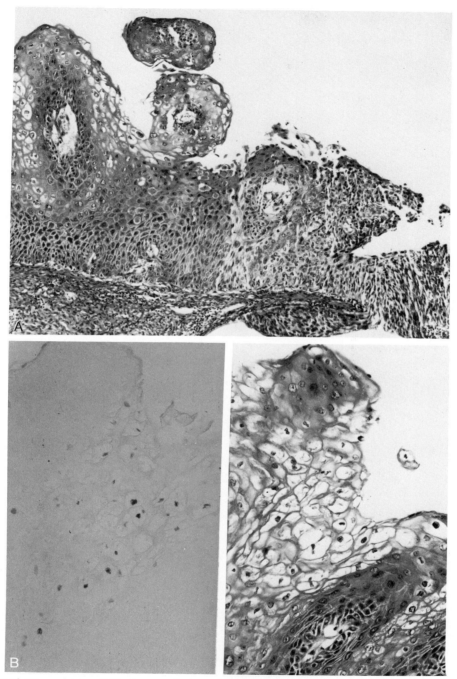

Figure 13–2. *A*, Exophytic condyloma *(left)* of exocervix immediately adjacent to carcinoma-in-situ, with gland involvement at the transformation zone. These two morphologically distinct lesions, both associated with human papillomavirus, in close apposition may reflect a variable response of different squamous epithelium to human papillomavirus infections. (From Kurman, R. J., Jenson, A. B., Sinclair, C., Lancaster, W. D.: *In* DeLellis, R. A.: Advances in Immunocytochemistry. New York, Masson, 1984.) *B*, Localization of human papillomavirus antigens within koilocytotic cells *(left)* of the exophytic condyloma seen in *A* (immunoperoxidase-PV antigens, no counterstain). *Right*, Hematoxylin and eosin stain of the same area showing portion of papillary fronds containing koilocytotic cells. This patient had been treated with steroids.

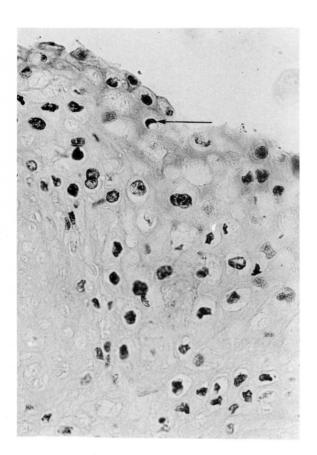

Figure 13–3. Human papillomavirus cytopathic effect in cervical dysplasias is best appreciated by observing morphologic changes in koilocytotic cells containing human papillomavirus antigen; koilocytotic cells negative for viral antigen but positive for human papillomavirus DNA show a similar cytopathic effect. The synthesis of viral capsid antigens occurs throughout the nucleus of permissive squamous cells, and positive immunologic stains outline the configuration of the entire nucleus. In this mild dysplasia, crescent-shaped nuclei (arrow), double nuclei, pyknotic nuclei, and enlarged nuclei with finely granular chromatin all stain positively for human papillomavirus antigens. At least two different types of human papillomavirus DNA were identified in this lesion (immunoperoxidase-PV common antigen, no counterstain). (From Kurman, R. J., Sanz, L. E., Jenson, A. B., Perry, S., Lancaster, W. D.: Int. J. Gynecol. Pathol. 1:17, 1982.)

Figure 13–4. Very mild dysplasia with early involvement of endocervical glands (arrow). The squamous cells show differentiation and evidence of human papillomavirus cytopathic effect, koilocytosis, nuclear wrinkling, and binucleation, but there is no proliferation of basal and parabasal cells.

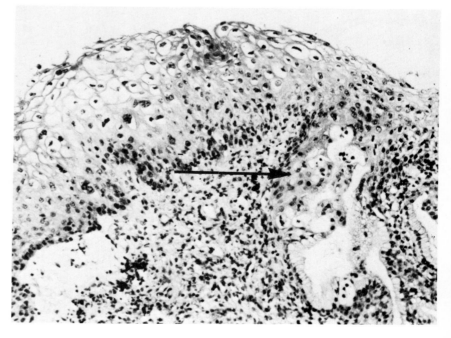

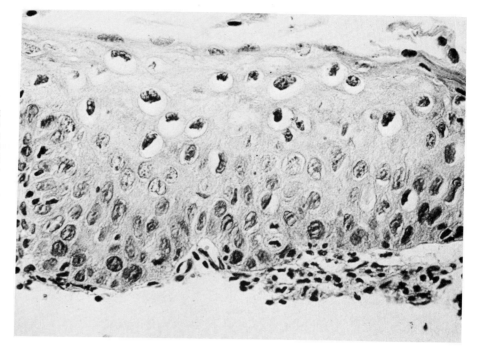

Figure 13–5. Mild dysplasia showing evidence of human papillomavirus infection characterized by koilocytosis with associated nuclear enlargement and wrinkling. In contrast to very mild dysplasia (Figure 13–4), there is proliferation of basal and parabasal cells. (From Kurman, R. J., Sanz, L. E., Jenson, A. B., Perry, S., Lancaster, W. D.: Int. J. Gynecol. Pathol. *1:*17, 1982.)

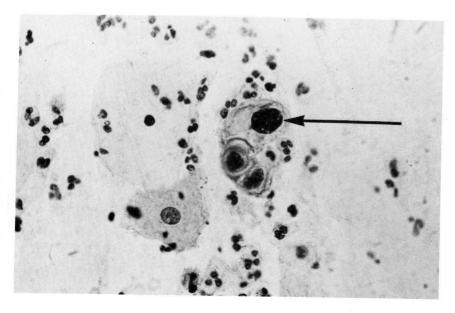

Figure 13–6. Cytologic smear stained for human papillomavirus capsid antigens from patient with mild cervical dysplasia. Human papillomavirus antigens *(arrow)* are seen in the nucleus of one of three koilocytotic cells; pyknotic nuclei in the other two cells of this cluster appear positive because of lack of contrast between the brown peroxidase precipitate and the hematoxylin staining of the nuclei (immunoperoxidase-PV common antigen; counterstain, Papanicolaou stain).

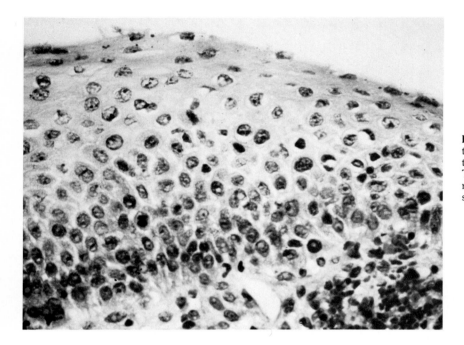

Figure 13–7. Moderate dysplasia characterized by proliferating cells that extend through half the thickness of epithelium. There is no apparent human papillomavirus cytopathic effect in this particular lesion.

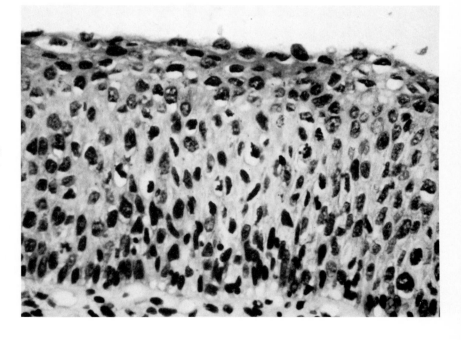

Figure 13–8. Severe dysplasia, showing greater than two thirds of the epithelium replaced by proliferating parabasal cells.

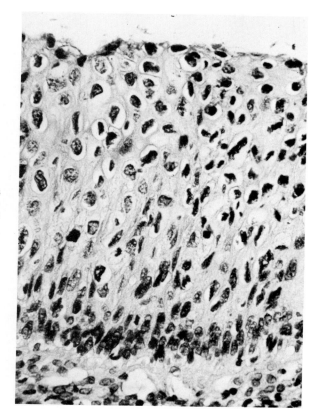

Figure 13–9. Severe dysplasia of the cervix, showing proliferating cells intermixed with degenerating cells displaying pyknotic nuclei and vacuolated cytoplasm; it is unclear whether the degenerative changes are occurring in proliferating cells or differentiating cells.

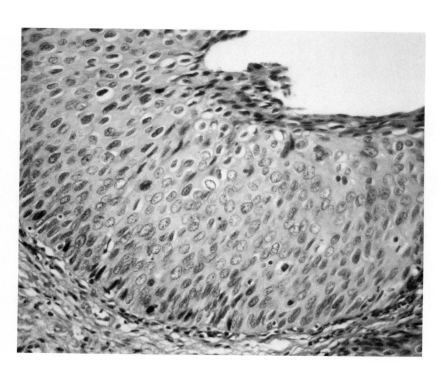

Figure 13–10. Severe dysplasia, showing proliferation of a relatively homogeneous cell type. The proliferation occupies four fifths the thickness of the epithelium.

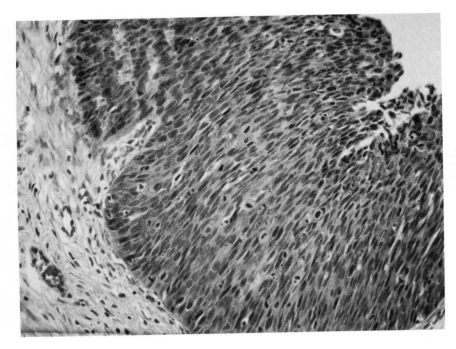

Figure 13–11. Carcinoma-in-situ composed of cells with spindle-shaped nuclei occurring throughout the full thickness of the epithelium.

Figure 13–12. Carcinoma-in-situ composed of cells with spindle-shaped nuclei that completely replace the squamous epithelium. This is similar to Figure 13–11 except that mitotic figures are not as obvious and the epithelium is not as thick.

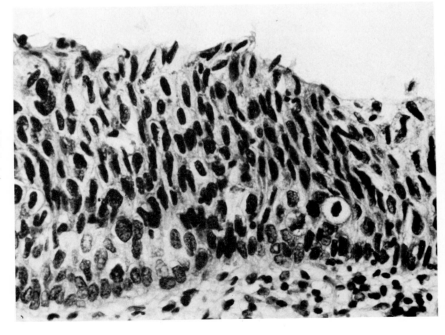

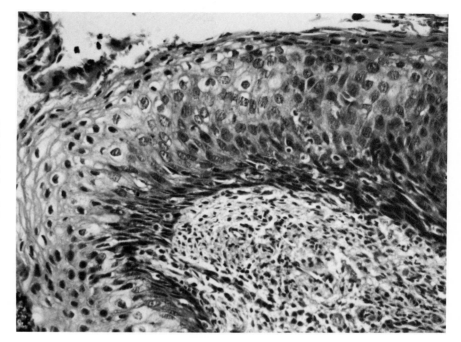

Figure 13–13. Morphologic continuum of mild dysplasia *(lower left)*, moderate dysplasia *(middle)*, and severe dysplasia *(right)*. The proliferating cells are composed of enlarged parabasal cells with hyperchromatic nuclei that occupy an increasing thickness of the epithelium. The dysplasia is graded according to the extent that the epithelium is replaced by these proliferating cells.

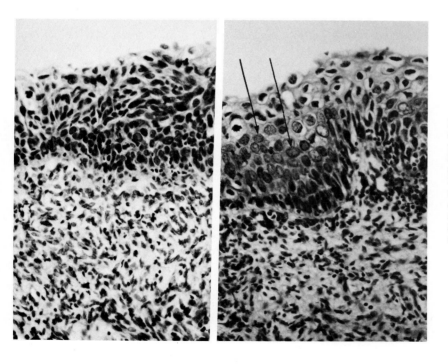

Figure 13–14. Two fields from the same cervical biopsy show the spectrum of dysplasia. The panel on the right shows mild to moderate dysplasia. The panel on the left shows severe dysplasia to carcinoma-in-situ. It is not unusual for the same lesion to show a morphologic continuum of dysplasia to carcinoma-in-situ with the proliferating cells showing different morphologic patterns. Some have large, homogeneous nuclei *(arrows)*, other nuclei are spindle-shaped.

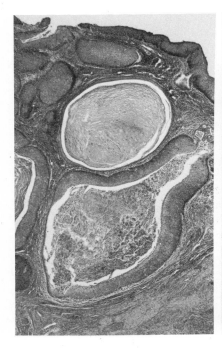

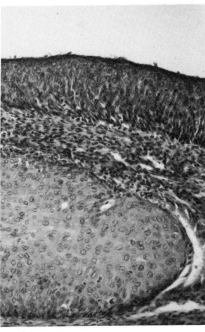

Figure 13–15. Low-power photomicrograph of carcinoma-in-situ with deep (5 to 6 mm) gland involvement. Cryotherapy with its limited depth of destruction would probably not completely eradicate this lesion.

proliferating cells appear to be "undifferentiated" basal/reserve cells that begin to mature near the surface. The undifferentiated cells vary considerably in size and shape; the nuclei are pleomorphic and hyperchromatic, exhibit coarse chromatin clumping, and have a disturbance of mitotic activity. In an attempt to quantify these changes, it was proposed that (1) mild dysplasia (Figs. 13–3 to 13–6) is a lesion composed of undifferentiated cells that occupy the deepest level but do not exceed one third of the thickness of the epithelium; (2) moderate dysplasia (Fig. 13–7) consists of undifferentiated cells that occupy between one half to three fourths of the thickness of the epithelium; and (3) severe dysplasia (Figs. 13–8 to 13–10 and 13–13 and 13–14) involves almost the full thickness of the epithelium, which is replaced by undifferentiated cells, except for the most superficial layer, which still shows some evidence of cell maturation.

It is well known that the biologic behavior of dysplastic lesions, especially less severe dysplasias, cannot be accurately predicted on the basis of their histologic appearance (Koss, 1979). The histologic criteria used for characterizing advanced dysplasias, however, seem to correlate with the biologic potential of lesions that progress to carcinoma-in-situ and invasive cancer. The best single histologic criterion for predicting which dysplasia will regress and which will progress is the presence of abnormal mitotic figures in the latter (Fu et al., 1981). The significance of abnormal mitotic figures was shown by measurement of the DNA chromosomal pattern of different intraepithelial lesions with microspectrophotometry. This technique determines whether a lesion is (1) euploid

(normal number of chromosomes) and therefore normal (or reactive); (2) polyploid (multiples of normal numbers of chromosomes), which is characteristic of reversible hyperplastic lesions; or (3) aneuploid, which is typical of invasive carcinomas. In a retrospective study, 85 percent of regressing dysplasias were euploid or polyploid, whereas 95 percent of dysplasias that persisted were aneuploid; all the lesions that progressed to invasive carcinoma were aneuploid (Fu et al., 1981). Histologically, it may be difficult if not impossible to distinguish lesions with high degrees of polyploidy from those that are aneuploid; however, microspectrometric studies have shown that those cells with abnormal mitotic figures have an aneuploid pattern of chromosomes. Therefore, one can make the diagnosis of an aneuploid lesion by identifying abnormal mitotic figures, which almost always are found in the zone of proliferating, undifferentiated cells of occasionally mild but usually moderate or severe dysplasias.

RELATIONSHIP OF CERVICAL DYSPLASIA TO HUMAN PAPILLOMAVIRUS (HPV)

Twenty-seven types of HPV have been identified in cutaneous and mucosal lesions (Table 13–1) (Jenson et al., 1985), with specific types HPV-6, HPV-11, HPV-16, HPV-18, and untyped HPV having preference for the cervix. It appears that some HPV types are preferentially associated with cervical lesions that are benign (HPV-6, HPV-11, and untyped HPV), whereas other types are associated with those that are malignant (HPV-16, HPV-18, and untyped HPV)

(Gissmann et al., 1984; Lancaster et al., 1985; Pfister, 1983). Previously, the inability to propagate the virus in tissue culture (Butel, 1972) or to transmit it to other species (Koller and Olson, 1972) were the main impediments to the study of the oncogenic potential of HPV. Our current knowledge of the role of HPV in cervical dysplasia and carcinoma is based on technical advances in immunocytochemistry and molecular virology that permit detection of HPV capsid antigens and DNA sequences (Gissmann et al., 1984; Lancaster et al., 1985; Pfister, 1983).

Most HPV-associated cutaneous and mucosal lesions have similar pathobiologic features (Howley, 1982; Jenson et al., 1984). The HPV genome appears to be in a stable form in the basal layer of the wart/papilloma, and early gene expression is associated with an increase in the stratum spinosum or prickle cell layer, acanthosis. This is followed by late gene expression, which is manifested by degenerative changes, HPV cytopathic effect in terminally differentiated squamous cells. The most prominent HPV cytopathic effect is cytoplasmic vacuolization (koilocytosis, which was first described by Koss and Durfee, 1956) with or without synthesis of intranuclear HPV capsid proteins and virion assembly in superficial prickle and/or granular squamous cells (Fig. 13–3). Other histologic changes include degenerative nuclear alterations, wrinkling and pyknosis, and production of excess keratin, hyperkeratosis. In exophytic lesions such as cutaneous warts and mucosal condylomas, acanthosis and hyperkeratosis expand the epithelial surface by causing papillary projections, referred to as "papillomatosis." Although flat lesions such as cervical dysplasias do not have a papillomatous surface, frequently epithelial spikes are evident histologically, thereby permitting recognition of HPV infection.

Kurman and colleagues (1983) reported that 95 percent of mild dysplasias, 77 percent of moderate dysplasias, 64 percent of severe dysplasias, and 44 percent of in-situ-carcinomas were associated with histologic evidence of HPV somewhere in the tissue

Table 13–1. **Classification of Human Papillomavirus Types and the Lesions with Which They Are Most Often Associated**

Type	Lesion
1, 4	Plantar warts
2	Common warts
3, 10	Flat warts
5, 8	Epidermodysplasia verruciformis (carcinomas)
6, 11	Laryngeal papillomas, anogenital warts
7	Butcher's warts
9, 12, 14, 15 17, 19–25	Epidermodysplasia verruciformis
13	Oral focal epithelial hyperplasia
16, 18	Cervical dysplasias, carcinomas; Bowenoid papulosis
26, 27	Immune deficiency, transplants

specimen. The histologic features that best correlated with HPV infection were koilocytosis and/or any two of the following: nuclear wrinkling, bi- and multinucleation, dyskeratosis, and papillary projections. When contiguous microscopic sections from the same paraffin block were examined by immunoperoxidase methods, papillomavirus antigens were present in nearly 30 percent of mild dysplasias, 16 percent of moderate dysplasias, and 3 percent of severe dysplasias, but never in carcinoma-in-situ or metaplastic squamous epithelium. HPV antigens were invariably intranuclear and confined to the upper layer of epithelium, mostly in koilocytotic cells (Fig. 13–3). Koilocytotic cells containing HPV antigen could not be distinguished morphologically from those that were negative for the capsid antigen. In 85 percent of cases with demonstrable HPV antigens, the positive cells were located over a zone of proliferating basal/parabasal cells showing varying degrees of nuclear atypia; capsid antigens were never expressed in the proliferating cells. From this study and others, it is known that the frequency of expression of HPV structural proteins in epithelium is inversely proportional to the extent of the underlying proliferation, which may explain why it is never seen in in-situ or invasive carcinomas. The presence of HPV antigens is synonymous with the assembly of infectious virions and indicates that the lesion is potentially contagious. We have referred to the proliferating cellular zone as "papillomavirus-associated hyperplasia" and to the HPV cytopathic changes in the differentiating cells as "papillomavirus-induced atypia." Together, these constitute the dysplastic lesion.

DNA hybridization studies on samples of cervical dysplasia reveal the presence of the HPV genome in nearly all cases of mild, moderate, and severe dysplasia and carcinomas-in-situ (Lancaster et al., 1983; Okagaki et al., 1983). Recently, HPV-16 was found in 61 percent of invasive and cervical cancers in German patients and in nearly 35 percent of similar cases from Kenya and Brazil (Durst et al., 1983). In contrast to its high prevalence in invasive carcinoma, HPV-16 has been found in only 16 percent of the cases of dysplasia, suggesting that it has a high carcinogenic potential. HPV-18, an HPV cloned from cervical cancer and subsequently found in cultured HeLa cells, has been detected in 25 percent of cervical cancers from patients in Africa and Brazil and in a small percentage of dysplasias in German patients (Boshart et al., 1984). Crum and coworkers (1984) correlated the presence of abnormal mitotic figures and aneuploidy in 80 percent of dysplastic lesions containing HPV-16. Thus, evidence is emerging that suggests that dysplastic lesions that progress to squamous cell carcinomas are preferentially associated with specific HPV types, such as HPV-16 and HPV-18.

There is precedence for the association of HPV with premalignant and malignant lesions of squamous epithelium. Epidermodysplasia verruciformis is a rare autosomal, recessive disease characterized by varying degrees of decreased cell-mediated immunity and increased susceptibility to HPV infection. It is manifested clinically by polymorphic skin lesions that resemble flat warts or macules (Jablonska et al., 1972; Lutzner, 1978; Orth et al., 1980). In approximately 25 percent of patients with epidermodysplasia verruciformis, malignant transformation occurs within the pityriasis-like lesions exposed to sunlight (actinic radiation), which apparently acts as a co-carcinogen. These hyperplasias progress through increasingly dysplastic changes, histopathologically similar to cervical dysplasia, before developing into carcinoma-in-situ, Bowen's disease, and eventually invasive squamous cell carcinoma. Only HPV-5 or HPV-8 can be identified in both primary and metastatic malignant lesions. Thus, it appears that the roles of HPV-5 and HPV-8 in dysplastic and neoplastic lesions in epidermodysplasia verruciformis may be analogous to the roles of HPV-16 and HPV-18 in dysplasias and squamous cell carcinomas of the cervix. In the latter lesion, circumstantial evidence suggests that herpes simplex virus infection (zur Hausen, 1982) or smoking (Vonka et al., 1984a) or both may act as co-carcinogens.

DYSPLASIA AS A PRECURSOR OF CANCER

Some epidemiologic studies have shown that patients with dysplasia have demographics that are similar to those of patients with carcinoma-in-situ and invasive carcinoma, thereby implicating dysplasia as a transitional stage in carcinogenesis. Other epidemiologic studies, however, show differences in the epidemiology of patients with dysplasia when compared with carcinoma-in-situ and invasive carcinoma. For example, in one representative study, women with carcinoma-in-situ or squamous carcinoma were younger at first coitus and at marriage than both the women in the control group and the patients with dysplasia (Terris et al., 1980). Data such as these suggest that carcinoma-in-situ and invasive cancer are different forms of the same disease but that dysplasia represents a heterogeneous group of diseases of which only some are precancerous. Conversely, all cases of carcinoma-in-situ and invasive cancer probably develop from dysplasias.

Although there is variation among different studies, it is generally accepted that the majority of mild and moderate dysplasias will regress or persist, whereas severe dysplasias or carcinomas-in-situ or both are more apt to persist or progress to invasive cancer. In a study by Richart and Barron (1969), over 90 percent of all grades of dysplasia progressed to carcinoma-in-situ if the patients were followed only by cytologic smears. It is known that biopsies and other trauma to the cervix may be therapeutic as well as diagnostic by causing lesions to regress or disappear. A long-term

follow-up by Nasiell and coworkers (1983) of 894 patients with moderate dysplasia is representative of many studies. Nasiell's group found that regression occurred in 54 percent, persistence in 16 percent, and progression in 30 percent. Progression occurred after a mean follow-up of 51 months. These statistics are not to be minimized and are important in understanding the biologic potential of dysplasias and neoplasia, but they do not offer guidelines for the pathologist, who frequently must make an evaluation based on one or two cytologic examinations and a subsequent single biopsy specimen.

PATHOLOGY CONSIDERATIONS IN MANAGEMENT

Correlation of cytology, colposcopy, and histology is essential to proper evaluation and treatment of precancerous lesions of the cervix. This requires close communication between the pathologist and gynecologist.

Screening for "clinically silent," premalignant cervical lesions by cytologic examination is rapid and relatively inexpensive. Mass cytology screening programs have been responsible for a dramatic decrease in cervical cancer, although the incidence of dysplasia has increased simultaneously. Unfortunately, there is a signficant false-negative rate of 5 to 50 percent (Gad and Koch, 1978), which for all practical purposes levels out at 20 percent. Half the false-negative cases are due to inadequate sampling, and half are due to misinterpretation of the smear by the cytologist. Inadequate sampling can be partially overcome by scraping the circumference of the cervix and then aspirating the endocervical canal to maximize the number of exfoliated cells in the sample. In clinical studies, the use of culposcopy in conjunction with cytology has reduced the false-negative rate to 3 percent (Vonka et al., 1984a). In an ongoing prospective study of women screened by cytology at Georgetown University, approximately 12 percent had HPV sequences detected in DNA isolated from exfoliated cervical cells, whereas only 6 percent showed abnormal cytology (Lorincz, et al., 1986), thus suggesting that the frequency of HPV infection of the cervix in the general population is much higher than anticipated and that hybridization may be twice as sensitive as standard cytology screening techniques.

The pathologist must pay particular attention to several factors when evaluating cervical biopsies, which can result in inadequate or inappropriate treatment if not brought to the attention of the gynecologist. For example, the presence of gland involvement in dysplastic and in-situ lesions (Fig. 13–15) should be stated in the pathology report because outpatient cryosurgery, the most common treatment of dysplasia, has a limited depth of destruction and may not completely eradicate deep intraepithelial lesions. Involvement of the margins of cone biopsies is associated with a high recurrence rate, and therefore this information also should be included in the pathology report. In addition, careful examination of endocervical curettings may identify fragments of a dysplasia that are not visible to the gynecologist, even with the aid of a colposcope. Finally, identification of HPV antigens by immunocytochemistry, particularly in less severe dysplasias, indicates the presence of infectious virus. Even if the lesion is adequately treated in positive cases, the male cohort has been shown to have a similar HPV-associated lesion, Bowenoid papulosis, which can reinfect the cervix. Therefore, the male partner should be evaluated carefully for the presence of papillomas on the shaft, corona, or urethra of the penis. Thus, most dysplasias should be treated as sexually transmitted diseases in which the infectious agent is still present.

ADENOCARCINOMA-IN-SITU

Adenocarcinoma-in-situ is an uncommon preinvasive lesion of the endocervical glands (Fig. 13–16). The average age of occurrence is 40 years. Its low incidence reflects that of invasive adenocarcinoma, which constitutes about 5 percent of all carcinomas arising in the cervix (Qizilbash, 1975). Interestingly, adenocarcinoma-in-situ frequently coexists with dysplasias

and carcinomas-in-situ of squamous epithelium (Friedell and McKay, 1953; Weisbrot et al., 1971). This coexistence has prompted various workers to suggest that the same etiologic agent or agents play a role in malignant transformation of the common analogue (subcolumnar reserve cell) of both metaplastic squamous epithelium and glandular endocervical cells (Christopherson et al., 1979). However, an epidemiologic evaluation of patients with adenocarcinoma-in-situ and invasive carcinoma has not been undertaken.

Several reasons have been given for designating adenocarcinoma-in-situ a "preinvasive lesion" (Abell and Gosling, 1962; Christopherson et al., 1979; Gloor and Ruzicka, 1982; Qizilbash, 1975): (1) Histologically, the lesion is identical with that of the well-differentiated invasive adenocarcinomas, except that it is confined to the endocervical glands; (2) cytologically, it is identical with adenocarcinoma cells; and (3) adenocarcinoma-in-situ is frequently seen at the margins of invasive adenocarcinomas. However, adenocarcinomas-in-situ must be distinguished from the hyperplasia associated with use of oral contraceptives (Taylor et al., 1967). Adenocarcinomas that metastasize to endocervical glands must also be excluded, particularly endometrial adenocarcinoma, by curettage or examination of hysterectomy specimens or by observation of a transition from normal endocervical epithelium to malignant epithelium (Maier and Norris, 1980). Dysplasias of endocervical glands have been described with histologic changes less severe than

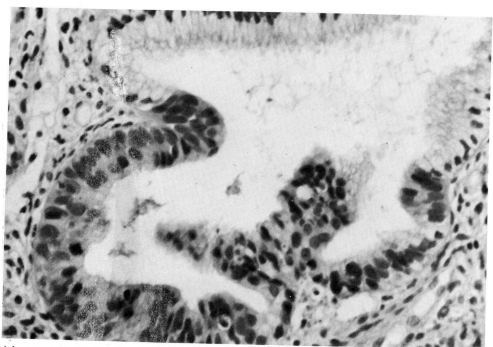

Figure 13–16. Adenocarcinoma-in-situ. Part of the normal endocervical gland epithelium is replaced by neoplastic cells, which form a small papillary projection. (Courtesy of Dr. Albores-Saavedra.)

those of well-differentiated adenocarcinomas—that is, the nuceli are less enlarged, chromatin is fine and evenly granular, and nucleoli are small and rounded (Bousfield et al., 1980).

Diagnosis of adenocarcinoma-in-situ has been made by cytology, endocervical curettage, cone biopsy, and hysterectomy (Bousfield et al., 1980; Christopherson et al., 1979; Gloor and Ruzicka, 1982; Qizilbash, 1974; Weisbrot et al., 1972). Because these lesions are focal and are frequently associated with squamous cell intraepithelial lesions, they are easily overlooked. Surgical removal of involved endocervical glands is a curative procedure, with most workers in the field suggesting hysterectomy as the procedure of choice. Awareness of the existence of adenocarcinoma-in-situ and careful examination of cytologic smears and biopsies of the cervix will lead to increased diagnosis and improved treatment of this particular preinvasive lesion.

References

Abell, M.R. and Gosling, J.R.G.: Gland cell carcinoma (adenocarcinoma) of the uterine cervix. Am. J. Obstet. Gynecol. 83:729, 1962.

Alexander, E.R.: Possible etiologies of cancer of the cervix other than herpesvirus. Cancer Res. 33:1485, 1973.

Boshart, M., Gissmann, L., Ikenberg, H., Kleinheinz, A., Scheurlen, W., zur Hausen, H.A.: New type of papillomavirus DNA, its presence in genital cancer biopsies and in cell lines derived from cervical cancer. EMBO J. 3:1151, 1984.

Bousfield, L., Pacey, F., Young, Q., Krumins, I., Osborn, R.: Expanded cytologic criteria for the diagnosis of adenocarcinoma in situ of the cervix and related lesions. Acta Cytol. 24:283, 1980.

Butel, J.: Studies with human papillomavirus modeled after known papovavirus systems. J. Natl. Cancer Inst. 48:285, 1972.

Christopherson, W.M., Nealon, N., Gray, L.A., Sr.: Noninvasive precursor lesions of adenocarcinoma and mixed adenosquamous carcinoma of the cervix uteri. Cancer 44:976, 1979.

Crum, C.P., Ikenberg, H., Richart, R.M., Gissman, L.: Human papilloma virus type 16 and early cervical neoplasia. N. Engl. J. Med. 310:880, 1984.

Durst, M., Gissman, L., Ikenberg, H., zur Hausen, H.J.: A new type of papillomavirus DNA from a cervical carcinoma and its prevalence in cancer biopsies from different geographic regions. Proc. Natl. Acad. Sci. 80:3812, 1983.

Editorial: Statement of caution. Interpretation of papillomavirus-associated lesions of the epithelium of uterine cervix. Am. J. Obstet. Gynecol. 146:125, 1983.

Friedell, G.H. and McKay, D.G.: Adenocarcinoma in situ of the endocervix. Cancer 6:887, 1953.

Fu, Y.S., Reagen, J.W., Richart, R.M.: Definition of precursors. Gynecol. Oncol. 12:S220, 1981.

Gad, C. and Koch, F.: The limitation of screening effect. A review of cervical disorders in previously screened women. Acta Cytol. 21:719, 1978.

Gissmann, L., Boshart, M., Dürst, M., Ikenberg, H., Wagner, D., zur Hausen, H.: Presence of human papillomavirus in genital tumors. J. Invest. Dermatol. 83:(Suppl.)26S, 1984.

Gissmann, L. and zur Hausen, H.: Personal communication.

Gloor, E. and Ruzicka, J.: Morphology of adenocarcinoma in situ of the uterine cervix. Cancer 49:294, 1982.

Howley, P.M.: The human papillomaviruses. Arch. Pathol. Lab. Med. 106:429, 1982.

Jablonska, S., Dabrowski, J., Jakubowicz, K.: Epidemodysplasia verruciformis as a model in studies on the role of papovavirus in oncogenesis. Cancer Res. 32:583, 1972.

Jenson, A.B., Kurman, R.J., Lancaster, W.D.: Human papillomaviruses. In Belsche, R. (ed.): Textbook of Human Virology. Littleton, MA, Wright-PSG, Inc., 1984, p. 951.

Jenson, A.B., Kurman, R.J., Lancaster, W.D.: Unpublished data.

Kessler, I.I.: Venereal factors in human cervical cancer. Cancer 39:1912, 1977.

Koller, L.D. and Olson, C.: Attempted transmission of warts from man, cattle and horses and of deer fibroma to selected hosts. J. Invest. Dermatol. 58:366, 1972.

Koss, L.G.: In Diagnostic Cytology and Its Histopathologic Bases, 3rd ed. Vol. 1. Philadelphia, J.B. Lippincott Co., 1979.

Koss, L.G. and Durfee, G.R.: Unusual patterns of squamous epithelium of the uterine cervix: cytologic and pathologic study of koilocytotic atypia. Ann. N.Y. Acad. Sci. U.S.A. 63:1235, 1956.

Kurman, R.J., Jenson, A.B., Lancaster, W.D.: Papillomavirus infection of the cervix. II. Relationship to intraepithelial neoplasia based on the presence of specific viral structural proteins. Am. J. Surg. Pathol. 7:39, 1983.

Kurman, R.J., Jenson, A.B., Sinclair, C., Lancaster, W.D.: Detection of human papillomaviruses by immunocytochemistry. In DeLelis, R.A. (ed.): Advances in Immunocytochemistry. New York, Masson Publishing, 1984, p. 201.

Kurman, R.J., Sanz, L.E., Jenson, A.B., Perry, S., Lancaster, W.D.: Papillomavirus infection of the cervix. I. Correlation of histology with specific structural antigens and DNA sequences. Int. J. Gynecol. Pathol. 1:17, 1982.

Kurman, R.J., Shah, K.H., Lancaster, W.D., Jenson, A.B.: Immunoperoxidase localization of papillomavirus antigens in cervical dysplasia and vulvar condylomas. Am. J. Obstet. Gynecol. 40:931, 1981.

Lancaster, W.D., Kurman, R.J., Jenson, A.B.: Papillomaviruses in anogenital neoplasms. In Loderer, W., et al.: Molecular Analysis and Diagnosis of Malignancy. Clifton, Humana Press, in press.

Lancaster, W.D., Kurman, R.J., Sanz, L.E., Perry, S., Jenson, A.B.: Detection of viral DNA sequences and evidence of molecule heterogeneity in dysplasias of the uterine cervix. Intervirology 20:202, 1983.

Lorincz, A.T., Lancaster, W.D., Kurman, R., Jenson, A.B., Temple, G.: Characterization of human papillomaviruses in cervical neoplasias and their detection in routine clinical screening. Proceedings, Banbury Conference, in press, 1986.

Lutzner, M.A.: Epidermodysplasia verruciformis: an autosomal recessive disease characterized by viral warts and skin cancer; a model for viral oncogenesis. Bull. Cancer 65:169, 1978.

Maier, R.C., Norris, H.J.: Coexistence of cervical intraepithelial neoplasia with primary adenocarcinoma of the endocervix. Obstet. Gynecol. 56:361, 1980.

Meisels, A. and Fortin, R.: Condylomatous lesions of the cervix and vagina: I. Cytologic patterns. Acta Cytol. 20:505, 1976.

Meisels, A., Fortin, R., Roy, M.: Condylomatous lesions of the cervix. II. Cytologic, colposcopic, and histopathologic study. Acta Cytol. 21:379, 1977.

Meisels, A., Roy, M., Fortier, M., Morin, C., Casas-Cordero, M., Shah, K.V., Turgeon, H.: Human papillomavirus infections of the cervix. The atypical condyloma. Acta Cytol. 25:7, 1981.

Nahmias, A. J., Josey, W. E., Naib, Z. M., Luce, C. F., Guest, B. A.: Antibodies to herpes virus hominis types 1 and 2 in humans. II. Am. J. Epidemiol. 91:747–752, 1970.

Nahmias, A. J., Naib, Z. M., Josey, W. E.: Epidemiological studies relating genital herpetic infection to cervical carcinoma. Cancer Res. 34:1111, 1974.

Nasiell, K., Nasiell, M., Vaclavinkova, V.: Behavior of moderate cervical dysplasia during long-term follow-up. Obstet. Gynecol. 61:609, 1983.

Okagaki, T.: Female genital tumors associated with human papillomavirus infection, and the concept of genital neoplasm—papilloma syndrome (GENPS). Pathol. Annu. Part 2:31, 1984.

Okagaki, T., Twiggs, L.B., Zachow, K.R., Lark, B.A., Ostrow, R.S., Faras, A.J.: Identification of human papillomavirus DNA in cervical and vaginal intraepithelial neoplasia and molecularly cloned virus-specific DNA probes. Int. J. Gynecol. Pathol. 2:153, 1983.

Orth, G., Jablonska, S., Breitburd, F., Favre, M., Croissant, O., Obalek, S., Jarzabek-Chorzelska, M., Rzesa, G.: Epidermodysplasia verruciformis: a model for viral oncogenesis in man. Cold Spring Harbor Conf. Cell Prolif. 7:259, 1980.

Pfister, H.: Biology and biochemistry of papillomaviruses. Rev. Physiol. Biochem. Pharmacol. 99:111, 1983.

Poulson, H.E., Taylor, C.H., Sobin, L.H.: Histological typing of female genital tract tumors. WHO Chron., 1975.

Purola, E. and Savia, E.: Cytology of gynecologic condyloma acuminatum. Acta Cytol. 21:26, 1977.

Qizilbash, A.H.: In situ and microinvasive adenocarcinoma of the uterine cervix: a clinical, cytologic and histologic study of 14 cases. Am. J. Clin. Pathol. 64:155, 1975.

Rawls, W.E., Tompkins, W.A.E., Melnick, J.L.: The association of herpes virus type 2 and carcinoma of the uterine cervix. Am. J. Epidemiol. 89:547, 1969.

Reagen, J.W., Seidemann, I.L., Saracusa, Y.: Cellular morphology of carcinoma in situ and dysplasia or atypical hyperplasia of uterine cervix cancer. Cancer 6:224, 1953.

Richart, R.M.: Natural history of cervical intraepithelial neoplasia. Clin. Obstet. Gynecol. 5:748, 1968.

Richart, R.M., Barron, B.A.: Follow-up study of patients with cervical dysplasia. Am. J. Obstet. Gynecol. 105:386, 1969.

Rotkin, I.A.: A comparison review of key epidemiological studies in cervical cancer related to current searches for transmissable agents. Cancer Res. 33:1353, 1973.

Spriggs, A.I.: Natural history of cervical dysplasia. Clin. Obstet. Gynecol. 8:65, 1981.

Syrjanen, K.J., Heinonen, U.-M., Kauraniemi, T.: Cytologic evidence of the association of condylomatous lesions with dysplastic and neoplastic changes in the uterine cervix. Acta Cytol. 25:17, 1981.

Taylor, H.B., Irey, N.S., Norris, H.J.: Atypical endocervical hyperplasia in women taking oral contraceptives. J.A.M.A. 202:637, 1967.

Terris, M., Wilson, F., Nelson, J.H., Jr.: Comparative epidemiology of invasive carcinoma of the cervix, carcinoma in situ, and cervical dysplasia. Am. J. Epidemiol. 112:253, 1980.

Vonka, V., Kanka, J., Hirsch, I., Zabadora, H., Krcmar, M., Suchankova, A., Rezacova, D., Broucek, J., Press, M., Domorazkova, E., Svoboda, B., Havrankova, A., Jelinek, J.: Prospective study on the relationship between cervical neoplasia and herpes simplex virus type-2 virus. II. Herpes simplex type-2 antibody presence in sera taken at enrollment. Int. J. Cancer 33:61, 1984b.

Vonka, V., Kanka, J., Jelinek, J., Subrt, I., Suchanek, A., Havrankova, A., Vachal, M., Hirsch, I., Domorazkova, E., Zavadora, H., Richterova, V., Naprstkova, J., Dvorakova, V., Svoboda, B.: Prospective study of the relationship between cervical neoplasia and herpes simplex type-2 virus. I. Epidemiological characteristics. Int. J. Cancer 33:49, 1984a.

Weid, G.L.: Proceedings of the First International Congress of Exfoliative Cytology (editorial): Vienna, Austria. Norwalk, CT, Appleton-Century-Crofts, 1962, p. 297.

Weisbrot, I.M., Stabinsky, C., Davis, A.M.: Adenocarinoma in situ of the uterine cervix. Cancer 29:1179, 1972.

Zur Hausen, H.: Human genital cancer: Synergism between two virus infections or synergism between a virus infection and initiating events? Lancet 2:1370, 1982.

ROBERT J. KURMAN
HENRY J. NORRIS

14 Endometrium

Proliferative endometrial lesions ranging from focal glandular crowding through hyperplasia and carcinoma form a morphologic continuum that is composed of an infinite number of discrete but overlapping stages. Since the 1930s, classifications have evolved in which degrees of proliferation are separately labeled, although criteria for them are subjective, ill defined, and highly variable. The absence of objective criteria, in and of itself, is an impediment to accurate histologic diagnosis, but the problem is compounded by a terminology that is consistent only in its lack of consistency (Gore, 1973). Different terms have been applied to similar lesions by various investigators; conversely, similar terms have been used to describe vastly different lesions. With diagnostic criteria mired in subjectivity and the nomenclature in chaos it should come as no surprise that knowledge about the behavior of these lesions is uncertain. The current problems in this area are as follows:

1. What are the histologic criteria in curettings by which a proliferative lesion with metastatic potential can be distinguished from one without metastatic potential?

2. What is the long-term behavior of the various forms of endometrial hyperplasia?

3. Within the spectrum of endometrial hyperplasia, which lesions have a high risk of progression to carcinoma?

4. What is the relationship of endometrial hyperplasia to carcinoma?

In this chapter, we will attempt to answer these questions and provide guidelines for the histologic diagnosis of various lesions in the proliferative spectrum. Our recommendations are based on two retrospective studies from the Armed Forces Institute of Pathology involving 374 patients in which a detailed correlation of morphologic patterns with biologic behavior was performed. The classification that developed as a result of these studies differs significantly from traditional classifications presently in use. Therefore, we have included a brief historical review of the nomenclature of the precursors of endometrial carcinoma in order to compare the various terms and the histologic patterns that they describe.

DEFINITIONS IN A HISTORICAL PERSPECTIVE

Cystic Hyperplasia. There is more agreement about the identification of this lesion, which is at the low end of the proliferative spectrum, than about the recognition of any of the others. It is the most common form of hyperplasia, is easily recognized, and is characterized by dilated glands of varying size lined by tall columnar or cuboidal epithelium that usually shows some degree of mitotic activity and stratification. The latter feature helps one distinguish the dilated glands of cystic hyperplasia from those lined by flattened epithelium that characterize cystic (senile) atrophy and the isolated dilated glands occasionally observed in normal proliferative or secretory endometrium.

Adenomatous Hyperplasia. The term "adenomatous hyperplasia" has been applied by different authors to describe widely differing patterns. Gusberg used it to include all categories of endometrial hyperplasia beyond cystic hyperplasia (Gusberg, 1947; Gusberg and Kaplan, 1963; Gusberg et al., 1954). He subdivided adenomatous hyperplasia into mild, moderate, and severe forms. Severe adenomatous hyperplasia corresponds to what other authors designate "atypical hyperplasia." In contrast, Hertig and colleagues (Hertig and Sommers, 1949; Hertig et al., 1949) used the term "adenomatous hyperplasia" to denote a histologic pattern that exhibits glandular projections and buds into the surrounding stroma. Vellios (1974) and Buehl and coworkers (1964) use the term in a similar fashion but restrict it to endometria with little or no atypia. Little is accomplished by adding the adjective "adenomatous" to "hyperplasia."

Atypical Hyperplasia. Novak and Rutledge (1948) introduced the term "atypical hyperplasia" to describe proliferative endometria characterized by a greatly increased number of glands with very little intervening stroma. Although they described the glandular pattern as closely resembling carcinoma and described the presence of moderately large uniform nuclei, they did not mention nuclear atypia. Campbell and Barter (1961) utilized a similar terminology but divided atypical hyperplasia into Types 1, 2, or 3 depending on how closely the lesion resembled carcinoma. They used complexity of the pattern rather than cytologic atypia as the basis for subdividing atypical hyperplasia. Vellios (1974), however, restricted the definition of "atypical hyperplasia" to endometria showing degrees of cellular atypia, even in the absence of glandular crowding. The discrepancy about what constitutes atypia persists in the literature. Some authors have used the term "atypical hyperplasia" to describe abnormally complex architectural patterns, regardless of cytologic atypia; others limit the term to describe endometria with cytologic atypia, regardless of the architectural pattern. The confusion between glandular complexity and cytologic atypia must be clarified.

Carcinoma-in-Situ. Hertig and colleagues (Hertig and Sommers, 1949; Hertig et al., 1949) introduced this term to describe a focal lesion with cytologic alterations in which glandular crowding was not usually a prominent feature. The cells were large with abundant amphophilic or eosinophilic cytoplasm that usually showed loss of polarity. The nuclei were pale, not hyperchromatic, but showed irregular nuclear membranes and fine granular chromatin. Intraglandular tufting was sometimes present. Buehl and associates (1964) and Vellios (1974) use the term to denote a process cytologically consistent with carcinoma. They distinguish carcinoma-in-situ from well-differentiated carcinoma on the basis of crowding. If glands having the characteristics of carcinoma-in-situ are crowded together to the point that "the likelihood of stromal invasion is high," the lesion is designated "invasive carcinoma." Welch and Scully (1977) use more precise criteria for distinguishing carcinoma-in-situ from well-differentiated carcinoma. "Carcinoma-in-situ" is defined as a small lesion that involves no more than five or six glands in which cytologic features of carcinoma are present but that demonstrates no evidence of invasion. If the change involves more than five or six glands, a diagnosis of "invasive carcinoma" is made. Welch and Scully acknowledge that invasion is often impossible to identify in areas of crowded glands. Tavassoli and Kraus (1978) distinguish an early carcinoma from atypical hyperplasia on the basis of the cytologically malignant-appearing cells in carcinoma that form intraglandular cribriform processes and intraglandular bridges without any recognizable stromal support in multiple levels of the block. They did not, however, identify an in-situ phase. Because of the uncertainty as to whether a significant and recognizable in-situ form exists and the absence of a uniform or accepted definition for the lesion, it is not included in the classification adopted by the World Health Organization (Poulson et al., 1975).

STROMAL INVASION IN THE DIFFERENTIATION OF ATYPICAL HYPERPLASIA–CARCINOMA-IN-SITU FROM WELL-DIFFERENTIATED CARCINOMA

To determine specific and reproducible criteria for distinguishing atypical hyperplasia and so-called carcinoma-in-situ from well-differentiated carcinoma in curettings, Kurman and Norris (1982) reviewed 204 curettings from the Armed Forces Institute of Pathology files. Cases showing the most severe forms of atypical hyperplasia, including examples of what have been regarded as carcinoma-in-situ and well-differentiated carcinoma, were selected and compared with the findings in non-irradiated hysterectomy specimens obtained within 1 month of the curettage. Degrees of cellular atypia, stratification, mitotic activity, and necrosis were recorded. An arbitrary definition of stromal invasion also was used. This proved the most useful criterion in predicting the presence of a biologically significant carcinoma in the uterus (a tumor that invaded the myometrium or metastasized) (King et al., 1984; Kurman and Norris, 1982).

Identification of stromal invasion, by arbitrary criteria, depends on the presence of one of the following: (1) an irregular infiltration of glands associated with an altered fibroblastic stroma or desmoplastic response; (2) a confluent glandular pattern in which individual glands, uninterrupted by stroma, merge and form a cribriform pattern; (3) an extensive papillary pattern; and (4) replacement of the stroma by masses of squamous epithelium. The processes that manifest the last three of the aforementioned features of invasion must be sufficiently extensive to involve half of a low-power field measuring 4.2 mm in diameter without intervening stroma (Kurman and Norris, 1982; Norris et al., 1983). These four features are discussed subsequently.

1. Infiltration of endometrial stroma by neoplastic glands frequently induces a desmoplastic or fibrous stromal response (Figs. 14–1 and 14–2). The altered stroma of invasion contains densely arranged parallel fibroblasts that disrupt the usual glandular pattern. The cells in the desmoplastic stroma are more spindle-shaped than the stromal cells of proliferative endometrium, and their nuclei are more elongated. The desmoplastic stroma demonstrates pronounced collagen, unlike proliferative and hyperplastic endometria, in which collagen is inconspicuous. The desmoplasia is frequently maintained when neoplastic glands invade the myometrium. The altered stroma associated with invasion may be contrasted to the stroma in atypical hyperplasia illustrated in Figure 14–3. Fragments of fibrous, relatively aglandular polyps or stroma from the lower uterine segment may obscure the picture, but the proximity of the lesion to normal fundal stroma should minimize the confusion. The atypical adenomyomatous polyp identified by Mazur (1981) is particularly difficult to distinguish from in-

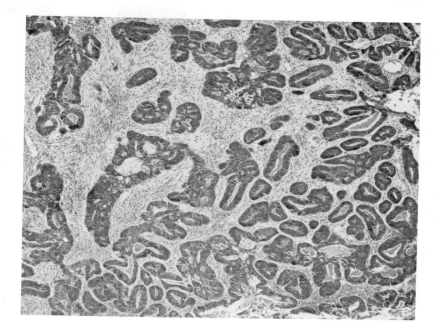

Figure 14–1. The desmoplastic response is a manifestation of stromal invasion. (From Kurman, R. J. and Norris, H. J.: Cancer 49:2547–2559, 1982.)

vasion of the myometrium. Usually, a basement membrane surrounds the atypical adenomyomatous polyp, but a basement membrane is not present in early stromal invasion. When a polyp is suspected or when fragments of lower uterine segment cannot be ruled out, features other than the altered stroma should be used to support the diagnosis of carcinoma.

2. Stromal invasion also is identified by the presence of a confluent glandular aggregate so extensive that it cannot be considered to result from crowded, hyperplastic glands. The point at which the proliferation reflects invasion is reached when half of a low-power field is occupied by a proliferation that lacks intervening stroma. Some proliferations are cribriform, resulting from proliferation and bridging of epithelium (Fig. 14–4); others are solid sheets. The epithelium lacks obvious cytologic features of carcinoma because frankly malignant cells identify a carcinoma, even when there is no invasion. Moderate and poorly differentiated carcinomas do not have a quantity requirement (i.e., greater than half a low-power field) for their diagnosis in curettings.

3. Complex papillary patterns represent stromal invasion if multiple branching fibrous processes lined

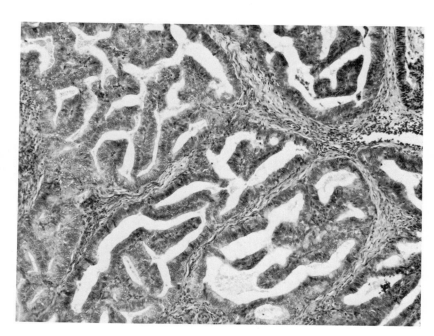

Figure 14–2. The endometrial stroma is altered and replaced by fibroblasts. Collagen is produced and results in retraction of tissue and a haphazard glandular pattern. (From Kurman, R. J. and Norris, H. J.: Cancer 49:2547–2559, 1982.)

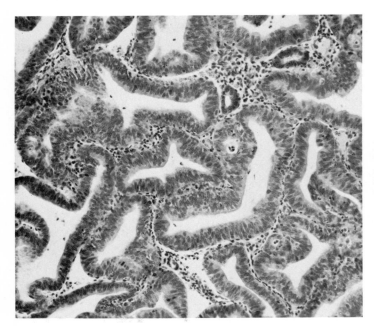

Figure 14–3. There is back-to-back glandular crowding in this atypical hyperplasia, but the stromal cells resemble those of proliferative endometrium; therefore, there is no evidence of stromal invasion. (From Kurman, R. J. and Norris, H. J.: Cancer 49:2547–2559, 1982.)

by epithelium involve at least half of a low-power field (Fig. 14–5). Hyperplasia may form papillary projections lined by stratified atypical epithelial cells, but these are confined within glandular lumina and lack fibrovascular cores.

4. A proliferation of squamous cells that fills, expands, and coalesces glands to form solid sheets of cells replacing the stroma represents invasion if it occupies at least half of a low-power field (Fig. 14–6). The squamous cells (morules or squamous metapla-

sia) need not have cytologic features of carcinoma (Fig. 14–7). This feature may be compared with that shown in Figure 14–8, in which squamous epithelium is confined within glandular lumina and occupies less than half of a low-power field. In contrast, cells with a high grade of nuclear atypia represent carcinoma of the endometrium, regardless of the area occupied by the cells.

Increasing degrees of nuclear atypia, mitotic activity, and stratification of cells in curettings were associated

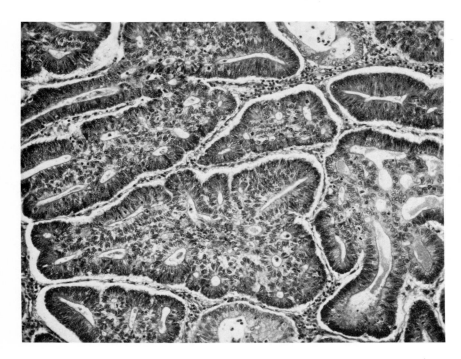

Figure 14–4. The cribriform pattern is a manifestation of stromal invasion if it occupies half of a low-power field. (From Kurman, R. J. and Norris, H. J.: Cancer 49:2547–2559, 1982.)

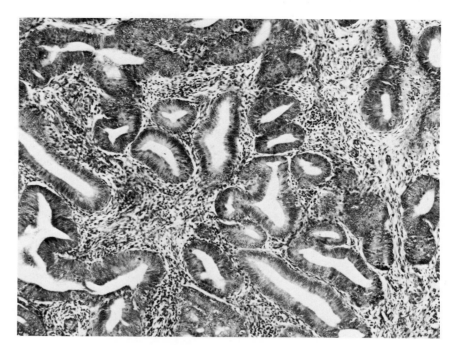

Figure 14–11. Simple hyperplasia with greater crowding than shown in Figure 14–11, but with minimal complexity.

with atypical hyperplasia progressed to carcinoma (p = 0.001) (Table 14–4) (Kurman et al., 1985).

In an effort to identify a subgroup of lesions with an increased risk of progression to carcinoma, further subdivision was based on the degree of glandular complexity and crowding. Thus, a proliferative lesion displaying no evidence of cytologic atypia and minimal to moderate glandular complexity and crowding was termed "simple hyperplasia" (Figs. 14–10 and 14–11), whereas one with marked glandular crowding was termed "complex hyperplasia" (Fig. 14–12). An endometrial proliferation displaying cytologic atypia without back-to-back crowding was designated "simple atypical hyperplasia" (Figs. 14–13 and 14–14), and one accompanied by marked crowding was designated "complex atypical hyperplasia" (Fig. 14–15). Progression to carcinoma occurred in only one (1 percent) of 93 patients with simple hyperplasia and in

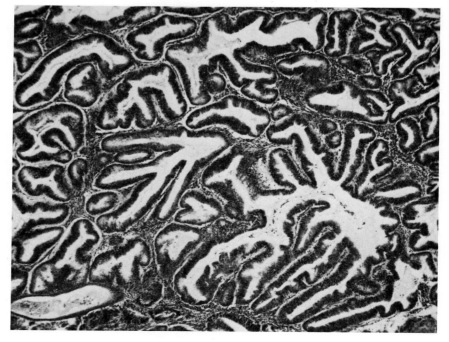

Figure 14–12. Complex hyperplasia characterized by crowded back-to-back glands with complex outlines.

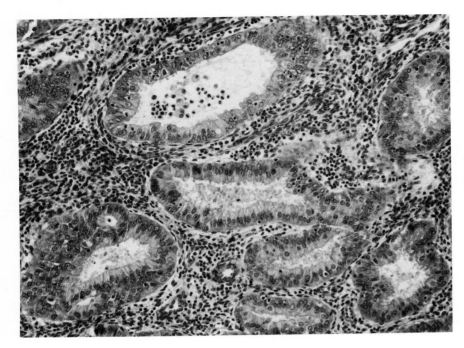

Figure 14–13. Simple atypical hyperplasia. Hyperplastic glands showing nuclear atypia are separated by abundant stroma.

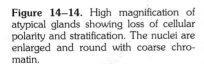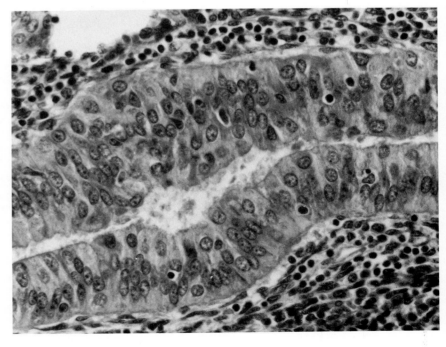

Figure 14–14. High magnification of atypical glands showing loss of cellular polarity and stratification. The nuclei are enlarged and round with coarse chromatin.

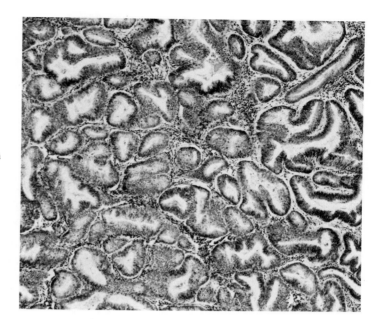

Figure 14–15. Complex atypical hyperplasia showing a complex crowded pattern.

only one (3 percent) of 29 patients with complex hyperplasia. In contrast, one (8 percent) of 13 patients with simple atypical hyperplasia and 10 (29 percent) of 35 patients with complex atypical hyperplasia progressed to carcinoma (Table 14–5). Thus, it is clear that cytologic atypia is the most useful criterion in the identification of a patient who has significantly increased risk of developing carcinoma, and the presence of superimposed glandular complexity and crowding places the patient at greater risk. In the future, non-invasive endometrial proliferations should be classified according to the presence of both cytologic and architectural abnormalities (Table 14–6).

RELATIONSHIP OF HYPERPLASIA TO CARCINOMA

The carcinomas that develop in patients with hyperplasia and atypical hyperplasia are relatively innocuous and stable. All but one of the carcinomas in our study were well-differentiated and confined to the endometrium. None of the patients who developed carcinoma died of the disease. The duration of progression from hyperplasia to carcinoma was 9.5 years;

from atypical hyperplasia to carcinoma it was 4.1 years. It has been shown that in 17 to 25 percent of women with atypical hyperplasia diagnosed in curettings, there will be a well-differentiated uterine carcinoma if hysterectomy is performed within 1 month of curettage (King et al., 1984; Kurman and Norris, 1982; Tavassoli and Kraus, 1978). In our long-term follow-up study (Kurman et al., 1985), 23 percent of women with atypical hyperplasia developed carcinoma if "untreated." In a similar study, Gusberg and Kaplan (1963) found that in their group of patients with "severe adenomatous hyperplasia," 20 percent had uterine carcinoma when hysterectomy was done shortly after curettage, but only 11 percent of those who were followed developed carcinoma. Several reasons may account for the relatively low rate of progression to carcinoma in patients with atypical hyperplasia who are followed. First, there is a general tendency for the highest grades of atypical hyperplasia to be treated by hysterectomy, with the milder degrees of atypia being managed with conservative interventions. Second, atypical hyperplasia may not be the precursor of all forms of endometrial cancer but only of a type that is slow-growing and not always progressive. This possibility is in accord with the view

Table 14–5. **Follow-up Comparing Cytologic and Architectural Abnormalities (170 Patients)**

Finding	Number of Patients	Regressed	Persisted	Progressed to Carcinoma
Simple hyperplasia	93	74 (80%)	18 (19%)	1 (1%)
Complex hyperplasia	29	23 (80%)	5 (17%)	1 (3%)
Simple atypical hyperplasia	13	9 (70%)	3 (23%)	1 (8%)
Complex atypical hyperplasia	35	20 (57%)	5 (14%)	10 (29%)

(Adapted from Kurman, R. J. et al.: Cancer 56:403–412, 1985.)

Table 14–6. Classification of Non-Invasive Endometrial Proliferations

I. Hyperplasia
   A. Simple hyperplasia
   B. Complex hyperplasia
II. Atypical hyperplasia
   A. Simple atypical hyperplasia
   B. Complex atypical hyperplasia

that there may be two forms of endometrial cancer (Bokhman, 1983). One form is low-grade, develops on a background of hyperplasia, is related to unopposed estrogenic stimulation, and occurs in young or perimenopausal women. This type of carcinoma grows slowly, may spontaneously regress, and has limited metastatic potential. Unopposed estrogenic stimulation appears to play an important role in the etiology of this disease: Nearly 30 percent of the young women in our study (Kurman et al., 1985) had evidence of polycystic ovarian disease and 14 percent of perimenopausal women had received exogenous estrogens. In this latter group of patients, cessation of estrogen therapy resulted in regression in 90 percent of women with hyperplasia and atypical hyperplasia. The second form of endometrial carcinoma is quite different. It arises de novo, is unrelated to hyperplasia or estrogenic stimulation, occurs in older women, and is more virulent. It is likely that the recently identified subtypes of endometrial carcinoma, which are associated with a poor prognosis—such as clear cell carcinoma (Christopherson et al., 1982), uterine papillary serous carcinoma (Hendrickson et al., 1982), and adenosquamous carcinoma (Alberhasky et al., 1982)—are included in this latter group because these neoplasms tend to arise in older women and are rarely associated with hyperplasia.

MANAGEMENT OF PATIENTS WITH NON-INVASIVE ENDOMETRIAL DYSPLASIA

Management of patients with non-invasive endometrial neoplasia should be based on several factors besides the histologic diagnosis. Women with hyperplasia (simple or complex), regardless of their age, can be treated conservatively because these lesions are associated with an extremely low risk (1 to 3 percent) of progressing to carcinoma. Appropriate management of women with atypical hyperplasia depends on the age of the patient. For young women who wish to remain fertile, hormonal treatment, either by suppression with progestins or by induction of ovulation, can be undertaken, but close follow-up is necessary. A conservative plan of management is justified: None of the patients in our study who progressed to carcinoma died of the tumor, and nearly one fourth of those who were under the age of 40 years later had normal term deliveries (Kurman et al.,

1985). In perimenopausal and menopausal women who are receiving exogenous estrogens, termination of estrogen therapy, even for atypical hyperplasia, suffices because these proliferations are iatrogenic and regress after the stimulus for their growth has been removed. In perimenopausal and postmenopausal women who are not receiving estrogens, a hysterectomy is indicated, even though one third of the lesions in women of this age group also regress.

In summary, endometrial proliferations display a continuum of overlapping histologic patterns. Biologically significant lesions with the capacity for deep myometrial invasion and metastasis can be identified in curettings by the presence of stromal invasion. Although stromal invasion has been arbitrarily defined, various authors have described this finding in detail and quantified it in order to enhance its reproducibility. One of the four components of endometrial stromal invasion (the desmoplastic reaction) may be a particularly accurate marker of a biologically significant lesion because it reflects the interaction between tumor growth and the host defense mechanism. If stromal invasion is identified, the lesion should be designated "well-differentiated carcinoma." A marked proliferative process in which there is cytologic atypia closely resembling well-differentiated carcinoma but in which stromal invasion cannot be demonstrated should be designated "atypical hyperplasia." If there is uncertainty about whether invasion is present, the lesion should not be designated "carcinoma." In view of the important role of endometrial stromal invasion in the identification of a significant endometrial lesion, future classification of endometrial neoplasia should differentiate non-invasive from invasive forms of the disease.

Non-invasive endometrial proliferations constitute a heterogeneous group of lesions that display a variety of cytologic and architectural alterations. Classification of the group according to the presence of cytologic atypia is the most useful criterion in predicting the likelihood of progression to carcinoma. Lesions lacking cytologic atypia are designated "hyperplasia"; those with cytologic atypia are designated "atypical hyperplasia." Progression to carcinoma occurs in 1 to 2 percent of patients with hyperplasia and in 23 percent of patients with atypical hyperplasia. Further categorization based on the degree of architectural abnormalities as manifested by complex glandular outlines and back-to-back crowding permits further discrimination. Hyperplasia and atypical hyperplasia displaying architectural abnormalities are designated "complex hyperplasia" and "complex atypical hyperplasia," respectively; proliferations with lesser degrees of architectural abnormalities are designated "simple hyperplasia" and "simple atypical hyperplasia." Progression to carcinoma occurs in 1 percent of patients with simple hyperplasia, in 3 percent with complex hyperplasia, in 8 percent with simple atypical hyperplasia, and in 29 percent with complex atypical hyperplasia. Future classifications of non-invasive lesions (hyperplasias) should therefore account for both cytologic and architectural abnormalities.

A morphologic recognizable precursor of endometrial cancer may exist for only a certain type of neoplasm. This tumor is low-grade, associated with unopposed estrogenic stimulation, and occurs in young and perimenopausal women. However, it appears that endometrial carcinomas in older women—including clear cell carcinoma, papillary serous carcinoma, and adenosquamous carcinoma—are more virulent, are not associated with estrogenic stimulation, and may arise de novo without a histologically identifiable precursor.

This study was supported in part by NCI Contract NO1-CM-17501.

References

Alberhasky, R.C., Connelly, P.J., Christopherson, W.M.: Carcinoma of the endometrium. IV. Mixed adenosquamous carcinoma. Am. J. Clin. Pathol. 77:655–664, 1982.

Beutler, H.K., Dockerty, M.B., Randall, L.M.: Precancerous lesions of the endometrium. Am. J. Obstet. Gynecol. 86:433–443, 1963.

Bokhman, J.V.: Two pathogenetic types of endometrial carcinoma. Gynecol. Oncol. 15:10–17, 1983.

Buehl, I.A., Vellios, F., Carter, J.E., Huber, C.P.: Carcinoma in situ of the endometrium. Am. J. Clin. Pathol. 42:594–601, 1964.

Campbell, P.E. and Barter, R.A.: The significance of atypical hyperplasia. J. Obstet. Gynaecol. Br. Commonw. 68:668–672, 1961.

Chamlian, D.L. and Taylor, H.B.: Endometrial hyperplasia in young women. Obstet. Gynecol. 36:659–666, 1970.

Christopherson, W.M., Alberhasky, R.C., Connelly, P.J.: Carcinoma of the endometrium: I. A clinicopathologic study of clear-cell carcinoma and secretory carcinoma. Cancer 49:1511–1523, 1982.

Gore, H.: Hyperplasia of the endometrium. *In* Norris, H., Hertig, A., Abell, M. (eds.): The Uterus. Baltimore, Williams & Wilkins Co., 1973, pp. 255–275.

Gusberg, S.B.: Precursors of corpus carcinoma. Estrogens and adenomatous hyperplasia. Am. J. Obstet. Gynecol. 54:905–927, 1947.

Gusberg, S.B. and Kaplan, A.L.: Precursors of corpus cancer. IV. Adenomatous hyperplasia as stage 0 carcinoma of the endometrium. Am. J. Obstet. Gynecol. 87:662–678, 1963.

Gusberg, S.B., Moore, D.B., Martin, F.: Precursors of corpus cancer. II. A clinical and pathological study of adenomatous hyperplasia. Am. J. Obstet. Gynecol. 68:1472, 1954.

Hendrickson, M., Ross, J., Eifel, P., Martinez, A., Kempson, R.: Uterine papillary serous carcinoma. A highly malignant form of endometrial adenocarcinoma. Am. J. Surg. Pathol. 6:93–108, 1982.

Hertig, A.T. and Sommers, S.C.: Genesis of endometrial carcinoma. I. Study of prior biopsies. Cancer 2:946–956, 1949.

Hertig, A.T., Sommers, S.C., Bengaloff, H.: Genesis of endometrial carcinoma. III. Carcinoma in situ. Cancer 2:964–971, 1949.

King, A., Seraj, I.M., Wagner, R.J.: Stromal invasion in endometrial carcinoma. Am. J. Obstet. Gynecol. 149:10–14, 1984.

Kurman, R.J., Kaminski, P.F., Norris, H.J.: The behavior of endometrial hyperplasia. A long term study of "untreated" hyperplasia in 170 patients. Cancer, 56:403–412, 1985.

Kurman, R.J. and Norris, H.J.: Evaluation of criteria for distinguishing atypical endometrial hyperplasia from well-differentiated carcinoma. Cancer 49:2547–2559, 1982.

Mazur, M.T.: Atypical polypoid adenomas of the endometrium. Am. J. Surg. Pathol. 5:473–482, 1981.

McBride, J.M.: Pre-menopausal cystic hyperplasia and endometrial carcinoma. J. Obstet. Gynaecol. Br. Emp. 66:288–296, 1959.

Norris, H.J., Tavassoli, F.A., Kurman, R.J.: Endometrial hyperplasia and carcinoma. Diagnostic considerations. Am. J. Surg. Pathol. 7:839–847, 1983.

Novak, E. and Rutledge, F.: Atypical endometrial hyperplasia simulating adenocarcinoma. Am. J. Obstet. Gynecol. 55:46–63, 1948.

Poulson, H.E., Taylor, C.W., Sobin, L.H.: Histologic Typing of Female Genital Tract Tumors. Geneva, WHO, 1975.

Tavassoli, F.A. and Kraus, F.T.: Endometrial lesions in uteri resected for atypical endometrial hyperplasia. Am. J. Clin. Pathol. 70:770–779, 1978.

Vellios, F.: Endometrial hyperplasia and carcinoma in situ. Gynecol. Oncol. 2:152–161, 1974.

Welch, W.R. and Scully, R.E.: Precancerous lesions of the endometrium. Hum. Pathol. 8:503–512, 1977.

ROBERT E. SCULLY

15 Ovary

Cancer of the ovary, the fifth most common form of fatal cancer in women (Silverberg, 1983), is a heterogeneous disease in terms of the diverse origins, different age distributions, and varying biologic characteristics of its subtypes (Scully, 1979). The three main forms of ovarian cancer are (1) the common epithelial carcinomas, which are thought to be derived ultimately from the surface "epithelium" (modified pelvic mesothelium) of the ovary; (2) tumors composed of steroid-hormone secreting cells, mostly granulosa cell tumors and Sertoli-Leydig cell tumors; and (3) malignant germ cell tumors. These three categories account for approximately 90, 6, and 3 percent of ovarian cancers, respectively. Precancerous and early cancerous lesions corresponding to the clinically evident forms of each of these subtypes of ovarian cancer require separate consideration.

COMMON EPITHELIAL CANCERS

Common epithelial tumors are divided into three categories according to their cytologic and architectural features, which correlate with their biologic behavior: benign, borderline (proliferating; of low malignant potential), and malignant (invasive) (Serov et al., 1973). Each of these categories is designated further according to its cell type as serous (resembling fallopian tube epithelium), mucinous (resembling endocervical or gastrointestinal epithelium), endometrioid (resembling endometrial epithelium), clear cell, and Brenner (resembling transitional epithelium). There is evidence that some mucinous tumors and Brenner tumors may have origins other than the surface epithelium (germ cells for both mucinous and Brenner tumors and rete ovarii additionally for the latter), but for convenience all the neoplasms in these two categories are classified within the common epithelial rubric. The evidence for the surface epithelial origin of common epithelial carcinomas is considerable:

1. The surface epithelium and its derivatives, surface epithelial inclusion glands (Fig. 15–1), may be characterized by any of the types of epithelium encountered in these neoplasms with differing degrees of frequency (common for serous and endometrioid epithelium and rare for mucinous, clear cell, and transitional epithelium).

2. Tumors containing various admixtures of the five types of epithelium may be encountered.

3. Precancerous changes have been identified rarely in the surface epithelium and its inclusion glands.

4. Tumor markers associated with common epithelial carcinomas have been demonstrated immunohistochemically in surface epithelial inclusion glands (Blaustein et al., 1981; Kabawat et al., 1983).

Precancerous lesions in the common epithelial category can be divided into three general groups: dysplasia and carcinoma-in-situ in the surface epithelium and its glands; similar lesions originating in a nonneoplastic but abnormal ovarian epithelium, such as that of endometriosis; and benign tumors of common epithelial type.

The surface epithelium of the ovary has not been studied adequately from the viewpoint of precancerous changes, partly because it is usually desiccated before fixation or has been rubbed off by whoever is handling the specimen. As a result, all that remains for microscopic examination is residual intact epithelium either in crevices below the surface or under the protective umbrella of fibrous adhesions. Only isolated examples of dysplasia or carcinoma-in-situ arising in surface epithelium (Figs. 15–2 and 15–3) have been reported (Graham and Graham, 1967; Graham et al., 1964; Graham et al., 1965). Those lesions were uncovered from patients in whom cul-de-sac puncture cytology had been positive for malignant cells and the excised ovaries were processed by a no-touch immediate-fixation technique and extensively sectioned (460 slides in one case). Problems with this procedure in detecting early ovarian cancer in asymptomatic women have been as follows: the low yield of positive results (Funkhouser et al., 1975; McGowan et al., 1966), the requirement of meticulous handling of the specimen, the necessity for extensive sampling in

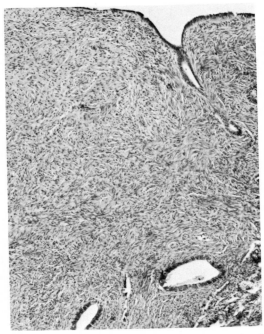

Figure 15–1. Surface epithelium and surface epithelial inclusion glands. One of the glands appears to have been formed by pinching off of the surface epithelium.

some cases, and the difficulty in interpreting the results in others.

Surface epithelial inclusion glands, which are generally considered the site of origin of the cystic forms of common epithelial carcinomas, are encountered in ovaries of patients of all ages, particularly older women, and are almost always well preserved in tissue sections. However, dysplastic changes and carcinoma-in-situ (Figs. 15–4 to 15–6) have been iden-

tified in them only very rarely and then often as part of a multifocal process that is frankly malignant elsewhere.

Although examination of ovaries removed prophylactically from women with a family history of ovarian cancer might be expected to disclose precancerous lesions in many cases, most investigators (Lurain and Piver, 1979; Piver et al., 1982) have not been able to identify such changes. Of those who have claimed to demonstrate them (Fraumeni et al., 1975; Graham et al., 1964; Gusberg and Deligdich, 1984), only the last authors, who studied the ovaries of identical twins of three women with ovarian cancer, have illustrated impressive degrees of epithelial dysplasia. Their photomicrographs reveal cellular stratification, nuclear pleomorphism, and loss of polarity within surface epithelial inclusion glands.

Endometriosis, a frequently encountered lesion of the ovary, is a proven site of origin of common epithelial cancers—particularly endometrioid and clear cell carcinomas—and rarely of other forms of common epithelial carcinoma, endometrioid stromal sarcomas, and malignant mesodermal mixed tumors (Mostoufizadeh and Scully, 1980; Scully et al., 1966). Endometrioid carcinoma has been reported to originate directly from endometriotic tissue in up to 24 percent of the cases in various series. Ipsilateral ovarian endometriosis has been detected in 11 to 17 percent, ovarian endometriosis of unspecified laterality in 9 to 20 percent, and pelvic endometriosis in 11 to 28 percent of cases of endometrioid carcinoma (Aure et al., 1971; Curling and Hudson, 1975; Czernobilsky et al., 1970; Fathalla, 1967; Kurman and Craig, 1972; Marry, 1971; Russell, 1979; Scully et al., 1966). Women whose endometrioid carcinoma has arisen in endometriosis have been a decade or more younger than those with endometrioid carcinoma of the ovary

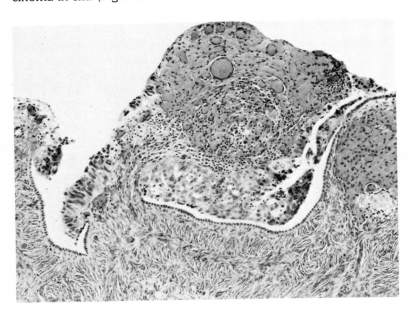

Figure 15–2. Surface growth of malignant epithelium associated with a fibrovascular adhesion.

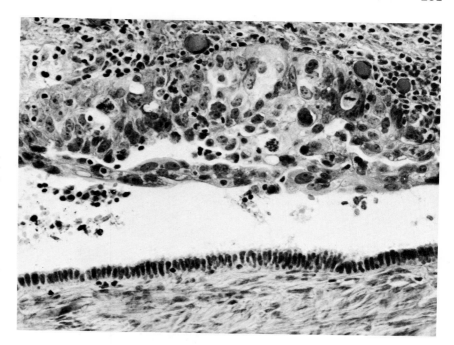

Figure 15–3. Close-up of surface carcinoma and underlying normal surface epithelium with which the carcinoma was continuous.

in general, providing supportive evidence for the precancerous role of this disorder.

Russell (1979) reported a 49 percent frequency of pelvic endometriosis in 33 cases of clear cell carcinoma of the ovary, and Aure and colleagues (1971) demonstrated a 24 percent frequency of ovarian endometriosis in 59 cases of the same type of tumor; both figures were surprisingly higher than figures given by the same authors for the association of endometriosis with endometrioid carcinoma (28 percent and 9 percent, respectively). Although isolated examples of serous and mucinous carcinoma have been reported to originate in endometriosis, the association of these tumors with that disorder is not significant.

Russell (1979) found only a 3 percent frequency of pelvic endometriosis in 233 cases of serous carcinoma and a 4 percent frequency in 69 cases of mucinous carcinoma. Aure and associates (1971) detected no ovarian endometriosis in 357 cases of serous carcinoma and found only a 0.5 percent frequency of that disorder in 203 cases of mucinous carcinoma.

Because carcinoma of the endometrium often arises on a background of hyperplasia with cytologic and architectural atypicality, one might expect that a proportion of carcinomas arising in endometriosis would have similar precursors. Atypical hyperplasia resembling that seen in the endometrium (Fig. 15–7), however, has been recorded in ovarian endometriotic

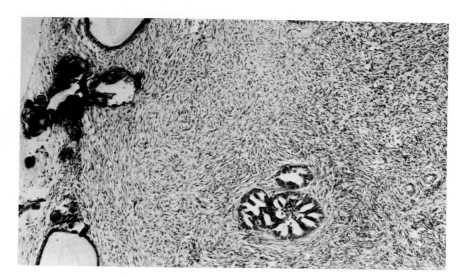

Figure 15–4. Superficial surface epithelial inclusion glands and calcifications *(left)* and severely dysplastic inclusion glands near center.

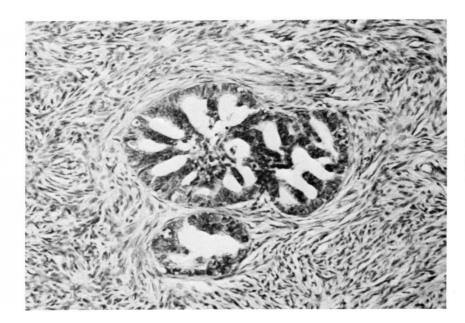

Figure 15–5. Close-up of severely dysplastic inclusion glands. (From Scully, R. E.: *In* Burghardt, E. and Holzer, E. (eds.): Clin. Oncol. 1:379–387, 1982.)

Figure 15–6. Dysplastic inclusion glands and small round almost solid nest of carcinoma-in-situ *(arrow)*.

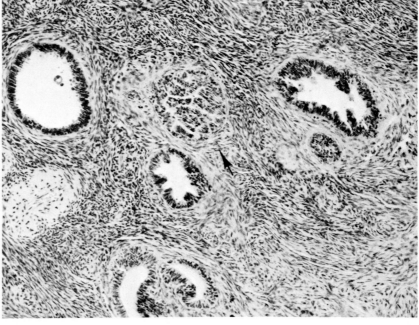

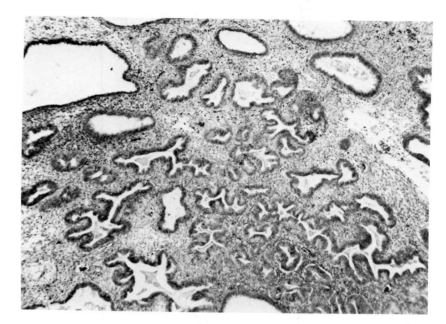

Figure 15–7. Cystic hyperplasia with architectural (adenomatous) atypicality in focus of endometriosis similar to a pattern encountered more often in the endometrium.

tissue only rarely (Czernobilsky and Morris, 1979; Mostoufizadeh and Scully, 1980; Scully, 1979), and its ultimate fate is unknown because either it has been found within a totally excised ovary or, if present within a partially resected specimen, its nature has not been elucidated by adequate follow-up data. One instructive case in which follow-up data were obtained involved a 55-year-old woman whose left ovary, which contained severely atypical endometriotic tissue (Fig. 15–8), had been dissected away from the pelvic wall. The patient was placed on estrogen therapy for 3 years. She then returned with an endometrioid adenocarcinoma that arose in the region where ovarian tissue had presumably been left behind (Fig. 15–9). The outcome in this case is interesting in light of one epidemiologic study that demonstrated a significant increase in the incidence of endometrioid carcinoma of the ovary in women on estrogen therapy (Cramer et al., 1983; Weiss et al., 1982).

Another atypical lesion that is encountered relatively often in endometriosis—but rarely, if ever, in the endometrium—is the lining of a cyst by a single row of large square cells with abundant, dense, eosinophilic cytoplasm and large, hyperchromatic, bizarre nuclei (Fig. 15–10) (Blaustein et al., 1982; Czernoblisky and Morris, 1979). The appearance of these

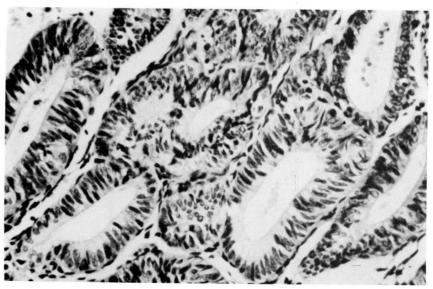

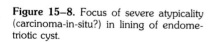

Figure 15–8. Focus of severe atypicality (carcinoma-in-situ?) in lining of endometriotic cyst.

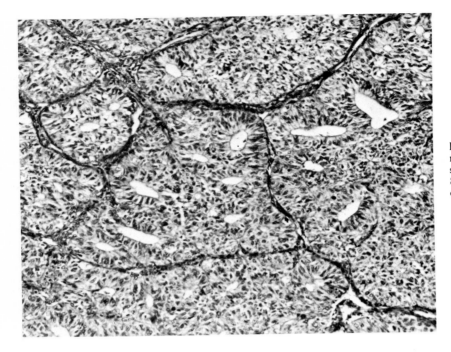

Figure 15–9. Endometrioid adenocarcinoma, Grade III, attached to pelvic wall at site where endometriotic cyst in Figure 15–8 had been dissected away 3 years previously.

nuclei suggests degeneration rather than precancerous atypia, but the significance of the alteration is currently unclear.

Whether common epithelial cancers arise in preexistent benign epithelial tumors of the same cell type and, if so, how often they do so are difficult to determine and warrant further investigation. Benign ovarian neoplasms are almost always removed as soon as they are detected, and therefore their natural history is largely unknown. Evidence of a benign to malignant transformation over a period of time is only circumstantial and rests on two arguments: (1) a generally observed older-age incidence associated with carcinomas in comparison with the age incidence reported for benign tumors of the same cell type, and (2) the frequent observation of various combinations

of benign, borderline, and invasive neoplasia within the same specimen.

The age distributions of benign, borderline, and invasive common epithelial tumors differ from one series to another for several possible reasons:

1. Variations exist in the diagnostic criteria for these three categories of neoplasia among individual pathologists.

2. Borderline tumors, which are usually not specifically designated "carcinomas" by reporting pathologists, are grossly under-represented in cancer registries as a result (Stalsberg, Bjarnason, et al., 1983; Stalsberg, de Carvalho, et al., 1983).

3. Conversely, tumors of this type, particularly those occurring in young women, are grossly over-represented in pathology-consultation material be-

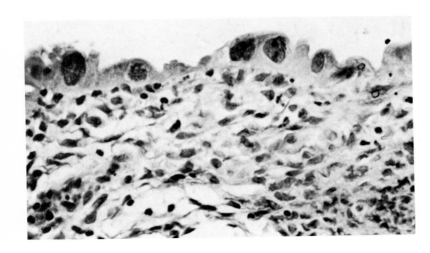

Figure 15–10. Endometriotic cyst lined by large cells with abundant cytoplasm and bizarre nuclei.

cause accurate diagnosis of these tumors is of great importance and their clinical management is controversial (Scully, personal observation).

Despite these problems, most investigators have reported progressively higher mean-age incidences for benign, borderline, and invasive tumors in both the serous and mucinous categories (Table 15–1). The differences between benign and invasive tumors are more significant than those between benign and borderline lesions and between borderline and invasive tumors. Parallel figures are not available for endometrioid and clear cell neoplasms because of the rarity of benign and borderline forms in those categories. Relatively few borderline and invasive Brenner tumors have been reported, but most of them have been

discovered in older women (average age for borderline, 60 years; for invasive, 63 years) (Hallgrímsson and Scully, 1972; Miles and Norris, 1972; Roth and Sternberg, 1971; Rybak et al., 1981; Woodruff et al., 1981; Yoonessi and Abell, 1979), among whom benign forms of this neoplasm are less common (average age, under 50 years) (Berge and Borglin, 1967; Ehrlich and Roth, 1971; Fox et al., 1972; Jorgensen et al., 1970; Silverberg, 1971; Waxman, 1979; Yoonessi and Abell, 1979). In summary, age-incidence data provide consistent but not conclusive evidence for progression of some benign common epithelial tumors to borderline or invasive neoplasms and of some borderline tumors to invasive forms.

Benign, borderline, and malignant neoplasias co-

Table 15–1. **Mean Age Incidences Associated With Three Types of Serous and Mucinous Tumors***

Authors	Type of Cases	No. Cases	Benign: Age (No. Cases)	Borderline: Age (No. Cases)	Invasive: Age (No. Cases)
Katsube et al., 1982, USA (population)	Serous	110 BBoM		43 (12)	56 (26)
	Muc	60 BBoM		35 (6)	59 (6)
Stalsberg, Bjarnason, et al., 1983, UICC (Cancer Registry)	Serous	1143 BoM		51 (63)	55 (1080)
	Muc	427 BoM		51 (61)	53 (366)
Russell, 1979, Australia (hospital)	Serous	460 BBoM	45 (227)	48 (70)	56 (163)
	Muc	362 BBoM	44 (293)	48 (52)	52 (17)
Chenevart and Gloor, 1980, Switzerland (hospital)	Serous	381 BBoM	49 (286)	46 (24)	60 (71)
	Muc	241 BBoM	45 (194)	51 (29)	62 (18)
Stalsberg, Blom, et al., 1983, Norway (hospital)	Serous	148 BBoM	48 (91)	56 (14)	53 (43)
	Muc	120 BBoM	42 (94)	55 (17)	64 (9)
Salazar, 1983, USA (hospital)	Serous	224 BBoM	42 (110)	40 (10)	59 (104)
	Muc	126 BBoM	43 (73)	48 (10)	45 (43)
Isarangkul, 1984, Thailand (hospital)	Serous	85 BBoM	42 (58)	42 (9)	58 (18)
	Muc	173 BBoM	37 (141)	38 (18)	50 (14)
Gronroos et al., 1969	All types	152 BoM		49 (61)	55 (91)
Aure et al., 1971, Norway (hospital)	All types	990 BoM		46 (161)	52 (829)
Bjorkholm et al., 1982, Sweden (hospital)	Serous	1310 BoM		50 (213)	56 (1097)
	Muc	344 BoM		53 (127)	55 (217)
Hart and Norris, 1973 (consult)	MucSt1	136 BoM		35 (97)	35 (39)

*Ages of affected patients are reported in years.
Abbreviations: B = benign; Bo = borderline; M = malignant; Muc = mucinous; St = stage.

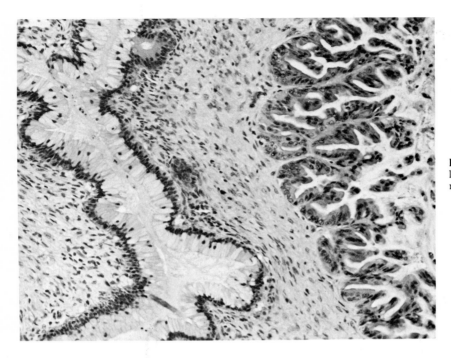

Figure 15–11. Mucinous cystadenoma on left and cystadenoma of borderline malignancy on right.

exist in varying combinations within common epithelial tumors—particularly those of mucinous, endometrioid, and clear cell types—and occasionally in serous and Brenner tumors as well (Figs. 15–11 to 15–13). From one end of the spectrum to the other, one may encounter the following: predominantly benign or borderline neoplasia with single or multiple microscopic foci of invasive carcinoma; benign or borderline neoplasia with large areas of carcinoma, which may be evident grossly; and predominant carcinoma with only minor components of benign or borderline neoplasia. Often, especially in mucinous tumors, a specimen may contain a haphazard mixture of all three forms of neoplastic growth. Although the presence of malignant foci within otherwise benign tumors is interpreted as cancerization of the benign element in most organs, there is no indisputable evidence that benign or borderline components of mixed common

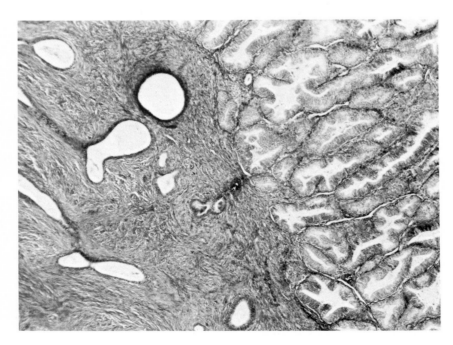

Figure 15–12. Endometrioid adenofibroma on left and adenocarcinoma on right.

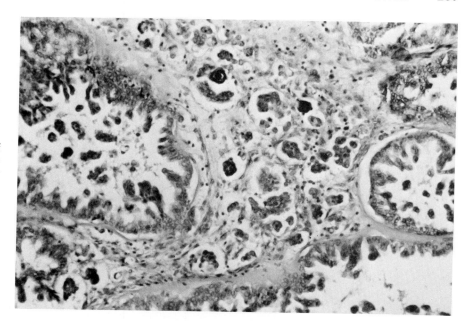

Figure 15–13. Central small focus of serous carcinoma in a tumor that otherwise was a uniform borderline malignancy.

epithelial carcinomas of the ovary are the forerunners of the malignant foci. An alternative interpretation is that the benign, borderline, and malignant elements develop more or less synchronously from the parent cells of the tumor, with each component having an independent potential for differentiation. Studies contrasting apparently pure common epithelial carcinomas with those that contain benign or borderline neoplastic elements in terms of their age incidences and other correlates might provide clues to the origin of these two forms of carcinoma. Possibly, the pure type arises de novo from surface epithelium or its glandular inclusions, whereas the mixed form develops from a pre-existing benign or borderline tumor of the same cell type.

SEX CORD–STROMAL TUMORS

The precursors of granulosa cell tumors and Sertoli-Leydig cell tumors are unknown. The discovery of the majority of granulosa cell tumors after menopause (Stenwig et al., 1979), when the ovary is presumably depleted of its follicles, suggests a possible origin in the ovarian stroma. Follicular granulosa cells that persist and proliferate within atretic follicles have been proposed as an alternative source of granulosa cell tumors (McKay et al., 1953). We have encountered such cells in the ovaries of both pregnant and non-pregnant women (Fig. 15–14). Study of granulosa cell tumors of microscopic size has not yielded histogenetic clues.

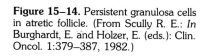

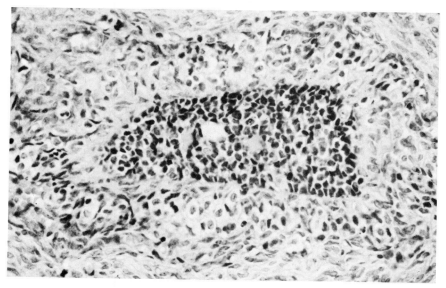

Figure 15–14. Persistent granulosa cells in atretic follicle. (From Scully R. E.: *In* Burghardt, E. and Holzer, E. (eds.): Clin. Oncol. 1:379–387, 1982.)

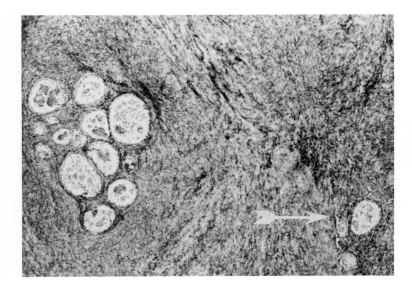

Figure 15–15. Two foci of sex cord tumor with annular tubules in ovarian cortex of patient with Peutz-Jeghers syndrome. (From Scully, R. E.: Cancer 25:1107–1121, 1970.)

Although male "remnants," hilus cells (hilar Leydig cells) and rete ovarii, are normally present in the ovarian hilus (Sternberg, 1949), they have not been linked to the development of Sertoli-Leydig cell tumors. However, the existence of transitions between the morphologic patterns of granulosa cell tumors and those of Sertoli-Leydig cell tumors—such as follicles merging with tubules and the rare finding of typical Leydig cells that contain crystalloids of Reinke within the ovarian stroma and its neoplasms (Sternberg and Roth, 1973)—suggests that at least some Sertoli-Leydig cell tumors arise from cells of female type rather than the male "remnants" in the ovarian hilus.

An ovarian tumor of great interest from the viewpoint of histogenesis of neoplasms in the sex cord–stromal group is the sex cord tumor with annular tubules (Scully, 1970; Young et al., 1982). This tumor, which is characterized by a predominance of ring-shaped tubules composed of Sertoli cells (Tavassoli and Norris, 1980), may contain additionally elongated, solid tubules indistinguishable from those of a typical Sertoli cell tumor as well as circumscribed aggregates with small cavities that resemble the islands of a microfollicular granulosa cell tumor. The sex cord tumor with annular tubules may occur as a large solitary lesion in an otherwise normal patient or, in approximately one third of cases, as typically multiple, bilateral tumorlets in a patient with Peutz-Jeghers syndrome (Figs. 15–15 and 15–16). The tumorlets develop within the ovarian stroma, presumably from follicles. They have not been reported to exceed 3 cm in diameter and have never been malignant, whereas the large solitary tumors are often malignant. Although there is no evidence that the multiple tu-

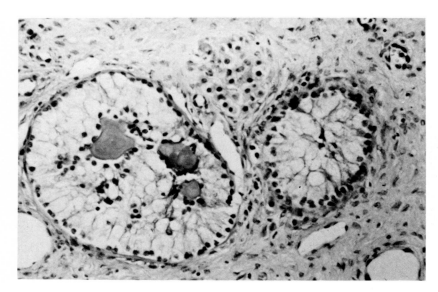

Figure 15–16. Sex cord tumor with annular tubules in patient with Peutz-Jeghers syndrome. (From Scully, R. E.: Cancer 25:1107–1121, 1970.)

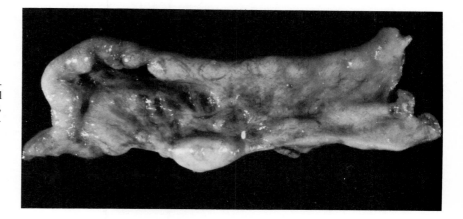

Figure 15–17. Ovoid nodule gonadoblastoma arising in barely visible gonadal streak below fallopian tube. (From Scully, R. E.: *In* Burghardt, E. and Holzer, E. (eds.): Clin. Oncol. 1:379–387, 1982.)

morlets give rise to large tumors with a malignant potential, they may be precursors of two types of sex cord–stromal tumor—both accompanied by isosexual pseudoprecocity—that have been reported to develop in children with the Peutz-Jeghers syndrome: two lipid-rich Sertoli cell tumors (folliculomes lipidiques) (Sohl et al., 1983) and two unusual sex cord–stromal tumors with a distinctive microscopic appearance (Young et al., 1983).

Other findings that indicate that granulosa cells and Sertoli cells as well as theca cells and Leydig cells are closely related morphologically and may be interchangeable in neoplasia are as follows: 1. Some women with the resistant ovary syndrome have alterations of their follicles that closely resemble the annular tubules of the sex cord tumor with annular tubules (Scully, personal observation). 2. Tubular transformation of graafian follicles is often seen in the canine ovary (Norris et al., 1970; Scully, personal observation).

MALIGNANT GERM CELL TUMORS

Lesions that predispose to malignant germ cell tumors in women include dysgenetic gonads associated with a karyotype that almost always contains a Y chromosome (Schellhas, 1974; Scully, 1970, 1981; Talerman, 1982) and dermoid cysts.

Approximately 25 percent of women with a Y chromosome–associated form of gonadal dysgenesis have a malignant germ cell tumor by the age of 30 years (Manuel et al., 1976). The most common form is the gonadoblastoma (Fig. 15–17), an in-situ germ cell tumor that contains immature sex cord elements and usually stromal derivatives (Leydig or lutein cells) as well as germ cells (Fig. 15–18) (Scully, 1970). An occasional gonadoblastoma arises in the gonad of a woman without a Y chromosome, who may be otherwise apparently normal. Rare patients, typically young children with what appear to be otherwise normal ovaries, have another type of germ cell–sex

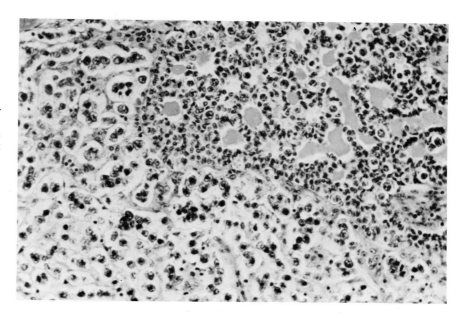

Figure 15–18. Gonadoblastoma *(upper right)* and dysgerminoma *(lower left)*. The gonadoblastoma contains numerous hyaline bodies composed of basement membrane material. (From Serov, S. F., Scully, R. E., Sobin, L. H.: International Histological Classification of Tumours No. 9, Histological Typing of Ovarian Tumours. Geneva, World Health Organization, 1973.)

cord tumor that resembles the gonadoblastoma but differs with respect to several histologic features. This lesion has been designated "germ cell–sex cord tumor, unclassified" (Talerman and van der Harten, 1977; Tavassoli, 1983).

The gonadoblastoma has not shown a capacity to metastasize per se, but in half the cases, by the time of its detection, its germ cells have escaped from their discrete compartments, shared with the sex cord elements of the tumor, and entered the stroma to form a germinoma (dysgerminoma, seminoma) (Fig. 15–18). In an additional 8 percent of the cases, another form of invasive germ cell cancer, usually of a higher grade of malignancy than the germinoma, has developed (Scully, 1970). Malignant germ cell tumors may also appear in dysgenetic gonads in the absence of evidence of an underlying gonadoblastoma, but it is possible in such cases that the latter was obliterated by the tumor or was missed as a result of inadequate sampling. Unclassified germ cell–sex cord tumors likewise have not been demonstrated to be malignant per se, but dysgerminomas and other primitive germ cell tumors have been encountered arising from them (Scully, personal observation).

Both dysgenetic gonads associated with a Y chromosome and gonadoblastomas, which can be recognized preoperatively in some cases as calcified pelvic masses, should be regarded as precancerous lesions requiring excision as soon as they have been detected. The gonadoblastoma is discussed in greater detail in Chapter 18.

The dermoid cyst is a teratoma composed of mature tissue with a predominance of skin and its appendages. In contrast to primitive germ cell tumors, which are almost always encountered in girls or women of reproductive age, the dermoid cyst is occasionally detected in postmenopausal women, whose ovaries

no longer contain recognizable germ cells. This finding is best interpreted as indicative of the leisurely growth rate of a tumor that originated years earlier. Approximately 2 percent of dermoid cysts contain adult-type malignant tumors, more than 80 percent of which are squamous cell carcinomas (Fig. 15–19) (Kelley and Scully, 1961; Peterson et al., 1956; Waxman and Deppisch, 1983). A few of these tumors have been detected in in-situ form within cutaneous or respiratory epithelium (Klionsky et al., 1972; Sobel, 1972; Waxman and Deppisch, 1983). The age-incidence data in Table 15–2 provide strong circumstantial evidence that the dermoid cyst is a precancerous lesion. In most cases, it is diagnosed during the third to fifth decades (Waxman and Deppisch, 1983); in contrast, squamous cell carcinomas arising in dermoid cysts are detected most often in the fifth to seventh decades; over 90 percent of these tumors have been found in women 40 years of age or older, and almost half of them have been discovered in women over 55 years of age. The relatively high frequency of squamous cell carcinomas in the postmenopausal period—during which, as already stated, dermoid cysts are not expected to develop de novo—provides convincing evidence that the latter are precancerous in a small proportion of cases. A variety of other malignant tumors arise less frequently within dermoid cysts. These include other cutaneous tumors, such as malignant melanoma and basal cell carcinoma, adenocarcinomas, carcinoid tumors, and sarcomas (Stamp and McConnell, 1983). These tumors, like squamous cell carcinomas, usually occur in older women, about half of whom are postmenopausal.

An important corollary of the preceding data, emphasized by Waxman and Deppisch (1983), is that whereas the frequency of malignant change in a dermoid cyst is less than 1 percent in patients under

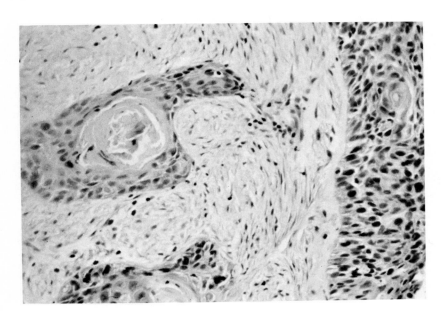

Figure 15–19. Carcinoma-in-situ lining dermoid cyst with underlying invasive squamous cell carcinoma. (From Scully, R. E.: *In* Burghardt, E. and Holzer, E.: Clin. Oncol. 1:379–387, 1982.)

Table 15–2. **Dermoid Cyst***

	Benign		Malignant (Squamous Cell Carcinoma)		
	Age Range	*Predominant Age*	*No. Cases*	*Age Range*	*Average Age*
Marcial-Rojas and Medina, 1958		86%: 11–50			
Caruso et al., 1971	10–80	80%: 15–45			
Salazar, 1983		61%: 21–40; average age 32			
Peterson et al., 1955, 1956	2–78	92%: 15–50; Most: 20–30	10	31–78	52
Gloor, 1979		80%: 20–59	6	44–61	52
Climie and Heath, 1968 (review)			18	33–68	54
Curling et al., 1979			10	46–73	60
Amérigo et al., 1979			5	45–59	51
Stamp and McConnell, 1983			18	36–76	56
Waxman and Deppisch, 1983 (review)			162†	30 to 10th decade	53

*Ages of affected patients are reported in years.
†Includes cases other than squamous cell carcinoma.

the age of 40 years, it is between 4 and 5 percent in the sixth and seventh decades and 15 percent in woman over 70 years of age. Therefore, dermoid cysts should be evaluated carefully for the possibility of cancerization, particularly in elderly patients.

References

Amérigo, J., Nogales, F.F., Jr., Fernandez-Sanz, J., Oliva, H., Valasco, A.: Squamous cell neoplasms arising from ovarian benign cystic teratoma. Gynecol. Oncol. 8:277, 1979.

Aure, J.C., Hoeg, K., Kolstad, P.: Carcinoma of the ovary and endometriosis. Acta Obstet. Gynecol. Scand. 50:63, 1971.

Aure, J.C., Hoeg, K., Kolstad, P.: Clinical and histological studies of ovarian carcinoma. Long-term follow-up of 990 cases. Obstet. Gynecol. 37:1, 1981.

Bell, D.A. and Scully, R.E.: Atypical and borderline endometrioid adenofibromas of the ovary: a report of 27 cases. Am. J. Surg. Pathol. 9:205, 1985.

Berge, T. and Borglin, N.E.: Brenner tumors. Histogenetic and clinical studies. Cancer 20:308, 1967.

Björkholm, E., Pettersson, F., Einhorn, N., Krebs, I., Nilsson, B., Tjernberg, B.: Long-term follow-up and prognostic factors in ovarian carcinoma. The Radiumhemmet series 1958 to 1973. Acta Radiol. Oncol. 21:413, 1982.

Blaustein, A.: Pelvic endometriosis. In Blaustein, A. (ed.): Pathology of the Female Genital Tract, 2nd ed. New York, Springer-Verlag, 1982, p. 464.

Blaustein, A.V., Kaganowicz, A., Wells, J.: Tumor markers in inclusion cysts of the ovary. Cancer 49:722, 1982.

Caruso, P.A., Marsh, M.R., Minkowitz, S., Karten, G.: An intense clinicopathologic study of 305 teratomas of the ovary. Cancer 27:343, 1971.

Chenevart, P., and Gloor, E.: Cystadénomes sereux et muqueux de l'ovaire a la limite de la malignité. Schweiz. Med. Wochenschr. 110:531, 1980.

Clement, P.B. and Scully, R.E.: Extrauterine mesodermal (mullerian) adenosarcoma. A clinicopathologic analysis of five cases. Am. J. Clin. Pathol. 69:276, 1978.

Climie, A.R.W. and Heath, L.P.: Malignant degeneration of benign cystic teratomas of the ovary. Review of the literature and report of a chondrosarcoma and carcinoid tumor. Cancer 22:824, 1968.

Cramer, D.W., Hutchison, G.B., Welch, W.R., Scully, R.E., Ryan, K.J.: Determinants of ovarian cancer risk. 1. Reproductive experiences. J. Natl. Cancer Inst. 71:711, 1983.

Curling, O.M. and Hudson, C.N.: Endometrioid tumours of the ovary. Br. J. Obstet. Gynaecol. 82:405, 1975.

Curling, O.M., Potsides, P.N., Hudson, C.N.: Malignant change in benign cystic teratoma of the ovary. Br. J. Obstet. Gynaecol. 86:399, 1979.

Czernobilsky, B. and Morris, W.J.: A histologic study of ovarian endometriosis with emphasis on hyperplastic and atypical changes. Obstet. Gynecol. 53:318, 1979.

Czernobilsky, B., Silverman, B.B., Mikuta, J.J.: Endometrioid carcinoma of the ovary. Cancer 26:1141, 1970.

Ehrlich, C.E. and Roth, L.M.: The Brenner tumor. A clinicopathologic study of 57 cases. Cancer 27:332, 1971.

Fathalla, M.F.: Malignant transformation in ovarian endometriosis. J. Obstet. Gynaecol. Br. Cwlth. 74:85, 1967.

Fox, H., Agrawal, K., Langley, F.A.: The Brenner tumour of the ovary. A clinicopathological study of 54 cases. J. Obstet. Gynaecol. Br. Cwlth. 79:661, 1972.

Fraumeni, J.F., Jr., Grundy, G.W., Creagan, E.T., Everson, R.B.: Six families prone to ovarian cancer. Cancer 36:364, 1975.

Funkhouser, J.W., Hunter, K.K., Thompson, N.J.: The diagnostic value of cul-de-sac aspiration in the detection of ovarian carcinoma. Acta Cytol. 19:538, 1975.

Gloor, E.: Tératomes matures benins avec tumeur maligne et tératomes monodermiques malins de l'ovaire. Présentation anatomo-clinique de 10 cas. Schweiz. Med. Wochenschr. 109:968, 1979.

Graham, J.B. and Graham, R.M.: Cul-de-sac puncture in the diagnosis of early ovarian carcinoma. J. Obstet. Gynaecol. Br. Cwlth. 74:371, 1967.

Graham, J.B., Graham, R.M., Schueller, E.F.: Preclinical detection of ovarian cancer. Cancer 17:1414, 1964.

Graham, R.M., Schueller, E.F., Graham, J.B.: Detection of ovarian cancer at an early stage. Obstet. Gynecol. 26:151, 1965.

Grönroos, M., Laurén, P., Lehto, J., Rauramo, L.: Ovarian cancer and its treatment. Ann. Chir. Gynaecol. Fenn. 58:83, 1969.

Gusberg, S.B. and Deligdish, L.: Ovarian dysplasia. A study of identical twins. Cancer 54:1, 1984.

Hallgrímsson, J. and Scully, R.E.: Borderline and malignant Brenner tumours of the ovary. Acta Pathol. Microbiol. Scand. 80:(suppl. 233):56, 1972.

Hart, W.R. and Norris, H.J.: Borderline and malignant mucinous tumors of the ovary. Histologic criteria and clinical behavior. Cancer 31:1031, 1973.

Isarangkul, W.: Ovarian epithelial tumors in Thai woman: a histological analysis of 291 cases. Gynecol. Oncol. 17:326, 1984.

Jorgensen, E.O., Dockerty, M.B., Wilson, R.B., Welch, J.S.: Clinicopathologic study of 53 cases of Brenner's tumors of the ovary. Am. J. Obstet. Gynecol. 108:122, 1970.

Kabawat, S.E., Bast, R.C., Jr., Bhan, A.K., Welch, W.R., Knapp, R.C., Colvin, R.B.: Tissue distribution of a coelomic-epithelium-related antigen recognized by the monoclonal antibody OC-125. Int. J. Gynecol. Pathol. 2:275, 1983.

Katsube, Y., Berg, J.W., Silverberg, S.G.: Epidemiologic pathology of ovarian tumors. Int. J. Gynecol. Pathol. 1:3, 1982.

Kelley, R.R. and Scully, R.E.: Cancer developing in dermoid cysts of the ovary. A report of 8 cases, including a carcinoid and a leiomyosarcoma. Cancer 14:989, 1961.

Klionsky, B.L., Nickens, O.J., Amortegui, A.J.: Squamous cell carcinoma in situ arising in adult cystic teratoma of the ovary. Arch. Pathol. 93:161, 1972.

Kurman, R.J. and Craig, J.M.: Endometrioid and clear cell carcinoma of the ovary. Cancer 29:1653, 1972.

Lurain, J.R. and Piver, M.S.: Familial ovarian cancer. Gynecol. Oncol. 8:185, 1979.

Manuel, M., Katayama, K.P., Jones, H.W., Jr.: The age of occurrence of gonadal tumors in intersex patients with a Y chromosome. Am. J. Obstet. Gynecol. 124:293, 1976.

Marcial-Rojas, R.A. and Medina, R.: Cystic teratomas of the ovary. A clinical and pathological analysis of two hundred sixty-eight tumors. Arch. Pathol. 66:577, 1958.

Marry, E.B.: Adenocarcinoma of endometriosis of the ovary. Am. J. Obstet. Gynecol. 110:783, 1971.

McGowan, L., Stein, D.B., Miller, W.: Cul-de-sac aspiration for diagnostic cytologic study. Am. J. Obstet. Gynecol. 96:413, 1966.

McKay, D.G., Hertig, A.T., Hickey, W.F.: The histogenesis of granulosa and theca cell tumors of the human ovary. Obstet. Gynecol. 1:125, 1953.

Miles, P.A. and Norris, H.J.: Proliferative and malignant Brenner tumors of the ovary. Cancer 30:174, 1972.

Mostoufizadeh, M. and Scully, R.E.: Malignant tumors arising in endometriosis. Clin. Obstet. Gynecol. 23:951, 1980.

Norris, H.J., Garner, F.M., Taylor, H.B.: Comparative pathology of ovarian neoplasms, IV. Gonadal stromal tumours of canine species. J. Comp. Pathol. 80:399, 1970.

Peterson, W.F., Prevost, E.C., Edmunds, F.T., Hundley, J.M., Jr., Morris, F.K.: Benign cystic teratomas of the ovary. Am. J. Obstet. Gynecol. 70:368, 1955.

Peterson, W.F., Prevost, E.C., Edmunds, F.T., Hundley, J.M., Jr., Morris, F.K.: Epidermoid carcinoma arising in a benign cystic teratoma. A report of 15 cases. Am. J. Obstet. Gynecol. 71:173, 1956.

Piver, M.S., Barlow, J.J., Sawyer, D.M.: Familial ovarian cancer: increasing in frequency? Obstet. Gynecol. 60:397, 1982.

Roth, L.M. and Sternberg, W.H.: Proliferating Brenner tumors. Cancer 27:687, 1971.

Roy, D.: Disseminated ovarian malignancy. Lancet 2:1054, 1982.

Russell, P.: The pathological assessment of ovarian neoplasms. I: Introduction to the common "epithelial" tumours and analysis of benign "epithelial" tumors. Pathology 11:5, 1979.

Rybak, B.J., Obert, W.B., Bernacki, E.G., Jr.: Malignant Brenner tumor of the ovary. Diagn. Gynecol. Obstet. 3:61, 1981.

Salazar, H.: Epidemiological observations on histologic types of ovarian tumours at Magee-Women's Hospital, a gynecological referral center in Pittsburgh, PA, USA. In Stalsberg, H. (ed.): An International Survey of Distributions of Histologic Types of Tumours of the Testis and Ovary. Geneva, UICC, 1983, p. 331.

Schellhas, H.F.: Malignant potential of the dysgenetic gonad. Part I. Obstet. Gynecol. 44:298, 1974.

Schellhas, H.F.: Malignant potential of the dysgenetic gonad. Part II. Obstet. Gynecol. 44:455, 1974.

Scully, R.E.: Personal observation.

Scully, R.E.: Gonadoblastoma. A review of 74 cases. Cancer 25:1340, 1970.

Scully, R.E.: Sex cord tumor with annular tubules. A distinctive ovarian tumor of the Peutz-Jeghers syndrome. Cancer 25:1107, 1970.

Scully, R.E.: Tumors of the ovary and maldeveloped gonads. Atlas of Tumor Pathology, 2nd series, fascicle 16. Washington, D.C., Armed Forces Institute of Pathology, 1979.

Scully, R.E.: Neoplasia associated with anomalous sexual development and abnormal sex chromosomes in the intersex child. Pediatr. Adolesc. 8:203, 1981.

Scully, R.E.: Minimal cancer of the ovary. Clin. Oncol. 1:379, 1982.

Scully, R.E., Richardson, G.S., Barlow, J.F.: The development of malignancy in endometriosis. Clin. Obstet. Gynecol. 9:384, 1966.

Serov, S.F., Scully, R.E., Sobin, L.H.: Histological typing of ovarian tumours. International Histological Classification of Tumours, No. 9, World Health Organization, 1973.

Silverberg, E.: Cancer statistics, 1983. CA 33:9, 1983.

Silverberg, S.: Brenner tumors of the ovary. A clinicopathological study. Cancer 28:588, 1971.

Sobel, H.J.: Bowen's disease and senile keratosis arising. Arch. Pathol. 94:372, 1972.

Sohl, H.M., Azoury, R.S., Najjar, S.S.: Peutz-Jeghers syndrome associated with precocious puberty. J. Pediatr. 103:593, 1983.

Stalsberg, H., Abeler, V., Blom, G.P., Bostad, L., Segadal, E., Westgaard, G.: Histologic types of ovarian cancer in Norway cancer registry material. In Stalsberg, H. (ed.): An International Survey of Distributions of Histologic Types of Tumours of the Testis and Ovary. Geneva, UICC, 1983, p. 242.

Stalsberg, H., Bjarnason, O., de Carvalho, A.R.L., Correa, P., Czernobilsky, B., Doctor, V.M., Hwang, W.S., Misad, O., Nathan, P., Parker, R.G.F., Salazar, H., Sampat, M.B., Sasano, N., Scully, R.E., Tulinius, H., Wade-Evans, T., Waterhouse, J.A.H., Williams, A.O.: International comparisons of histologic types of ovarian cancer in cancer registry material. In Stalsberg, H. (ed.): An International Survey of Distributions of Histologic Types of Tumours of the Testis and Ovary. Geneva, UICC, 1983, p. 247.

Stalsberg, H., Blom, P.G., Bostad, L.H., Westgaard, G.: Ovarian tumours and endometriosis in Norway General Hospital material. In Stalsberg, H. (ed.): An International Survey of Distributions of Histologic Types of Tumours of the Testis and Ovary. Geneva, UICC, 1983, p. 307.

Stalsberg, H., de Carvalho, A.R.L., Correa, P., Czernobilsky, B., Doctor, W.M., Parker, R.G.F., Sasano, N., Wade-Evans, T., Waterhouse, J.A.H.: International comparisons of histologic types of benign and malignant ovarian tumours in general hospital material. In Stalsberg, H. (ed.): An International Survey of

Distributions of Histologic Types of Tumours of the Testis and Ovary. Geneva, UICC, 1983, p. 313.

Stamp, G.W.H. and McConnell, E.M.: Malignancy arising in cystic ovarian teratomas. A report of 24 cases. Br. J. Obstet. Gynaecol. 90:671, 1983.

Stenwig, J., Hazekamp, J.T., Beecham, J.B.: Granulosa cell tumors of the ovary. A clinicopathological study of 118 cases with long-term follow-up. Gynecol. Oncol. 7:136, 1979.

Sternberg, W.H.: The morphology, androgenic function, hyperplasia and tumors of the human ovarian hilus cells. Am. J. Pathol. 25:493, 1949.

Sternberg, W.H. and Roth, L.M.: Ovarian stromal tumors containing Leydig cells. 1. Stromal-Leydig cell tumor and non-neoplastic transformation of ovarian stroma to Leydig cells. Cancer 32:940, 1973.

Stolk, J.G., Baak, J.P.A., van der Putten, H.W., Kurver, P.H.S.: Premalignancy of the ovary. Gynecol. Obstet. Proc. IX World Congress Gynecol. Obstet. Tokyo, Exerpta Med, Elvesier-North Holland, 1979.

Talerman, A.: Germ cell tumors of the ovary. In Blaustein, A. (ed.): Pathology of the Female Genital Tract, 2nd ed. New York, Springer-Verlag, 1982, p. 602.

Talerman, A. and van der Harten, J.J.: A mixed germ cell sex-cord stromal tumor of the ovary associated with isosexual precocious puberty in a normal girl. Cancer, 40:889, 1977.

Tavassoli, F.A.: A combined germ cell-gonadal stromal-epithelial tumor of the ovary. Am. J. Surg. Pathol. 7:73, 1983.

Tavassoli, F.A. and Norris, H.J.: Sertoli tumors of the ovary. A clinicopathologic study of 28 cases with ultrastructural observations. Cancer 46:2281, 1980.

Tobacman, J.K., Tucker, M.A., Kase, R., Greene, M.H., Costa, J., Fraumeni, J.F., Jr.: Intraabdominal carcinomatosis after prophylactic oophorectomy in ovarian-cancer-prone families. Lancet 2:795, 1982.

Waxman, M.: Pure and mixed Brenner tumors of the ovary. Clinicopathologic and histogenetic observations. Cancer 43:1830, 1979.

Waxman, M. and Deppisch, L.M.: Malignant alteration in benign teratomas. In Damjanov, I., Knowles, B., Solter, D. (eds.): The Human Teratomas. Experimental and Clinical Biology. Clifton, N.J., Humana Press, 1983.

Weiss, N.S., Lyon, J.L., Krishnamurthy, S., Dretert, S.E., Liff, I.M., Daling, J.R.: Non-contraceptive estrogen use and the occurrence of ovarian cancer. J. Natl. Cancer Inst. 68:95, 1982.

Woodruff, J.D., Dietrich, D., Genadry, R., Parmley, T.H.: Proliferative and malignant Brenner tumors. Review of 47 cases. Am. J. Obstet. Gynecol. 141:118, 1981.

Yoonessi, M. and Abell, M.R.: Brenner tumors of the ovary. Obstet. Gynecol. 54:90, 1979.

Young, R.H., Dickersin, G.R., Scully, R.E.: A distinctive sex-cord stromal tumor causing sexual precocity in the Peutz-Jeghers syndrome. Am. J. Surg. Pathol. 7:233, 1983.

Young, R.H., Dickersin, G.R., Scully, R.E.: Juvenile granulosa cell tumor of the ovary. A clinicopathological analysis of 125 cases. Am. J. Surg. Pathol. 8:575, 1984.

Young, R.H., Welch, W.R., Dickersin, G.R., Scully, R.E.: Ovarian sex-cord tumors with annular tubules. Cancer 50:1384, 1982.

GILBERT H. FRIEDELL
ILEANA R. HAWKINS
GEORGE K. NAGY

16 Urinary Bladder

Carcinomas of the urinary bladder are similar in many ways to carcinomas of certain other mucous membranes, notably those of the uterine cervix, the bronchial tree, the oral cavity, and others. All these cancers generally arise within, or in association with, areas of carcinoma in situ, each of which in turn develops within a field of atypical epithelium. There are, however, differences between cancers of the bladder and cancers at the other sites just mentioned. Bladder cancers are predominantly transitional cell tumors, while squamous cell carcinomas predominate at the other sites. Moreover, bladder tumors for the most part are papillary or have a significant papillary component, a feature which does not hold true at the other sites. An even more important difference between the classification of bladder cancer and carcinoma of most other organs is that papillary, epithelial neoplasms of the bladder are generally designated as "carcinoma" even if they are *not* invasive at the time of diagnosis.

This terminological practice by urologists and pathologists poses a problem for us in discussing preneoplastic bladder lesions, because, by accepted convention and definition, these lesions are *not* called preneoplastic sites, but neoplastic. In the United States, approximately 25 to 35 percent of all new bladder tumors seen by urologists are of this variety. Moreover, those patients with Grade 1 non-invasive papillary transitional cell carcinomas will probably never have invasive cancer in their bladders, although superficial lesions might recur. Patients with Grade 2 or Grade 3 papillary transitional cell carcinomas are more likely to have recurrences and to have subsequent truly invasive cancer.

Within the TNM classification system, papillary noninvasive neoplastic-appearing transitional cell epithelium is designated as Ta, while noninvasive flat carcinoma is designated as TIS. It is of some interest that both varieties of non-invasive lesions—papillary as well as flat—are generally associated either in space or in time with some degree of nonpapillary epithelial "field change."

In dealing with small papillary lesions that are resected at cystoscopy, it is essential to remember that any attempt to predict the behavior of bladder epithelium must of necessity be a prediction of the behavior of the epithelium remaining in the bladder after the biopsy or other type of resection of bladder epithelium. Thus, a prediction of the biologic changes associated with the development of bladder cancer presumes that the same malignant potential is present in the residual epithelium. There is the possibility that removal or disruption of a circumscribed lesion has completely eliminated the only problem area.

In other words, when we discuss the prognosis of bladder cancer, we are discussing the *prognosis of a patient* rather than that of a particular tumor.

We will now move to discuss flat carcinoma-in-situ and lesser degrees of urothelial atypia. Our diagnosis of carcinoma-in-situ, and of preneoplastic lesions is generally based on criteria similar to those used in other organs. Our definitions follow.

In *carcinoma-in-situ* there is proliferation of epithelial cells with morphologic cellular characteristics similar to those seen in carcinoma originating in the same organ, but without evidence of invasion of the subepithelial tissue. This lesion is related in space or time to carcinoma of the same histologic type, and—if untreated—will progress to an invasive neoplasm of the same histologic type in *a significantly high percentage of cases*. It may not progress during the lifetime of the patient (although our assumption is that it would do so if the patient lived long enough), but only rarely does it spontaneously regress. Invasion will presumably be a function of the tumor-host interaction, as well as the "virulence" of the neoplastic epithelium.

In *preneoplastic lesions* there is proliferation of epithelial cells with nonneoplastic histologic features, associated in space or time with the development of in-situ or invasive carcinoma of the same histologic type. The constituent cells are atypical, but *individually and collectively they do not reach the degree of cellular abnormality of carcinoma-in-situ*. The lesion, if not entirely removed by biopsy, can either persist

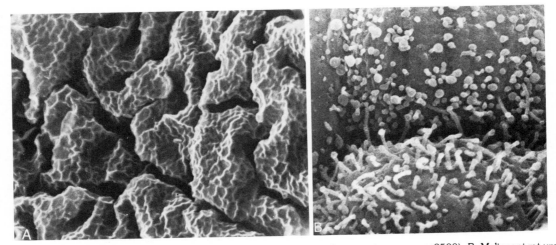

Figure 16–1. *A*, Normal rat urothelium showing regular microridges (scanning electron microscopy, ×9500). *B*, Malignant rat urothelium showing pleomorphic microvilli (scanning electron microscopy, ×9300). (Courtesy of Dr. Jerome B. Jacobs, Worcester, MA.)

in this form or progress to in-situ or to invasive carcinoma.

The identification of preneoplastic lesions as such is based on both their morphologic characteristics and their biologic characteristics. The problem is that for any morphologic entity, we may be able to describe the microscopic characteristics, but we may not have any meaningful information about its biology—or the biologic potential of the residual bladder epithelium. Or, we may be confronted with morphologic "look-alikes" with very different biologic behaviors.

We would like to mention that scanning electron microscopy might provide us with such a tool. It has been shown that the presence of pleomorphic microvilli on bladder epithelial cell surfaces, revealed by scanning electron microscopy (Figs. 16–1 and 16–2), may be a marker for severe proliferative abnormality of the cells in question, and may even indicate the malignant potential of the epithelium from which these cells arose (Jacobs et al., 1976). However, until more data from such studies or other techniques for predicting biologic behavior have been developed, we will have to accept the fact that a given morphologic picture may represent either truly preneoplastic epithelium or atypical but not preneoplastic epithelial proliferation. Despite this difficulty, we believe it will

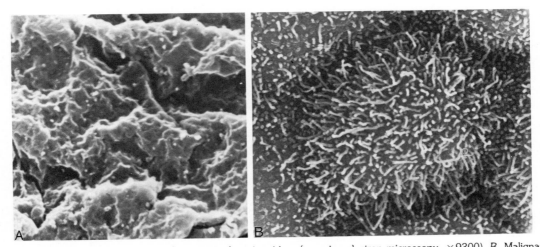

Figure 16–2. *A*, Normal human urothelium showing regular microridges (scanning electron microscopy, ×9300). *B*, Malignant human urothelium showing pleomorphic microvilli (scanning electron microscopy, ×4500). (Courtesy of Dr. Jerome B. Jacobs, Worcester, MA.)

be of value to illustrate the kinds of epithelial changes which fall into the category of preneoplastic lesions.

Although biological and biochemical methods, such as karyotyping, tumor antigen examination, isoenzyme studies, and red blood cell adherence have a great potential, presently the definitive diagnosis of urothelial changes rests upon histology. We, therefore, describe the morphology of premalignant and potentially premalignant changes in detail. Most of these changes are well represented in our photomicrographs. As a baseline, we include a description of normal urothelium.

NORMAL UROTHELIUM

Although Henle's term, "transitional epithelium," implies that the epithelium lining the urinary tract (urothelium) is a transition between squamous and columnar types, it is generally agreed that it is a highly differentiated tissue in its own right, even though it retains the capability to produce squamous or columnar epithelium under special circumstances (Mostofi, 1954). It has two particularly important functions: (1) it forms a barrier between the urine and the interstitial fluid of the body, preventing rediffusion of waste products, and (2) it is distensible, allowing the bladder to adapt to the changing volume of urine without impairment of the barrier function.

Morphologically, the urothelium, even in a flattened state, as seen in the distended bladder, appears to be at least three layers thick (Fig. 16–3). The surface cells are large, frequently multinucleate, and because of their peculiar shape and size are often referred to

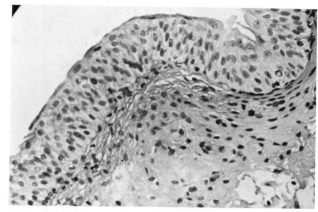

Figure 16–3. Normal human urothelium in a contracted state, showing about six "nuclear layers." On the surface, large so-called "umbrella cells" are seen.

as "umbrella cells." They represent one of the rare normal tetraploid cell types in the mammalian body. The ultrastructure of their luminal surface is composed of characteristic scalloped asymmetric, concave plaques (Fig. 16–4) that appear as troughs and are joined by symmetric interplaque unit membranes (Koss, 1969). The concave plaques show an asymmetry of the inner and outer dense lines, the outer line being thicker than the inner. In the umbrella cells, there are so-called discoidal cytoplasmic vesicles which seem to be communicating with the surface, suggesting that they provide a reserve of the luminal plasma membrane required during distention of the bladder. There are hemidesmosomes attaching the

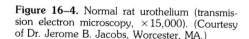

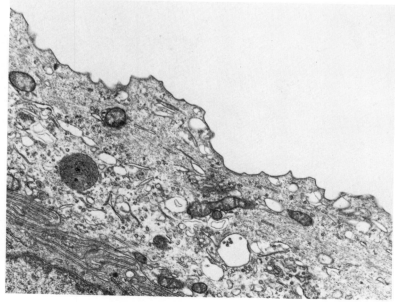

Figure 16–4. Normal rat urothelium (transmission electron microscopy, ×15,000). (Courtesy of Dr. Jerome B. Jacobs, Worcester, MA.)

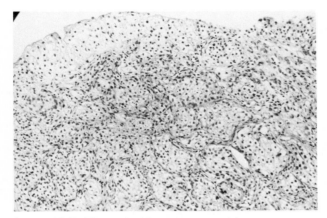

Figure 16–5. Massive proliferative cystitis, with numerous von Brunn's nests deep in the suburothelial connective tissue. The urothelial cells in the nests are well differentiated and similar to the cells of the surface epithelium.

basal cells to the underlying basement membrane. Bundles of filaments are also found, which are probably identical with the tonofilaments of squamous cells. The number of desmosomes between urothelial cells is smaller than that found in squamous epithelia.

PROLIFERATIVE CYSTITIS

One of the most frequently encountered lesions in bladder biopsy material is "proliferative cystitis" (Figs. 16–5, 16–6, and 16–7), which includes the morphologic entities of "von Brunn's nests," or "cystitis cystica," or "cystitis glandularis." Since there is a substantial overlap between these entities, particularly between von Brunn's nests and "cystitis cystica," we recommend usage of the term "proliferative cystitis." As indicated in Figures 16–5, 16–6, and 16–7, von Brunn's nests in the subepithelial connective tissue are composed of buds of urothelial cells which may or may not retain their connections to the surface urothelium. Cystitis cystica appears to be a variant of von Brunn's nests with the urothelial components replaced by one or more cysts lined by columnar or cuboidal epithelium. Unfortunately, the diagnostic threshold of individual pathologists for each of these lesions can be quite different, and the degree of cystic dilatation sometimes figures in the diagnosis. Cystitis glandularis by definition must contain intestinal type columnar epithelium, and often has goblet cells (Fig. 16–7), but it is considered by many to be a variant of cystitis cystica rather than a separate entity.

The malignant potential of proliferative cystitis appears to be very low. However, the prognosis of cystitis glandularis may be somewhat more ominous since it can be found associated with primary adenocarcinomas of the bladder. The number of von Brunn's nests increases with advancing age, and therefore it is not surprising that there is a frequent association between proliferative cystitis and bladder tumors, also a disease of older age groups.

Under some circumstances it can be difficult to differentiate between massive proliferative cystitis (Figs. 16–5, 16–6, and 16–7) and inverted papilloma (see Fig. 16–17), although the differentiation is not crucial since both entities are considered benign.

Dysplastic urothelial changes, including carcinoma-in-situ, may appear in von Brunn's nests (Fig. 16–8). It is important to recognize this phenomenon, and to

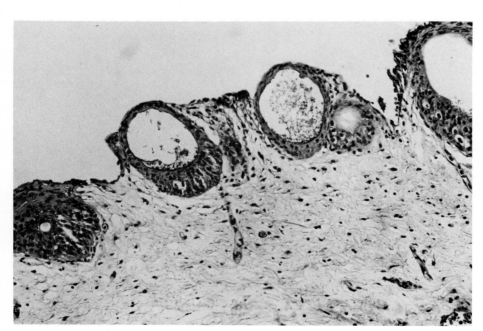

Figure 16–6. Proliferative cystitis with von Brunn's nests and beginning cystitis cystica. This picture demonstrates that the cysts develop from von Brunn's nests.

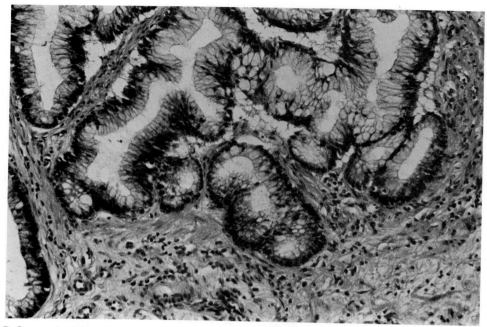

Figure 16–7. Cystitis glandularis. It is rarer than the other forms of proliferative cystitis. The glands are "colonic" in appearance.

distinguish it from invasion of carcinoma into the suburothelial connective tissue.

DIFFUSE PAPILLOMATOSIS OF BLADDER

This uncommon lesion, depicted in Figure 16–9, consists of innumerable small, short, papillary structures with minimal branching, lining a substantial portion of the inner surface of the bladder (Mostofi, 1968). The surface of the papillae is covered by rather well-differentiated, focally hyperplastic urothelium, not unlike that of papillomas. Since the lesion is rare, little is known about its malignant potential.

SQUAMOUS CHANGE OF UROTHELIUM

This urothelial abnormality, sometimes referred to as "squamous transformation" or "squamous metaplasia," is common. Non-keratinizing, stratified, non-neoplastic-appearing squamous epithelium, similar to that found in the esophagus and vagina, replaces the urothelium (Fig. 16–10). This phenomenon is so frequent in the bladder trigone of females that some investigators consider it to be physiological. Under certain circumstances, it is even possible to determine the hormonal status within the menstrual cycle of women by examining urine cytology specimens, since this squamous epithelium undergoes the same hor-

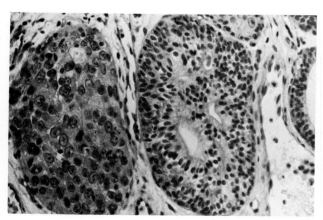

Figure 16–8. Epithelial dysplasia in von Brunn's nest. This is moderate dysplasia and not carcinoma-in-situ. Carcinoma-in-situ in von Brunn's nest must be distinguished from invasion.

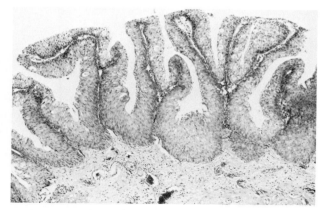

Figure 16–9. Diffuse papillomatosis of bladder. The inner surface of the bladder is lined by papillary structures covered by minimally dysplastic, frequently columnar-shaped transitional cells. The malignant potential of this rare lesion is not well known.

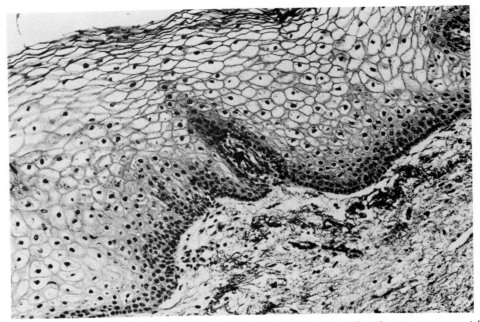

Figure 16–10. Squamous change of urothelium. This type of metaplasia is frequently found in the trigonum, especially in females. Its malignant potential, if any, is low.

monal changes as its counterpart in the uterine cervix. It is a rare urinary cytology specimen which does not contain at least a few squamous cells, although, of course, the origin of these cells is not necessarily a squamous change inside the bladder, since squamous cells can also come from the distal parts of both the female and male urethra. Squamous changes are frequently found in association with transitional or squamous cell carcinomas of the urinary tract, but this can be largely coincidental. If the squamous change is induced by an independent factor such as a bladder stone, diverticulum, or cyclophosphamide treatments (these associations are quite frequent), then the change probably represents a more ominous transitional state toward the development of squamous cell carcinoma.

RADIATION CHANGE AND CHEMOTHERAPY EFFECTS

Radiation and chemotherapy profoundly affect the morphologic appearance of urothelium. We know more about the effects of thiotepa than those of other agents because this drug has been widely used in the intravesical treatment of bladder cancer (Murphy et al., 1981). Cyclophosphamide effects have also been studied extensively since this drug is concentrated in urine and frequently causes hemorrhagic cystitis and urothelial disturbances (Wall and Clausen, 1975).

Radiation also induces substantial epithelial and connective tissue changes in the bladder wall (Gowing, 1960; Fajardo and Berthrong, 1978). As far as the urothelial effects are considered, radiation and some chemotherapeutic agents, for example, Thiotepa, produce lesions morphologically similar to the "dysplastic" changes which we will describe. At times it is difficult to ascertain whether the epithelial changes are part of the disease or the result of therapy. Further studies of the tissue in question by scanning electron microscopy might be of help.

Moreover, since radiation and some anti-cancer drugs have a cancerogenic potential, we cannot rule out the possibility that these treatment modalities, under some circumstances, contribute to or enhance the neoplastic process. Thus, the epithelial change

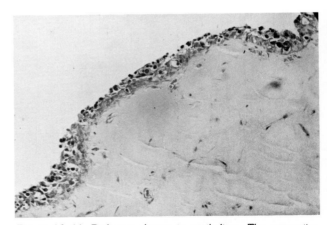

Figure 16–11. Radiation change in urothelium. The connective tissue is severely edematous. The presence of large, atypical fibroblasts is also characteristic. The urothelium shows marked atypia. In such cases, it is difficult and frequently impossible to decide whether the urothelial abnormalities are related to the original neoplastic diathesis or to the irradiation.

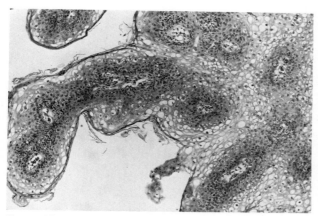

Figure 16–12. Squamous cell papilloma of the bladder. This very rare lesion has a delicate connective tissue core which is covered by well-differentiated squamous epithelium. No dysplasia is present.

might reflect not just persistence of cancer despite therapy but modification of the neoplastic epithelium due to the therapy's functioning as a promoting agent.

Our Figure 16–11 shows irradiated bladder mucosa with widespread urothelial and connective tissue changes. The urothelium itself demonstrates many features of moderate dysplasia, to be described below.

SQUAMOUS CELL PAPILLOMA

This lesion, like diffuse papillomatosis of the urinary bladder, is so uncommon that most pathologists will probably never encounter one. It is comparable in appearance to benign squamous papilloma of the skin or palate. It consists of a delicate, branching connective tissue core covered by many layers of well-differentiated, stratified squamous epithelium, not unlike that of the "squamous change of bladder" (Fig. 16–12). Because of its rarity we do not know much about its biologic potential, except that it has exhibited a tendency to epithelial proliferation by developing a papillary form. The relationship between the flat squamous change and the squamous papilloma of bladder mucosa may be similar to the relationship between non-papillary urothelial hyperplasia and papilloma or Grade 1 papillary transitional cell "carcinoma," in which the papillary nature of the latter suggests a greater proliferative tendency than that possessed by the flat hyperplastic lesion.

TRANSITIONAL CELL PAPILLOMA

This lesion is relatively uncommon and, if we accept the WHO definition, comprises only about one percent of all bladder tumors. The WHO definition (Mostofi et al., 1973) notes that the transitional cell papilloma is ". . . . . a papillary tumor with a delicate fibrovascular stroma covered by regular transitional epithelium indistinguishable from that of the normal bladder and not more than six layers thick" (Figs. 16–13 and 16–14). Focally, there may be more than six cell layers present owing to tangential sectioning of the tissue, but for the most part the epithelial cell layers will vary between three and six in number (Fig. 16–13).

The distinction between a papilloma and a papillary non-invasive transitional cell carcinoma may be diffi-

Figure 16–13. Transitional cell papilloma. It is ". . .a papillary tumor with a delicate fibrovascular stroma covered by regular transitional epithelium indistinguishable from that of the normal bladder and not more than six layers thick." In this picture, more than six urothelial cell layers are seen focally, but this is the consequence of tangential cutting. The illustrations in the cited reference are similar.

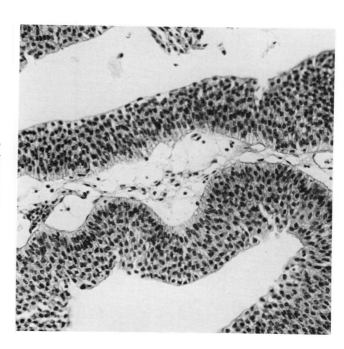

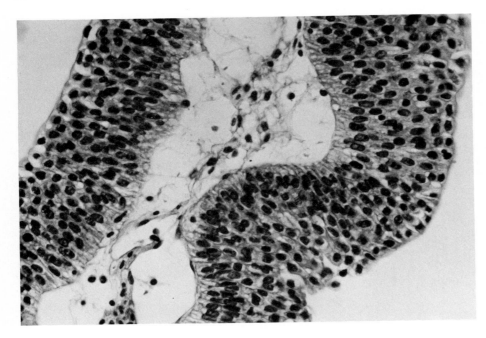

Figure 16–14. Transitional cell papilloma, higher power.

cult to make if there are only a few more than six cell layers present and if there is minimal nuclear pleomorphism. However, since the prognosis of low-grade non-invasive transitional carcinomas is good, the penalty for error is minimal.

Another entity which must be differentiated from transitional cell papilloma is the rare inflammatory papillary cystitis (Pugh, 1973) (Fig. 16–15).

UROTHELIAL HYPERPLASIA

This flat lesion is characterized by the presence of more than six layers of epithelium without any change in nuclear-cytoplasmic ratio, nuclear size, shape, po-

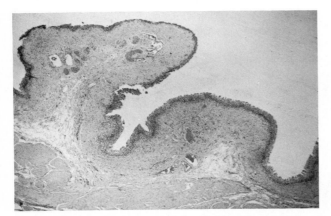

Figure 16–15. Papillary cystitis of the bladder. The edematous, slightly inflamed mucosa forms thick folds which are covered by normal urothelium. Note the difference between this lesion and the transitional cell papilloma shown in Figures 16–13 and 16–14.

larization, or chromatin content (Fig. 16–16). If the lesion occurs associated with low-grade tumors and/or urothelial dysplasia, it is the latter lesions which take precedence in determining the biologic potential of the abnormal bladder epithelium (Koss, 1974).

TRANSITIONAL CELL PAPILLOMA, INVERTED TYPE

This is also a rare lesion, and most pathologists believe it is the endophytic counterpart of the benign, exophytic transitional cell papilloma. It is characterized by anastomosing cords of urothelium in the subepithelial connective tissue covered by thin, normal bladder mucosa (Fig. 16–17). Another rather consistent feature is the presence of cystic structures in the urothelial masses, a finding not seen in exophytic papillomas (DeMeester et al., 1975). In the vast majority of cases, the inverted papilloma is undoubtedly benign. We have seen several cases, however, in which the histologic similarities to a low-grade transitional cell carcinoma were so great as to necessitate the diagnosis of Grade 1 transitional cell carcinoma, despite the architectural resemblance to an inverted papilloma.

NEPHROGENIC ADENOMA

This rare lesion occurs mostly in the bladder exposed to chronic irritation or trauma, and appears to originate in the urothelium (Kaswick et al., 1976; Bhagawan et al., 1981). It consists of glandular structures resembling renal tubules (Fig. 16–18). In spite of its morphologic resemblance to the so-called adenoma-

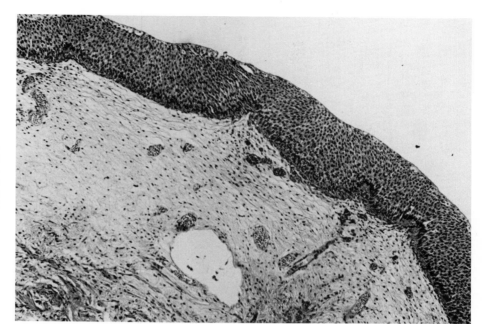

Figure 16–16. Urothelial hyperplasia. There are about 15 "nuclear layers" of otherwise regular, well-polarized urothelial cells. Hyperplasia is found mostly in bladders with other lesions (low-grade tumors and dysplasias).

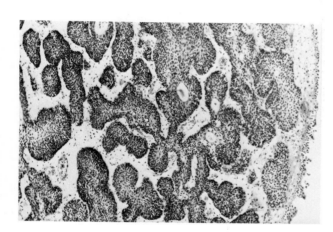

Figure 16–17. Inverted papilloma of bladder. The anastomosing epithelial cords consist of cells closely resembling normal urothelium. Another important histologic feature is the presence of microcysts within the cords.

Figure 16–18. Nephrogenic adenoma. A rare lesion, usually associated with inflammation, possibly metaplastic in origin. Its malignant potential seems to be low.

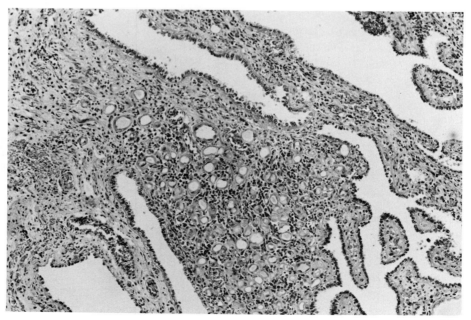

toid tumor, a neoplasm of the male and female pelvic and genital organs, the latter is probably of mesothelial and not urothelial origin. Neither is there any evidence that the nephrogenic adenoma of the bladder is related to the mesonephros or the metanephros. It is generally accepted that the nephrogenic adenoma is benign. We, however, think that this lesion very rarely might be a precursor of an adenocarcinoma, although possibly only under very special circumstances. Structures resembling nephrogenic adenomas are seen frequently in untreated cases of exstrophy of the bladder, a condition in which the development of adenocarcinoma is a significant problem.

PREMALIGNANT LESIONS

Farrow and Utz (1983) state that ". . . . . if definability and reproducibility of subjective morphologic criteria are difficult to achieve with in-situ carcinoma, any less well developed epithelial abnormality such as dysplasia will present even greater difficulties, both in the recognition and the interpretation of clinical significance." We demonstrated that on the basis of strictly defined morphologic criteria a rather high degree of consensus can be achieved among pathologists in the morphologic evaluation of these lesions (Nagy et al., 1982). It remains to be seen, however, just how useful this morphologic classification will be for the pathologist, the urologist, and the patient.

Despite the fact that terminology itself can evoke emotional responses among pathologists, we use the term "dysplasia" which seems to have gained acceptance in recent literature (Murphy and Soloway, 1982). We are aware of the fact that complicated biologic processes cannot be completely characterized by a word or by a combination of several words. We use the term "dysplasia" as a code word for the observed phenomena, without attributing any philosophical meaning to it. The term "bronchopneumonia" is also a code word which has been widely accepted although it does not express the complexities of the underlying pathologic processes.

In the following, we delineate in tabular form the histologic criteria for classifying flat premalignant urothelial lesions (Nagy et al., 1982). We used four categories (mild, moderate, and severe dysplasia and carcinoma-in-situ), not because we are convinced that there are four distinct groups of lesions—each with different biologic behavior and prognosis—but because we believe that initially in data collection it is better to start with more categories than might prove at a later date to be necessary. Once follow-up information for each morphologic entity is available, it is a simple matter to combine two or more categories which are found to have similar biologic potential. Collecting the data on which to base this combination of categories is the difficult problem.

In the interpretation of premalignant lesions in another organ, the uterine cervix, this "lumping" procedure has been going on for some time, although not all investigators agree with the results. Richart's cervical intraepithelial neoplasia (CIN) concept, for example, stresses that the premalignant lesions of the

Table 16–1. Definitions Used in Interpretation of Flat, Noninvasive Lesions of Urothelium (Histology)

Terms	Definitions
Urothelial thickening	At least seven nuclear layers present in areas sectioned perpendicular to the basal lamina.
Polarization	A. *Normal:* The basal cells are columnar. Almost all nuclei, except those in the superficial layer, are arranged perpendicular to the basal layer and/or the surface. B. *Altered:* The nuclei of intermediate cells are no longer arranged with their long axes perpendicular to either the surface of the basal lamina. This disorientation varies in degree. In general, more loss of polarity occurs in more severe lesions.
Nuclear crowding	A focal increase in number of nuclei per unit space. Often this is manifested by overlapping of nuclei in relatively thin sections (4μ). Nuclear crowding probably reflects increases in nuclear-cytoplasmic ratios. Care should be taken to avoid interpretation of cells in invaginated areas or areas of compression.
Nuclear border irregularity	Angular indentations of nuclear border with tendency toward lobulation of nuclei. The indentations may vary from one to three and may be so marked that the nuclei appear folded. In general, more severe lesions have more nuclear irregularity.
Increased nuclear size	Nuclei larger than those of normal intermediate cells. There is some variation in nuclear size and shape among cells.
Chromatin	Evaluation of the chromatin structure is very subjective. The apparent composition and distribution are dependent upon fixation and staining. Nevertheless, some guidelines in the interpretation of chromatin are offered. A. *Normal:* Very finely granular (dusty) with a tendency toward peripheral concentration. B. *Abnormal:* The granules are more distinct and may be either fine or coarse. As the lesion becomes more severe, the chromatin tends to be less peripherally concentrated and more irregularly distributed throughout the nuclei.

Table 16–2. **Criteria for Mild Dysplasia**

Description	Urothelium with slight nuclear irregularities, not more pronounced than the features acceptable in ''Grade 1 Transitional Cell Carcinoma'' (WHO). Lesions may or may not be full thickness. In the past, this lesion has often been interpreted as normal.
Mandatory features	
Polarization	Slight and/or focal alteration.
Superficial cells	Usually present and normal.
Nuclear size	Slight variation from normal.
Nuclear crowding	Slight.
Nuclear irregularity	Slight.
Chromatin	Finely granular and evenly distributed.
Noncritical features	
Mitoses	Rare.
Connective tissue	Inflammation may or may not be present.

cervix form a continuous morphologic and biologic spectrum (Richart, 1973). In the concept, ''severe dysplasia'' and ''carcinoma-in-situ'' are not separate entities. We know less about the premalignant lesions of urothelium than about the premalignant lesions of the cervix, since the cervix has been more thoroughly studied. Our four categories for urothelial premalignant lesions definitely do not imply that we think they are separate and distinct processes, but at this time ''splitting'' seems to be a better approach than ''lumping.'' In the accompanying tables we have listed our

Table 16–3. **Criteria for Moderate Dysplasia**

Description	Urothelium with unequivocal nuclear irregularities, corresponding to changes in ''Grade 2 Transitional Cell Carcinoma'' (WHO). Lesions involve most or all of intermediate cell layers.
Mandatory features	
Polarization	Altered.
Superficial cells	Usually present and normal.
Nuclear size	More variation than in mild dysplasia.
Nuclear crowding	Present and more prominent than in mild dysplasia.
Nuclear iregularity	Prominent.
Chromatin	Predominantly finely granular and evenly distributed. Some nuclei with coarsely granular chromatin may occur.
Noncritical features	
Mitoses	Not unusual.
Nucleoli	May be prominent.
Connective tissue	Same as in mild dysplasia.

Table 16–4. **Criteria for Severe Dysplasia**

Description	Urothelium with severe cellular irregularities, corresponding to changes in a ''Grade 3 Transitional Cell Carcinoma'' (WHO). The lesion involves basal and intermediate cells but tends to spare the superficial layer. These changes are very similar to those of carcinoma-in-situ and may represent only a slight variation of the latter. The differentiation is particularly difficult if there is extensive denudation of the superficial layers.
Mandatory features	
Polarization	Markedly altered.
Superficial cells	Present but may be abnormal.
Nuclear size	Variable. Bizarre nuclei may occur.
Nuclear crowding	Present.
Nuclear irregularity	Present. Indentations and angularities of the nuclear borders are prominent.
Chromatin	Coarsely granular and irregularly distributed.
Noncritical features	
Mitoses	Common.
Nucleoli	Often prominent.
Connective tissue	Same as in mild dysplasia.

guidelines and definitions for flat urothelial premalignant lesions, modified from Nagy et al., 1982.

Examples of different degrees of dysplasias and carcinoma-in-situ are depicted in Figures 16–19 to 16–28.

Table 16–5. **Carcinoma-In-Situ**

Description	Urothelium with nuclear irregularities corresponding to changes in ''Grade 3 Transitional Cell Carcinoma'' (WHO). The lesions extend from the basal layer to the surface and include the superficial layer. Lesions need not be hyperplastic.
Mandatory features	
Polarization	Lost.
Superficial cells	Absent.
Nuclear size	Same as in severe dysplasia.
Nuclear crowding	Same as in severe dysplasia.
Nuclear irregularity	Same as in severe dysplasia.
Chromatin	Same as in severe dysplasia.
Noncritical features	
Mitoses	Common.
Nucleoli	Same as in severe dysplasia.
Connective tissue	Significant hyperemia is usual. Inflammation may be marked.
Denudation	Common.

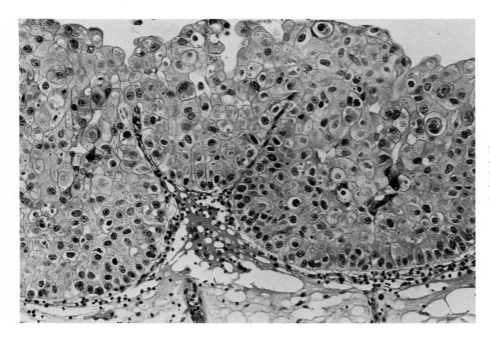

Figure 16–19. Moderate dysplasia of urothelium. There are obvious nuclear irregularities and thickening of urothelium with a "squamoid" appearance.

Figure 16–20. Marked epithelial dysplasia. The degree of nuclear abnormalities is more pronounced than in the previous figure. The flattening of cells on the surface indicates maturation, which is why we do not classify this lesion as carcinoma-in-situ.

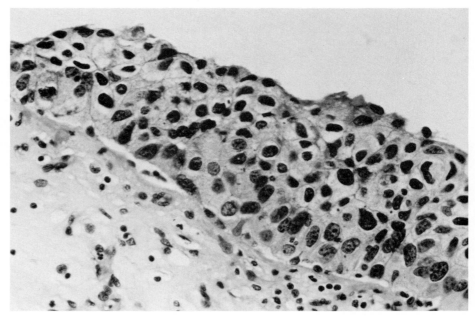

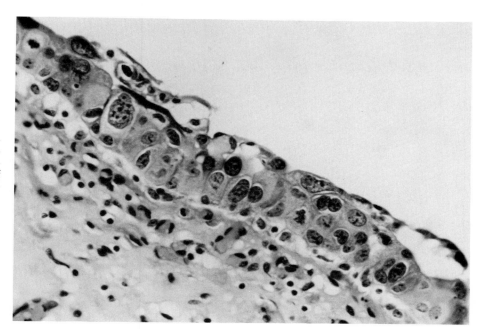

Figure 16–21. Transitional cell carcinoma-in-situ, showing all the classic features. The urothelium is relatively thin, possibly because of increased fragility and desquamation.

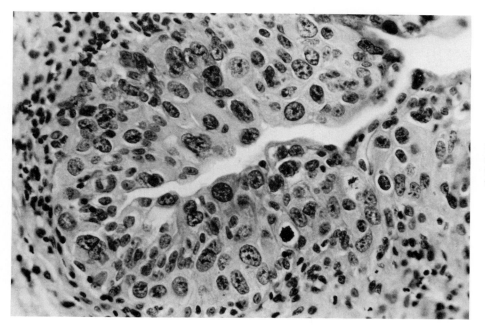

Figure 16–22. Transitional cell carcinoma-in-situ, much thicker than the lesion in Figure 16–21. Note the mitotic forms.

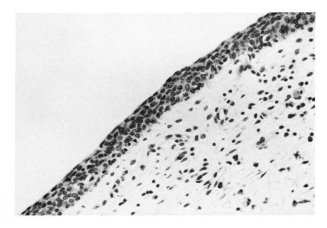

Figure 16–23. Mild urothelial dysplasia. The urothelium is no thicker than usual; the polarity of the urothelial cells is, however, disturbed, and the nuclei are large, hyperchromatic, and slightly variable in shape. No "umbrella cells" have been formed.

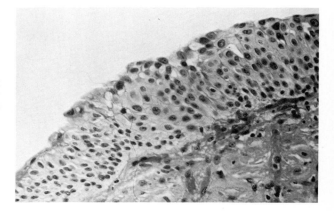

Figure 16–24. Mild urothelial dysplasia with slight hyperplasia. About two thirds of the urothelium shown here is slightly hyperplastic, since it contains approximately ten "nuclear layers." Nuclear abnormalities are also present (compare the normal and abnormal urothelial areas). The surface differentiation is well retained.

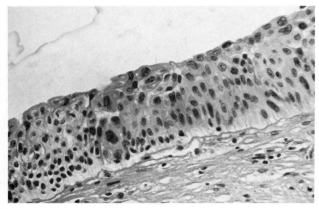

Figure 16–25. Mild and moderate urothelial dysplasia. The nuclear abnormalities in the central portion of the area shown are beyond the stage of mild dysplasia. One third of urothelium is hyperplastic and does not reveal dysplasia.

Figure 16–26. Moderate urothelial dysplasia. There is marked nuclear variability and hyperchromasia, but the nuclear-cytoplasmic ratio is only slightly changed, and traces of polarity and differentiation toward the surface can still be recognized.

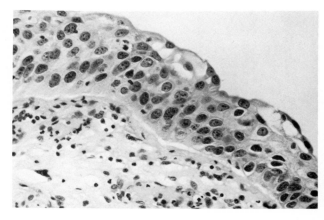

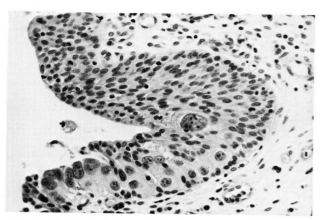

Figure 16–27. Marked urothelial dysplasia. The focal nuclear abnormalities are beyond the stage of moderate dysplasia. In a small focus, the dysplastic changes extend to the surface. Hyperplasia is also present.

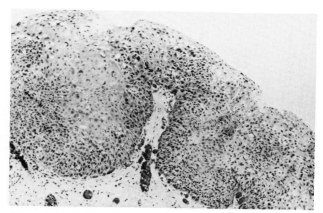

Figure 16–29. Squamous carcinoma-in-situ in urothelium. This low-power picture demonstrates that the basement membrane is intact, that is, the process is confined to the urothelium.

SQUAMOUS CELL CARCINOMA-IN-SITU

Since our system encompasses only premalignant changes in urothelial cells, it is proper to say a few words about the infrequently encountered squamous cell carcinoma-in-situ (Figs. 16–29 and 16–30). Urothelial cells and squamous cells share many cytologic and ultrastructural features, so that classification of cells into the urothelial or squamous category may become arbitrary, especially if the cells become more dysplastic and lose their ability to produce intact and specialized organelles ("dedifferentiation"). That may be the reason why in cases of poorly differentiated carcinoma-in-situ the cells do not exhibit specialized structures, and automatically are categorized into the urothelial group. Rarely, however, it occurs that in spite of a certain degree of dedifferentiation the cells focally retain their capability to produce tonofilaments and desmosomes and to proceed with some keratin-

ization, which renders them recognizable as squamous cells by light microscopy. We demonstrate one such case in Figures 16–29 and 16–30. No data are available for the prognostic implications of this lesion. We assume that the implications are similar to those of urothelial carcinoma-in-situ.

CYTOLOGIC DIAGNOSIS

The most valuable test for the detection of in-situ carcinoma is a properly conducted and accurately interpreted exfoliative cytologic examination of the urine (Farrow and Utz, 1983; Murphy et al., 1984). The cytologic diagnosis of premalignant urothelial lesions becomes, however, increasingly difficult with the decreasing severity of urothelial changes, since the lower the grade of dysplasia, the greater will be the cytologic similarities between normal and altered urothelial cells. The difficulty in interpretation also includes the problem of applying the same criteria to specimens obtained under different circumstances, for

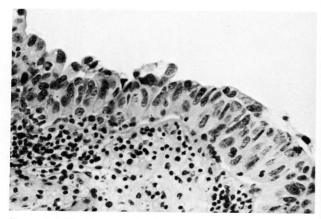

Figure 16–28. Transitional cell carcinoma-in-situ. The cells are markedly dysplastic and the entire thickness of urothelium is involved. The connective tissue is inflamed and contains dilated vessels.

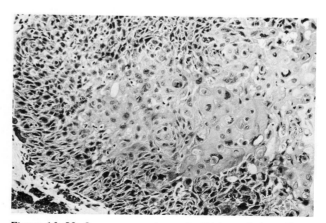

Figure 16–30. Squamous carcinoma-in-situ in urothelium. Detail of the previous picture, revealing unmistakable squamous changes.

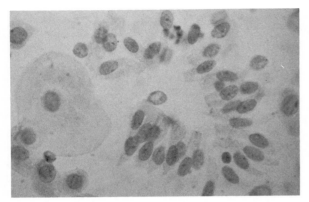

Figure 16–31. Normal urine cytology, bladder washing specimen. One large, well-differentiated squamous cell, many columnar-shaped cells and normal transitional cells (Papanicolaou stain).

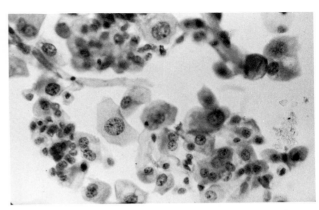

Figure 16–32. Reactive transitional cells, bladder washing. Slight nuclear irregularities are seen. The specimen is cellular (Papanicolaou stain).

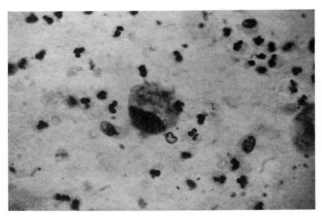

Figure 16–33. "Decoy cell"—a large, degenerated cell with dense nucleus imitating a malignant cell. The cytoplasm is also degenerated. No nuclear detail can be recognized (Papanicolaou stain).

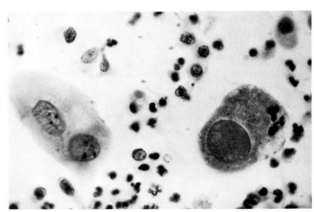

Figure 16–34. Eosinophilic inclusion body. It is found almost exclusively in degenerated cells and is not related to any specific disease (Papanicolaou stain).

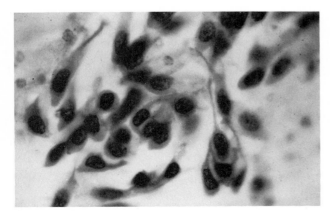

Figure 16–35. Transitional cell carcinoma, Grade I. A very difficult cytologic diagnosis, because the tumor cells are uniform, well differentiated, and similar to normal transitional cells. In such cases, histologic confirmation should always be sought (Papanicolaou stain).

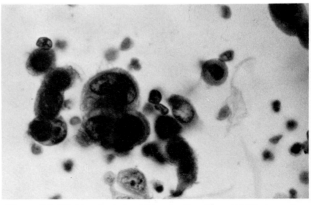

Figure 16–36. Dysplastic transitional cells with variability in nuclear size, shape, and chromatin structure. Histologically, moderate degree of dysplasia was found (Papanicolaou stain).

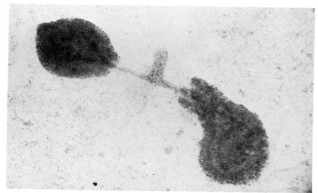

Figure 16–37. Papillary "frond" with branching connective tissue core from a catheterized urine. This is irrefutable evidence of a low-grade papillary carcinoma. Unfortunately, entire papillary fragments are found extremely rarely in cytologic specimens (Papanicolaou stain).

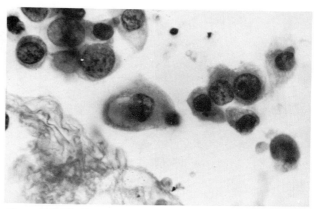

Figure 16–38. Transitional cell carcinoma-in-situ. High nuclear-cytoplasmic ratio, hyperchromatism, and variability in nuclear size. The diagnosis was histologically confirmed (Papanicolaou stain).

example, voided urine, catheterized urine, or bladder washings. The situation is complicated even more by the fact that some investigators are willing to use the so-called "expanded criteria" in the diagnosis of pre-malignant and malignant urothelial lesions in high risk groups (Harris et al., 1971). This approach is justified on the basis of Bayesian predictive value theory.

In Figures 16–31 to 16–38 we show normal cytologic features, reactive changes, and some pitfalls in urinary specimens. As mentioned, the cytologic diagnosis of low-grade papillary carcinoma is difficult. The usual cellular alterations characteristic of malignancy are not seen in cells exfoliated from these lesions. Exfoliated cells from cases with slight and moderate dysplasia are similar to those from cases of papillary transitional cell carcinoma, Grade 1, since the severity of cellular changes in these lesions as we define them should parallel low-grade papillary carcinomas (Fig. 16–36). Rarely, a specific papillary configuration of cells seen on the slide of a urine sample can solve diagnostic problems (Fig. 16–37). Finally, we have illustrated the cytologic changes found in urothelial carcinoma-in-situ (Fig. 16–38), a picture which should not cause difficulties for the experienced cytologist.

References

Bhagawan, B.S., Tiamson, E.M., Wenk, R.E., Berger, B.W., Hamamoto, G., Eggleston, J.C.: Nephrogenic adenoma of the urinary bladder and urethra. Human Pathol. 12:907–916, 1981.

DeMeester, L.J., Farrow, G.M., Utz, D.C.: Inverted papillomas of the urinary bladder. Cancer 36:505–513, 1975.

Fajardo, L.F., Berthrong, M.: Radiation injury in surgical pathology, Part I. Am. J. Surg. Pathol. 2:159–199, 1978.

Farrow, G.M., Utz, D.C.: Carcinoma in situ. In: Bryan, G.T., and Cohen, S.M. (Eds): The Pathology of Bladder Cancer, Vol. I., p. 47. Boca Raton, Florida, CRC Press, 1983.

Gowing, N.F.C.: Pathological changes in the bladder following irradiation. Br. J. Radiol. 33:484–487, 1960.

Harris, M.J., Schwinn, C.P., Morrow, J.D., Gray, R.L., Browell, B.M.: Exfoliative cytology of the urinary bladder irrigation specimen. Acta Cytol. 15:385–399, 1971.

Jacobs, J.B., Arai, M., Cohen, S.M., Friedell, G.H.: Early lesions in experimental bladder cancer: 2. Scanning electron microscopy of cell surface markers. Cancer Res. 36:2512–2517, 1976.

Kaswick, J.A., Weisman, J., Goodwin, W.E.: Nephrogenic metaplasia (adenomatoid tumors) of bladder. Urology 8:283–286, 1976.

Koss, L.G.: Tumors of the Urinary Bladder. Atlas of Tumor Pathology, Second Series, Fascicle 11. Washington, D.C., Armed Forces Institute of Pathology, 1974.

Koss, L.G.: The asymmetric unit membranes of the epithelium of the urinary bladder of the rat. An electron microscopic study of a mechanism of epithelial maturation and function. Lab. Invest. 21:154–168, 1969.

Mostofi, F.K.: Potentialities of the bladder epithelium. J. Urol. 71:705–713, 1954.

Mostofi, F.K.: Pathological aspects and spread of carcinoma of bladder. J.A.M.A. 206:1764–1769, 1968.

Mostofi, F.K., Sobin, L.H., Torloni, H. (Eds.): Histological Typing of Urinary Bladder Tumours. International Histological Classification of Tumours, No. 10, WHO, Geneva, 1973.

Murphy, W.M., Soloway, M.S.: Urothelial dysplasia. J. Urol. 127:849–854, 1982.

Murphy, W.M., Soloway, M.S., Finebaum, P.J.: Pathologic changes associated with topical chemotherapy for superficial bladder cancer. J. Urol. 126:461–464, 1981.

Murphy, W.M., Soloway, M.S., Jukkola, A.F., Crabtree, W.N., Ford, K.S.: Urinary cytology and bladder cancer. The cellular features of transitional cell neoplasms. Cancer 53:1555–1565, 1984.

Nagy, G.K., Frable, W.J., Murphy, W.M.: Classification of premalignant urothelial abnormalities. A Delphi study of the National Bladder Cancer Collaborative Group A. Pathol. Annual 17:219–233, 1982.

Pugh, R.C.B.: The pathology of cancer of the bladder. Cancer 32:1267–1274, 1973.

Richart, R.M.: Cervical intraepithelial neoplasia. Pathol. Annual 8:301–328, 1973.

Wall, R.L., Clausen, K.P.: Carcinoma of the urinary bladder in patients receiving cyclophosphamide. New Engl. J. Med. 293:271–273, 1975.

MYRON TANNENBAUM
MICHAEL J. DROLLER

17 Prostate Gland

Prostatic cancer is a common occurrence when prostate glands from autopsy specimens are serially blocked. This observation has been confirmed many times. As a result many approaches have been tried for the earlier detection of prostatic cancer. These include the time-tested approaches of measuring serum prostatic acid phosphatase and the use of newer diagnostic modalities such as ultrasonography and computed tomography for the detection of extraprostatic cancer spread. All of these newer modalities, however, depend on *tissue diagnosis* for final confirmation.

What then is the earliest morphologic pattern indicative of biologically active prostatic cancer? In the last decade there has been an impasse because of the different measuring rods for detecting prostatic cancer. To the urologist, it is the presence of a rectally detectable nodule. Hopefully this means a finger-felt nodule that is clinically a stage B lesion—that is, the tumor is limited to the prostate and has not spread beyond the capsule of the prostate gland. Unfortunately, many urologists are well aware that when the radically removed prostate gland is examined pathologically, the cancer is a stage higher than they suspected clinically. Consequently, there is a greater need to detect this cancer at an earlier stage. Therefore, biopsies are often obtained when there is a suspicious or indurated area in any one of the lobes of the prostate gland.

Unfortunately, many of the prostatic cancers that are seen are at a later stage clinically and are usually detected as incidental cancers in tissue obtained by either transurethral resection (TURP) or open prostatectomy from patients with obstruction. This means that there are many patients who have clinically active prostatic cancer that the urologist cannot detect rectally. These figures approach those of the autopsy incidence. There are two to three chances in ten that men, when they reach the age of 65, will have some form of prostatic cancer. Histologically, many of these cancers will be biologically active. Many glands that are architecturally benign may have areas in which

there are cytologic findings identical to those seen in areas of cancer. If we were to use these criteria alone as indicators for prostatic cancer, then our incidence would double, that is, six to seven chances in ten of having a morphologic form of prostatic cancer.

What would be the incidence of prostatic cancer if we were to use the tools of the molecular biologist and measure conformational membrane changes? With what measurement do we equate the initiation of therapy such as orchiectomy, radical prostatectomy, chemotherapy, or radiotherapy? Let us now consider some of the various morphologic stages that are used in the evaluation of prostatic cancer.

ATYPICAL EPITHELIAL HYPERPLASIA

For decades, there was considerable difficulty in distinguishing the many benign atypical glandular alterations from prostatic cancer. Franks (1954b) tried to differentiate the proliferation of small glands from those seen in connection with glandular atrophy classified as *postatrophic hyperplasia of the prostate gland.* However, irregular or *atypical epithelial hyperplasia* is often found in association with benign hypertrophied glands in tissue obtained from transurethral resections or suprapubic prostatectomy specimens (Fig. 17–1).

Dysplasia of the prostate gland was a term introduced by Kastendieck (1976). There are four different types: (1) cribriform patterns, (2) papillary patterns, (3) tubular patterns, and (4) adenomatous patterns (Figs. 17–2 to 17–5). These patterns or structures may serve to identify the possible precursor stages of the various cancerous patterns (Gleason grades) found in the prostate gland. In essence, the fundamental morphologic criteria found in Kastendieck's prostatic dysplasia (Kastendieck, 1980) as well as Tannenbaum's *atypical epithelial hyperplasia* (Tannenbaum, 1977) are: cytologic atypia, irregular glandular architecture, and a disorganization of the mor-

313

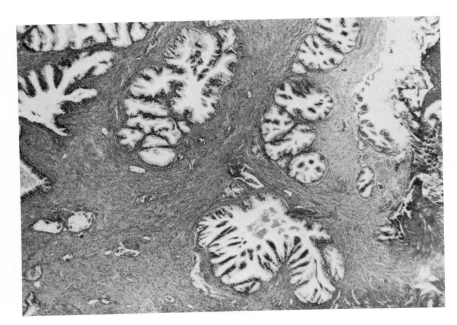

Figure 17–1. Primary atypical epithelial (ductal papillary) hyperplasia. No fibrovascular cores in papillary projections.

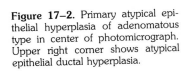

Figure 17–2. Primary atypical epithelial hyperplasia of adenomatous type in center of photomicrograph. Upper right corner shows atypical epithelial ductal hyperplasia.

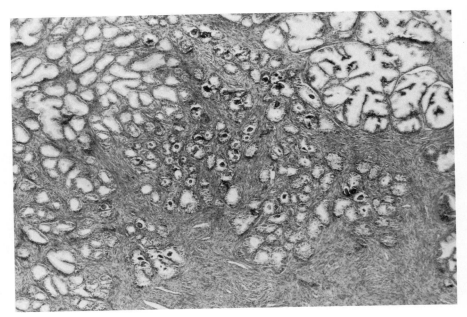

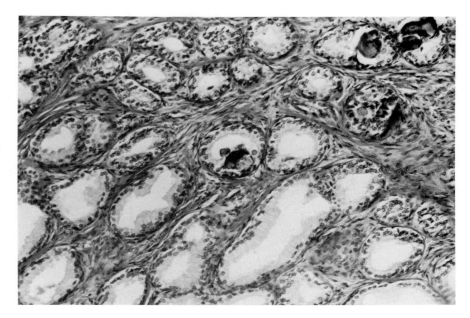

Figure 17–3. Higher power of Figure 17–2 with cell secretions in lumen of gland; double layer of cells. Cells have pleomorphic nuclei, but no nucleoli.

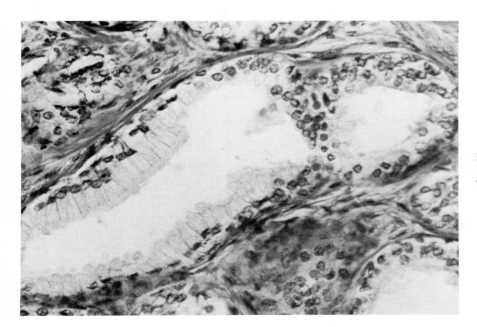

Figure 17–4. Higher power of Figure 17–2 with two glands. Note variability of nuclear size.

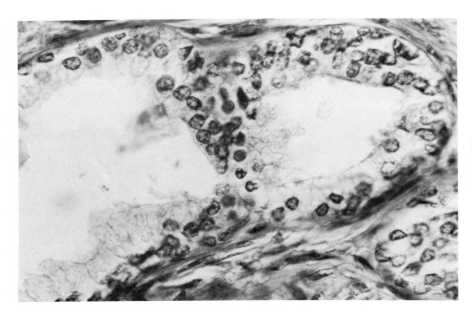

Figure 17–5. Even higher power of Figure 17–2 with atypical nuclei. Some nuclei are beginning to have onset of nucleoli formation.

phologic integrity between the glandular epithelium and the stroma. Here, there is an epithelial-stromal border which may be indistinct and the proliferating glands simulate an invasive growth pattern.

There are instances when the epithelial glandular configurations are extremely difficult to differentiate from prostatic cancer. Histologically, these foci are found quite frequently in prostatic chips obtained by transurethral resection as well as in tissue sections from suprapubic prostatectomies. These atypical glandular proliferations are found not only in prostatic tissue with glandular atrophy but more commonly in association with areas of benign prostatic hypertrophy.

The fundamental morphologic criteria for the *atyp-ical epithelial hyperplasia* would therefore include: (1) varying degrees of cytologic atypia, (2) irregular glandular architecture, and (3) architectural disorganization of the epithelial-mesenchymal interface. These atypical epithelial hyperplasias are found in different percentages of tissue depending upon the extent of the prostatic cancer. There is an inverse relationship between tumor size and the volume of primary atypical epithelial hyperplasia. Kastendieck (1980) showed that very small cancers occupied less than 10 percent of the volume of the prostate gland, whereas small tumors occupy from 11 to 30 percent, middle-sized tumors 31 to 50 percent, and large carcinomas more than 50 percent of the prostate tissue. Two or more

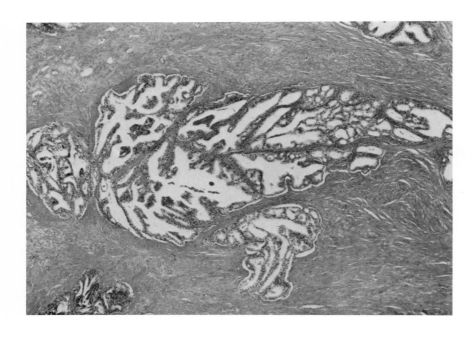

Figure 17–6. Low-power photomicrograph of primary atypical epithelial hyperplasia with pseudocribriform pattern in ducts.

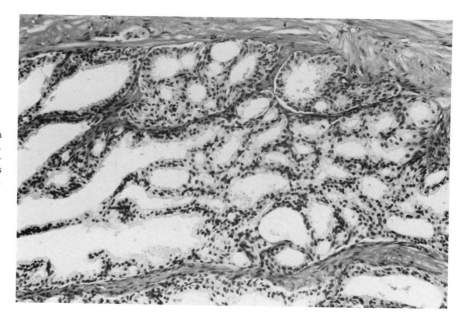

Figure 17–7. Pseudocribriform pattern extending from ducts into terminal acini. Possible precursor form of cribriform pattern of prostatic carcinoma. Note glands within glands and no fibrovascular stalks.

clearly separated tumor foci were considered to be representative of a multifocal carcinoma. When there is a diffuse carcinoma of the prostate, it tends to spread throughout the gland. In these cases, the determination of a definite focus of carcinoma is not possible.

The labeling of a specific glandular proliferation as atypical epithelial hyperplasia (atypical primary hyperplasia), in the sense of dysplasia, can be based on both histologic and cytologic features. These areas consist of irregular epithelial proliferations showing tubular, papillary, and/or pseudocribriform structures (Figs. 17–6 to 17–8). The prostatic epithelium can be multilayered and may reveal cytologic atypia with pleomorphic nuclei (Figs. 17–3 and 17–8) and slightly prominent small nucleoli. These latter structures may be, in some instances, as large as those found in the more invasive carcinomas of the prostate gland. In addition, there may be total disarray of the normal interrelationship between the basal portions of the glands and the surrounding stroma. This epithelial-mesenchymal transition zone may be indistinct. As a result the glands may simulate an invasive pattern.

Kastendieck also established a relationship between atypical epithelial hyperplasia and carcinoma of the prostate gland with respect to tumor stage, tumor size

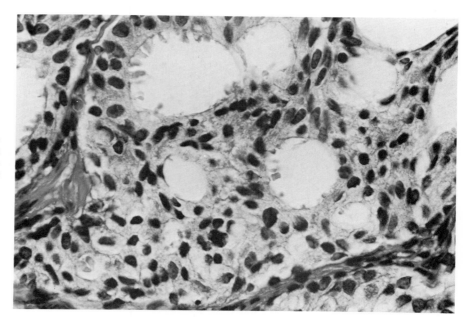

Figure 17–8. Higher-power photomicrograph of part of cribriform pattern in Figure 17–6. Note pleomorphic nuclei and apocrine snouts to apical areas of the surface cells.

(volume fraction), number of tumor foci, and the extent of histologic differentiation (Kastendieck, 1980). Briefly, we will consider tumor stage and tumor size.

Tumor Stage

A total of 180 carcinoma specimens were divided into three stages: P1, P2, and P3. There were 12 P1 cases (6.7 percent), 36 P2 (20 percent), and 132 P3 (73.3 percent) cases. It was also found expedient to subdivide the P3 cases into a capsular-penetrating stage or transitional stage, P2–3, where there were 40 cases (22.2 percent). There were 92 cases (51.1 percent) which demonstrated unequivocal capsular penetration. Of these, there were 36 (20 percent) which also demonstrated seminal vesicle infiltration. The earlier stages of prostatic carcinoma also demonstrated a greater degree of involvement by primary atypical epithelial hyperplasia of the remaining glandular structures. P1 cases had 93 percent involvement by primary atypical epithelial hyperplasia, whereas P2 had 83.3 percent, P2-3 had 65 percent, and P3 had 43.5 percent.

Tumor Size

Most carcinomas were classified as relatively small when the volume of tissue involvement was between 10 and 30 percent (99/180 = 55 percent). The second most commonly found tumors were the large neoplasms which occupied at least half, often far more, of the prostate gland (46/280 = 25.5 percent). In contrast, intermediate size carcinomas were rarely seen (14/180 = 7.8 percent). Twenty-one cases (10 percent) were listed as very small carcinomas where the volume of tumor was less than 10 percent. There was an inverse relationship between tumor size and the volume of primary atypical epithelial hyperplasia. The larger tumor sizes had smaller areas of tissue involved with the atypical hyperplasias, whereas the prostate glands with smaller tumor volume had larger areas of atypical epithelial hyperplasia. Does this observation imply that there is recruitment from the atypical epithelial hyperplasia into carcinoma? Or have the larger carcinomas simply obliterated much of the atypical epithelial hyperplasia?

Helpap has also studied the relationship between primary atypical epithelial hyperplasia and carcinoma of the prostate (Helpap, 1980). In 4341 tissue biopsies, he found 122 cases of atypical epithelial hyperplasia without carcinoma. In these cases, there was a microglandular (Fig. 17–9), papillary clear cell (Fig. 17–10), or adenomatous or cribriform pattern (Fig. 17–11). Of these, 38 percent showed slight cellular atypia. Moderate atypia was observed in 36 percent of the cases, and marked cellular and structural atypia were found in 14 percent. A small number of cases (12.4 percent) showed a transition from severe atypical epithelial hyperplasia to carcinoma after further serial sectioning of the paraffin blocks. Helpap was also able to demonstrate that the most common histologic patterns in primary atypical epithelial hyperplasia were the microglandular and papillary clear cell patterns. There were no statistically significant differences between cases of slight, moderate, and severe atypia.

A histologic analysis of 524 cases of prostatic carcinoma was also performed. There was a correlation between the different histologic patterns of prostatic carcinoma and the patterns of the primary atypical epithelial hyperplasia. Differentiated adenocarcinomas were most frequently found in association with slight

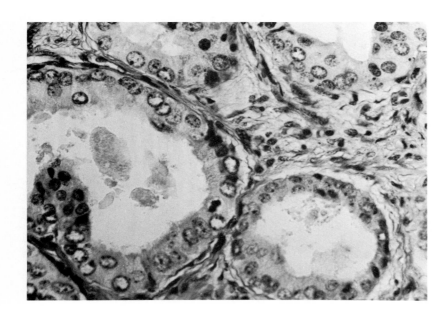

Figure 17–9. Light microscopic photograph of the glandular pattern of carcinoma similar to the adenosis of atypical epithelial glandular hyperplasia.

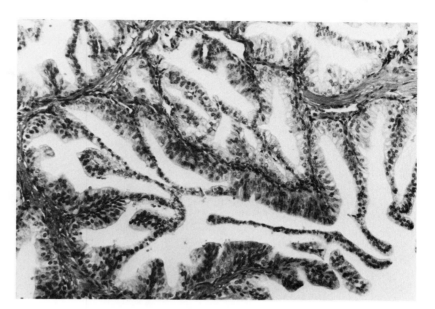

Figure 17–10. Photomicrograph of the papillary carcinoma that can arise from atypical papillary hyperplasia.

or moderate microglandular clear cell or papillary atypical epithelial hyperplasia. In contrast, there was a high correlation of severe atypical epithelial hyperplasia with the cribriform pattern and the solid anaplastic types of carcinoma.

Cell Kinetics of Primary Atypical Epithelial Hyperplasia

Mitotic figures are extremely rare in histologic sections of primary atypical epithelial hyperplasias, (less than 0.01 percent). In severe atypical epithelial hyperplasias, the average mitotic index is 0.06 percent. Glandular carcinomas reveal mitotic indices of 0.02 percent and cribriform carcinomas of 0.04 to 0.06 percent.

The average labeling index in 65 cases of simple glandular hyperplasia was 0.49 (0.4 percent). These cases demonstrated no significant difference from three cases which had an accompanying nonspecific chronic inflammation with a labeling index of 0.60 (0.04 percent). In postatrophic hyperplasia without carcinoma, 11 cases revealed a labeling index of 1.60 (0.8 percent). However, in primary atypical epithelial hyperplasia where there was marked structural atypia in the vicinity of adenocarcinoma, a labeling index of 1.50 (0.84 percent) was found. The single values ranged from 0.2 to 4.1 percent. This labeling index is similar to that of the poorly differentiated (Gleason score 8 to 10) adenocarcinomas of the prostate (0.2 to 2.4 percent) as well as to that of the cribriform

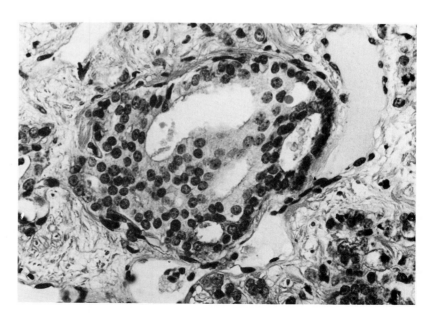

Figure 17–11. Light microscopic photomicrograph of the commonly found cribriform pattern of carcinoma, somewhat similar to the pseudocribriform pattern of primary atypical epithelial hyperplasia.

patterns of carcinoma (0.4 to 5.7 percent). Helpap also determined that the average duration of the DNA-synthesis phase (S-phase) was 9.5 hours, which is not significantly different from that of simple and primary atypical epithelial hyperplasia or from carcinoma. It was concluded from the autoradiographic studies that the labeling index of primary atypical epithelial hyperplasia was three times higher than that of simple hyperplasia. However, the labeling index of primary atypical epithelial hyperplasia was similar to that of the poorly differentiated adenocarcinomas and/or the cribriform patterns of carcinoma of the prostate. The similar labeling indexes of primary atypical epithelial hyperplasia and carcinoma suggest that the former is a precursor for carcinoma of the prostate. Clinically, therefore, those patients with only primary atypical epithelial hyperplasia with marked cellular and structural atypia but without definitive carcinoma in the needle biopsy or transurethral resection material should be reexamined periodically.

EARLY DETECTION OF PROSTATIC CANCER OR MINIMALLY INVASIVE CANCER BY CYTOLOGY

Until now, there has been a great reluctance on the part of many American pathologists to examine aspiration biopsies of the prostate. Most urologists prefer the traditional transperineal Vim-Silverman needle biopsy, and so most American pathologists have had little opportunity to examine thin-needle aspiration biopsies for carcinoma of the prostate (Tannenbaum, 1983).

In the Scandinavian countries as well as throughout other parts of Europe, transrectal fine-needle aspiration biopsy is the preferred method for the diagnosis of prostatic carcinoma (Epstein, 1976; Esposti, 1966; Sparwasser, 1970; Ventura et al., 1977). Unfortunately, little attention has been paid to this type of biopsy in the American literature. Only Rheinfrank and Nulf (1969) and Kline and coworkers (1977) have reported using this technique. The diagnosis of prostatic carcinoma by aspiration biopsy was first described by Ferguson in 1930. Although at first he intended to obtain a small core of tissue, instead he made smears and stained them with hematoxylin and eosin, as has been the practice at Memorial Center for Cancer since the advent of the needle aspiration biopsy at that institution (Ferguson, 1930). No results were given in Ferguson's paper, and the method was not used again until 1960, when Franzen and colleagues published a report describing their preliminary results with the transrectal biopsy.

Biopsy Site

Carcinoma of the prostate can produce solitary nodules, local induration, or nodular and diffuse enlarge-

ments, all resulting in abnormal palpable masses that are targets for aspiration biopsy.

For purposes of obtaining material for aspiration cytology, the concept of the biopsy site being the posterior (dorsal) lobe is the most practical. Transrectal digital palpation of the posterior "lobe" and formulation of a clinical impression are the initial diagnostic maneuvers (Emmet et al., 1962). The prostate gland will then be considered normal, pathologic with benign changes, suspicious for malignancy, or clinically malignant.

In several studies in which the palpatory findings, including stony induration, were judged suspicious or malignant, the diagnosis was correct in 50 percent of the cases (Emmet et al., 1962; Jewett, 1956; Sika and Lindquist, 1963). Emmet has summarized almost 2800 cases in which the preoperative clinical evaluation indicated benign disease. From 4.6 percent to 29.4 percent were found to be carcinoma. In a more recent study, digital rectal examination was found to have a higher degree of accuracy. By carefully grouping palpatory findings, Esposti, a clinical cytopathologist, was able to increase the accuracy of digital examination (Esposti, 1974). He divided his clinical cases into the following four groups:

Group I—Clinically benign
Group II—Cancer, slightly probable
Group III—Cancer, probable
Group IV—Clinically cancer

Consequently, he was able to demonstrate cytomorphologically the percentages of cancer to be 62.4 percent and 89.0 percent in Groups III and IV, respectively. In Group I, only 1 of 175 tumors was cytologically cancer.

Urinary cytology of exfoliated cells, expressed by massaging a clinically suspicious gland, can provide diagnostic cells. This procedure is considered to be of only limited value (Kaufman and Schultz, 1962).

Adequacy of Tissue Sample

Aspiration cytology of the prostate gland was first reported by Ferguson in 1930. He used a sterile Record syringe with a 15 cm. 18 gauge needle and obtained a representative tissue sample in 70 percent of the patients using the transperineal approach. This material was evaluated cytologically, but the diagnostic procedure did not receive general acceptance (Ferguson, 1930). It was not until 1960 that a flexible transrectal fine-needle method was introduced by Franzen and colleagues. Since then, many reports of its use have appeared and thousands of biopsies have been performed (Alfthan et al., 1970; Bishop and Oliver, 1970; Epstein, 1976; Esposti, 1966; Esposti, 1974; Franzen et al., 1960; Williams et al., 1967).

Clinical selection of patients determines the yield of carcinoma. At the Karolinska Hospital, approximately 30 percent of the patients are diagnosed as having carcinoma. In contrast, Linsk, who receives all his referrals from one urology source, finds that well over 60 percent of patients have cancer.

Where slides are submitted for cytologic evaluation, clinical data supplied by the clinician are helpful. More important, however, is the assurance that the aspiration and the smears are technically satisfactory. Fixation of tissue free from artifact is especially important because of the small number of aspirated cells that are obtained from the prostate. Technical problems can be minimized if there is cooperation between the cytologist and the clinician.

What is Observed?

Granulomatous Prostatitis. Chronic inflammation may produce localized or diffuse induration that becomes a target for puncture. Granulomatous inflammation may also produce localized induration. This type of inflammation was clinically confused with cancer in 69 percent of cases on initial examination (Taylor et al., 1977).

Normal prostate epithelium may be absent, although islands of benign epithelium, often atypical, may be scattered through the inflammatory exudate. Individual cells, often stripped or degenerated, may be present in the background and can be confused with poorly differentiated cancer cells. The nuclear chromatin pattern is fine and ill-defined. Nucleoli are rarely or faintly seen. Sheets of benign cells may be accompanied by prostatic debris, usually inspissated secretions within glandular structures.

Malignant Lesions. The aspirate from prostate carcinoma will contain many cells if the needle has been well placed. Cancer is usually quite evident, and scanning is usually not necessary. In experienced hands, isolated clusters of tumor cells in a predominantly benign smear may be enough to define the diagnosis as malignant. Cancer cells may be grossly crowded together, and, under high power, careful examination at the edge of a dense cluster will reveal the cytologic changes of cancer. However, stripped nuclei should be considered cautiously, and only in the context of the entire smear. Distorted benign nuclei may simulate cancer cells. In the hands of a trained cytopathologist, the diagnosis of carcinoma emerges with the recognition of cytologic variations from normal epithelium.

Can Malignancy be Graded?

Grading of prostatic carcinoma correlates with survival when the cytologic changes in the sections form the basis for the grading (Kahler, 1939). This parallels cytologic grading. An attempt at histologic grading based on growth pattern was unsuccessful because of variation within the section (Vickery and Kerr, 1963).

Cytologic grading of malignancy has great clinical significance, since it serves as a guide for the clinician in the choice of therapy (Esposti, 1971 and 1974). Patterns have been established by Esposti, although other observers do not agree (Epstein, 1976; Esposti, 1974).

Grade I: Well-Differentiated Cancer. Identification of Grade I cancer is simplified by the presence of numerous adenomatous structures on the smear. Nuclear chromatin is irregular, and nucleoli of varying size and shape may be seen. Atypia in the absence of the adenomatous changes is considered insufficient alteration for the specific diagnosis of well-differentiated carcinoma.

Grade II: Moderately Differentiated Cancer. In Grade II carcinoma there is some retention of the microadenomatous structure but with greater cellular atypia, larger nucleoli, and, in general, a greater deviation from benign morphology.

Grade III: Poorly Differentiated Cancer. Cells are enlarged, irregular in size and shape, and dissociated.

Are There False Negative and False Positive Results?

False negative results occur in most reported cytologic series as well as in core histologic biopsy series (Kaufman et al., 1954; Lin et al., 1979; Shepard, 1968). They vary from 10 percent to 30 percent. In experienced hands, they are primarily the result of nonrepresentative sampling, especially with small lesions. They may also result from underestimation of atypical cellular findings (DeGaetani and Trentini, 1978). The results of core biopsy for tissue parallel those of fine needle aspiration biopsy, and it is unusual to request core biopsy because of negative fine needle aspiration (Alfthan et al., 1970; Epstein, 1976; Kline et al., 1977). Concomitant core biopsy and fine needle aspiration have been suggested but appear unwarranted because of the ease and convenience of the fine needle and the resulting minimal additional diagnostic yield that simultaneous use would provide.

False positive cytologic diagnoses, that is, cases not confirmed by histologic examination, have been reported (Ekman et al., 1967; Lin et al., 1979; Ventura et al., 1977). Several morphologic changes can be confused with carcinoma. These occur in the following disorders and situations.

1. *Atypical epithelial hyperplasia.* Atypical epithelial hyperplasia is one pitfall in the diagnosis of cancer. Indeed, such a benign proliferation may be mistaken for poorly differentiated cancer and result in a false positive diagnosis (De Gaetani and Trentini, 1978). Criteria that can be used to identify carcinoma include coarse, uneven chromatin, large irregular nucleoli, and irregular hyperchromatic nuclei.

2. *Granulomatous prostatitis.* Atypical epithelium

suspicious for carcinoma has been reported in granulomatous prostatitis (Taylor et al., 1977).

3. *Seminal vesicle puncture.* Atypical and bizarre cells are seen in seminal vesicle punctures and must be distinguished from cancer (Koivuniemi and Tyrkko, 1976).

Hormonal Effects Can Be Measured

Administration of female hormones may produce cellular alteration in hormonally sensitive tumors (well- and moderately differentiated types) (Williams et al., 1967; Zajieck, 1979). Large glycogen or squamoid cells are often attached to intact clusters of tumor cells. This response may take several months and may be complete or incomplete on follow-up puncture. Failure to convert to glycogen in the cells is evidence that the tumor is not hormonally responsive.

Nonprostatic Epithelium Is Observed

Transitional Cell Carcinoma. Malignant transitional epithelium is infrequently obtained by transrectal aspiration. These tumors arise from the prostatic urethra or prostatic ducts and grow in the central portion of the prostate gland. Deep penetration of the needle will reach such tumors. Adenocarcinoma may occur simultaneously, and a mixture of transitional and adenocarcinoma cells may be seen on the smear. Transitional cells can be recognized by an eccentric nucleus and well-defined cytoplasm, which may assume a pointed geometric pattern. The majority of these malignant tumors of the urethra and the periurethral prostatic ducts are generally detected preoperatively by cytologic examination of freshly voided urine.

Seminal Vesicle Epithelium. If seminal vesicle epithelium does occur, it may yield large atypical cells that must be identified and distinguished from poorly differentiated prostatic cancer.

Clinical Application

Transrectal core biopsy failed to gain general acceptance for years because of fear of infection or fistula and, presumably, because of inertia (Emmet et al., 1962). With the fine-needle technique, fistula formation is nonexistent and infection is not clinically significant. This technique provides diagnostic material in inflammatory and neoplastic diseases of the prostate with a high degree of specificity. The procedure is essentially atraumatic, and repeat punctures are accepted by patients. It is particularly useful as an outpatient screening procedure.

Results of Prostatic Aspirations

The number of reported series is insufficient to make an accurate assessment of the results of fine-needle aspiration biopsy. For example, rates of accuracy reportedly range from 63 percent (Sunderland and Lederer, 1971) to 91 percent (Rheinfrank and Nulf, 1969). Only one report states a false negative rate (17.7 percent) in hormonally treated patients (Schulte-Wissermann and Luchtrath, 1971). Two others report false positive rates of 2 percent and 28 percent (Ventura et al., 1977). From some of these reports, it is not possible to determine how many cases were actually biopsied.

Table 17–1 summarizes four series in which there are sufficient data to calculate both sensitivity and specificity.

All authors agree that the ease and convenience of the fine-needle aspiration makes it the preferred initial biopsy procedure for the diagnosis of prostatic cancer. If clinical suspicion of tumor remains after a negative needle aspiration, then either a repeat aspiration or a tissue needle biopsy should be recommended. Several authors also note that performing multiple aspirations not only of the nodule but also of other areas of the prostate at the same examination may increase diagnostic accuracy (Ekman et al., 1967; Staehler et al., 1975).

MORPHOLOGIC GRADING OF MINIMAL INVASIVE PROSTATIC CARCINOMA

There have been many attempts to grade prostatic cancer. Some of these attempts have also included a combination of the morphologic grade with the clinical staging especially noting the degree of lymph node

Table 17–1. **Results of Selected Series of Fine-needle Aspiration Biopsies of Prostate***

Reference	True Positive	False Positive	True Negative	False Negative	Sensitivity (%)	Specificity (%)	Unsatisfactory
Faul et al.	24	1	81	4	86	99	16
Esposti	60	4	101	5	92	96	4
Bishop and Oliver	37	1	113	1	97	99	30
Williams et al.	33	0	15	3	91	100	12

*See Frable, 1983.

involvement. Some attempts have been made to even predict clinical invasiveness, that is, the breakout from tissue glandular architecture and/or metastases to lymph nodes, by exclusively utilizing the morphologic glandular architecture and assigning a numerical grade to the various glandular patterns (Tannenbaum, 1983).

The histologic grading of prostatic cancer is considered to be of great clinical significance, and consequently it has assumed a primary position in the histologic evaluation of surgically removed tissue (Murphy, 1978). Clinical decisions may be influenced by the histologic grading, particularly if the primary cancer is considered to be aggressive and should be treated at an earlier stage. For many years it was thought that the greater the degree of dedifferentiation of the primary prostatic tumor, the greater is its invasive ability or the more likely it will be associated with an advanced clinical stage (Murphy, 1979). As a consequence, several major grading systems have been devised by pathologists and urologists. The Gleason system has been adopted as a histologic reference for classifying patients with this disease (Murphy, 1979).

Gleason Classification or Histologic Grading of Carcinoma of the Prostate

The Gleason system depends on histologic patterns rather than on the nuclear details of the glands prevalent within the small biopsies obtained. The system is used by several institutions because it appears to have some predictability as to the extent of lymph node involvement. The Gleason score (Gleason, 1977) is based on the histologic evaluation of the prostatic tissue obtained by biopsy. First, we determine the primary pattern, that is, the morphologic pattern of the tumor glandular configuration that is most prevalent within the piece or pieces of tissue obtained. In addition to the primary pattern, we must ascertain a secondary pattern, which is the second most prevalent type found within the same tissue. The primary and secondary patterns are added to obtain the Gleason score. This system of grading does not necessarily reflect what are the ''best'' and ''worst'' forms of the cancer but rather those patterns that predominate within the biopsy or tissue obtained.

A brief description of the various five Gleason patterns is presented here. All these patterns are tabulated in Table 17–2.

Pattern 1. This is a well-differentiated pattern in which the tumor consists of single, separated, round-to-oval glands that are uniform in size.

Pattern 2. The tumor is well differentiated and made up of single, but separate, round-to-oval glands. These glands are similar in size and shape to those found in Pattern 1, but in Pattern 2 they are more variable. There is also some stromal spacing between the glands.

Pattern 3. This pattern of carcinoma is moderately well differentiated; it is the most common pattern found and consists of two distinctive appearances. One exhibits the papillary or cribriform variety of tumor that is confined in a smooth and sharply delimited rounded mass. The second variety may be either of a small-gland or a large-gland variety. These glands demonstrate a marked variation in size and shape and are usually separated by more than one gland diameter. The boundary of the tumor is usually poorly defined. These patterns are usually associated with invasion of the stroma and may not be detected clinically. However, they may be detected initially in transurethral resection chips. In terms of invasion, this is one form of the *minimally invasive type of prostatic cancer.*

Pattern 4. This form of prostate tumor is poorly

Table 17–2. **Histologic Patterns of Adenocarcinoma of the Prostate***

Pattern	Margins of Tumors Areas	Gland Pattern	Gland Size	Gland Distribution	Stromal Invasion
1	Well defined	Single, separate, round	Medium	Closely packed	Minimal, expansile
2	Less definite	Single, separate, rounded, but more variable	Medium	Spaced up to one gland diameter, average	Mild, in larger stromal planes
3 or	Poorly defined	Single, separate, more irregular	Small, medium, or large	Spaced more than one gland diameter, rarely packed	Moderate, in larger or smaller stromal planes
3	Poorly defined	Rounded masses of cribriform or papillary epithelium	Medium or large	Rounded masses with smooth sharp edges	Expansile masses
4	Ragged infiltrating	Fused glandular masses or ''hypernephroid''	Small	Fused in ragged masses	Marked, through smaller planes
5 or	Ragged, infiltrating	Almost absent, few tiny glands or signet ring cells	Small	Ragged anaplastic masses of epithelium	Severe, between stromal fibers or destructive
5	Poorly defined	Few small lumina in rounded masses of solid epithelium central necrosis?	Small	Rounded masses and cords with smooth, sharp edges	Expansile masses

*See Gleason, 1977.

differentiated. The tumor may consist of irregular masses of fused glands. This means that the glands are not single and separated: that is, they are coalesced and branching. There may also be single glands that form lumens and glands with ragged and irregular edges. These patterns consist definitely of infiltrating glands and invariably constitute the condition clinically of *minimal invasive carcinoma of the prostate.* It is important to define this condition, and the Gleason classification is certainly helpful. As a result, there have been attempts to use the Gleason classification as a predictor of lymph node metastases, a point that is discussed later.

Pattern 5. This pattern consists of poorly differentiated prostatic cancer. In this instance, the cancer usually demonstrates minimal differentiation. It consists of a very raggedly infiltrating mass of epithelial cells with only a very few demonstrating occasional, poorly formed glandular lumen or signet ring cells, confirming that this is a primary prostatic adenocarcinoma. All of these patterns are tabulated in Table 17–2.

CLINICAL STAGING

Carcinomas of the prostate can also be grouped into four clinical stages. Clinical experience has shown a relationship of stage with the histologic progression of the tumor (Bailar et al., 1966).

Stage I Prostatic Cancer (Stage A). Usually, Stage I prostatic cancer refers to a latent or occult carcinoma, and histologically it represents a microscopic focal lesion within the prostate gland. It is not uncommon to further divide occult cancer of the prostate into stages A_1 and A_2. The distinction of A_2 disease depends on whether the tumor is found in less than, or more than, three high-power microscopic fields (Murphy et al., 1980). Commonly, these Stage I lesions consist of a Grade 1 tumor that is usually a well-differentiated adenocarcinoma (Gleason Grades 1 and 2). On careful examination of surgical pathology material, it appears that these types of cancer are usually found in men over the age of 45. In Grade I prostatic cancers (Gleason Grades 1 and 2), these latent foci are usually 80 times or more histologically prevalent than the palpable or symptomatic clinical prostatic cancer (Ashley, 1965; Mostofi and Price, 1973). These well-differentiated Grade I, Stage I carcinomas are usually not associated with elevated levels of serum prostatic acid phosphatase.

Stage II Prostatic Cancer (Stage B). Clinically this stage represents a nodule that is histologically and anatomically confined to the prostate gland and which is detected on rectal examination. Tumors are usually histologic Grade I or II (Gleason Grades 1, 2, and 3) (Culp, 1968; Kirchheim et al., 1966). These types of cancer are usually not associated with a rise in the serum prostatic acid phosphatase. There are subdivisions in the B category in which the cancers are subdivided into Stages B_1 and B_2. Stage B_1 denotes that the tumor is a small discrete nodule that is confined to a single lobe of the prostate, and Stage B_2 consists of larger areas or multiple nodules of tumor confined to the prostate.

Stage III Prostatic Cancer (Stage C). These types are usually associated with *clinical signs of invasion* of an adjacent organ such as the seminal vesicle. Clinical Stage C_1 means that there is an invasive tumor that is not actually involving the seminal vesicle but is still localized within the prostate gland, whereas Stage C_2 involves the seminal vesicle. Frequently, there are mixtures of various grades of malignancy and a tumor may contain Grades II, III (Gleason Grade 4), and sometimes even a Grade IV (Gleason Grade 5). Histologic grades other than the Gleason are defined in detail later. Patients with these types may or may not have elevated levels of serum prostatic acid phosphatase.

Stage IV Prostatic Cancer (Stage D). In clinical Stage D disease, the cancers are clinically manifested by metastases to regional or distant lymph nodes. There may be pelvic node metastases sometimes associated with ureteral obstruction and hydronephrosis. Metastases to organs such as bone, liver, and so on do occur. Serum prostatic acid phosphatase is usually elevated.

Gleason Grading and Lymph Node Metastases

Prostatic cancer spreads via hematogenous routes as well as through lymphatic channels. As a consequence, there has been a tendency to correlate clinical staging with the percentage of lymph node involvement as well as using the Gleason classification alone as the sole predictor of the percentage of lymph node metastases. This will be discussed subsequently. Even when the lesions are in the Stage A category (more specifically the Stage A_2), and apparently confined to the prostate, in more than three high-power microscopic fields, there is still some predictability that lymph node metastases will occur (see Table 17–3) (Murphy, 1981). We will also consider combining the Gleason histologic grading with staging, but first let us review the data which have been obtained using the Gleason system alone in predicting lymph node involvement.

Recently, Kramer et al. have used the Gleason grading in an attempt to evaluate what percentage of their surgical staged cases had lymph node metastases. They have stated that clinical staging is inaccurate as a predictor of the biologic potential of prostate cancer and, consequently, they were prompted to evaluate this type of cancer by other means. They reviewed 228 patients with prostatic adenocarcinoma who were seen over a period of four years. Of these

Table 17–3. **Incidence of Positive Lymph Nodes in Relation to Clinical Stage‡**

Clinical Stage	Percentage of Lymph Nodes Positive	
A$_1$	0*	0†
A$_2$	24	18
B$_1$	15	11
B$_2$	38	22
C	47	33

*Material discussed by Dr. R. Correa, Virginia Mason Hospital, Jan. 14, 1979 (343 cases).

†Material discussed by Dr. E. Carlton, Baylor University, Jan. 14, 1979 (295 cases).

‡See Murphy, 1981.

228 patients, 144 had no detectable bone disease and as a result underwent pelvic lymphadenectomy staging, with or without preliminary bilateral pedal lymphangiography. The primary prostatic biopsies were classified by the Gleason grading system of tumor differentiation. Of the patients with Gleason scores 8, 9, or 10, 93 percent had regional lymph node metastases, regardless of the preliminary clinical stage. Furthermore, no patient with a Gleason score of 2 to 4 had lymph node metastases. The incidence of falsely positive and falsely negative lymphangiograms was 29 and 35 percent respectively, reflecting the unreliability of pedal lymphangiography in predicting lymph node involvement in patients with prostatic cancer. They concluded that the Gleason system was reliable and reproducible and provided a more accurate prediction of the surgical stage of the disease.

On the other hand, Gaeta has also tried to correlate the Gleason patterns with surgical staging of the disease. He found that there were patients with Gleason scores of 3 or 4 who had lymph node metastases. They constituted approximately 33 percent of the stage D disease cases. Consequently, Gaeta devised his own system of grading that assesses glandular profiles as well as cellular nuclear patterns.

In all of these studies, the Gleason classification has been used extensively as a reference. Gleason has also studied the extent of the tumor in transurethral resection and prostatectomy specimens. Interestingly, Gleason's data reveal that the higher grade tumors (scores of 7 to 10) involve, in most instances, more than 50 percent of the tissue, whereas the lower grade tumors (2 to 5) involve less than 50 percent. The higher grade tumors (scores 8 to 10) were noted to involve lymph nodes in 93 percent of cases (Kramer, 1980). From both these studies, can it then be inferred that a critical volume of tumor is needed before metastasis can occur?

Gleason has also tried to correlate the extent of tumor in the transurethral resection specimens with the histologic pattern scores (Table 17–4). The higher grade tumors tend to involve a larger portion of the resected tissue than the lower grade tumors. There was also a correlation between death rates and the extent of the tumor, but this was less significant than the correlation between the extent of the tumor and tumor grade.

Gleason Grading of Prostatic Cancer and Acid Phosphatase Secretion

There are varying degrees of differentiation in adenocarcinomas of the prostate. The clinical behavior of these cancers demonstrates a broad spectrum of variation in different individuals. Prostatic cancer may remain localized for many years without clinical manifestations or it may spread to various organs and cause enzyme elevations in the blood (Gutman and Gutman, 1938). In many patients, the cancer cells maintain their synthetic activity and continue to be dependent on androgens for their secretory function, as well as for structural differentiation and growth (Brandes et al., 1964). It is important that some type of structural-functional organization of the prostatic cancer cell be established and correlated with its secretory ability (that is, the release of prostatic acid phosphatase either into the lumen of the gland or into the blood stream where the elevated levels can be detected). At the present time there is no immunohistochemical correlation with the various histologic patterns—that is, the Gleason classification for prostatic carcinoma and prostatic acid phosphatase secretion—nor have many ultrastructural studies of prostatic cancer been conducted to determine whether such patterns might relate to prostate grade and clinical aggressiveness (Brandes and Kirchheim, 1977).

Table 17–4. **Extent of Tumor by Histologic Pattern Score (TUR and Prostatectomy Specimens, Only)***

Pattern Score	Percent Area Involved by Tumor					
	< 5%	5–9%	10–19%	20–49%	≥ 50%	Total (%)
2–3	40	40	17	3	0	100
4–5	17	25	22	23	13	100
6	7	12	11	27	43	100
7–8	4	5	5	20	66	100
9–10	4	3	4	19	70	100

*See Gleason, 1977.

Gleason Grading and Ultrastructural Features of Prostatic Cancer Cells

Nonmalignant glands are usually characterized by the presence of well-developed glandular lumens. However, prostatic carcinomas may also form lumens. Therefore, other criteria are needed to evaluate the degree of malignancy in those carcinomas that form glands. By light microscopy, the presence of prominent eosinophilic nucleoli has been considered indicative of prostatic malignancy. In fact this histologic finding has been especially useful in distinguishing well-differentiated prostatic cancers from normal glands (Tannenbaum, 1977; Totten et al., 1953). Furthermore, for prostatic cancer, some light microscopic grading systems have used nucleolar prominence as a criterion for higher grade disease (Harada et al., 1966; Mostofi, 1970).

With these facts in mind, Tannenbaum et al. (1982) investigated nucleolar ultrastructure and size as an indicator of tumor aggressiveness. A retrospective study was conducted on 52 patients with localized and metastatic carcinomas of the prostate. Nucleolar surface area measurements were made by stereologically analyzing pictures obtained by the backscattered electron imaging (BEI) attachment to a scanning electron microscope (SEM). The data obtained were compared with the Gleason grading system, which is based on light microscopic glandular patterns. In patients with no evidence of disease three years or more after radical prostatectomy, the initial biopsy demonstrated nucleolar surface areas that averaged 1.28 μm^2 (range 0.60 to 2.27 μm^2), whereas patients with metastases or those dying of their cancer exhibited an average nucleolar surface area of 5.17 μm^2 (range 2.49 to 10.01 μm^2). With only one exception, progressive disease was always associated with nucleolar measurements larger than 2.40 μm^2. Nucleolar surface measurements exhibited a close correlation between the initial biopsy and the radical prostatectomy specimen. In contrast, the Gleason grades varied by more than 30 percent between the initial and final specimens in 70 percent of cases. Only 9 of 16 patients with aggressive disease ever demonstrated Gleason grades above 6. The development of a nucleolar grading system may provide a means of determining prognosis in prostatic cancer that complements the Gleason light microscopic grading system.

There are other ultrastructural features that exhibit changes when the different grades or Gleason patterns are reexamined. The major ultrastructural specializations of the secretory apparatus of the prostate, that is, the Golgi apparatus and its secretory vacuoles, are located in the apical and supranuclear regions of each nonmalignant prostatic luminal surface cell. These cells line the acini as well as many of the branching prostatic ducts. By means of immunoperoxidase techniques, these secretory regions can be seen to contain prostatic acid phosphatase. Each acinus is surrounded by an abundant amount of connective tissue stroma as well as an occasional smooth muscle cell. Beneath the surface cells, the non-secretory small basal cell or reserve cells can be found interposed between the basement membrane and the surrounding connective tissue stroma. These basal cells are usually attached to the basement membrane. The basement membrane forms a continuous layer or external wall at the nonluminal outer surface of the plasma membrane of the basal cell.

Histochemical examination of prostatic tissue reveals that there are alterations of several enzymes that are, most likely, connected with the secretory mechanisms of the gland. A significant decrease or deletion of these mechanisms occurs in the prostate cancer cell. This can be shown ultrastructurally as well as immunohistochemically, and the phenomenon appears to be related to the degree of dedifferentiation. In normal prostatic epithelial surface cells that line the lumen, prostatic acid phosphatase is localized in the supranuclear region. This corresponds to the region of the Golgi apparatus as well as to the area that is occupied by secretory vacuoles and lysosomes (Kirchheim et al., 1974). These enzymes are normally secreted into the lumen of the acini. Histochemically, there is a decreased intensity of staining for these enzymes in moderately differentiated adenocarcinomas. There is even a greater loss of activity in the more poorly differentiated and invasive prostatic cancer cells. To a great degree, the magnitude of this physiological and anatomic dedifferentiation can be related ultrastructurally to the grade of the tumor and, in many instances, also to the stage of the tumor.

Grade I Prostatic Carcinoma (Gleason Grade 1 or 2). By means of light microscopy, it can be seen that the glandular architecture of these cells does not significantly differ from that of adjacent normal glands. In many instances, these cells will have prominent nucleoli of varying size. In Grade I tumors (Gleason Grades 1 or 2) there are no ultrastructural changes that are readily discernible in terms of cytoplasmic dedifferentiation. The cells retain their normal secretory polarity and are arranged around a central lumen. As in normal cells, the secretory vacuoles and Golgi elements are concentrated in the apical pole of the surface cell.

Grade II Prostatic Carcinoma (Gleason Grade 3). The basal cells are conspicuously absent and the central lumens of the acini are replaced by more rudimentary slitlike structures that are probably not connected with the secretory duct. The glands are in a back-to-back arrangement, and there is usually deletion of the interstitial connective tissue and smooth muscle cells that are normally found between the glands. The basement membrane is lost, and the loss of polarity is reflected in terms of ultrastructural cellular displacement of the Golgi complex and secretory vacuoles from the supranuclear region and location toward other areas of the cell. This is *ultrastructurally the minimal invasive form of prostatic cancer.*

Grade III Prostatic Cancer (Gleason Grade 4). Lumen formation is frequently seen by light microscopy and, ultrastructurally, the lumen may be seen as thin narrow spaces. The polarity of secretion of the Golgi apparatus is completely lost even though the secretory vacuoles may be abundant and scattered throughout the cytoplasm. There is thus a lack of supranuclear polarity that is usually exhibited by normal cells.

Grade IV Prostatic Carcinoma (Gleason Grade 5). Here the tumor cells are arranged in cords and clusters, and they extensively infiltrate the surrounding stroma as well as the periprostatic lymphatic channels. Ultrastructural lumen formation can be seen only as intracellular lumina which are reminiscent of the early fetal stages described in other glands (Shepard, 1968). The cells retain only a few secretory features such as secretory vacuoles and bizarre cisternal spaces that are probably of Golgi origin. The carcinoma cells that lie within the lymphatic channels show total loss of polarity, and their secretory vacuoles probably empty into the surrounding space. This feature possibly explains the elevated serum prostatic acid phosphatase levels in those cases in which the tumor is both invasive and metastastic.

References

Alfthan, O., Klintrup, H.E., Koivuniemi, A., et al.: Cytological aspiration biopsy and Vim-Silverman biopsy in the diagnosis of prostatic carcinoma. Ann. Chir. Gynaecol. 59:226–229, 1970.

Ashley, D.J.B.: On the incidence of carcinomas of the prostate. J. Pathol. Bacteriol. 90:217–224, 1965.

Bailar, J.C., III, Mellinger, G.T., Gleason, D.F.: Survival rates of patients with prostatic cancer, tumor stage, and differentiation. Cancer Chemotherapy Rep. 50:129–136, 1966.

Bishop, D., and Oliver, J.A.: A study of transrectal aspiration biopsies of the prostate with particular regard to prognostic evaluation. J. Urol. 117:313–315, 1977.

Brandes, D., Kirchheim, D., Scott, W.W.: Ultrastructure of the human prostate: Normal and neoplastic. Lab. Invest. 13:1541–1560, 1964.

Brandes, D., Kirchheim, D.: Histochemistry of the prostate, *In*: Tannenbaum, M. (Ed.), Urologic Pathology: The Prostate. Philadelphia, 1977, Lea & Febiger, pp. 99–128.

Culp, O.S.: Radical perineal prostatectomy. J. Urol. 98:618–626, 1968.

DeGaetani, C.F., Trentini, G.P.: Atypical hyperplasia of the prostate: A pitfall in the cytologic diagnosis of carcinoma. Acta Cytol. 22:483–486, 1978.

Ekman, H., Hedberg, K., Persson, P.S.: Cytological versus histological examination of needle biopsy specimens in the diagnosis of prostatic cancer. Br. J. Urol. 39:544–548, 1967.

Emmet, J.L., Barber, K.W., Jr., Jackman, R.J.: Transrectal biopsy to detect prostatic carcinoma. J. Urol. 87:460–466, 1962.

Epstein, N.A.: Prostatic biopsy: A morphological correlation of aspiration cytology and needle biopsy histology. Cancer 38:2078–2087, 1976.

Esposti, P.: Cytologic diagnosis of prostatic tumors with the aid of transrectal aspiration biopsy. A critical review of 1,110 cases and a report of morphologic and cytochemical studies. Acta Cytol. 10:182–186, 1966.

Esposti, P.L.: Cytologic malignancy grading of prostatic carcinoma by transrectal aspiration biopsy. Scand. J. Urol. Nephrol. 5:199–209, 1971.

Esposti, P.L.: Aspiration biopsy cytology in the diagnosis and management of prostatic carcinoma. Stockholm, 1974, Stähl and Accidens Tryck.

Faul, P., Klosterhalfen, H., Schmiedt, E.: Erfahrungen mit der feinnadebiopsie (Saug-bzw aspirationsbiopsie nach Franzen) der prostata. Urologe 10:120–129, 1971.

Ferguson, R.S.: Prostatic neoplasms, their diagnosis by needle puncture and aspiration. Am. J. Surg. 9:507–511, 1930.

Frable, W.J.: Thin-needle aspiration biopsy. Philadelphia, 1983, W.B. Saunders Co., pp. 275–285.

Franks, L.M.: Atrophy and hyperplasia in the prostate proper. J. Path. Bacteriol. 68:617–622, 1954b.

Franzen, S., Giertz, G., Zajicek, J.: Cytological diagnosis of prostatic tumours by transrectal aspiration biopsy. Br. J. Urol. 32:193–196, 1960.

Gaeta, J.F.: Glandular profiles and cellular patterns in prostatic cancer grading. Urology 17:33–37, 1981.

Gleason, D.F.: Histologic grading and clinical staging of prostatic carcinoma. *In*: Tannenbaum, M. (Ed.), Urologic Pathology: The Prostate. Philadelphia, 1977, Lea & Febiger, pp. 177–198.

Gutman, A.B., Gutman, E.B.: An 'acid' phosphatase occurring in the serum of patients with metastasizing carcinoma of the prostate gland. J. Clin. Invest. 17:473–478, 1938.

Harada, M., et al.: Preliminary studies of histologic prognosis in cancer of the prostate. Cancer Treat. Rep. 61:223–227, 1966.

Helpap, B.: The biological significance of atypical hyperplasia of the prostate. Virchows Arch. Path. Anat. Histol. 387:307–317, 1980.

Jewett, H.J.: Significance of the palpable prostatic nodule. J.A.M.A. 160:838–839, 1956.

Kahler, J.E.: Carcinoma of the prostate gland: J. Urol. 41:557–561, 1939.

Kastendieck, H.: Correlations between atypical primary hyperplasia and carcinoma of the prostate. Path. Res. Pract. 169:366–387, 1980.

Kastendieck, H., Altenähr, E., Hüsselman, H., Bressel, M.: Carcinoma and dysplastic lesions of the prostate. A histomorphological analysis of 50 total prostatectomies by step-section technique. Z. Krebsforsch. 88:33–54, 1976.

Kaufman, J.J., Rosenthal, M., Goodwin, W.E.: Methods of diagnosis of carcinoma of the prostate: A comparison of clinical impression, prostatic smear, needle biopsy, open perineal biopsy and transurethral biopsy. J. Urol. 72:450–465, 1954.

Kaufman, J.J., Schultz, J.L.: Needle biopsy of the prostate. A re-evaluation. J. Urol. 87:164–167, 1962.

Kirchheim, D., Brandes, D., Bacon, R.L.: Fine structure and cytochemistry of human prostatic carcinoma. *In*: Brandes, D. (Ed.), Male Accessory Sex Organs: Structure and Function in Mammals. New York, 1974, Academic Press, pp. 397–405.

Kirchheim, D., Niles, N.R., Frankus, E., et al.: Correlated histochemical and histological studies on thirty radical prostatectomy specimens. Cancer 19:1683–1696, 1966.

Kline, T.S., Kelsey, D.M., Kohler, F.P.: Prostatic carcinoma and needle aspiration biopsy. Am. J. Clin. Pathol. 67:131–136, 1977.

Koivuniemi, A., Tyrkko, J.: Seminal vesicle epithelium in fine-needle aspiration biopsies of the prostate as a pitfall in the cytologic diagnosis of carcinoma. Acta Cytol. 20:116–119, 1976.

Kramer, A.S., Spahr, J., Brendler, C.B., et al.: Experience with Gleason's histopathologic grading in prostate cancer. J. Urol. 124:223–225, 1980.

Lin, B.P.C., Davies, W.E.L., Harmata, P.A.: Prostatic aspiration cytology. Pathology 11:607–614, 1979.

Linsk, J.A., Franzen, S.: Clinical Aspiration Cytology. Philadelphia, 1983, J.B. Lippincott, pp. 243–266.

Mostofi, F.K.: Carcinoma of the prostate. *In*: Riches, E. (Ed.), Modern Trends in Urology, London, 1970, Butterworths, pp. 231–263.

Mostofi, F.K., Price, E.B.: Tumors of the Male Genital System, 2nd series, Fascicle 8. Washington, D.C., Armed Forces Institute of Pathology, 1973.

Murphy, G.P.: Prostate cancer: Progress and change. Ca-A Cancer J. Clinicians 28:104–115, 1978.

Murphy, G.P., Whitmore, W.F., Jr.: A report of the workshops on the current status of the histologic grading of prostate cancer. Cancer 44:1490–1494, 1979.

Murphy, G.P., Gaeta, J.F., Pickren, J., et al.: Current status of classification and staging of prostate cancer. Cancer 45: 1889–1985, 1980.

Murphy, G.P.: Prostate cancer: Continuing progress. Ca-A Cancer J. Clinicians 31:96–110, 1981.

Rheinfrank, R.E., Nulf, T.H.: Fine needle aspiration biopsy of the prostate. Endoscopy 1:27–32, 1969.

Schulte-Wissermann, H., Luchtrath, H.: Aspirationsbiopsie und cytologie beim prostatacarcinom. Virchows Arch. Pathol. Anat. Physiol. 352:122–129, 1971.

Shepard, T.H.: Development of the human fetal thyroid. Gen. Comp. Endocrinol. 10:174–181, 1968.

Sika, J.V., Lindquist, H.D.: Relationship of needle biopsy diagnosis of prostate to clinical signs of prostatic cancer. J. Urol. 69:737–741, 1963.

Sparwasser, K., Luchtrath, H.: Die transrectale saugbiopsie der prostata. Urologe 9:281–285, 1970.

Staehler, W., Ziegler, H., Volter, D. et al.: Zytodiagnostik der prostata. Stuttgart, 1975, Schattauer.

Sunderland, H., Lederer, H.: Prostatic aspiration biopsy. Br. J. Urol. 43:603–607, 1971.

Tannenbaum, M.: Histopathology of the prostate gland. In: Urologic Pathology: The Prostate, Tannenbaum, M. (Ed.). Philadelphia, 1977, Lea & Febiger, pp. 303–397.

Tannenbaum, M.: Urologic Pathology: The Prostate, Philadelphia, 1977, Lea & Febiger, pp. 365–367.

Tannenbaum, M., Tannenbaum, S., DeSanctis, P.N., et al.: Prognostic significance of nucleolar surface area in prostate cancer. Urology 19:546–551, 1982.

Tannenbaum, M.: Aspiration biopsy of the prostate: The pathologist's viewpoint. In: Seminars in Urology, Vaughan, E.D., Jr. (Ed.), Prostate Cancer: Current concepts and controversies, Part I (Olsson, C.A. Guest Ed.). New York, 1983, Grune & Stratton, pp. 172–175.

Tannenbaum, M.: Prostate cancer grading: Light and electron microscopy. In: Seminars in Urology, Vaughan, E.D., Jr. (Ed.), Prostate cancer: current concepts and controversies, Part I, Olsson, C.A. (Guest Ed.). New York, 1983, Grune & Stratton, pp. 186–192.

Taylor, E.W., Wheeler, R.F., Correa, R.J., Jr., et al.: Granulomatous prostatitis: Confusion clinically with carcinoma of the prostate. J. Urol. 117:316–319, 1977.

Totten, R.S., et al.: Microscopic differential diagnosis of latent carcinoma of the prostate. Arch. Pathol. 55:131–136, 1953.

Ventura, M., Barasolo, E., Morano, E., et al.: Franzen needle transrectal prostatic biopsy in the cytologic diagnosis of prostatic cancer. J. Urol. Nephrol. (Paris) 83:858–862, 1977.

Vickery, A.L., Kerr, W.S.: Carcinoma of the prostate treated by radical prostatectomy. Cancer 16:1598–1607, 1963.

Williams, J.P., Still, B.M., Pugh, R.C.B.: The diagnosis of prostatic cancer. Cytological and biomechanical studies using the Franzen biopsy needle. Br. J. Urol. 39:549–554, 1967.

Zajicek, J.: Aspiration biopsy cytology. II. Cytology of intradiaphragmatic organs. In: Monographs on Clinical Cytology, Wied, G.L. (Ed.). Basel, 1979, S. Karger.

ROBERT E. SCULLY

18 Testis

Classification

Precancerous lesions of the testis can be divided into three main categories: intratubular germ cell neoplasia, the apparent forerunner of invasive germ cell tumors in adults; gonadoblastomas, which occur almost exclusively in individuals who have dysgenetic gonads and whose sexual development has been abnormal; and intratubular Sertoli cell neoplasia, the precursor of certain types of Sertoli cell tumor that are only rarely malignant.

INTRATUBULAR GERM CELL NEOPLASIA

This term was adopted by a committee of pathologists who convened at the International Symposium on Human Testicular Cancer, Mouse Teratocarcinoma and Oncofetal Proteins in Minneapolis in 1980 to discuss the classification and nomenclature of testicular tumors (Scully, 1982).* The designation includes all forms of atypical and malignant lesions of germ cells confined to the lumens of testicular tubules as well as similar lesions accompanied by microinvasion (Table 18–1).

By far the most common form of intratubular germ cell neoplasia, which is termed "unclassified" in the Minneapolis classification and which has also been designated "carcinoma in situ" (Skakkebaek, 1972) and "intratubular atypical germ cells" (Mark and Hedinger, 1965), involves focal proliferation of cells resembling closely those of the seminoma within tubules. In the earliest stage of this lesion, which is only occasionally observed, large rounded cells with abundant clear cytoplasm and central nuclei containing one or a few prominent nucleoli appear focally along the basement membranes of tubules in which evidence of spermatogenic activity remains (Schulze and Holstein, 1977; Skakkebaek et al., 1982).

*Eadie Heyderman, M.D.; Robert J. Kurman, M.D.; F. K. Mostofi, M.D.; Lucien E. Nochomovitz, M.D.; Juan Rosai, M.D.; Robert E. Scully, M.D.

In the more commonly encountered later stages of development (Figs. 18–1 to 18–4) spermatogenic cells have disappeared, larger numbers of atypical cells are found at the periphery of the tubules, and Sertoli cells have been displaced toward the center of the lumens; mitotic figures are common in the atypical germ cells, which may extend into the rete testis. The lamina propria may be thickened and hyalinized.

The atypical germ cells have been demonstrated to have an aneuploid nuclear DNA pattern (Müller et al., 1981), to contain glycogen in their cytoplasm (Coffin et al., 1984) (Fig. 18–5), to stain immunohistochemically for placenta-like alkaline phosphatase (Aguirre et al., 1985) and for ferritin in some cases (Jacobsen et al., 1980; Sigg and Hedinger, 1984), and to have ultrastructural characteristics similar to those of prespermatogonial cells and seminoma cells (Albrechtsen et al., 1982; Gondos et al., 1983; Nielsen et al., 1974; Schulze and Holstein, 1977; Sigg and Hedinger, 1984) (Table 18–2). Staining for alpha-fetoprotein and chorionic gonadotropin has been negative (Sigg and Hedinger, 1984).

The term "intratubular germ cell neoplasia, unclassified" (IGCNU) was preferred by the Minnesota committee over "carcinoma in situ" for the lesion described above because follow-up studies have revealed that either a nonseminomatous germ cell tumor or a seminoma may develop from it if an orchiectomy is not performed (Table 18–3) (Andres et al., 1980;

Table 18–1. **Classification of Intratubular Germ Cell Tumors**

Intratubular germ cell neoplasia, unclassified
Intratubular germ cell neoplasia, unclassified with extratubular infiltration
Intratubular seminoma:
a. Classic
b. Spermatocytic
Intratubular embryonal carcinoma
Intratubular germ cell neoplasia, other forms
Seminoma with syncytiotrophoblast cells
Syncytiotrophoblast cells
Yolk sac tumor

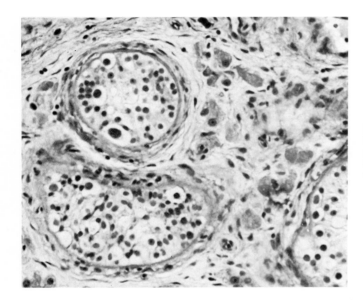

Figure 18–1. Intratubular germ cell neoplasia, unclassified, in several tubules within testicular scar of 30-year-old man with metastatic retroperitoneal seminoma. There is slight thickening and hyalinization of the lamina propria of the tubules. Leydig cells are present in the scar tissue.

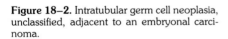

Figure 18–2. Intratubular germ cell neoplasia, unclassified, adjacent to an embryonal carcinoma.

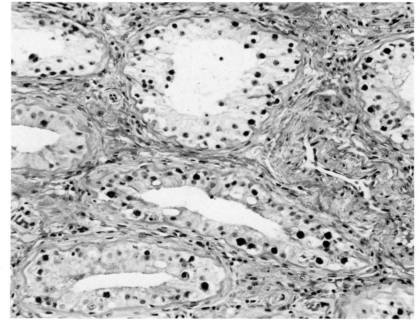

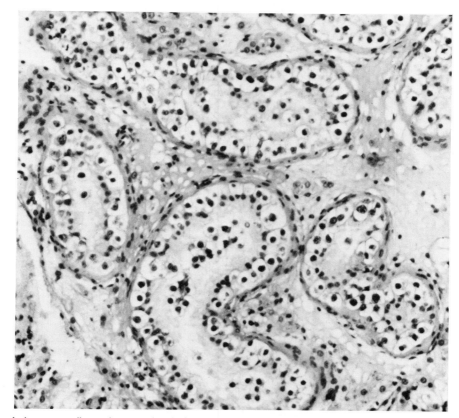

Figure 18–3. Intratubular germ cell neoplasia, unclassified, an incidental finding in a biopsy specimen from a 24-year-old infertile man. See also Figures 18–4 and 18–10.

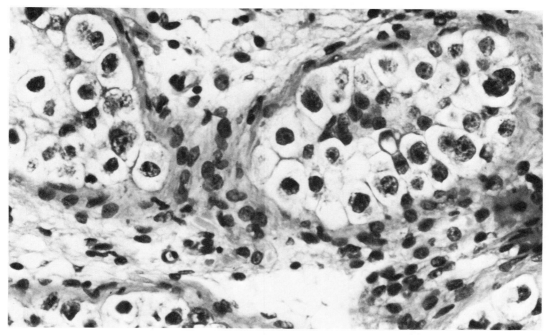

Figure 18–4. High-power view of Figure 18–3. The atypical germ cells have abundant clear cytoplasm and hyperchromatic nuclei with prominent nucleoli. See also Figures 18–3 and 18–10.

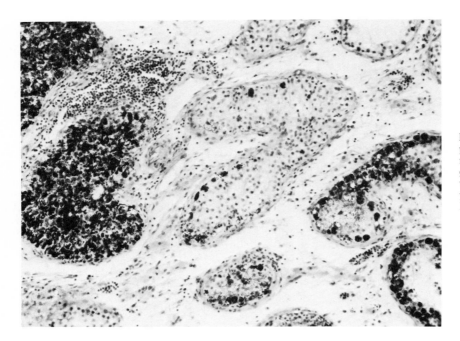

Figure 18–5. Intratubular germ cell neoplasia, unclassified, and intratubular seminoma (adjacent to non-seminomatous germ cell tumor) stained for glycogen by the periodic acid-Schiff method. The neoplastic cells are strongly positive. See also Figures 18–8 and 18–9.

Berthelsen et al., 1982; Pryor et al., 1983; Sigg and Hedinger, 1981; Skakkebaek, 1978; Skakkebaek et al., 1981), and these invasive forms of germ cell cancer are not carcinomas in the strict sense of the term.

The atypical intratubular cells may penetrate the lamina propria and infiltrate the stroma focally in the form of single cells or small clusters (Figs. 18–6 and 18–7), giving rise to the lesion designated "intratubular germ cell neoplasia, unclassified, with extratubular infiltration" or microinvasive germ cell tumor (Eyben et al., 1981). Whether the extratubular atypical germ cells are committed to developing into a seminoma or may also evolve into a non-seminomatous germ cell tumor is not known.

When the atypical germ cells proliferate to the extent that they obliterate the Sertoli cell element and fill the tubules (Figs. 18–5, 18–8, and 18–9), the term "intratubular seminoma" (of the classic type) is used. Although there is no certainty that this lesion invariably gives rise to a seminoma if it becomes invasive, it has been designated seminoma because, except for its location, it is identical to the invasive form of the tumor even to the extent that it may be infiltrated by lymphocytes.

Intratubular germ cell neoplasia, unclassified, and intratubular seminoma must be differentiated from several other lesions they may resemble superficially. The very rare intratubular spermatocytic seminoma is characterized by neoplastic cells with distinctive features, which will be described below. Viral orchitis, as well as other forms of orchitis, is an occasional source of confusion. In these disorders the tubules are distended with cells having the characteristics of inflammatory cells of various types (Morgan, 1976); in granulomatous orchitis Langhans-type giant cells are present within the tubules in one-quarter of the cases. In addition, orchitis is generally characterized by a prominent infiltrate of inflammatory cells in the interstitial tissue. Lymphoma involving the testis grows within tubules in about one-third of the cases (Gowing, 1976). The tumor cells, however, have the appearance of malignant lymphoid cells with nuclear features unlike those of germ cells and generally scanty cytoplasm, which is free of glycogen. Also, in cases of lymphoma the interstitial tissue between the involved tubules is heavily infiltrated by a proliferation of neoplastic cells.

Intratubular germ cell neoplasia, unclassified, with or without extratubular infiltration, has been reported in the parenchyma adjacent to invasive germ cell

Table 18–2. **Ultrastructural Features of Intratubular Germ Cell Neoplasia, Unclassified**

Nuclei
Large
Prominent nucleoli
Cytoplasm
Glycogen
Polarization of organelles
Microfilaments, peripheral
Microtubules
Nuages*
Dense-core vesicles†
Annulate lamellae
No intercellular bridges

*Accumulations of finely granular, moderately electron-dense material lying free in cytoplasm.

†Homogeneous electron-dense material in the centers of otherwise empty-appearing vesicles.

Table 18–3. **Follow-up Data on Patients with Intratubular Germ Cell Neoplasia, Unclassified**

Authors	Number of Cases	Less than 1 Year		1 to Less than 5 Years		5 Years or More	
		*No Invasive Tumor**	*Invasive Tumor*	*No Invasive Tumor**	*Invasive Tumor*	*No Invasive Tumor**	*Invasive Tumor*
Sigg and Hedinger (1981)	10	2	2	2	1	2	1
Berthelsen et al. (1982)	12†	5		6	1		
Skakkebaek (1978)	6			2	4		
Pryor et al. (1983)	8	1	2		2	1	2
Total	36	8	4	10	8	3	3

*Either no clinical evidence of invasive tumor or no invasive tumor in orchiectomy specimen.
†Thirteenth case eliminated because of identity with one in column below.

tumors as well as in testes without invasive neoplasms. Its presence has been recorded adjacent to seminomas in 64 to 89 percent of the cases and outside non-seminomatous germ cell tumors in 97 to 100 percent of the cases (Figs. 18–2, and 18–5) (Jacobsen et al., 1981; Sigg and Hedinger, 1980; Skakkebaek, 1975). Intratubular seminoma, in contrast, has been encountered in a similar location in only 44 percent of cases of seminoma and 27 percent of those of non-seminomatous germ cell tumors (Figs. 18–5, 18–8, 18–9) (Sigg and Hedinger, 1980). Both IGCNU (Fig. 18–1) and intratubular seminoma have also been identified within or adjacent to scars in the testes of patients with metastatic seminomas and non-seminomatous germ cell tumors in the absence of clinical evidence of testicular involvement (Azzopardi et al., 1961; Azzopardi and Hoffbrand, 1965). The experience with occult primary testicular cancers has been too limited and incompletely documented to give figures for the frequency of occurrence of these intratubular lesions in cases of this type.

In testes containing tumors or scars of involuted tumors, it is difficult to be certain whether the intratubular changes described above are precancerous or in-situ lesions, have resulted from intratubular penetration by invasive tumor cells, or reflect a reaction of spermatogenic epithelium to one or more products of the adjacent neoplasm. In the last decade, however, Skakkebaek, Berthelsen, and their associates (1981, 1982) and other investigators (Andres et al., 1980; Pryor et al., 1983; Sigg and Hedinger, 1981) have provided strong evidence based on testicular biopsy and follow-up data that the intratubular lesions described, particularly the unclassified form, are truly precancerous in at least a proportion of the cases. Such lesions have been found in the apparent absence of invasive neoplasms in biopsy specimens of cryptorchids (Figs. 18–6 and 18–7), the testes of infertile men (Figs. 18–3 and 18–4), which are usually of small volume and associated with oligospermia or azoospermia, and testes contralateral to germ cell tumors. Biopsies of cryptorchids, most of which had

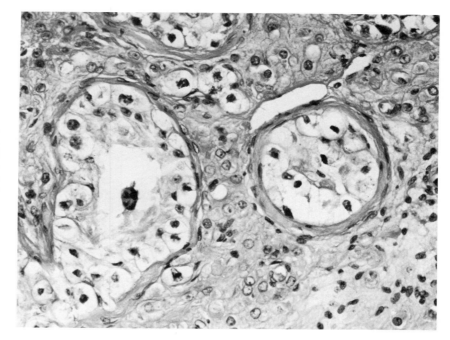

Figure 18–6. Intratubular germ cell neoplasia, unclassified, with extratubular infiltration in biopsy specimen of 22-year-old man with bilateral cryptorchidism. Malignant cells lie singly and in clumps in the interstitial tissue. The lamina propria of the tubules is slightly thickened and hyalinized. See also Figure 18–7.

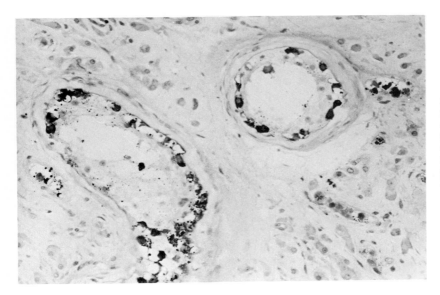

Figure 18–7. Intratubular germ cell neoplasia, unclassified, with extratubular infiltration in orchiectomy specimen of 22-year-old man with bilateral cryptorchidism stained for glycogen by the periodic acid-Schiff method. The neoplastic cells within the tubules and in the stroma are strongly positive. See also Figure 18–6.

Figure 18–8. Intratubular seminoma adjacent to non-seminomatous germ cell tumor. See also Figures 18–5 and 18–9.

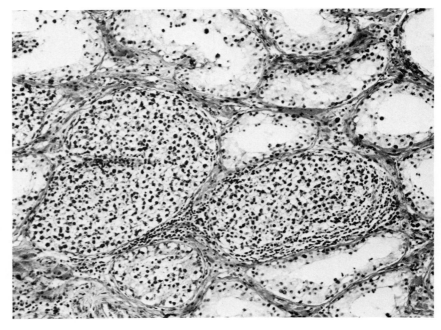

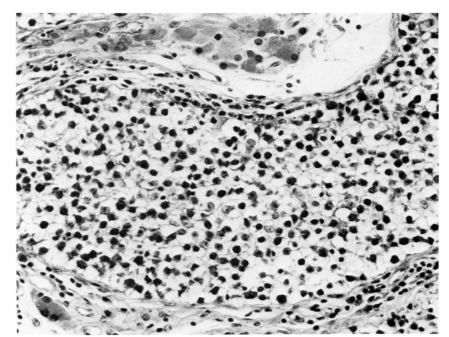

Figure 18–9. High-power view of Figure 18–8. The intratubular cells have the typical appearance of classic seminoma cells. A minor degree of lymphocytic infiltration is present. Leydig cells are seen near the top of the field. See also Figures 18–5 and 18–8.

been treated by orchidopexy, have yielded one of these lesions in 2 to 8 percent of the cases (Krabbe et al., 1979), biopsies of testes from sterile men in 0.4 to 1 percent of the cases, and biopsies of testes contralateral to germ cell tumors in 5 percent of the cases (Berthelsen et al., 1982). Testes in the last two categories were often cryptorchid (or previously cryptorchid) or small or both.

Since approximately one-third of patients with the androgen insensitivity syndrome, whose testes are typically undescended, have a testicular germ cell tumor, usually a seminoma, by the age of 50 years (Manuel et al., 1976), it is not surprising that IGCNU has been encountered in them as well (Müller and Skakkebaek, 1984; Scully, personal observation; Skakkebaek, 1979). We have also seen IGCNU in the testis of a patient with dysgenetic male pseudohermaphroditism and an intratubular gonadoblastoma, and the lesion has also been illustrated by several authors in the testes of virilized phenotypic females with mixed gonadal dysgenesis; intratubular gonadoblastomas have also been present in these cases (Coco et al., 1975; Josso et al., 1969; Teter et al., 1964). Finally, IGCNU has been described in both testes of a phenotypic male with a uterus, a unilateral seminoma and embryonal carcinoma, and a contralateral cryptorchid (Nistal et al., 1980).

The age distribution of IGCNU reflects to a large extent that of the patients whose testes have been investigated specifically for the presence of this lesion. In the testicular tumor study groups the ages of the patients have ranged from 15 to 69 years, but the age span of those with positive findings has not been recorded. Guinand and Hedinger (1981) were unable to identify the lesion in the testes of 25 children with testicular germ cell tumors (yolk sac tumors and mature teratomas), 6 months to 6 years of age, suggesting the possibility that prepubertal spermatogonia can evolve directly into neoplasms without passing through a stage of IGCNU. Most of the patients without tumors have been in the third or fourth decade, although one man with a previously removed tumor of the contralateral testis was 48 years of age at the time of diagnosis. Muffly et al. (1984) were unable to demonstrate the lesion in 113 biopsy specimens of cryptorchids from 102 patients 3 months to 16 years of age. Nevertheless, isolated examples of IGCNU have been encountered in young patients. Two boys in whom one of bilateral cryptorchids contained the lesion were 13 and 10 years of age (Dorman et al., 1979; Müller et al., 1984). We have seen the lesion in a 9-year-old boy with sexual precocity associated with localized Leydig cell hyperplasia (? early neoplasia) and focal spermatogenesis. Finally, IGCNU has been identified in a 10-year-old patient with mixed gonadal dysgenesis (Coco et al., 1975) and in three young patients with the incomplete androgen insensitivity syndrome (aged 2 months to 14 years) (Müller and Skakkebaek, 1984).

Follow-up studies on men in whom IGCNU has been discovered on biopsy have established the precancerous nature of the lesion. In the four largest series in the literature (Berthelsen et al., 1982; Pryor et al., 1983; Sigg and Hedinger, 1981; Skakkebaek, 1978), 36 patients have had follow-up examinations (Table 18–3). Four of the 12 patients who were followed for less than a year were discovered to have invasive tumors (three seminomas, one microinvasive,

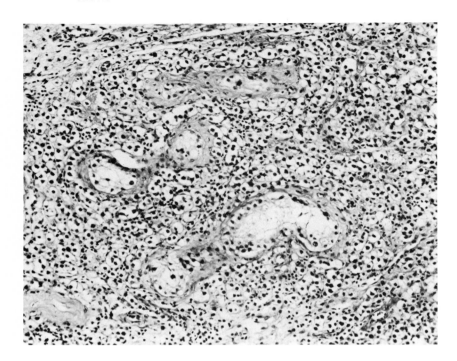

Figure 18–10. Seminoma, one of two 0.1-cm foci of tumor in orchiectomy specimen of 24-year-old infertile man whose biopsy specimen is illustrated in Figures 18–3 and 18–4. Several tubules containing atypical germ cells are surrounded by tumor.

and one "teratocarcinoma"), which very likely had been present but undetected at the time of biopsy (Fig. 18–10); eight of the 18 patients followed for one to less than five years had invasive tumors ("undifferentiated"; embryonal carcinoma; teratoma; teratoma and yolk sac tumor; two seminomas; and two intratubular germ cell neoplasias with extratubular infiltration [microinvasive seminomas]), which may have been present but undetected in some of the cases at the time of biopsy, whereas the remaining 10 had no evidence of invasive tumor; finally, of the six patients followed for five or more years, seminoma developed in three (at six, six, and nine years), but three others were still free of clinical evidence of tumor at six, seven, and eight years. One man, not included in the above unselected series of followed patients, had an embryonal carcinoma seven years after a biopsy had shown intratubular atypical germ cells (Andres et al., 1980), and another had IGCNU with extratubular infiltration 10½ years after a biopsy performed at the age of 10 years had shown only intratubular involvement (Müller et al., 1984).

Because of lack of follow-up data in the rare cases of intratubular seminoma that have been detected on biopsy, it has not been established whether it invades exclusively as seminoma or in some instances progresses to a non-seminomatous invasive germ cell tumor. The aforementioned finding that it is associated synchronously with invasive seminomas more often than with invasive non-seminomatous tumors, the converse of IGCNU, suggests that it may have a greater commitment to progress into invasive seminoma than the IGCNU.

Masson (1946) in his original description of the spermatocytic seminoma noted the presence of intratubular tumor in the testicular parenchyma uninvolved by neoplasia in one of his cases. He pointed out that this finding could not be ascribed to intratubular extension of the invasive tumor because of its distance from the latter. Subsequent investigators (Rosai et al., 1969; Scully, 1961; Talerman, 1980) have made similar observations. We are not aware of a single clearly documented case of intratubular spermatocytic seminoma unaccompanied by invasive tumor. but have encountered one example of it, a 1.5 mm in diameter cluster of involved tubules discovered in an atrophic testis that was removed from a 49-year-old man because of adjacent infection (Figs. 18–11, 18–12). The lesion, like invasive spermatocytic seminoma, was characterized by cells with hyperchromatic, round nuclei of varying sizes, which differed from those of intratubular germ cell neoplasia, unclassified, and classic seminoma by their lack of both abundant clear cytoplasm rich in glycogen and uniform nuclei with prominent nucleoli; the lesion was focally calcified. Intratubular germ cell neoplasia, unclassified, was present elsewhere in the testis (Fig. 18–13).

Intratubular embryonal carcinoma (Akhtar and Sidiki, 1979; Azzopardi et al., 1961; Mostofi, 1980; Mostofi and Price, 1973) is much rarer than intratubular germ cell neoplasia, unclassified, and intratubular classic seminoma and has not been described in biopsy specimens. It has been seen occasionally in the parenchyma adjacent to germ cell tumors and in relation to scars of occult testicular tumors that have metastasized. Intratubular embryonal carcinoma, like its invasive counterpart, is characterized by cells containing nuclei that are larger and more atypical than

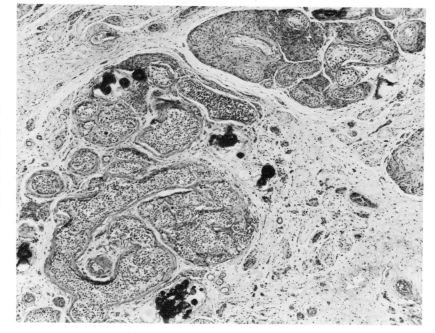

Figure 18–11. Intratubular spermatocytic seminoma in orchiectomy specimen from 49-year-old man with small testes in upper part of scrotum. Most of the tubules are shrunken and hyalinized, but several in a large cluster in the left half of the field are filled with neoplastic cells and show focal calcification. A prominent irregular nest of Leydig cells is present in the upper part of the field between tubules containing Sertoli cells. See also Figures 18–12 and 18–13.

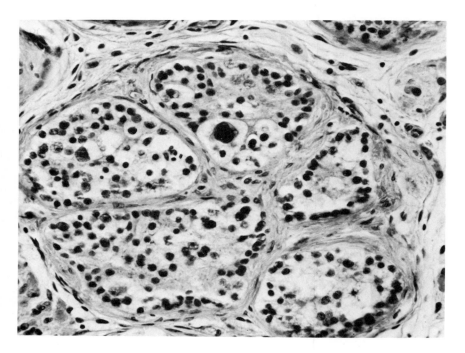

Figure 18–12. High-power view of intratubular spermatocytic seminoma. The nuclei are rounded and vary in size. See also Figures 18–11 and 18–13.

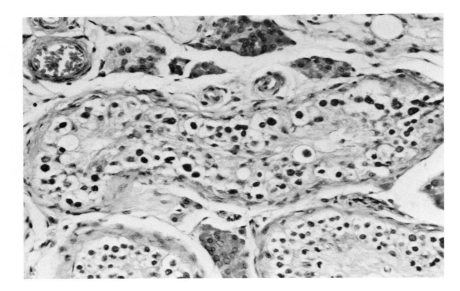

Figure 18–13. Intratubular germ cell neoplasia, unclassified, from atrophic testis of 49-year-old man whose intratubular spermatocytic seminoma is illustrated in Figures 18–11 and 18–12.

those of the seminoma (Fig. 18–14). The lesion is prone to undergo a caseation type of necrosis, with the necrotic material often acquiring an affinity for hematoxylin (Fig. 18–15) (Azzopardi et al., 1961). On occasion yolk sac tumor (endodermal sinus tumor) has been encountered within tubules in cases of invasive yolk sac tumors in infants (Teilum, 1976), and syncytiotrophoblast cells have been found within tubules accompanied by atypical germ cells or intratubular seminoma (Mostofi, 1980; Mostofi and Price, 1973). Whether these rare types of intratubular germ cell neoplasia are incipient forms of invasive cancer is not known. Intratubular teratoma has not yet been reported in the human testis.

GONADOBLASTOMA

The gonadoblastoma (Scully, 1970, 1981) is a tumor composed of germ cells similar to those of the seminoma and dysgerminoma, sex cord elements, consistent with immature Sertoli or granulosa cells, and in approximately two-thirds of the cases cells of Leydig or lutein-cell type, which do not contain crystalloids of Reinke. The germ cells and sex cord elements are enclosed within discrete nests surrounded by basement membranes and arranged in one or more of three distinctive patterns. The germ cells may form the center of a nest with sex cord cells in single file along the periphery or they may be enveloped by sex

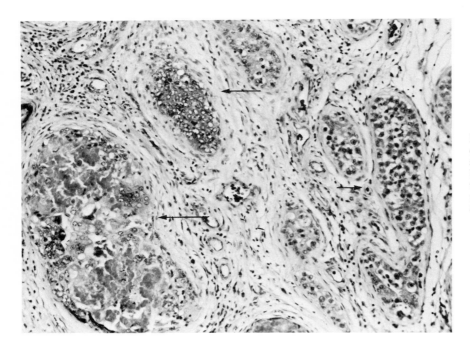

Figure 18–14. Intratubular embryonal carcinoma *(long arrows)* and intratubular seminoma *(short arrow)* adjacent to embryonal carcinoma and teratoma. In one tubule the embryonal carcinoma has undergone caseation-type necrosis. See also Figure 18–15.

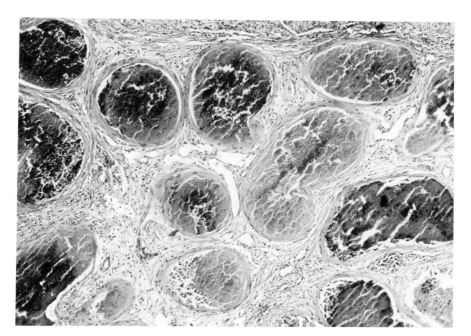

Figure 18–15. Hematoxylinophilic deposits in centers of tubules containing necrotic embryonal carcinoma.

cord cells, much as primordial ova are surrounded by coronas of immature granulosa cells (follicular epithelium); thirdly, the sex cord cells may be arranged around hyaline bodies containing basement membrane material and merging focally with the basement membrane at the periphery of the nest (Fig. 18–16). Several changes may occur in a gonadoblastoma that alter its microscopic appearance. The hyaline bodies may coalesce to form large masses; and laminated calcific deposits may appear in the hyaline bodies and may merge to form complex mulberry-like structures.

Finally, in half the cases the germ cells within the nests penetrate the basement membranes and invade the stroma to form a germinoma. In less than 10 percent of the reported cases another type of germ cell tumor, almost always more malignant than the seminoma, has arisen on the background of a gonadoblastoma. Gross examination of a gonadoblastoma reveals a discrete nodule that may be soft or hard depending in part on its content of calcium. In some cases the calcification is so extensive that it can be seen on x-ray films. If a seminoma or some other

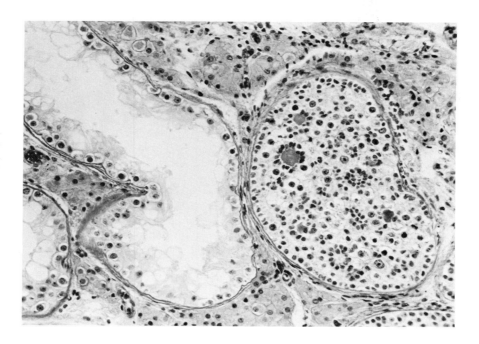

Figure 18–16. Intratubular gonadoblastoma in dysgenetic testis of 13-year-old phenotypic female with mixed gonadal dysgenesis. An adjacent tubule contains atypical germ cells. The contralateral streak gonad also contained a gonadoblastoma.

type of malignant germ cell tumor has developed, its gross features are superimposed on those of the gonadoblastoma.

Gonadoblastomas are encountered in otherwise normal testes only on exceptionally rare occasions. In over 80 percent of the cases these tumors develop in phenotypic females, who are usually virilized to some degree. In the remaining cases they are found in phenotypic males, who almost always have hypospadias, cryptorchidism, and some development of müllerian duct derivatives and who often have gynecomastia. Although it is generally impossible to determine the nature of a gonad that has been replaced by a gonadoblastoma, one can identify a remnant of streak gonad composed of ovarian-type stroma in approximately 20 percent of the cases and a remnant of dysgenetic testis in a similar proportion. Patients with gonadoblastoma almost always have either a 46 XY, a 45 XO/46 XY, or another form of mosaic karyotype containing a Y chromosome. The forms of intersexual disorder that predispose to this type of tumor in the phenotypic male are dysgenetic male pseudohermaphroditism and mixed gonadal dysgenesis, which are classified as variants of the same disease by some investigators (Rajfer and Walsh, 1981).

The gonadoblastoma may be clearly intratubular without distortion of testicular architecture, but even when it has grown to form confluent masses of germ cells and sex cord elements, it retains the characteristics of an in-situ or precancerous lesion. It has never been reported to metastasize as such, although I have seen a case of a phenotypic female in whom an isolated "implant" was found in the cul-de-sac several months after biopsy of a gonadoblastoma. The precancerous nature of this lesion is evidenced by its strong association with invasive germ cell tumors. Although the latter are usually discovered synchronously, in an occasional case one appears in a conserved contralateral gonad years after the removal of an apparently unilateral gonadoblastoma.

Two tumors may be confused with a gonadoblastoma. One is the extremely rare sex cord–germ cell tumor, unclassified (Talerman, 1980). It is composed of a mixture of germ cells, which are usually more mature than those of the gonadoblastoma, and sex cord elements arranged in patterns that typically differ from those within a gonadoblastoma; hyaline bodies and calcification are rarely present. Also, this tumor is encountered in the testes (and ovaries) of individuals who have undergone normal sexual development. The other neoplasm from which the gonadoblastoma must be differentiated in the ovary is the sex cord tumor with annular tubules (Young et al., 1982), which resembles it except for a lack of germ cells. This differential diagnosis should not create a problem in the testis, however, since the sex cord tumor with annular tubules is extremely rare in this site. Non-neoplastic clusters of immature tubules pop-

ulated by Sertoli cells, which are encountered commonly in cryptorchids and occasionally in descended testes, sometimes contain small numbers of spermatogonia, creating a superficial resemblance to a gonadoblastoma The absence of the characteristic architectural patterns of the latter, however, enable one to exclude the diagnosis.

INTRATUBULAR SERTOLI CELL NEOPLASIA

Since the Sertoli cell normally occupies a position within the testicular tubule, it is logical to assume that intratubular Sertoli cell neoplasia precedes the development of invasive Sertoli cell tumors. Intratubular large-cell calcifying Sertoli cell tumors (Fig. 18–17) appear to be the forerunners of the more common extratubular forms of the neoplasm (Proppe and Scully, 1980), which may be associated with a variety of endocrine and other syndromes. With one exception, however, the recorded examples of these tumors have been clinically benign. Sertoli cell neoplasms of other types have not been reported to be confined to tubules, but it would not be surprising if they occasionally exist in this location. We have seen one example of a juvenile granulosa cell tumor of an infant testis in which intratubular neoplasia was present adjacent to the invasive tumor.

DISCUSSION

Largely as a result of the investigations of Skakkebaek and his coworkers (1972–1984) there is strong evidence that biopsy of testes known to be at risk for the development of cancer may reveal intratubular germ cell neoplasia, which in an unknown, but significant proportion of the cases will progress to clinical cancer. Preliminary studies have indicated that this lesion typically has a diffuse distribution and that one or two biopsy specimens 3 mm in diameter will usually be sufficient for its recognition (Berthelsen and Skakkebaek, 1981).

Knowledge of the frequency with which such biopsies will reveal incipient cancer in susceptible subjects requires investigation of a larger number of cases than has been described so far and, of greater importance, a refinement of the criteria for selecting patients for biopsy. Those subjected to this procedure to date have fallen into three overlapping categories of patients known from epidemiologic and clinical studies to be at increased risk for testicular cancer: those with unilateral or bilateral cryptorchidism, either current or corrected by hormonal or surgical therapy (Batata et al., 1982; Morrison, 1976; Skakkebaek et al., 1982); those with a history of cancer of the contralateral testis (Aristizabal et al., 1978; Cockburn et al., 1983); and those presenting with infertility, particularly a subgroup with oligospermia and testes of small vol-

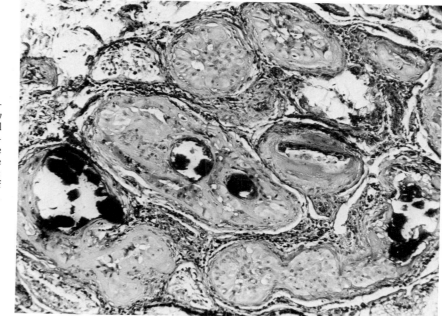

Figure 18–17. Intratubular large cell calcifying Sertoli cell tumor in orchiectomy specimen of 11-year-old boy with sexual precocity and pituitary gigantism. The patient also had an extratubular tumor of the same type and a steroid cell tumor of the testis. (From Proppe, K., and Scully, R. E.: Large-cell calcifying Sertoli cell tumor of the testis. Am. J. Clin. Pathol. 74:607, 1980, Fig. 5).

ume (Berthelsen and Skakkebaek, 1983). Some of the patients who have been included in the last group in various investigations have also had cryptorchidism or a history of cancer of the contralateral testis.

Although precancerous changes have been recorded in approximately 0.4 to 1.0 percent of infertile patients who have had testicular biopsies (Pryor et al., 1983; Sigg and Hedinger, 1981; Skakkebaek, 1978), such biopsies have been performed in many centers for a variety of testicular and extratesticular disorders of both known and unknown causation. Therefore, it can be anticipated that the frequency of a positive finding will increase once higher-risk subgroups within the category of sterile men are defined more precisely. A precancerous tubular lesion was found in three of 49 adult subjects who had been treated for cryptorchidism or had spontaneous but delayed testicular descent and agreed to having a biopsy in one series of cases (Krabbe et al., 1979), but was identified on multiple sectioning of orchiectomy specimens in only one of 39 adult subjects with current cryptorchidism in another study (Fritjofsson and Busch, 1981). Obviously, larger numbers of cases of cryptorchidism must be investigated before assessing the value of biopsy and determining the possible role of the age of orchidopexy in the subsequent development of cancer.

Since testicular cancer is bilateral much more often metachronously than synchronously, in 1 to 2 percent of cases (Aristizabal et al., 1978; Cockburn et al., 1983), it is not surprising that biopsy of the testis contralateral to a cancer was positive for a precancerous lesion in over 5 percent of 250 cases (Berthelsen et al., 1982). The testis was of small volume or had been previously cryptorchid, or both, in 85 percent

of the positive cases. It is also of interest that four of 17 patients with IGCNU in a biopsy specimen of one testis (23 percent) had the same lesion in the biopsy specimen of the contralateral testis (Sigg and Hedinger, 1982; Skakkebaek, 1978; Skakkebaek et al., 1982).

Patients with a family history of testicular cancer (Gulley et al., 1974; Zevallos et al., 1983) have not been investigated by testicular biopsy, but appear to be appropriate candidates for this procedure, particularly if cryptorchidism, oligospermia, or a reduced testicular volume is found.

The recorded follow-up of patients with positive biopsies (Table 18–2) has been too scanty to permit confident conclusions about optimal management; both orchiectomy (Skakkebaek and Berthelsen, 1978) and conservation with careful follow-up (Sigg and Hedinger, 1981) have been recommended. If the latter approach is selected, the problem should be explained to the patient, he should be instructed to examine his testes at regular intervals, and he should be seen every few months by his physician, who may perform additional biopsies. Serum radioimmunoassays for alpha-fetoprotein, chorionic gonadotropin, and other markers may be of value, but cannot be relied upon for the detection of early invasive disease (Scully, 1982).

Although it seems probable that intratubular germ cell neoplasia, unclassified, is the most common forerunner of invasive testicular cancer, its absence in the vicinity of yolk sac tumors of children, the occasional finding of intratubular yolk sac tumor and embryonal carcinoma in the vicinity of invasive tumors of those types, and the common finding of intratubular seminoma near invasive seminomas suggest that these forms of neoplasia may evolve directly within the tubules without passing through a stage of intratubular germ cell neoplasia, unclassified. In addition, although the latter lesion may be found in the dysgenetic testes of individuals who have undergone abnormal sexual development, the intratubular gonadoblastoma appears to be a precursor of a number of invasive germ cell tumors in this population of patients. There is rarely a need to biopsy gonads from phenotypic males with dysgenetic male pseudohermaphroditism or mixed gonadal dysgenesis to detect a precancerous lesion since these organs are usually removed in toto because of the high risk of malignant change; exceptions may be cases in which a unilateral well-developed testis lies in the scrotum or is undescended but correctible by orchidopexy.

References

Aguirre, P., Scully, R.E., Dayal, Y., DeLellis, R.A.: Placenta-like alkaline phosphatase in germ cell tumors of the ovary and testis. Lab. Invest. 52:2a, 1985.

Akhtar, M., Sidiki, Y.: Undifferentiated intratubular germ cell tumor of the testis: Light and electron microscopic study of a unique case. Cancer 43:2332, 1979.

Albrechtsen, R., Nielsen, M.H., Skakkebaek, N.E., Wewer, U.: Carcinoma in situ of the testis. Some ultrastructural characteristics of germ cells. Acta Pathol. Microbiol. Scand. Sect. A 90:301, 1982.

Andres, T.L., Trainer, T.D., Leadbetter, G.W.: Atypical germ cells preceding metachronous bilateral testicular tumors. Urology 15:307, 1980.

Aristizabal, S., Davis, J.R., Miller, R.C., Moore, M.J., Boone, M.L.M.: Bilateral primary germ cell testicular tumors: Report of four cases and review of literature. Cancer 42:591, 1978.

Azzopardi, J.G., Hoffbrand, A.V.: Retrogression in testicular seminoma with viable metastases. J. Clin. Pathol. 18:135, 1965.

Azzopardi, J.G., Mostofi, E.K., Theiss, E.A.: Lesions of testes observed in certain patients with widespread choriocarcinoma and related tumors. Am. J. Pathol. 38:207, 1961.

Batata, M.A., Chu, F.C.H., Hilaris, B.S., Whitemore, W.F., Golbey, R.B.: Testicular cancer in cryptorchids. Cancer 49:1023, 1982.

Berthelsen, J.G., Skakkebaek, N.E.: Value of testicular biopsy in diagnosing carcinoma in situ of testis. Scand. J. Urol. Nephrol. 15:165, 1981.

Berthelsen, J.G., Skakkebaek, N.E.: Distribution of carcinoma-insitu in testes from infertile men. Int. J. Androl. Suppl. 4:171, 1981.

Berthelsen, J.G., Skakkebaek, N.E.: Gonadal function in men with testis cancer. Fertil. Steril. 39:68, 1983.

Berthelsen, J.G., Skakkebaek, N.E., von der Maase, H., Sorensen, B.L.: Screening for carcinoma in situ of the contralateral testis in patients with germinal testicular cancer. Brit. Med. J. 285:1683, 1982.

Cockburn, A.G., Vugrin, D., Batata, M., Hajdu, S., Whitmore, W.F.: Secondary primary germ cell tumors in patients with seminoma of the testis. J. Urol. 130:357, 1983.

Coco, R., Chemes, H., Bergada, C.: Asymmetrical gonadal differentiation and gonadoblastoma. Acta Endocrinol. 80:753, 1975.

Dorfman, S., Trainer, T.D., Lefke, D., Leadbetter, G.: Incipient germ cell tumor in a cryptorchid testis. Cancer 44:1357, 1979.

Eyben, F.E.v., Mikulowski, P., Busch, C.: Microinvasive germ cell tumors of the testis. J. Urol. 126:842, 1981.

Fritjofsson, Busch: Discussion of Skakkebaek et al., 1981. Int. J. Androl. Suppl. 4:160, 1981.

Gondos, B., Bethelsen, J.G., Skakkebaek, N.E.: Intratubular germ cell neoplasia (carcinoma in situ): A preinvasive lesion of the testis. Ann. Clin. Lab. Sci. 13:185, 1983.

Gowing, N.F.C.: Malignant lymphoma of the testis. In: Pathology of the Testis, Pugh, R.C.B., Ed. Oxford, England, Blackwell Scientific, 1976, pp. 334–355.

Guinand, S., Hedinger, C.: Cellules germinales atypiques intratubulaires et tumeurs germinales testiculaires de l'enfant. Ann. Pathol. 1:251, 1981.

Gulley, R.M., Kowalski, R., Neuhoff, C.F.: Familial occurrence of testicular neoplasms: A case report. J. Urol. 112:620, 1974.

Jacobsen, G.K., Henriksen, O.B., Der Maase, H.V.: Carcinoma in situ of testicular tissue adjacent to malignant germ-cell tumors: A study of 105 cases. Cancer 47:2660, 1981.

Jacobsen, G.K., Jacobsen, M., Clausen, P.P.: Ferritin as a possible marker protein of carcinoma-in-situ of the testis. Lancet 2:533, 1980.

Josso, N., Nezelof, C., Picon, R., deGrouchy, J., Dray, F., Rappaport, R.: Gonadoblastoma in gonadal dysgenesis: a report of two cases with 46XY/45X mosaicism. J. Pediat. 74:425, 1969.

Krabbe, S., Skakkebaek, N.E., Berthelsen, J.G., Eyben, F.V., Volsted, P., Mauritzen, K., Eldrup, J., Nielsen, A.H.: High incidence of undetected neoplasia in maldescended testes. Lancet 1:999, 1979.

Manuel, M., Katayama, K.P., Jones, H.W. Jr.: The age of occurrence of gonadal tumors in intersex patients with a Y chromosome. Am. J. Obstet. Gynecol. 124:293, 1976.

Mark, G.J., Hedinger, C.: Changes in remaining tumor-free testicular tissue in cases of seminoma and teratoma. Virchows Arch. Pathol. Anat. 340:84, 1965.

Masson, P.: Etude sur le seminome. Rev. Can. Biol. 5:361, 1946.

Morgan, A.D.: Inflammation and infestation of the testis and paratesticular structures. In: Pathology of the Testis, Pugh, R.C.B., Ed. Oxford, England, Blackwell Scientific, 1976, pp. 79–138.

Morrison, A.S.: Cryptorchidism, hernia and cancer of the testis. J. Nat. Cancer Inst. 56:731, 1976.

Mostofi, F.K.: Pathology of germ cell tumors of testis: A progress report. Cancer 45:1735, 1980.

Mostofi, F.K., Price, E.B. Jr.: Tumors of the Male Genital System. Washington, D.C., Armed Forces Institute of Pathology, 1973.

Muffly, K.E., McWhorter, C.A., Bartone, F.E., Gardner, P.J.: The absence of premalignant changes in the cryptorchid testis before adulthood. J. Urol. 131:523, 1984.

Müller, J., Skakkebaek, N.E.: Testicular carcinoma in situ in children with the androgen insensitivity (testicular feminisation) syndrome. Brit. Med. J. 288:1419, 1984.

Müller, J., Skakkebaek, N.E., Lundsteen, C.: Aneuploidy as a marker for carcinoma-in-situ of the testis. Acta Path. Microbiol. Scand. Sect. A 89:67, 1981.

Müller, J., Skakkebaek, N.E., Nielsen, O.H., Graem, N.: Cryptorchidism and testis cancer. Atypical germ cells followed by carcinoma in situ and invasive carcinoma in adulthood. Cancer 54:629, 1984.

Nielsen, H., Nielsen, M., Skakkebaek, N.E.: The fine structure of a possible carcinoma-in-situ in the seminiferous tubules in the testis of four infertile men. Acta Path. Microbiol. Scand. 82:235, 1974.

Nistal, M., Paniagua, R., Isorna, S., Mancebo, J.: Diffuse intratubular undifferentiated germ cell tumor in both testes of a male subject with a uterus and ipsilateral testicular dysgenesis. J. Urol. 124:286, 1980.

Proppe, K., Scully, R.E.: Large-cell calcifying Sertoli cell tumor of the testis. Am. J. Clin. Pathol. 74:607, 1980.

Pryor, J.P., Cameron, K.M., Chilton, C.P., Ford, T.F., Parkinson, M.C., Sinokrot, J., Westwood, C.A.: Carcinoma in situ in testicular biopsies from men presenting with infertility. Brit. J. Surg. 55:780, 1983.

Rajfer, J., Walsh, P.C.: Mixed gonadal dysgenesis-dysgenetic male pseudohermaphroditism. In: Pediatric Adolescent Endocrinology, Vol. 8. The Intersex Child. Basel, Switzerland, S. Karger, 1981, pp. 105–115.

Rosai, J., Silber, I., Khodadoust, K.: Spermatocytic seminoma. 1. Clinicopathologic study of six cases and review of the literature. Cancer 24:92, 1969.

Schulze, C., Holstein, A.F.: On the histology of human seminoma: Development of the solid tumor from intratubular seminoma cells. Cancer 39:1090, 1977.

Scully, R.E.: Spermatocytic seminoma of the testis. A report of 3 cases and review of the literature. Cancer 14:788, 1961.

Scully, R.E.: Gonadoblastoma. A review of 74 cases. Cancer 25:1340, 1970.

Scully, R.E.: Neoplasia associated with anomalous sexual development and abnormal sex chromosomes. *In*: Pediatric Adolescent Endocrinology, Vol. 8. The Intersex Child. Basel, Switzerland, S. Karger, 1981, pp. 203–217.

Scully, R.E.: Intratubular germ cell neoplasia (carcinoma in situ): What it is and what should be done about it. World Urology Update Series. 1: Lesson 17, 1982.

Scully, R.E. Personal observations.

Sigg, C., Hedinger, C.: Keimzelltumoren des hodens und atypische keimzellen. Schweiz. Med. Wschr. 110:801, 1980.

Sigg, C., Hedinger, C.: Atypical germ cells in testicular biopsy in male sterility. Int. J. Androl. Suppl. 4:163, 1981.

Sigg, C., Hedinger, C.: Atypical germ cells of the testis. Comparative ultrastructural and immunohistochemical investigations. Virchows Arch. (Pathol. Anat.) 402:439, 1984.

Skakkebaek, N.E.: Possible carcinoma in-situ of the testis. Lancet 2:516, 1972.

Skakkebaek, N.E.: Atypical germ cells in the adjacent "normal" tissue of testicular tumours. Acta Pathol. Microbiol. Scand. 83:127, 1975.

Skakkebaek, N.E.: Carcinoma in situ of the testis: Frequency and relationship to invasive germ cell tumours in infertile men. Histopathology 2:157, 1978.

Skakkebaek, N.E.: Carcinoma in situ of the testis in testicular feminization syndrome. Acta Pathol. Microbiol. Scand. (A) 87:87, 1979.

Skakkebaek, N.E., Berthelsen, J.G.: Carcinoma-in-situ of testis and orchiectomy. Lancet 2:204, 1978.

Skakkebaek, N.E., Berthelsen, J.G., Müller, J.: Carcinoma-in-situ of the undescended testis. Urol. Clin. North Am. 9:377, 1982.

Skakkebaek, N.E., Berthelsen, J.G., Visfeldt, J.: Clinical aspects of testicular carcinoma-in-situ. Int. J. Androl. Suppl. 4:153, 1981.

Talerman, A.: Gonadoblastoma associated with embryonal carcinoma in an anatomically normal male. J. Urol. 113:355, 1975.

Talerman, A.: The pathology of gonadal neoplasms composed of germ cells and sex cord stroma derivatives. Pathol. Res. Pract. 170:24, 1980.

Talerman, A.: Spermatocytic seminoma. Clinicopathological study of 22 cases. Cancer 45:2169, 1980.

Teilum, G.: Special Tumors of Ovary and Testis. Comparative Pathology and Histological Identification. Philadelphia, Pennsylvania, J.B. Lippincott, 1976, pp. 408–414.

Teter, J., Philip, J., Wecewicz, G.: "Mixed" gonadal dysgenesis with a gonadoblastoma in situ. Am. J. Obstet. Gynecol. 90:929, 1964.

Young, R.H., Welch, W.R., Dickersin, G.R., Scully, R.E.: Ovarian sex cord tumor with annular tubules. Cancer 50:1384, 1982.

Zevallos, M., Snyder, R.N., Sadoff, L., Cooper, J.F.: Testicular neoplasm in identical twins. J.A.M.A. 250:645, 1983.

B.E. BUCK
K.E. BOVE

19 Wilms' Tumor

Observations in newborn infants (Potter, 1961) and careful searches of both nephrectomy specimens and the contralateral kidney in cases of Wilms' tumor have revealed a number of associated lesions which are generally regarded as precursors (Bove, Koffler, and McAdams, 1969; Bove and McAdams, 1976). These observations are supported by findings in a larger study (National Wilms' Tumor Study III) (Bonadio, Kiviat, and Beckwith, 1981). Pertinent data may be summarized as follows:

1. Nodular remnants of the metanephric blastema are an incidental finding in sections of kidney in 0.25 to 1 percent of autopsies performed on infants (Bennington and Beckwith, 1975; Bove and McAdams, 1978). This microscopic finding is often associated with trisomy 18 (Bove, Koffler, and McAdams, 1969).

2. At least one fifth of kidneys removed for Wilms' tumor have remnants of aberrant metanephric differentiation in the form of nodular renal blastema, metanephric hamartoma, or multifocal nephroblastomatosis. Most of these lesions occupy the subcapsular cortex or column of Bertin, the site of the original nephrogenic zone. Another form of precursor lesion, located within lobules and called intralobar nephroblastomatosis, is also associated with Wilms' tumor. All of these lesions may be considered embryonal hamartomas, defined as persistent tumor-like masses of imperfectly developed tissue derived from and often containing blastema which is normal for the site.

3. Grossly visible Wilms' tumorlets and small classic Wilms' tumors may be found within or immediately adjacent to the embryonal hamartomas in a kidney removed for Wilms' tumor. This finding supports the idea that Wilms' tumors may develop in such lesions.

4. The vast majority of bilateral Wilms' tumors are associated with such hamartomas (Bove and McAdams, 1976) and have an excess of associated malformations (Bond, 1975).

5. Patients with solitary Wilms' tumor plus multifocal precursors are also more likely to have associated malformations (LeMasters and Bove, 1980) and have a small risk of developing a Wilms' tumor in the contralateral kidney.

6. The putative precursors are rare as incidental findings at autopsy or in nephrectomy specimens from older children or adults (Scharfenberg and Beckman, 1984).

Nodular renal blastema is typically in the subcapsular renal cortex or in the central portions of the columns of Bertin. The lesions are often multiple and are usually between 100 and 300 micra in diameter. They have either no capsule or only a thin delicate fibrous peripheral layer. Fetal-type glomeruli are often seen at the edges of the nodules and may be derived from them. Rosettes and/or primitive tubules may be seen within the nodules of blastema. The blastemal cells are primitive in appearance, with ovoid, deeply chromatic nuclei showing little polymorphism. Cytoplasm is scant and mitotic figures are rare (Figs. 19–1 and 19–2). Nodular renal blastema is very common in trisomy 18 (Bove, Koffler, and McAdams, 1969), and Wilms' tumor (Fig. 19–3) has occurred in the small number of babies with trisomy 18 who have survived infancy (Geiser and Shindler, 1969).

Metanephric hamartomas occur typically in the subcapsular renal cortex. They may be recognized grossly on the external surface as slight irregularities. They often have a depressed profile on the cut surface but may contain discrete nodules. They vary from microscopic size to lesions up to 2 to 3 cm in diameter. They contain islands of blastema as well as small, well-developed tubules in a variable amount of dense fibrous stroma (Figs. 19–4 to 19–6). Tubular epithelial cells are small, ovoid, and contain deeply chromatic nuclei surrounded by scant cytoplasm. The epithelium may be arranged in papillary fronds and psammoma bodies may be numerous. Hamartomas which contain abundant stroma and sparse tubules are common in older patients, suggesting that regression may occur, although the mechanism is unknown.

Wilms' tumorlets are discrete, nodular, grossly visible lesions composed of proliferating embryonal renal

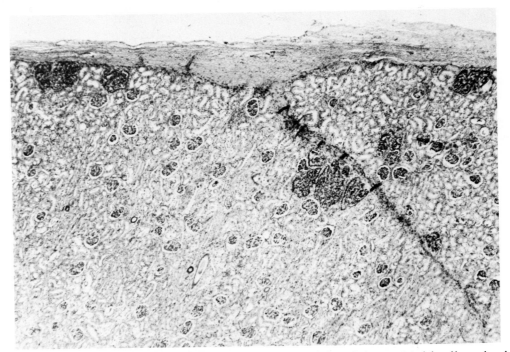

Figure 19–1. Nodular renal blastema beneath the capsule of the kidney and along an interlobar fibrous band.

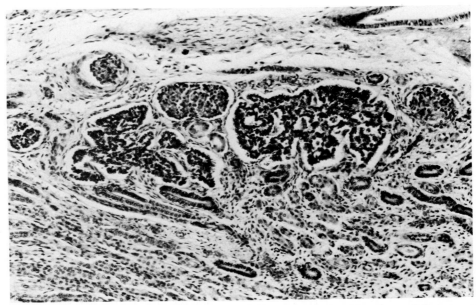

Figure 19–2. Nodular renal blastema along an interlobar fibrous band. Notice the two immature glomeruli that seem to have developed from the blastematous focus, and perhaps as many as three others in early stages of development.

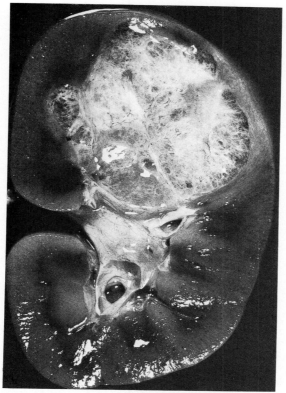

Figure 19–3. Wilms' tumor within the kidney of a patient with trisomy 18.

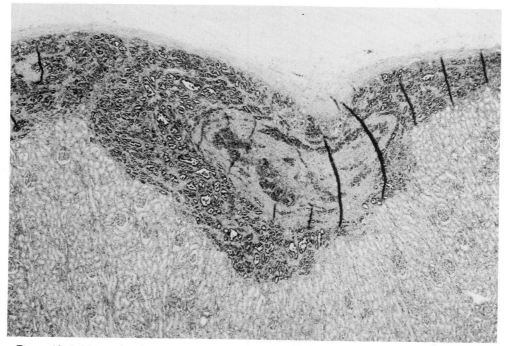

Figure 19–4. Metanephric hamartoma with partial sclerosis. The surface indentation was noted grossly.

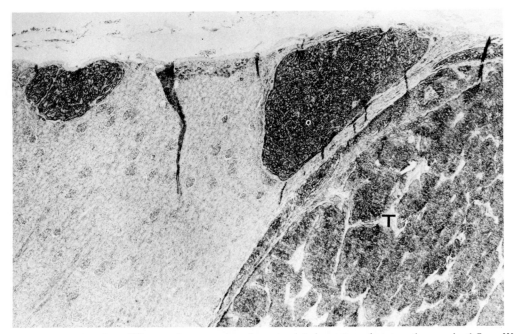

Figure 19–5. Two large nodules of renal blastema have a region of metanephric hamartoma between them and a 1.5-cm Wilms' tumorlet *(T)* nearby.

blastema. These lesions may be up to several centimeters in diameter and, though usually monomorphous, may show focal incomplete tubular differentiation. Most commonly, these lesions are subcapsular in location and appear to be developing within metanephric hamartomas (Figs. 19–5 and 19–6), distorting the superficial profile of the kidney. A second type of Wilms' tumorlet develops independently of the subcapsular cortex within the renal lobule (Fig. 19–7). These are usually polymorphous lesions with a prominent cystic component. Such lesions were noted by Bove and McAdams in their survey of lesions associated with Wilms' tumors (1976) and have recently been more extensively discussed by Kiviat and

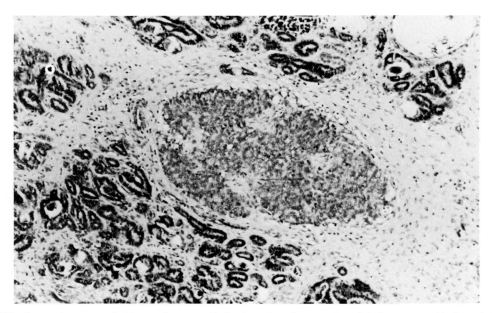

Figure 19–6. Wilms' tumorlet surrounded by, and presumably having arisen from, metanephric hamartoma. Both epithelial and stromal components are recognizable within the tumorlet. Psammoma bodies and sclerotic stroma are present focally in the hamartoma.

Beckwith, J.B., Palmer N.F.: Histopathology and prognosis of Wilms' tumor: results of the First National Wilms' Tumor Study. Cancer 41:1937–1948, 1978.

Bennington, J.L., Beckwith, J.B.: Tumors of the kidney, renal pelvis and ureter. *In:* Atlas of Tumor Pathology, 2nd series, Sect. 2, Fasc. 12. Washington, D.C., Armed Forces Institute of Pathology, 1975, pp. 32–40.

Bonadio, J.F., Kiviat, N., Beckwith, J.B.: Nephrogenic rests, multicentric Wilms' tumor and nephroblastomatosis: the NWTS experience. Presented at Interim Meeting, Pediatric Pathology Club, Duke University, October 23, 1981.

Bond, J.V.: Bilateral Wilms' tumor. Lancet 2:482–484, 1975.

Bove, K.E., Koffler, H., McAdams, A.J.: Nodular renal blastema: definition and possible significance. Cancer 24:323–332, 1969.

Bove, K.E., McAdams, J.: The Nephroblastomatosis Complex and Its Relationship to Wilms' Tumor: A Clinicopathologic Treatise. *In:* Perspectives in Pediatric Pathology, Rosenberg H.S., Bolande R.P. (Eds.), Vol. 3, Chicago, Year Book Medical Publishers, Inc., 1976, pp. 185–223.

Bove, K.E., McAdams, J.: Multifocal nephroblastic neoplasia. J. Natl. Cancer Inst. 61:285–294, 1978.

Breslow, N.E., Beckwith, J.B.: Epidemiological features of Wilms' tumors: Results of the National Wilms' Tumor Study. J. Natl. Cancer Inst. 68:429–436, 1982.

Buck, B.E., Claflin, A.J., Malinin, T.I.: Comparison of methodologies for the preparation of human fetal kidney cell cultures. (Abstract). Fed. Proc. (FASEB), 42:602, 1983.

Chatten, J.: Epithelial differentiation in Wilms' tumor: A clinicopathologic appraisal. *In:* Perspectives in Pediatric Pathology, Rosenberg, H.S., and Bolande, R.P. (Eds.), Volume 3. Chicago, Year Book Medical Publishers, Inc., 1976, pp. 225–254.

de Chadarevian, J.P., Fletcher, B.D., Chatten, J., Rabinovitch, H.H.: Massive infantile nephroblastomatosis. A clinical, radiological, and pathological analysis of four cases. Cancer 39:2294–2305, 1977.

Fearon, E.R., Volgelstein, B., Feinberg, A.P.: Somatic deletion and duplication of genes on chromosome 11 in Wilms' tumours. Nature 309:176–178, 1984.

Geiser, C.F., Schindler, A.M.: Long survival in a male with 18-trisomy syndrome and Wilms' tumor. Pediatrics 44:111–116, 1969.

Green, D.M., Fine, W.E., Li, F.P.: Offspring of patients treated for unilateral Wilms' tumor in childhood. Cancer 49:2285–2288, 1982.

Hethcote, H.W., Knudson, A.G.: Model for the incidence of embryonal cancers: application to retinoblastoma. Proc. Natl. Acad. Sci. U.S.A. 75:2453–2457, 1978.

Hou, L.T., Holman, R.L.: Bilateral nephroblastomatosis in a premature infant. J. Pathol. Bacteriol. 82:249–255, 1961.

Kiviat, N.B., Beckwith, J.B.: Intralobar nephrogenic rests and related Wilms' tumors. Presented at Interim Meeting, Pediatric Pathology Club, Duke University, October 23, 1981.

Knudson, A.G.: Mutation and cancer: statistical study of retinoblastoma. Proc. Natl. Acad. Sci. U.S.A. 68:820–823, 1971.

Knudson, A.G.: Mutation and cancer: neuroblastoma and pheochromocytoma. Am. J. Hum. Genet. 24:514–532, 1972.

Knudson, A.G., Strong, L.C.: Mutation and cancer: A model for Wilms' tumor of the kidney. J. Natl. Cancer Inst. 48:313–324, 1972.

Knudson, A.G., Meadows, A.T.: Developmental genetics of neuroblastoma, J. Natl. Cancer Inst. 57:675–682, 1976.

Knudson, A.G., Hethcote, H.W., Brown, B.W.: Mutation and childhood cancer: a probabilistic model for the incidence of retinoblastoma. Proc. Natl. Acad. Sci. U.S.A. 72:5116–5120, 1975.

Kondo, K., Chilcote, R.R., Maurer, H.S., Rowley, J.D.: Chromosome abnormalities in tumor cells from patients with sporadic Wilms' tumor. Cancer Res. 44:5376–5381, 1984.

Koufos, A., Hansen, M.F., Lampkin, B.C., Workman, M.L., Copeland, N.G., Jenkins, N.A., Cavenee, W.K.: Loss of alleles at loci on human chromosome 11 during genesis of Wilms' tumour. Nature 309:170–172, 1984.

LeMasters, G.K., Bove, K.E.: Genetic/environmental significance of multifocal nodular renal blastema. Am. J. Pediat. Hematol. Oncol. 2:81–87, 1980.

Matsunaga, E.: Genetics of Wilms' tumor. Hum. Genetics 57:231–246, 1981.

Meadows, A.T., Lichtenfeld, J.L., Koop, C.E.: Wilms's tumor in three children of a woman with congenital hemihypertrophy. N. Engl. J. Med. 291:23–24, 1974.

Nicholson, G.W.: An embryonic tumor of the kidney in a foetus. J. Pathol. Bacteriol. 34:711–730, 1931.

Nowell, P.C.: The clonal evolution of tumor cell populations. Science 194:23–28, 1976.

Nowell, P.C.: Cytogenetics. *In:* Cancer, A Comprehensive Treatise, 2nd edition, Becker, F.F. (Ed.). New York, Plenum Press, 1982, pp. 3–46.

Orkin, S.H., Goldman, D.S., Sallan, S.E.: Development of homozygosity for chromosome 11p markers in Wilms' tumour. Nature 309:172–174, 1984.

Potter, E.L., Thierstein, S.T.: Glomerular development in the kidney as an index of fetal maturity. J. Pediat. 22:695–706, 1943.

Potter, E.L.: Pathology of the Fetus and Newborn, 2nd edition, Chicago, Year Book Medical Publishers, Inc., 1961, p. 199.

Reeve, A.E., Housiaux, P.J., Gardner, R.J.M., Chewings, W.E., Grindley, R.M., Millow, L.J.: Loss of a Harvey *ras* allele in sporadic Wilms' tumour. Nature 309:174–176, 1984.

Riccardi, V.M., Sujanski, E., Smith, A.C., Francke, V.: Chromosomal imbalance in the aniridia-Wilms' Tumor association: 11 p interstitial deletion. Pediatrics 61:604–610, 1978.

Scharfenberg, J.C., Beckman, E.N.: Persistent renal blastema in an adult. Hum. Pathol. 15:791–793, 1984.

Solomon, E.: Recessive mutation in aetiology of Wilms' tumour. Nature 309:111–112, 1984.

Turleau, C., de Grouchy, J., Tournade, M-F., Gagnodoux, M-F., Junien C.: Del 11 p/aniridia complex. Report of three patients and review of 37 observations from the literature. Clin. Genet. 26:356–362, 1984.

JUAN E. OLVERA-RABIELA

20 Central Nervous System

The incipient or early neoplasms in the central nervous system can give rise to clinical manifestations if they are situated in strategic locations. At the other extreme, they may be asymptomatic and first discovered incidentally at autopsy. The local pressure effects of an intracranial tumor upon vital structures makes the neoplastic entity biologically malignant, irrespective of its histologic type. For example, the obstructive effect of a tumor in the ventricular system causes hydrocephalus and intracranial hypertension, which, if not treated in time, can cause death, even if the tumor is histologically benign and quite small.

Morphologic precursors of central nervous system (CNS) tumors are unknown. Thus, only the small but well-established neoplasms can be discussed. There are, however, a number of systemic diseases, some of which are genetically determined, that are associated with a high incidence of CNS tumors. These diseases include neurofibromatosis, von-Hippel Lindau syndrome, which is associated with hemangioblastomas of the cerebellum, and tuberous sclerosis. Likewise, a definite risk of neoplasia exists in patients receiving central nervous system irradiation, although at present it is not possible to predict this risk for one individual because of the many variables (Anderson and Treip, 1984).

In this chapter, some examples of early neoplasms which originate from neuroepithelial tissue, nerve sheath cells, meningeal and related tissues, germ cells, blood vessels, and malformative and choristomatous tumors are considered.

Fibrillary Astrocytomas. They may arise in various sites within the central nervous system at any age. In childhood and adolescence the cerebellum, brain stem, and hypothalamus are usually involved. In adult life the cerebral hemispheres are more commonly affected. The tumor is poorly demarcated, firm, and gives an increased opacity to involved structures (Davis, 1971) (Fig. 20–1).

Before these fibrillary astrocytomas cause intracranial hypertension, they may manifest themselves by

epilepsy if they affect the cortex of the frontal, parietal, or temporal lobes. When small they can be treated successfully by surgery (Pool and Kamrin, 1966).

Glioblastoma Multiforme. The glioblastoma multiforme is the most common neoplasm of neuroectodermal derivation. It is usually encountered between the ages of 50 and 70 (Earle et al., 1957; Jellinger, 1978). Most of them occur in the cerebral white matter, but often the central gray matter is also involved. The histologic malignancy is usually correlated with a rapid progression of mental symptoms, motor deficits, seizures, and cranial hypertension.

These tumors are rarely removed surgically. Occasionally they are discovered at autopsy in the early stage, when death is due to other causes (Fig. 20–2).

Astrocytoma of the Cerebellum. Astrocytomas are more common in the first two decades. Very often, these tumors are circumscribed and cystic (Fig. 20–3). In general, they can be treated surgically with a greater rate of success than the cerebral astrocytomas (Gol and McKissock, 1978). In most cystic tumors the neoplasm may be represented as a mural nodule (Ringertz and Nordenstam, 1951). In these cases the resection of the nodule and aspiration of the cyst can be curative.

Subependymal Giant Cell Astrocytoma. This tumor may or may not be associated with tuberous sclerosis. It often occupies the walls of a lateral ventricle over the basal ganglia. It is usually well defined and can cause obstruction of one foramen of Monro (Fig. 20–4). It may be calcified and contain dilated blood vessels. It is composed of large gemistocytic astrocytes with abundant eosinophilic cytoplasm and thick processes. These tumors have a slow growth in spite of the presence of giant cells (Kapp et al., 1967). The prognosis is good following total or partial resection, as patients have survived many years without recurrence (Cooper, 1971).

Oligodendroglioma. This is a rather uncommon neuroectodermal tumor, mainly found in young adults. The large majority grow slowly in the cerebral

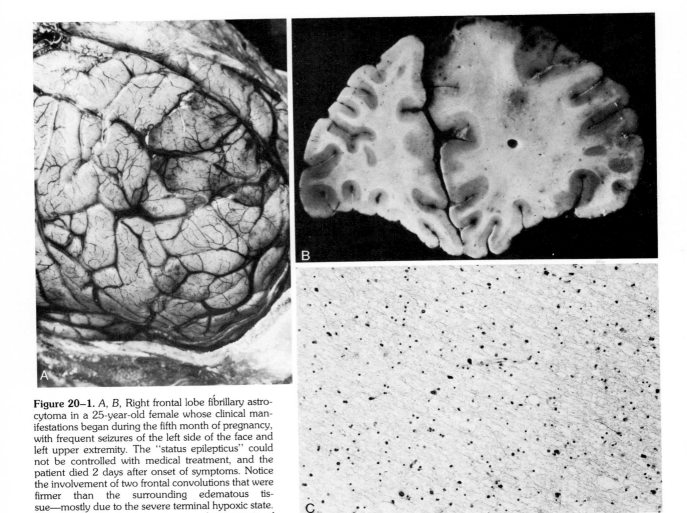

Figure 20–1. *A, B,* Right frontal lobe fibrillary astrocytoma in a 25-year-old female whose clinical manifestations began during the fifth month of pregnancy, with frequent seizures of the left side of the face and left upper extremity. The "status epilepticus" could not be controlled with medical treatment, and the patient died 2 days after onset of symptoms. Notice the involvement of two frontal convolutions that were firmer than the surrounding edematous tissue—mostly due to the severe terminal hypoxic state. The increased consistency is very characteristic of fibrillary astrocytomas. The poor demarcation and the infiltration of the cortex can be observed in the coronal section. *C,* Fibrillary astrocytoma. A moderate increase in the number of astrocytes, some of which show minimal hyperchromatism. Glial fibrils are abundant.

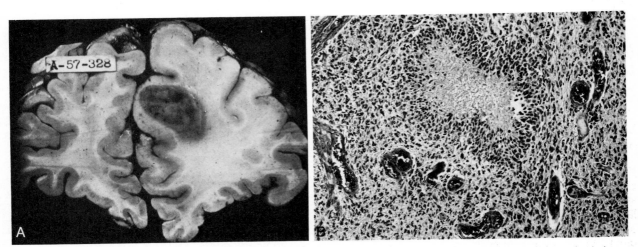

Figure 20–2. *A,* A 45-year-old male who had alternating periods of depression and euphoria died after a session of electroshock therapy. A well-circumscribed and highly vascularized neoplasm is located in the rostromedial portion of the left frontal lobe white matter. This is indeed an early stage in the growth of a glioblastoma multiforme. *B,* Histologically, a well-defined area of necrosis with nuclear palisading is noted. Capillary proliferation is prominent.

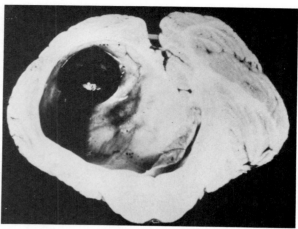

Figure 20–3. Cystic astrocytoma of the right cerebellar hemisphere with a highly vascularized mural nodule. This 17-year-old boy had signs and symptoms of cerebellar dysfunction for a few weeks. He was admitted to a hospital because of manifestations of increased intracranial pressure. Pneumoventriculography was performed, and a posterior fossa craniotomy was planned for the next day. The patient died a few hours after the injection of air into the ventricular system, because of herniation of the cerebellar tonsils.

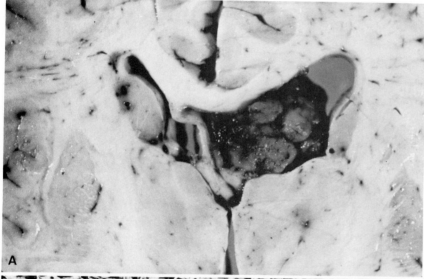

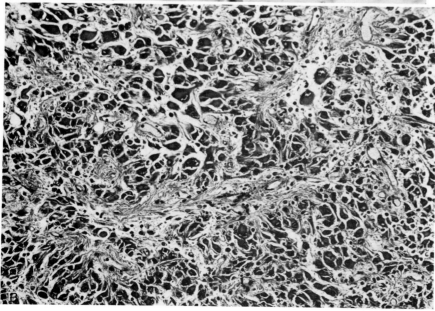

Figure 20–4. *A,* A rather small subependymal giant cell astrocytoma found in a 9-year-old boy who had the typical manifestations of tuberous sclerosis. This neoplasm had already obstructed the left foramen of Monro, and the dilated left lateral ventricle with the tumor is readily apparent. *B,* Most cells are gemistocytic in type and have an abundant eosinophilic cytoplasm. Numerous blood vessels and a fibrillary background are also present.

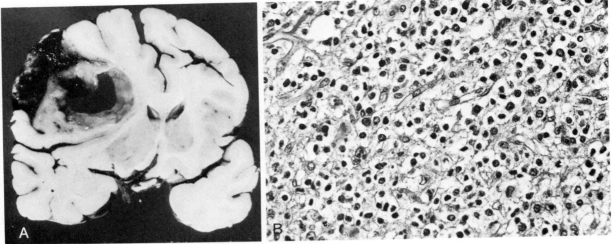

Figure 20–5. *A,* A left frontal lobe oligodendroglioma that has infiltrated the cortex and has a cystic portion. This is the smallest tumor of this type in the files of our pathology unit. The history was that of a 55-year-old male who had had seizures of the grand mal type for several weeks with some speech difficulties. Calcifications were visible on x-ray films and histologically. Only a small portion of the tumor was obtained at surgery because of profuse bleeding. Death occurred a few hours after the operation.

A smaller oligodendroglioma found at surgery or at autopsy would be a rarity. The possible explanation for this is the fact that most grow slowly and attain a rather large size before they give rise to clinical manifestations. *B,* The tumor is composed of cells with a round hyperchromatic nucleus and a prominent perinuclear halo.

hemispheres and as a rule are a cause of epilepsy when they reach the cortex. It would be a rarity to find a small oligodendroglioma at surgery or at autopsy. Most are easily detected radiographically or with computed tomography. Visible calcifications in roentgenograms far exceed the ones seen in astrocytomas. The external surface of the affected lobe has one or more enlarged convolutions and the cut surface is generally pink and occasionally cystic (Fig. 20–5).

The microscopic diagnosis of oligodendroglioma, and in particular the differentiation from astrocytoma, should present no problems in most cases. The round nuclei, the presence of perinuclear halos, the monotonous small size and angular configuration of the vessels, the invariable presence of calcospherites, the lack of fibrillar background, and in pure oligodendrogliomas the negative results for glial fibrillary acidic protein should favor the diagnosis of this neoplasm.

There are well documented examples of the development of malignancy in this tumor (Barnard, 1968). The results of surgical treatment and radiotherapy are also well analyzed in a large series (Weir and Elvidge, 1968).

Subependymoma. It is a variant of ependymoma characterized by the proliferation of both subependymal astrocytes and ependymal cells. They arise more commonly in the fourth ventricle and sometimes they are found at necropsy (Boykin et al., 1954). Some are associated with granular ependymitis due to chronic leptomeningitis. Occasionally they grow to a large size. At surgery they are firmly attached to the site of origin, even when they are small (Scheithauer, 1978) (Fig. 20–6).

Ependymoma. Ependymomas can appear in any site lined by ependymal cells and in the central canal of the spinal cord (Fig. 20–7, *A* and *B*). For unknown reasons, they are somewhat more common in the fourth ventricle, where they usually grow from the floor and soon cause obstruction to the cerebrospinal fluid. Therefore, they do not have to achieve a large size, as do the supratentorial ones, to cause intracranial hypertension (Fig. 20–7,*C*). In any location they are sharply demarcated from the neighboring tissue, either grossly or microscopically,

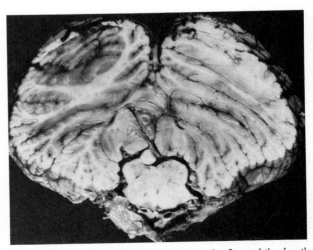

Figure 20–6. A small subependymoma on the floor of the fourth ventricle. The patient, a 44-year-old man, had basal leptomeningitis and granular ependymitis due to cysticercosis. Could this neoplasm by itself, have given manifestations of obstruction to the flow of cerebrospinal fluid? If detected, its resection would have been easily accomplished and obstruction of the fourth ventricle would have been avoided.

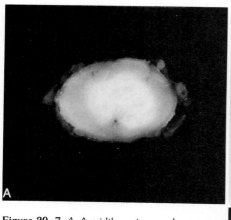

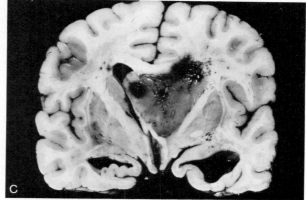

Figure 20–7. *A,* A midthoracic ependymoma of the spinal cord found in a middle-aged female who had von Recklinghausen's neurofibromatosis. Many other neoplasms were found as part of the disease, among them bilateral acoustic schwannomas and a large number of intracranial meningiomas. The clinical manifestations that this spinal cord ependymoma could have given were probably overshadowed by the ones produced by the other neoplasms. *B,* A section of the tumor illustrated in *A* stained with luxol fast blue. *C,* A 28-year-old male had a few weeks history of intracranial hypertension. The diagnosis of ependymoma of the right lateral ventricle was made clinically and at surgery. The patient died shortly after a craniotomy and biopsy of the tumor, because of intraneoplastic bleeding (not shown in photograph). Ependymomas of the lateral ventricle of smaller size than the one illustrated here may not give signs and symptoms of intracranial hypertension, unless one of the foramina of Monro is obstructed. (*A* courtesy of Dr. Haruo Okazaka, Mayo Clinic, Rochester, MN.)

and this feature helps in the distinction from other primary tumors of the central nervous system, especially astrocytomas.

The most common histologic feature in ependymomas is the presence of acellular areas around blood vessels in which one finds fibrillar material, which is identified immunohistochemically as glial fibrillary acidic protein. The nuclei of ependymoma cells are hyperchromatic as compared to those of well-differentiated astrocytomas or oligodendrogliomas. Typical ependymal rosettes are not always found and the formation of tubules and papillae are even more difficult to find. The small PTAH-positive structures known as blepharoplasts are characteristic but difficult to identify especially in surgical material; their absence, however, should not make one change the diagnosis of ependymoma if other features are present.

Ependymomas have to be considered in the differential diagnosis in some particular locations. Occasionally a medulloblastoma may be confused with an ependymoma but, as a general rule, the former is a more primitive neuroectodermal tumor, has more mitotic activity, and rarely forms rosettes.

The astrocytomas of the cerebellum and brain stem can invade the fourth ventricle and, especially at surgery, they can be confused with ependymomas.

The pathologist should have no difficulty in diagnosing an astrocytoma if fibrillar material and piloid astrocytes are present. On rare occasions the differentiation between a third ventricle ependymoma and a pituitary adenoma may be a problem, but if the tumor is radiologically found in the sella turcica one can practically rule out a tumor originating in the ependymal lining of the third ventricle.

Medulloblastoma. This is a poorly differentiated neoplasm of neuroectodermal origin and restricted to the cerebellum. It is more common in the first and second decades but is also found in adults (Rubinstein and Northfield, 1964; Olvera-Rabiela and Poucell, 1974).

In children most tumors are found in or near the vermis (Fig. 20–8). It is unfortunate that this tumor may spread early along the cerebrospinal pathway and have distant metastatic implants, even when the primary is relatively small.

Surgery and radiotherapy to the entire neuraxis are used to increase the five-year survival rate (McFarland et al., 1969; Mealey and Hall, 1977).

Acoustic Schwannoma. The acoustic schwannoma takes origin from the eighth nerve near the internal auditory meatus. Small tumors expand the internal auditory orifice, and this can be detected

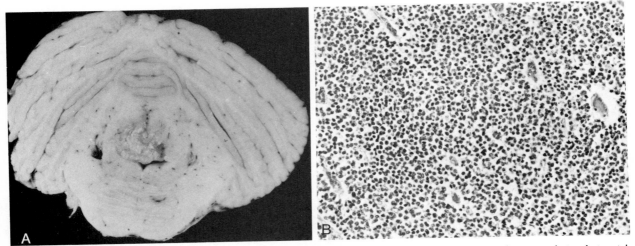

Figure 20–8. *A,* A small medulloblastoma in the cerebellar vermis of a 5-year-old boy. There was no intracranial pressure, but unfortunately many subarachnoid implants were found, especially on the lower spinal cord and nerve roots of the cauda equina. Many different clinical diagnoses were made, and death was due to intercurrent infections. *B,* Sheets of small undifferentiated round cells with hyperchromatic nuclei and scant cytoplasm are noted. The small amount of stroma contains a few blood vessels.

radiographically. Larger neoplasms inevitably compress the pons, cerebellum, and other cranial nerves.

It is well known that medium and large tumors have a high surgical morbidity and mortality (Cushing, 1917). A common complication of surgery is the ischemic lesion in the region supplied by the superior cerebellar artery. In small tumors (Fig. 20–9) surgery can be performed without the dreadful ischemic lesions and permanent damage to neighboring cranial nerves and pons (Kasantikul et al., 1980).

Sphenoidal Ridge and Olfactory Meningiomas. Meningiomas that arise from the sphenoidal ridge usually project into the middle fossa, though occasionally they may spread forward into the anterior fossa as well. They may extend along the sphenoid

ridge and into the Sylvian fissure and may even surround the internal carotid artery as it emerges from the cavernous sinus, constricting it in an annular fashion, sometimes to the point where the blood supply to the hemisphere is reduced to a clinically significant degree (Boldrey, 1971). Small tumors located in the middle or lateral thirds of the ridge (Fig. 20–10) can be cured by surgery (Horning and Kernohan, 1950).

Olfactory meningiomas originate from the ethmoid plate and the olfactory groove. The differentiation between this meningioma and the one from the tuberculum sellae is sometimes difficult to establish. The involved nervous system structures may be the same, depending on the direction of the growth. The

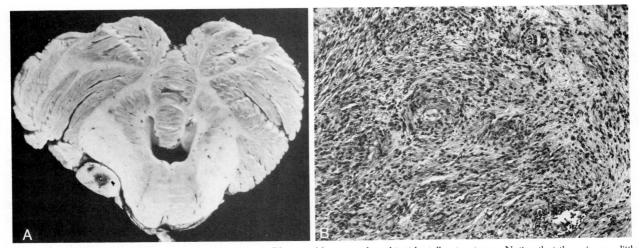

Figure 20–9. *A,* A small eighth nerve schwannoma in a 78-year-old woman found incidentally at autopsy. Notice that there is very little compression of the left middle cerebellar penduncle. Tumors of this size (less than 1 cm) usually are associated with a short history of decreased hearing loss and tinnitus. Microscopically, the tumor was rather cellular and composed of fascicles of Schwann cells interspersed with some foam cells.

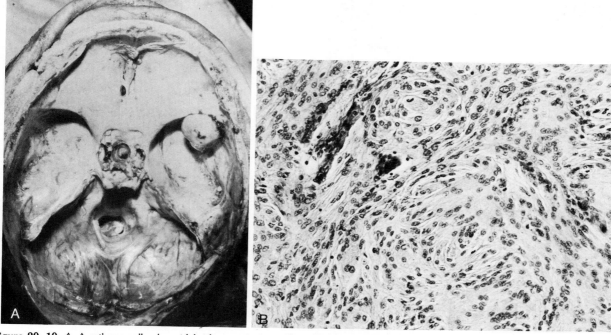

Figure 20–10. *A,* A rather small sphenoidal ridge meningioma, laterally located and therefore easier to treat surgically. This 71-year-old woman had another meningioma attached to the falx, between the parietal lobes, that was unsuccessfully resected because of profuse bleeding. The one illustrated here was an autopsy finding. *B,* Meningothelial meningioma. The tumor is composed of whorls of meningothelial cells.

small meningiomas that have caused olfactory tract compression (Fig. 20–11) and slightly larger ones with minor visual field deficits can be operated upon with excellent results (Bakay and Cares, 1972).

Germinal Tumors. Most neoplasms in or near the pineal gland are germinal tumors, indistinguishable on histologic grounds from those that occur in the gonads and in other extragonadal sites (Jellinger, 1973).

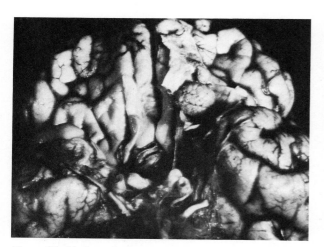

Figure 20–11. A small olfactory groove meningioma in a 55-year-old woman, which had compressed the olfactory bulb and nerve. It was an autopsy finding. The tumor has been removed from its bed, which is seen on the right gyrus rectus.

There is general agreement that pineal germinomas are more common in males and suprasellar ones in females, but male preponderance is striking. As is also evident in the published series, they are clinically recognized more often between the ages of 15 and 25 years (Dayan et al., 1966; Donat et al., 1978).

Tumors that originate in or near the pineal soon produce aqueductal compression and invade the quadrigeminal plate. A careful neurologic examination can detect this neoplasm in the incipient stage (Fig. 20–12).

Hemangioblastoma of the Cerebellum. This is a vascular neoplasm that appears predominantly in the cerebellum and, as a rule, can be treated surgically with a great rate of success (Horax, 1954; Obrador and Martin-Rodriguez, 1977). Most cerebellar hemangioblastomas are small mural nodules in a cyst, very similar and sometimes grossly indistinguishable from cystic astrocytomas (Fig. 20–13). The tumor is composed of small vessels, with prominent endothelial cells and a variable component of cells, usually referred to as "stromal cells," which may contain abundant lipid material. Nothing in this tumor indicates histologic malignancy; perhaps the best name would be hemangioendothelioma, but the term hemangioblastoma seems hard to abandon.

On frozen section this neoplasm can be confused with an astrocytoma if the tissue in the immediate vicinity of the nodule is examined. The presence here of gliosis with Rosenthal fibers can be misleading. The

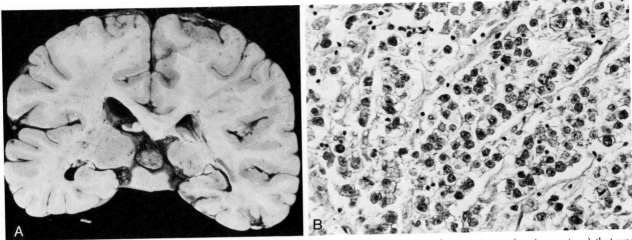

Figure 20–12. *A,* The pineal gland is enlarged about three times because of the presence of a germinoma (seminoma type) that was found to infiltrate the parenchyma of the gland. The patient, a 19-year-old male, had a similar tumor that compressed the hypothalamus. The quadrigeminal plate compression from the enlarged pineal gland manifested itself by impeded upward gaze. *B,* Cords of neoplastic cells having abundant clear cytoplasm and vesicular nuclei with prominent nucleoli are present in this germinoma.

demonstration of neutral fat in the stromal cells is very helpful in diagnosis. Quite often a metastatic renal cell carcinoma in the cerebellum is confused with a hemangioblastoma. The presence of glycogen in the clear cells of the renal carcinoma is also a helpful diagnostic aid.

Craniopharyngioma. The large majority of these neoplasms are suprasellar and soon give rise to manifestations secondary to compression of the pituitary gland, hypothalamus, and optic chiasm. The radiographic, tomographic, gross and histologic characteristics are well known. Occasionally the pathologist may have to differentiate a craniopharyngioma from an epidermoid cyst, especially when the surgical material shows very little epithelium which is not of the

adamantinomatous type. The cells of the epidermoid cyst lining usually show keratinization and rest on fibrous connective tissue.

It is difficult to accomplish a total excision of this neoplasm, especially when the external surface is already adherent to the neighboring structures. The incomplete resection is usually complemented with radiotherapy, but the length of survival is unpredictable (Kramer et al., 1961; Shapiro et al., 1979). With a small craniopharyngioma (Fig. 20–14), it is easier to avoid surgical morbidity.

Lipoma. This is a neoplasm of choristomatous nature that is infrequently encountered intracranially. The corpus callosum (Fig. 20–15), the cerebellum and the quadrigeminal plate are the usual sites. The

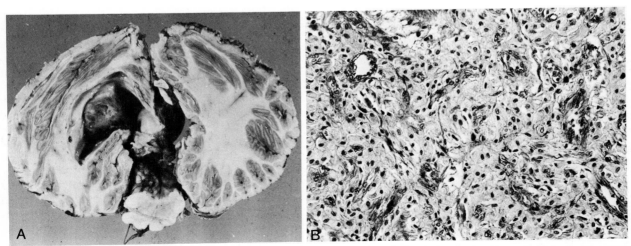

Figure 20–13. *A,* Hemangioblastoma. A 48-year-old man with a short history of cerebellar dysfunction and increased intracranial pressure died after ventriculography with contrast material. There is a small mural nodule in a cyst that occupies the right cerebellar hemisphere and part of the vermis. *B,* Stromal cells with a foamy appearance are seen between proliferating capillaries.

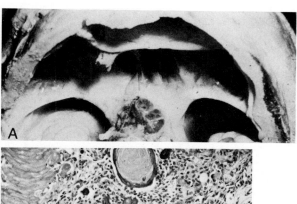

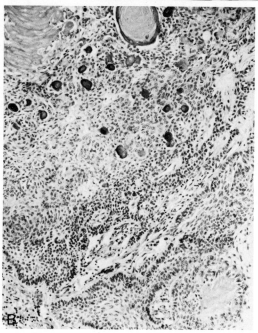

Figure 20–14. *A,* A small craniopharyngioma in a 17-year-old boy, which had produced pituitary dysfunction and minor visual field deficits. Death was due to an unrelated cause. The almost complete or total resection of this tumor would have been much easier than in the ones with their capsule firmly fixed to neighboring structures. *B,* Islands of basaloid epithelium and numerous foci of calcification are present.

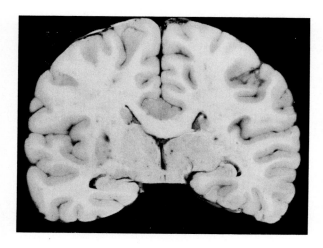

Figure 20–15. A small well-circumscribed lipoma over the corpus callosum in a 10-year-old girl who died during surgical correction of a defect in the nose. No clinical manifestations attributable to this tumor were known.

large majority of intracranial lipomas are autopsy findings, but some have been diagnosed by computed tomography (Kazner et al., 1980). These malformative tumors, because of their location, are difficult to excise completely, but in some cases, the cerebrospinal fluid obstruction can be treated by shunting procedures (Kazner et al., 1980).

Epidermoid Cysts. The cerebellopontine angle and the parapontine area (Fig. 20–16) are common sites. They grow slowly, but even when not yet large, rupture is not uncommon and complicates surgical treatment (Guidetti and Gagliardi, 1977). There are several reports of their malignant transformation (Davidson and Small, 1960; Fox and South, 1965).

Intraspinal Neurilemmoma (Schwannoma). Most intraspinal neurilemmomas are found on the dorsal roots, at any spinal segment, and not associated with other components of von Recklinghausen's disease. Some are located inside the dura mater and others pass through the intervertebral foramina (Fig. 20–17). At surgery the tumor can be dissected away from the spinal root, as this is not incorporated in the neoplasm. Microscopically these tumors exhibit predominantly Antoni A tissue and palisading of nuclei. The distinction from meningiomas, either grossly or microscopi-

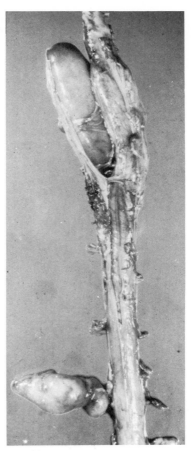

Figure 20–17. A 20-year-old woman with von Recklinghausen's disease had several intraspinal schwannomas. The large cervical neoplasm had caused motor deficit in upper and lower extremities, and death was due to edema of the cervical segment of the cord. The tumor could not be resected because of inadequate surgical approach. There are several other nerve sheath tumors in lower spinal roots, one with a classic dumb-bell shape, and smaller ones in other dorsal roots that by themselves could have given signs of radicular compression.

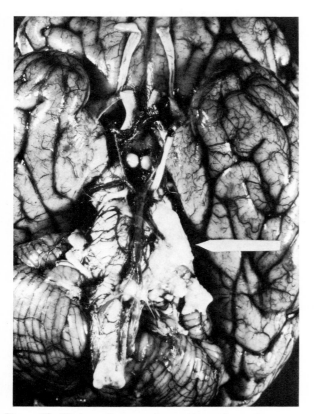

Figure 20–16. A small parapontine epidermoid cyst that was an incidental finding at autopsy in a 53-year-old man. The slow growth of this lesion probably explains the onset of symptoms when they attain a larger size.

cally, presents no problems. The meningioma is found firmly fixed to the dura mater, not as round and smooth as the neurilemmoma and contains a large number of psammoma bodies which can be felt when sectioned.

Neurilemmomas which have not attained a large size can be easily and completely excised (Love and Dodge, 1952).

References

Anderson, J.R., Treip, C.S.: Radiation-induced intracranial neoplasms. A report of three possible cases. Cancer 53:426–429, 1984.

Bakay, L., Cares, H.L.: Olfactory meningiomas. Report on a series of twenty-five cases. Acta Neurochiur. 26:1–2, 1972.

Barnard, R.O.: The development of malignancy in oligodendrogliomas. J. Pathol. Bacteriol. 96:113–123, 1968.

Boldrey, E.: The Meningiomas. *In:* Pathology of the Nervous System, Vol. 2. Minckler, J. (Ed.). New York, McGraw-Hill, 1971, pp. 2125–2142.

Boykin, F.C., Cowen, D., Iannuci, C.A.J., Wolf, A.: Subependymal glomerate astrocytomas. J. Neuropath. Exp. Neurol. 13:30–49, 1954.

Cooper, J.R.: Brain tumors in hereditary multiple system hamartomatosis (tuberous sclerosis). J. Neurosurg. 34:194–202, 1971.

Cushing, H.: Tumors of the Nervus Acusticus and the Syndrome of the Cerebellopontine Angle. Philadelphia, W.B. Saunders Company, 1917.

Davidson, S.E., Small, J.M.: Malignant change in an intracranial epidermoid. J. Neurosurg. Psychiat. 23:176–178, 1960.

Davis, H.L.: Astrocytomas. *In:* Pathology of the Nervous System, Vol. 2. Minckler, J. (Ed.). New York, McGraw-Hill, 1971, pp. 2007–2025.

Dayan, A.D., Marshall, A.H.E., Miller, A.A., Pick, F.J., Rankin, N.E.: Atypical teratomas of the pineal and hypothalamus. J. Pathol. Bacteriol. 92:1, 1966.

Donat, J.F., Okazaki, H., Gomez, M.R., Reagan, T.J., Baker, H.L., Laws, E.R., Jr.: Pineal tumors. A 53-year experience. Arch. Neurol. 35:736–740, 1978.

Earle, K.M., Rentschler, E.H., Snodgrass, S.R.: Primary intracranial neoplasms. Prognosis and classification of 513 verified cases. J. Neuropathol. Exp. Neurol. 16:321–331, 1957.

Fox, E., South, E.A.: Squamous cell carcinoma developing in an intracranial epidermoid cyst (cholesteatoma). J. Neurol. Neurosurg. Psychiat. 28:276–281, 1965.

Gol, A., McKissock, W.: The cerebellar astrocytomas. A report of 98 verified cases. J. Neurosurg. 16:287–296, 1978.

Guidetti, B., Gagliardi, F.M.: Epidermoid and dermoid cysts. Clinical evaluation and late surgical results. J. Neurosurg. 47:12–18, 1977.

Horax, G.: Benign (favorable) types of brain tumor. The end result (up to twenty years) with statistics of mortality and useful survival. N. Engl. J. Med. 240:981–984, 1954.

Horning, E.D., Kernohan, J.W.: Meningiomas of the sphenoidal ridge. A clinicopathological study. J. Neuropathol. Exp. Neurol. 9:373–384, 1950.

Jellinger, K.: Glioblastoma multiforme: morphology and biology. Acta Neurochir. 42:5–32, 1978.

Kapp, J.P., Paulson, G.W., Odom, G.L.: Brain tumors with tuberous sclerosis. J. Neurosurg. 26:191–202, 1967.

Kassantikul, V., Netsky, N.G., Glasscock, M.E., Hays, J.W.: Acoustic neurilemmoma. Clinicoanatomic study of 103 patients. J. Neurosurg. 52:28–35, 1980.

Kazner, E., Stochdorph, O., Wende, S., Grume, T.: Intracranial lipoma. Diagnosis and therapeutic considerations. J. Neurosurg. 52:234–245, 1980.

Kramer, S., McKissock, W., Concannon, J.P.: Craniopharyngiomas. Treatment by combined surgery and radiation therapy. J. Neurosurg. 18:217–226, 1961.

Love, J.G., Dodge, H.W., Jr.: Dumbbell (hourglass) neurofibromas affecting the spinal cord. Surg. Gynecol. Obstet. 94:161–172, 1952.

McFarland, D.R., Horowitz, H., Saenger, E.L., Bahr, G.K.: Medulloblastoma: a review of prognosis and survival. Br. J. Radiol. 42:198–214, 1969.

Mealey, J., Jr., Hall, P.V.: Medulloblastoma in children. Survival and treatment, J. Neurosurg. 46:56–64, 1977.

Obrador, S., Martin-Rodriguez, J.G.: Biologic factors involved in the clinical features and surgical management of cerebellar hemangioblastomas. Surg. Neurol. 7:79–85, 1977.

Olvera-Rabiela, J.E., Poucell, S.: El meduloblastoma desmoplásico. Revisión de algunos conceptos a propósito de 10 casos en sujetos adultos. Patología. 12:99–111, 1974.

Pool, J.L., Kamrin, R.P.: The treatment of intracranial gliomas by surgery and radiation. Prog. Neurol. Surg. 1:258–299, 1966.

Ringertz, N., Nordenstam, H.: Cerebellar astrocytoma. J. Neuropath. Exp. Neurol. 10:343–367, 1951.

Rubinstein, L.J., Northfield, D.W.: Medulloblastoma and the so-called "arachnoidal cerebellar sarcoma." A critical re-examination of a nosological problem. Brain. 87:379–412, 1964.

Scheithauer, B.W.: Symptomatic subependymoma. J. Neurosurg. 49:689–696, 1978.

Shapiro, K., Till, K., Grant, D.N.: Craniopharyngiomas in childhood. A rational approach to treatment. J. Neurosurg. 50:617–623, 1979.

Walker, R., Lieberman, A.N., Pinto, R., George, A., Ransohoff, J., Trubek, M., Wise, A.: Transient neurologic disturbances, brain tumors and normal computed tomography scans. Cancer 52:1502–1506, 1983.

Weir, B., Elvidge, A.R.: Oligodendrogliomas. An analysis of 63 cases. J. Neurosurg. 29:500–505, 1968.

JORGE ALBORES-SAAVEDRA

21 Soft Tissue

The preinvasive stage of many carcinomas which arise in squamous or glandular epithelia is well established, but the precursor lesions of nearly all soft-tissue sarcomas are unknown. As a rule, benign soft-tissue tumors do not become malignant. In fact, we are aware of only a few sarcomas that arise in pre-existing benign lesions. For instance, malignant schwannomas may be a late complication of neurofibromatosis; lymphangiosarcomas appear almost exclusively in long-standing chronic lymphedema; certain types of sarcomas develop in previously radiated tissues, and Kaposi's sarcoma has been observed in immunosuppressed individuals. At present, it is not possible to predict from either clinical or morphologic grounds those patients who will go on to develop a malignant tumor. However, close follow-up of these high-risk patients may lead to the detection of small malignant tumors, especially those located in superficial soft tissues.

NEUROFIBROMATOSIS AND MALIGNANT SCHWANNOMA

In regard to neurofibromatosis, it is estimated that 2 to 10 percent of patients develop a malignant schwannoma. The latent period, defined as the time between the appearance of neurofibromatosis and the diagnosis of schwannoma, is, on the average, 15 years; and, therefore, the majority of patients with malignant schwannoma and neurofibromatosis are between 20 and 50 years of age (Guccion and Enzinger, 1979). The tumor arises from either a large deep-seated nerve trunk or from a neurofibroma (Figs. 21–1 and 21–2). Sudden enlargement of a pre-existing mass in a patient with von Recklinghausen's neurofibromatosis should alert the physician to consider a diagnosis of malignant schwannoma.

Malignant schwannomas that complicate von Recklinghausen's neurofibromatosis are histologically similar to those that are not associated with this genetically determined disorder. They are composed of spindle cells arranged in a herringbone pattern (Fig. 21–3).

Perivascular concentration of tumor cells and myxoid areas are constant features, whereas nuclear palisading is uncommon. A contiguous neurofibromatous component with atypical changes that has been interpreted as representing transition between the pre-existing benign lesion and the malignant neurogenic tumor is helpful in the diagnosis (Fig. 21–4). The neoplastic cells share some light and electron microscopic features with those of normal Schwann cells (Chitale and Dickersin, 1983). The occasional demonstration of immunocytochemical markers for Schwann cells, such as myelin basic protein and S-100 protein, has provided additional support for the Schwann cell origin (Mogollon et al., 1984; Nakajima et al., 1982). A small proportion of malignant schwannomas contain rhabdomyoblasts, cartilage, osteoid, bone, and even glandular structures with mucin (Woodruff et al., 1973; Takahara et al., 1979) (Figs. 21–5 to 21–7). These heterologous elements, however, do not influence the clinical presentation and do not change the poor prognosis associated with these tumors (Guccion and Enzinger, 1979). Neoplastic Schwann cells may become facultative melanocytes and produce melanin (Burns et al., 1983). I have seen an unusual example of malignant schwannoma having areas of an angiosarcoma, which was confirmed by the presence of Factor VIII-related antigen (FVIII R Ag) positive cells. Pure rhabdomyosarcomas, angiosarcomas, and liposarcomas have also been reported in patients with neurofibromatosis (D'Agostino et al., 1963; Millstein et al., 1981).

GARDNER'S SYNDROME AND FIBROMATOSIS

Gardner's syndrome, another genetically determined condition, is often complicated with locally aggressive fibromatosis and less frequently with various types of sarcomas (Weary et al., 1964). Inherited as an autosomal dominant trait, the syndrome is characterized by intestinal polyposis, epidermal cysts, and osteomas which arise mainly in the skull and facial bones

Text continued on page 372

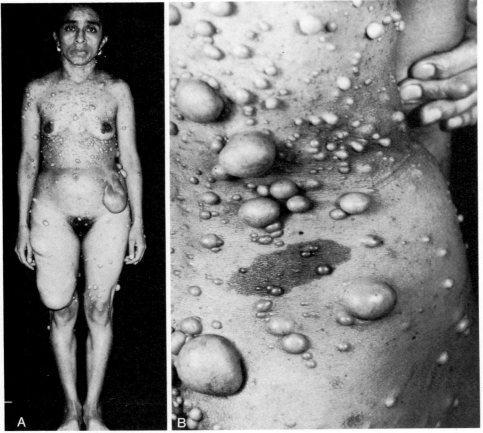

Figure 21–1. *A,* This 38-year-old patient with multiple neurofibromatosis developed a rapidly growing mass in the anterior aspect of the lower portion of the right thigh that proved to be a malignant schwannoma arising from a neurofibroma. *B,* Detail of neurofibromas and café au lait spots in the abdominal wall of the same patient.

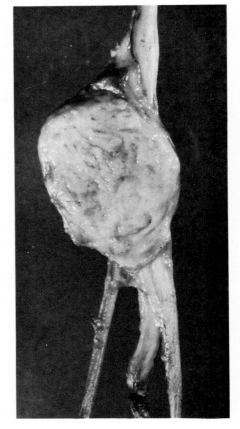

Figure 21–2. Malignant schwannoma that arose from the median nerve in a patient with multiple neurofibromatosis. The tumor, which was composed of gray-white tissue, extended along the nerve and invaded soft tissues.

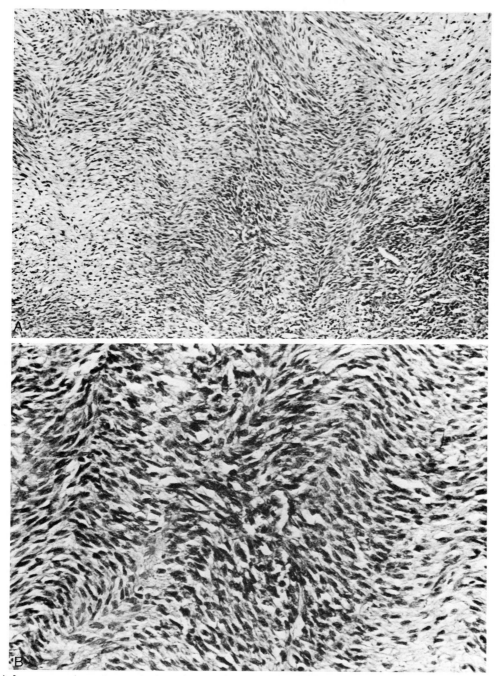

Figure 21–3. *A,* Low-power photomicrograph of a malignant schwannoma depicting the herringbone pattern and myxoid areas. *B,* Higher magnification of *A,* showing a cellular area in which fascicles of spindle-shaped cells with hyperchromatic nuclei are seen.

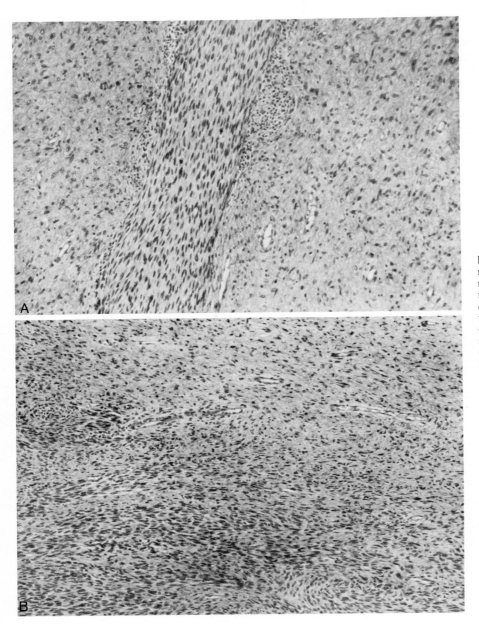

A

B

Figure 21–4. *A,* A fascicle of malignant schwannoma traversing a neurofibroma from which it arose. The neurofibroma contains a few atypical cells. *B,* Another photomicrograph of the same tumor shown in *A.* Most of the tumor represents malignant schwannoma, but in the right upper quadrant, areas of atypical neurofibroma can still be recognized.

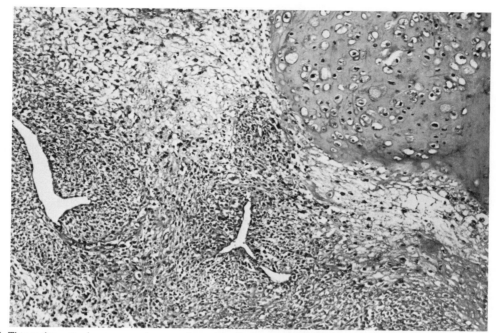

Figure 21–5. This malignant schwannoma shows malignant cartilage, myxoid areas, and perivascular concentration of neoplastic cells.

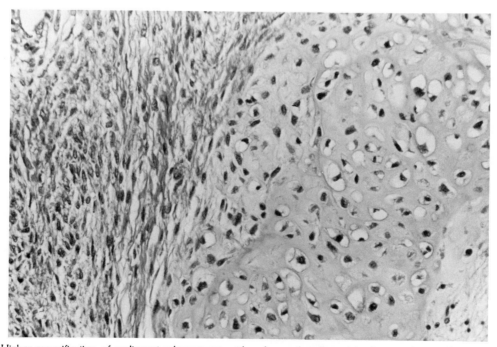

Figure 21–6. Higher magnification of malignant schwannoma with a focus of malignant hyaline cartilage and a fascicle of neoplastic Schwann cells.

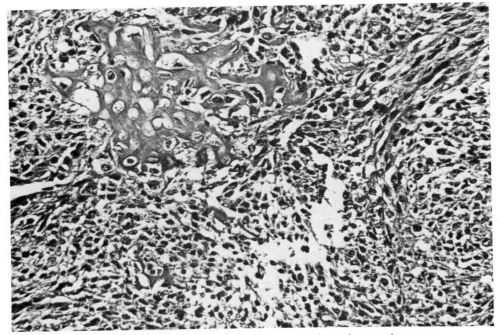

Figure 21–7. A microscopic focus of osteoid is seen in this malignant schwannoma.

(Gardner, 1982.) Malignant transformation of the intestinal adenomas commonly occurs in the periampullary region of adult patients (Bussey, 1978). Foci of carcinoma-in-situ can be found in the adenomas (Scully et al., 1982), and remnants of adenoma and carcinoma-in-situ are often present in the infiltrating adenocarcinomas. About one-half of the patients develop mesenteric or retroperitoneal fibromatosis or less frequently fibromatosis in the abdominal wall, usually months or years following intestinal resection for adenomas or carcinoma. Some cases of fibromatosis, however, are unrelated to surgical trauma (Simpson et al., 1964). As a rule, the fibromatosis appears 10 to 15 years after the onset of osteomas

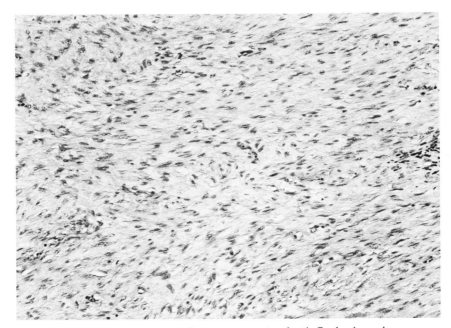

Figure 21–8. Retroperitoneal fibromatosis associated with Gardner's syndrome.

and epidermal cysts, which are discovered during childhood or adolescence. The mesenteric or retro-peritoneal fibromatosis may grow slowly and be asymptomatic or may rapidly reach a large size and cause pain or intestinal obstruction due to compression or invasion of the intestine. The microscopic picture of fibromatosis in Gardner's syndrome is similar to that of sporadic fibromatosis in other anatomic sites (Fig. 21–8). Liposarcomas, chondrosarcomas, osteosarcomas, and other malignant tumors, including cutaneous and thyroid carcinomas, have also been reported in association with Gardner's syndrome (Fraumeni et al., 1968; Camiel et al., 1968).

Werner's syndrome, a rare and autosomal recessive disorder characterized by shortness of stature and premature aging, is often complicated with a variety of malignant tumors, including soft-tissue sarcomas. Leiomyosarcomas, fibrosarcomas, and malignant fibrous histiocytomas have all been reported (Usui et al., 1984).

CHRONIC LYMPHEDEMA AND LYMPHANGIOSARCOMA

The lymphangiosarcoma is usually a complication of long-standing lymphedema of the upper extremities in patients subjected to radical mastectomy for breast cancer (Stewart and Treves, 1948). In fact, it has been estimated that 90 percent of all lymphangiosarcomas associated with chronic lymphedema occur following radical mastectomy for breast carcinoma (Woodward et al., 1972). However, only 0.4 percent of 894 women surviving five years after mastectomy developed this malignant tumor (Shirger, 1962). The patients are usually elderly females with a significant degree of lymphedema in the arm. The average time interval between the appearance of lymphedema and the development of the tumor is 10 years. I have seen one case of postmastectomy lymphangiosarcoma in a male and another that arose in an edematous leg of a woman following radical hysterectomy and radiotherapy for carcinoma of the uterine cervix. There is one case report of a lymphangiosarcoma occurring in a lower extremity in a patient with chronic lymphedema caused by filarial infection (Sordillo et al., 1981). Several examples of lymphangiosarcomas located in the extremities or in the abdominal wall in patients with congenital, traumatic, or idiopathic chronic lymphedema have also been documented (Mackenzie, 1971; Dubin et al., 1974): These patients are usually 10 to 20 years younger than those with lymphedema secondary to radical mastectomy. Furthermore, the lymphedema is of longer duration and any extremity may be affected.

It is not clear how lymphedema leads to neoplastic transformation. Chronic lymphatic obstruction is known to stimulate proliferation of lymphatic vessels, which may be the first step in the development of the tumor. However, lymphangiosarcoma rarely occurs in patients with lymphedema due to filaria. A localized defect in cellular immunity that has been demonstrated in lymphedematous extremities (Schreiber et al., 1979) may also play a role in the genesis of the tumor. Radiotherapy may also be an important contributing factor in some patients.

Clinically the tumor is papuloid or macular or appears as a cutaneous nodule with a bluish-red color. It is slightly elevated above the skin surface and may be painful. As the tumor grows, satellite nodules, either isolated or confluent, form plaques or larger masses, which tend to ulcerate. Sometimes the tumor growth is so widespread that it can cover an entire upper extremity and even part of the thoracic wall.

Prior to the development of lymphangiosarcoma, there is a dermal proliferation of small lymphatic channels which are lined by normal-appearing or slightly atypical endothelial cells (Fig. 21–9, A). The term lymphangiomatosis has been applied to this proliferative lesion (Woodward et al., 1972). When the lesion occurs in the vicinity of a lymphangiosarcoma, its small lymphatic vessels usually merge imperceptibly with other vascular channels that are lined by endothelial cells with obvious features of malignancy. Moreover, lymphangiomatosis may progress to lymphangiosarcoma. For these reasons lymphangiomatosis is considered to be a preneoplastic change which provides support for the endothelial lymphatic origin of these tumors. If dermal nodules of lymphangiomatosis are discovered before the appearance of a clear-cut lymphangiosarcoma, the therapeutic decision becomes difficult. Local excision of the skin nodules and close follow-up of the patients are recommended.

The fully developed lymphangiosarcoma is composed of small, dilated, often anastomosing lymphatic channels lined by large endothelial cells with hyperchromatic or vesicular nuclei (Figs. 21–9, B, and 21–10). However, some vessels are lined by flat normal-appearing endothelial cells. The vessel lumen may be empty, filled with clear fluid, or even contain erythrocytes. Collections of lymphocytes are occasionally present, in or around the walls of the lymphatic channels. Endothelial cells may appear poorly differentiated and grow as solid nests, sheets, or cords, a histologic picture reminiscent of carcinoma. These poorly differentiated areas have led some pathologists to believe that lymphangiosarcomas probably represent retrograde metastases from the original breast carcinoma (Salm, 1968). However, recent immunohistologic studies have shown that cells from lymphangiosarcomas stain for FVIII R Ag and for Ulex europaeu I-lectin (UEA I), which are markers for endothelial cells (Miettinen et al., 1983). Only the better differentiated areas of the lymphangiosarcoma are FVIII R Ag–positive, whereas most neoplastic cells from these tumors react with UEA I. To further substantiate the mesenchymal origin of these neo-

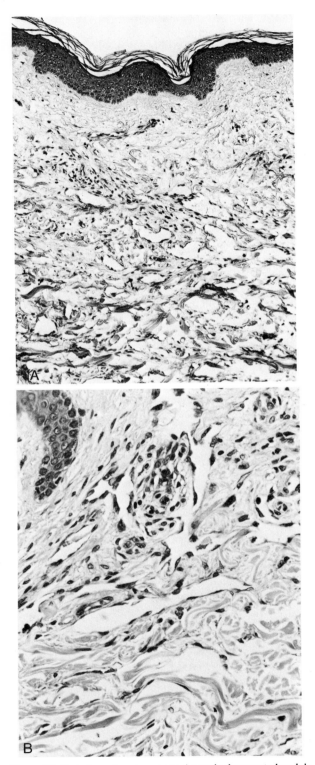

plasms, it should be noted that they are keratin-negative but vimentine positive (Miettinen et al., 1983).

LIPOMA AND LIPOSARCOMA

Malignant transformation of lipomas has occasionally been reported (Huvos, 1985). However, it is almost impossible to prove this contention because most liposarcomas show a mixture of mature fat cells and lipoblasts and also because of the slow growth and long clinical evolution of these tumors, especially the well differentiated types.

POSTRADIATION SARCOMAS

A variety of soft tissue sarcomas may develop following radiation for benign and malignant conditions (Bentley et al., 1975; Gray, 1983; Adam and Reif, 1977; Ducatman, 1983; Hardy et al., 1978; Kim et al., 1979; Sagerman et al., 1969). The average latent period is 10 years. In most patients there is no correlation between the dose of radiation and the subsequent development of sarcoma. Moreover, in some patients the sarcoma may arise from tissues that were not included within the field of radiation. The

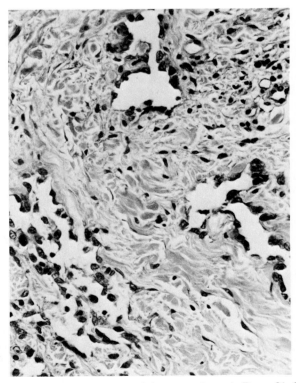

Figure 21–9. A, Lymphangiomatosis. A poorly demarcated nodule of lymphatic vessels is seen in the dermis. The patient was a 56-year-old female 7 years after radical mastectomy for breast carcinoma. B, Postmastectomy lymphangiosarcoma in a male. Empty lymphatic vascular channels are lined by either normal-appearing or slightly atypical endothelial cells.

Figure 21–10. Another area of the tumor shown in Figure 21–9. Here the vascular channels are lined by atypical endothelial cells having large, hyperchromatic nuclei. (Courtesy of Dr. Hector Santiago.)

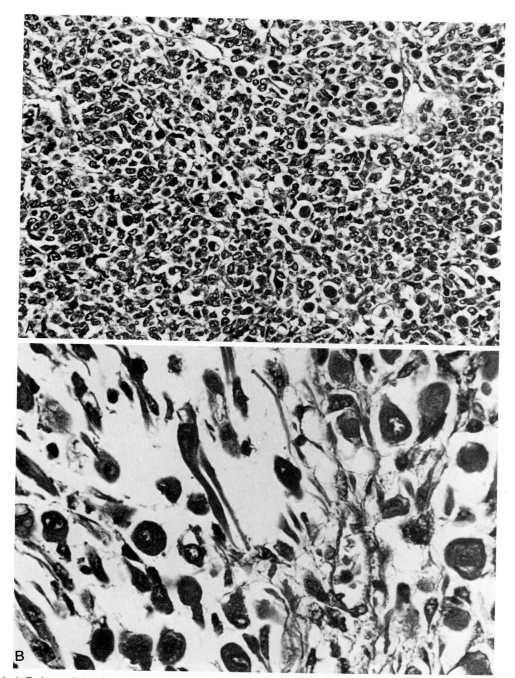

Figure 21–11. *A,* Embryonal rhabdomyosarcoma that arose in the soft tissues of the orbit 6 years after radiation therapy for retinoblastoma. Although most cells are round and appear undifferentiated, some show rhabdomyoblastic differentiation. *B,* Another area of the tumor shown in *A* in which most cells are differentiated rhabdomyoblasts, some with cross striations.

most frequent histologic types reported have been fibrosarcomas, malignant schwannomas, rhabdomyosarcomas, and malignant fibrous histiocytomas (Fig. 21–11). These sarcomas do not differ in structure and clinical behavior from those that arise spontaneously. Fibrosarcomas should be distinguished from postradiation fibromatosis by the same criteria that are used to separate spontaneous fibrosarcoma from fibromatosis (Petit et al., 1954). Occasionally, however, drawing lines of separation between these two postradiation lesions is exceedingly difficult owing to the high cellularity, increased mitotic activity, and marked degree of atypia in some cases of postradiation fibromatosis.

PREVIOUS SURGERY, CHRONIC INFLAMMATION, AND MALIGNANT FIBROUS HISTIOCYTOMA

In recent years, at least three malignant fibrous histiocytomas have been described at sites of previous surgery. The first tumor appeared in the aorta one year after the insertion of a Dacron thoracic aortic graft (Weinberg ad Maini, 1980). Another malignant fibrous histiocytoma developed in an amputation stump six years following an above-knee amputation for gangrene, and the third tumor originated in the groin two years after a hernioplasty for a left inguinal hernia (Inoshita and Youngberg, 1984). I have re-

cently seen a malignant fibrous histiocytoma that arose in the testis of a 74-year-old man with chronic orchiepididymitis of six years' duration (Fig. 21–12). The exuberant fibrohistiocytic reaction seen in association with different types of foreign material, including silica (Weiss et al., 1978) and suture material, should be distinguished from the malignant fibrous histiocytomas that arise at surgical sites. However, these tumors show considerable cellular pleomorphism and atypical mitotic figures, which are not present in the nonneoplastic fibrohistiocytic foreign body reactions. Since the process of repair and scarring involves histiocytes, fibroblasts, and primitive mesenchymal cells, it has been postulated that on rare occasions

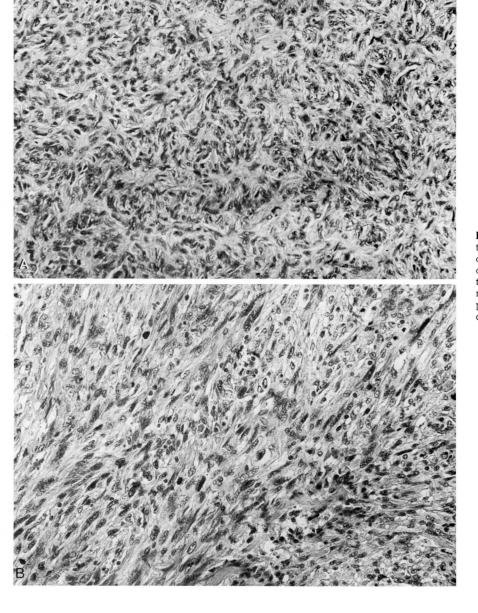

Figure 21–12. Malignant fibrous histiocytoma that arose from the testis of a 74-year-old man with chronic orchiepididymitis of 6 years' duration. *A,* Prominent cartwheel pattern reminiscent of dermatofibrosarcoma protuberans. *B,* Fibrosarcomatous component showing mitotic figures.

Illustration continued on opposite page

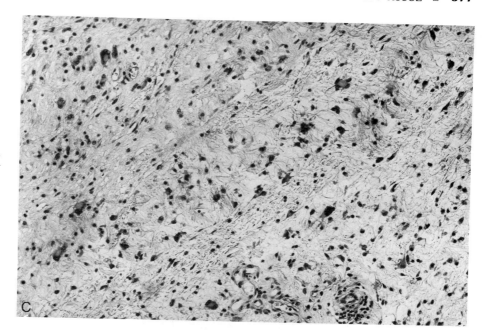

Figure 21–12 *Continued. C,* Myxoid area with several Touton-type giant cells.

such a process may predispose to malignant transformation. At present, however, the possibility that previous surgery and the development of malignant fibrous histiocytoma are coincidental cannot be excluded.

IMMUNOSUPPRESSION AND KAPOSI'S SARCOMA

In recent years we have seen an epidemic of Kaposi's sarcoma—chiefly in young homosexual men with the new viral disease known as acquired immune deficiency syndrome (AIDS). According to reports, Kaposi's sarcoma occurs in 33 to 90 percent of patients with AIDS. The anatomic distribution of the lesions and the biologic behavior of this sarcoma differ from those of the ordinary sporadic type, but are similar to those of the tumor that occurs endemically in Africa. The Kaposi's sarcoma in patients with AIDS is characterized by an aggressive clinical course with frequent involvement of the alimentary tract, lymph nodes, and lungs (Reichert et al., 1983; Finkbeiner et al., 1982). Kaposi's sarcoma has also been reported in immunosuppressed patients following organ transplantation (Penn, 1979). The incidence of Kaposi's sarcoma in organ transplant recipients with different types of tumors has been estimated at around 5 percent. Visceral involvement is common in these patients and when present the prognosis of Kaposi's sarcoma is poor. However, discontinuation of immunosuppressive therapy has resulted in prolonged remissions.

The association of multicentric Castleman's disease and Kaposi's sarcoma is well documented (Frizzera et al., 1980). These two rare lesions may appear simultaneously and may even coexist in the same lymph node (Rywlin et al., 1983). A recent study has suggested that Kaposi's sarcoma and Castleman's disease may in fact represent different tissue reactions to the same causative agent (Rywlin et al., 1983). Kaposi's sarcoma has been linked to cytomegalovirus infection (CMV). In the colon we have seen marked endothelial proliferation closely simulating Kaposi's sarcoma in association with CMV infection. Furthermore, the frequent occurrence of the tumor in young homosexuals, the elevated titers of antibodies to CMV, and the demonstration of the virus genome in cells from Kaposi's sarcoma strongly support this linkage (Drew et al., 1982).

Histologically, the early lesions of Kaposi's sarcoma are difficult to recognize because the capillary proliferation and the spindle-shaped endothelial cells are usually obscured by an inflammatory infiltrate rich in lymphocytes and plasma cells (Fig. 21–13). This inflammatory stage of Kaposi's sarcoma is often confused with granulation tissue, especially in the skin. In lymph nodes, inflammatory Kaposi's sarcoma may be confused with angioimmunoblastic lymphadenopathy. As the tumor progresses the inflammatory component disappears or decreases considerably and the spindle-cell areas and slit-like vascular spaces become more prominent, making the diagnosis easy to establish (Fig. 21–14). However, in patients with AIDS, there is often no progressive evolution of inflammatory Kaposi's sarcoma to the classic type (Moskowitz et al., 1984). For this reason, these authors believe that inflammatory Kaposi's sarcoma is only a morphologic variant of the tumor and not a precursor or early stage.

Finally, most sarcomas, regardless of their histomorphology, when deeply located, are quite large and

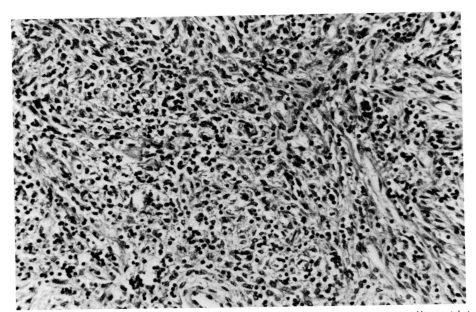

Figure 21–13. Small vascular channels and spindle-shaped cells are obscured by a dense inflammatory infiltrate rich in lymphocytes and plasma cells. Inflammatory phase of Kaposi's sarcoma from a patient with acquired immune deficiency syndrome. (Courtesy of Dr. George Hensley, University of Miami.)

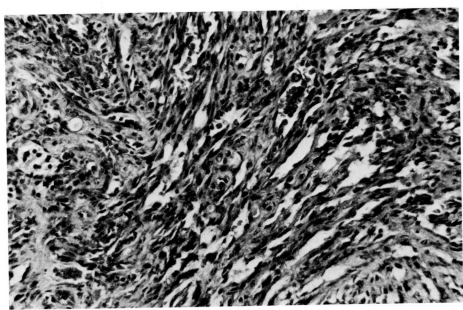

Figure 21–14. The characteristic slit-like vascular spaces and spindle-shaped cells of Kaposi's sarcoma are seen in this pulmonary nodule from a patient with acquired immune deficiency syndrome.

presumably of long duration at the time of diagnosis. On the other hand, the sarcomas that arise in the superficial soft tissues may be discovered early in their course and consequently are often small and perhaps of short duration. Included in this latter group are the epithelioid sarcomas, dermatofibrosarcoma protuberans, angiomatoid variants of fibrous histiocytomas, angiosarcomas, leiomyosarcomas, and malignant schwannomas. We have had the opportunity to examine several of these tumors, some of which measured only a few millimeters, but their structure was similar to that of the larger, fully developed sarcomas. Despite an intentional search, we were not able to demonstrate any precursor lesions in the vicinity of these small tumors.

References

Adam, Y.G., Reif, R.R.: Radiation-induced fibrosarcoma following treatment of breast cancer. Surgery 8:421–425, 1977.

Bentley, S.J., Davis, P., Jason, M.I.V.: Neurofibrosarcoma following radiotherapy for ankylosing spondylitis. Ann. Rheum. Dis. 34:536–538, 1975.

Burns, D.K., Silva, F.G., Forde, K. A., Mount, P. M., Clark, B.: Primary melanocytic schwannoma of the stomach. Cancer 52:1432–1441, 1983.

Bussey, H.J.R., Veale, A.M.O., Morson, B.C.: Genetics of gastrointestinal polyposis. Gastroenterology 74:1325–1330, 1978.

Camiel, M.R., Mule, J.E., Alexander, L.L., et al.: Association of thyroid carcinoma with Gardner's syndrome in siblings. N. Engl. J. Med. 278:1056, 1968.

Chitale, A.R., Dicersin, R.: Electron microscopy in the diagnosis of malignant schwannomas. Cancer 51:1448–1461, 1983.

D'Agostino, A.N., Soule, E.H., Miller, R.H.: Primary malignant neoplasms of nerves (malignant neurilemmomas) in patients without manifestations of multiple neurofibromatosis (von Recklinghausen's disease). Cancer 16:1003–1014, 1963.

D'Agostino, A.N., Soule, E.H., Miller, R.H.: Sarcoma of the peripheral nerves and somatic soft tissues associated with multiple neurofibromatosis (von Recklinghausen's disease). Cancer 16:1015–1027, 1963.

Drew, W.L., Connant, M.A., Miner, R.C., Huang, E.S., Ziegler, J.L., Groundwater, J.R., Gullet, J.H., Volberding, P., Abrams, D.I., Mintz, L.: Cytomegalovirus and Kaposi's sarcoma in young homosexual men. Lancet 2:125–127, 1982.

Dubin, H.U., Creehan, E.P., Headington, J.T.: Lymphangiosarcoma and congenital lymphedema of the extremity. Arch. Dermatol. 110:608–612, 1974.

Ducatman, B.S., Scheithauser, B.W.: Post-irradiation neurofibrosarcoma. Cancer 51:1028–1033, 1983.

Finkbeiner, W.E., Eghert, B.M., Groundwater, J.R., Sagebiel, R.W.: Kaposi's sarcoma in young homosexual men: A histopathologic study with particular reference to lymph node involvement. Arch. Pathol. Lab. Med. 106:261–264, 1982.

Fraumeni, J.F. Jr., Vogel, C.L., Easton, J.M.: Sarcomas and multiple polyposis in a kindred. A genetic variety of hereditary polyposis. Arch. Int. Med. 121:57, 1968.

Frizzera, G., Rosai, J., Banks, P.M., Bayrd, E.D., Massarelli, G.: A multicentric lymphoproliferative disorder with the morphologic features of Castleman's disease. A clinicopathologic study of ten patients. Lab. Invest. 42:22, 1980.

Gardner, E.J.: Follow-up study of a family group exhibiting dominant inheritance for a syndrome including intestinal polyps, osteomas, fibromas and epidermal cysts. Am. J. Hum. Genet. 14:376, 1982.

Gray, G.R.: Fibrosarcoma. A complication of interstitial radiation

therapy for benign hemangioma occurring after 18 years. Br. J. Radiol. 47:60, 1983.

Guccion, J.G., Enzinger, F.M.: Malignant schwannoma with von Recklinghausen's neurofibromatosis. Virchows Arch. (Pathol. Anat. Histol.) 383:43–57, 1979.

Harcy, T.J., An, T., Brown, P.W., Terz, J.J.: Post-irradiation sarcoma (malignant fibrous histiocytoma) of axilla. Cancer 42:118–124, 1978.

Huvos, A.G.: The spontaneous transformation of benign into malignant soft tissue tumors. Am. J. Surg. Pathol. 9:7–20, 1985.

Inoshita, T., Youngberg, G.A.: Malignant fibrous histiocytoma in previous surgical sites. Report of two cases. Cancer 53:176–183, 1984.

Kim, J.H., Chu, F.C., Woodard, H.Q., Melamed, M.R., Huvos, A., Cantin, J.: Radiation-induced soft tissue and bone sarcoma. Radiology 129:501–508, 1979.

Mackenzie, D.H.: Lymphangiosarcoma arising in chronic congenital and idiopathic lymphedema. J. Clin. Pathol. 24:524–528, 1971.

Miettinen, M., Letho, V., Virtanen, I.: Post-mastectomy angiosarcoma (Stewart-Treves syndrome). Am. J. Surg. Pathol. 7:329–339, 1983.

Millstein, D.I., Tang, C., Campbell, E.: Angiosarcoma developing in a patient with neurofibromatosis (von Recklinghausen's disease) Cancer 47:950–954, 1981.

Mogollon, R.J., Penneys, N.S., Ziegels-Weissman, J., Albores-Saavedra, J., Nadji, M.: Malignant schwannoma presenting as skin mass. Confirmation by the demonstration of myelin basic protein within tumor cells. Cancer 53:1190–1193, 1984.

Moskowitz, L.B., Hensley, G.T., Gould, E.W., Weiss, S.D.: The frequency and anatomical distribution of lymphadenopathic Kaposi's sarcoma in the acquired immune deficiency syndrome. An autopsy series. Hum. Pathol. 16:447–456, 1985.

Nakijama, T., et al.: An immunoperoxidase study of S-100 protein distribution in normal and neoplastic tissues. Am. J. Surg. Pathol. 6:715–727, 1982.

Penn, I.: Kaposi's sarcoma in organ transplant recipients: Report of 20 cases. Transplantation 27:8–11, 1979.

Petit, V.D., Chamness, J.T., Ackerman, L.V.: Fibromatosis and fibrosarcoma following irradiation therapy. Cancer 7:149–157, 1954.

Reichert, C.M., O'Learly, T.J., Levens, D.L., Simrell, C.R., Macher, A.A.: Autopsy pathology in the acquired immune deficiency syndrome. Am. J. Pathol. 112:357–382, 1983.

Rywlin, A.A., Rosen, L., Cabello, B.: Coexistence of Castleman's disease and Kaposi's sarcoma. Report of a case and a speculation. Am. J. Dermatopathol. 5:277–281, 1983.

Sagerman, R.H., Cassady, J.R., Tretter, P., Ellsworth, R.M.: Radiation induced neoplasia following external beam therapy for children with retinoblastoma. Am. J. Roentgenol. 105:529–535, 1969.

Salm, R.: The nature of the so-called post-mastectomy lymphangiosarcoma. J. Pathol. Bacteriol. 85:445–456, 1968.

Schreiber, H., Barry, F.M., Russell, W.C., et al.: Stewart-Treves syndrome: A lethal complication of post-mastectomy lymphedema and regional immune deficiency. Arch. Surg. 114:82–85, 1979.

Scully, R.E., Mark, E.J., McNeely, B.U.: Villous adenoma with focal carcinoma in-situ, periampullary, with extension into common bile duct (Gardner's syndrome), with polyposis of small and large intestine. N. Engl. J. Med. 307:1566–1573, 1982.

Shirger, A.: Postoperative lymphedema. Etiologic and diagnostic factors. Med. Clin. North. Am. 46:1045–1050, 1962.

Simpson, R.D., Harrison, E.G., Mayo, C.W.: Mesenteric fibromatosis in familial polyposis. Cancer 17:526, 1964.

Sordillo, E.M., Sordillo, P.P., Hadju, S.I., Good, R.A.: Lymphangiosarcoma after filarial infection. J. Dermat. Surg. Oncol. 7:235–239, 1981.

Stewart, F.M., Treves, N.: Lymphangiosarcoma in post-mastectomy lymphedema: A report of six cases of elephantiasis chirurgica. Cancer 1:64–73, 1948.

Takahara, O., Nakayama, I., Yokoyama, S., et al.: Malignant neurofibroma with glandular differentiation (glandular schwannoma). Acta Pathol. Jpn. 29:597–606, 1979.

Usui, M., Ishui, S., Yamawaki, S., Hirayama, T.: The occurrence of soft tissue sarcomas in three siblings with Werner's syndrome. Cancer 54:2580–2586, 1984.

Weary, P.P.E., Linthicum, A., Cawley, E.P., et al.: Gardner's syndrome. A family group and review. Arch. Dermatol. 90:20, 1964.

Weinberg, D.S., Maini, B.S.: Primary sarcoma of the aorta associated with a vascular prosthesis. A case report. Cancer 46:398–402, 1980.

Weiss, S.W., Enzinger, F.M., Johnson, F.B.: Silica reaction simulating fibrous histiocytoma. Cancer 42:2738–2743, 1978.

Woodruff, J.M., Chermik, N.L., Smith, M.C., Millet, W.B., Fotte, F.F., Jr.: Peripheral nerve with rhabdomyosarcomatous differentiation (malignant Triton's tumors). Cancer 32:426–439, 1973.

Woodward, A.H., Ivings, J.J., Soule, E.H.: Lymphangiosarcoma arising in chronic lymphedematous extremities. Cancer 30:562–572, 1972.

BRUCE D. RAGSDALE
DONALD E. SWEET

22 Bone

As in other organ systems, it has become clear that not all malignant tumors arising from bone are de novo. In proportion to the available data, benign antecedents for many malignant tumors can be demonstrated. Prior to reviewing some of the antecedents now known to confer a risk of malignancy, it is necessary to explore some general concepts.

The skeleton, by virtue of its structural dynamics and mineral content, affords the opportunity to demonstrate change over time through a correlation of clinical history, sequential radiographs, and histologic footprints of altered remodeling. Clinically, the development of symptoms referable to a known bone lesion indicates altered biologic activity and warns of possible malignant change. Radiographic clues of antecedent lesions include patterns of altered density, internal margins, and periosteal reactions. Histologic clues of antecedent benign lesions include remnants of such lesions, relative proportions and arrangement of cartilage, bone type (lamellar versus woven), and orientation of cement lines.

An appreciation of the relationships between bone lesions requires an understanding of normal bone physiology, especially the details of growth, development, maintenance, and changes associated with age. Equally important is the integration of clinical data, such as sex, age of onset, anatomic location, radiographic patterns, histologic composition, and natural history (the tendency of bone lesions to undergo morphologic modification over time). Accordingly, most diagnostic pitfalls can be avoided and causal relationships recognized by insisting on the opportunity to correlate clinical, radiologic, and pathologic data relating to the individually unique characteristics reflected in each patient's lesion. By this method it becomes clear that certain benign bone lesions should be removed if technically and medically possible.

CLINICAL IMPLICATIONS OF TERMS

If a lesion is benign but is known to have the capacity to undergo malignant transformation, then one expects complete removal will be curative. If it is a "low-grade sarcoma," one hopes for cure following complete removal but cannot be nearly as certain because metastases may be slow to appear. A tumor should not be designated as "low-grade sarcoma" unless one believes that without further change in histology the tumor can metastasize. The morphologic borderline between "active" benign lesions versus low-grade malignant lesions is an individual matter among pathologists but directly influences the frequency of diagnosing malignant change in a benign antecedent lesion.

Subtotal removal of a benign lesion may or may not be followed by clinical recurrence; the possibility of malignant transformation of the residuum can be monitored by follow-up, including radiographs. The decision to follow a patient or perform a second procedure is based on factors that include anatomic site, level of patient activity, projected longevity, propensity of a particular lesion to recur or transform, and so on. Subtotal or piecemeal removal of a "low-grade malignant lesion" assures local regrowth. Generally the histologic grade of sequential "recurrences" tends to increase because the progeny of more rapidly proliferative clones may predominate in successive regrowths.

BENIGN ANTECEDENTS OF BONE SARCOMAS

Antecedent benign lesions serving as the origin for malignant tumors are becoming increasingly recognized in various organ systems. In bone, some of these entities are well accepted; others are controversial or as yet undefined. Some of the latter will be mentioned in this chapter. The rising incidence of bone sarcomas in bone after middle age is largely accounted for by sarcomatous transformation of antecedent benign conditions, in our opinion. Five of the seven basic categories of disease readily offer examples: (1) trauma and repair—irradiated bone; (2)

inflammatory—osteomyelitis; (3) circulatory—infarct; (4) anomaly—osteochondroma and enchondroma; (5) benign neoplasia—osteoblastoma and giant cell tumor. The other two, (6) metabolic and (7) neuromechanical, may not be exempt. It seems likely the numerically more common "de novo" sarcomas of bone may also have their origins in aberrations of normal growth and development.

When malignant change occurs, the only item of importance to patient care is the presence of malignancy. Specific benign lesions are not limited to a single histologic direction of malignant change. Not infrequently, more than one malignant pattern in a single tumor complicates classification. A more informative alternative to diagnosis by malignant pattern (for example "osteosarcoma") is to apply a name emphasizing the antecedent lesion (for example, "bone infarct with high-grade sarcomatous change"). Nor can it be assumed sarcomas arising in relation to antecedent benign lesions will behave the same as de novo sarcomas of similar pattern. Accordingly, unless attention is called to the phenomenon of malignant transformation, a case is likely to appear in a series with de novo tumors and may significantly modify results. This is an important initial step in understanding this area of oncology and in determining which benign lesions deserve removal or close clinical follow-up.

At times, local recurrence or distant metastases may contain histologic elements not found in the original tumor. For example, osteoid may be produced in the pulmonary metastases from what was clearly sarcomatous change of an enchondroma. For consistency in reporting and understanding pathobiology, such findings should not lead to a change in the original diagnosis, for example, under the assumption "the problem was osteosarcoma all along." Bone tumors are named for their dominant most differentiated appearance at their site of origin. The patterns in metastases and soft tissue extensions are not always valid for naming, since not uncommonly the morphology is modified as the tumor grows in a different environment.

Clues to an antecedent benign lesion may be histologic (for example, benign lesional tissue mixed with sarcoma); gross, for example, radiographic: remnants of original internal margins, deformation of bone outline by aberrant remodeling or slow periosteal reaction, and/or characteristic residual patterns of mineralization; or clinical, as in a benign lesion known to be present for decades, a history of polyostotic fibrous dysplasia, or work at hyperbaric pressure. Malignant transformation of a benign lesion should be considered when no simple conventional diagnostic term will cover an unusual clinical evolution, radiographic sequence, or complexity of histologic patterns.

Insight concerning potential for malignant transformations is facilitated by insistence on complete data, including extended radiographic sequences, and laboratory support capable of producing whole mount histologic sections. Whole mount sections, originally produced by a colloidin technique and adapted to paraffin at the Armed Forces Institute of Pathology (AFIP), are a means of displaying antecedent benign conditions and permit precise radiologic-pathologic correlations (Madewell et al., 1981; Ragsdale et al., 1981; Sweet et al., 1981).

SARCOMA-IN-SITU

In parallel with the concept of intraepithelial carcinoma, the idea of sarcoma-in-situ is a useful designation to communicate the presence of minimal cytologic malignancy, with the implication that the sarcoma will have a slow but definite tendency to progress and accelerate, eventually becoming overtly malignant and capable of giving rise to distant metastases. As with the epithelial concept (for example, polyp with carcinoma-in-situ), a hallmark of sarcoma-in-situ is cellular crowding and atypia, that is, variation in size, shape, and stain intensity exceeding the range of benign morphology. The latter features are the usual morphologic deviations of malignant cells common to cytology and histology. For cartilage lesions, where this concept is most useful, cellular variation combines with close spacing and also loose, watery-appearing matrix in focal patches that stand out distinctly against the more basophilic hyalin cartilage. In contrast to epithelial lesions, there is no basement membrane to serve as a defining boundary of invasiveness. Areas of sarcoma-in-situ within or around a benign lesion do not yet show a tendency for growth into surrounding marrow, overlying soft tissue, or vascular invasion. Accepting this diagnosis recognizes that a limited sample may not be totally representative and might lead to an underestimation of the malignant component. Close clinical-radiologic-pathologic correlation, including postoperative x-rays, is essential in evaluating such lesions.

As with intraepithelial carcinoma, complete removal of a bone tumor with "in-situ sarcoma" should be curative in most instances. However, a therapeutic obstacle to accomplishing this is inherent in the common orthopedic approach of attempting to remove or biopsy bone tumors by going through them during curettage as opposed to en bloc resection. This is especially true for cartilage lesions where part of the picture of early malignancy is a loose, watery matrix that readily spills into tissue planes exposed by surgery. The likelihood of cure by curettage would seem enhanced by adjuncts such as phenol cautery of the defect or liquid nitrogen freezing of the margins.

HISTOLOGIC PATTERNS OF SECONDARY SARCOMAS

The names of malignant bone tumors are variously derived from their cellular products, for example, chondrosarcoma, osteosarcoma, liposarcoma, angiosarcoma; their cytologic characteristics, for instance, spindle cell sarcoma, round cell sarcoma, malignant giant cell tumor; or by eponyms, such as Ewing's sarcoma. In addition to these patterns, secondary bone sarcomas can present with extreme pleomorphism bringing to mind metastatic carcinoma, a range in cell size that mimics lymphoma, and commonly a combination of malignant spindle and xanthoma cells, malignant fibroxanthoma.

Malignant Fibroxanthoma. The original term for malignant tumors composed of fibroblasts and xanthoma cells, often with "storiform" pattern, was malignant fibrous xanthoma (O'Brien and Stout, 1964). The concept of the histiocytic nature of this malignancy was founded upon tissue culture results (Ozzello, Stout, and Murray, 1963). Canonization of malignant fibrous histiocytoma as the preferred synonym occurred subsequently (Stout and Lattes, 1967). We prefer the descriptive designation malignant fibroxanthoma over the term "malignant fibrous histiocytoma" because the latter implies a histiocytic origin, based upon the assumption that all cells containing small xanthomatous vacuoles are functional macrophages. This ignores the fact that normal fat cell development can include both spindle cells and xanthoma cells. Furthermore, to some degree, fibroblasts are motile and not uncommonly contain small fat droplets. Many cells other than histiocytes have been shown capable of phagocytosis. Thus the 1963 tissue culture observations that form the cornerstone of the fibrous histiocytoma concept can be challenged. Since malignant fibroxanthoma is such a common secondary sarcomatous pattern in many antecedent benign lesions, for example, radiation osteitis, bone infarct, and enchondroma, the latter should be carefully excluded when the former is found, especially in adults.

Lymphoma. Rarely, lymphoma can be superimposed on chronic osteomyelitis. Indolent (sclerosing) lymphomas commonly evoke dense bone with a mosaic pattern, an index of chronically accelerated remodeling activity due to the tumor. These may be difficult to distinguish from the rare Paget's disease complicated by lymphoma since the bone outline tends to be widened in both.

SPECIFIC LESIONS ASSOCIATED WITH MALIGNANCY, DISCUSSED BY DISEASE CATEGORY

Trauma and Repair

Fracture. Long ago the similarity between bone tumors and fracture repair, or callus, gave rise to the idea bone tumors were "repair awry" (Codman, 1924). This statement is insightful if one's concept of repair includes the remodeling activity that attends growth and the increased turnover associated with

many benign bone lesions. However, cases suspected to represent malignant transformation of fracture callus almost always turn out to be pathologic fractures due to occult bone sarcomas. Jaffe could find no documented case of "osteogenic sarcoma" developing at the site of fracture in a previously normal bone (Jaffe, 1974). Verification of the sequence requires exclusion of tumor at the time of fracture by review of the radiographs and a history of trauma adequate to fracture normal bone. The secondary malignant patterns we have seen superimposed on old fracture sites are osteosarcoma, malignant fibroxanthoma (Fig. 22–1), and leiomyosarcoma.

The hyperplastic callus of osteogenesis imperfecta and hyperphosphatasia can mimic osteosarcoma (see Fig. 27–29). True osteosarcoma arising in callus of osteogenesis imperfecta is now documented (Klenerman, et al., 1967) (see Fig. 27–30).

Orthopedic Devices and Foreign Bodies. The number of cases where a bone sarcoma has arisen around an endoprosthesis are in the anecdotal range (Fig. 22–2). However, use of endoprosthetic devices is only now reaching the two and three decade mark, the time at which many other conditions reach their maximum for secondary malignancy.

If a malignant tumor is found in association with a prosthetic device, we know of no way a cause-and-effect relationship can be proved, but it can frequently be disproved. The reason for the original procedure must be determined to have been benign, and the absence of a malignant process at that time verified by radiologic-pathologic correlation of pre- and post-operative radiographs and adequate, complete specimen material.

Malignant tumors arising in relation to foreign bodies other than orthopedic devices are extremely rare and of two types. Those with coexistent chronic infection are more appropriately discussed under the heading of osteomyelitis. The remainder are more likely related to cicatrix (Fig. 22–3) than the object itself, for example, retained missiles (Fig. 22–4).

Irradiated Bone (Fig. 22–5). Ionizing radiation is the only environmental agent known to produce bone sarcomas (Fraumeni, 1975). Malignancy can follow external beam irradiation applied for benign bone tumors, for example, giant cell tumor (see Fig. 22–31), non-neoplastic problems (tuberculous arthritis), and malignant tumors near bone, for example, lymphomas and breast (Fig. 22–6) and gynecologic carcinomas. Bone sarcomas can also follow internal radiation from occupational (such as radium) or medicinal (for instance, thorium and radium) use. Postradiation sarcomas tend to be aggressive high-grade tumors that may or may not produce matrix. The latent period is quite variable, from a few years to a few decades, and this may be dose related.

No excess of bone cancer has been reported from whole body irradiation among atomic bomb survivors in Japan (Yamamoto and Wakabayshi, 1969), perhaps because the lethal dose is well below the thresh-

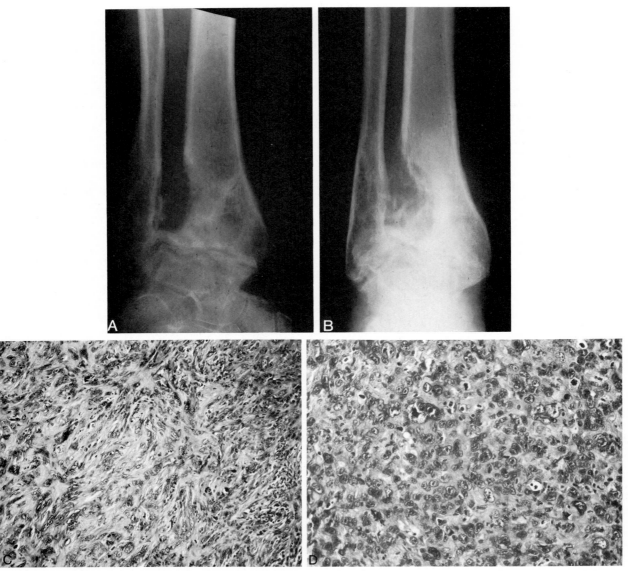

Figure 22–1. Malignant fibroxanthoma complicating an old fracture site. *A 55 year old man complained of progressive pain and swelling for 8 months at the site of a healed fracture sustained when a crate fell on the ankle 27 years previously. A,* The initial radiograph confirms healed oblique fractures through the distal tibia and fibula. *B,* Lytic change afflicts the facing surfaces of these bones and progresses, particularly in the tibia, during the 1 month interval between views. *C,* The yellow cheeselike material and "fish-flesh" substance removed at open biopsy consist of pleomorphic malignant cells in a storiform pattern. *D,* Some of the large malignant cells have markedly irregular nuclear contours and enormous nucleoli.

Figure 22–2. Sarcomatous change in relation to an intramedullary rod. *Six years after internal fixation of the left femur after a mortar shell fragment fracture of the left femur, pain and fever and a 10 × 10 cm medial thigh mass developed in a 43 year old veteran.* A, The admission radiograph indicates diaphyseal lucency surrounding the intramedullary rod. Along the proximal medial surface are osteophytic remnants of remodeled fracture callus. Beneath a medial soft tissue thigh mass, the distal fracture fragment has sharp edges that bespeak an active process superimposed on the fracture site. When a preoperative course of antibiotics did not change the symptoms, an above-knee amputation was performed through the lesser trochanter level under a presumed clinical diagnosis of septic nonunion. The intramedullary nail was withdrawn through the greater trochanter rather than through the amputated stump end.

B, A whole mount section of the distal fragment shows a dark staining rim of malignant cellular tissue toward its proximal end. C, Moderately pleomorphic stellate and spindle-shaped cells (upper right) impinge on antecedent lamellar bone stimulating a front of osteoclasia. Fibrin precipitates in the tumor mimic tumor osteoid (upper left corner). A diagnosis of pleomorphic osteolytic sarcoma was issued. *The patient died 17 months after amputation from an infected massive stump recurrence treated with radiotherapy. No distant metastases were detected at autopsy.*

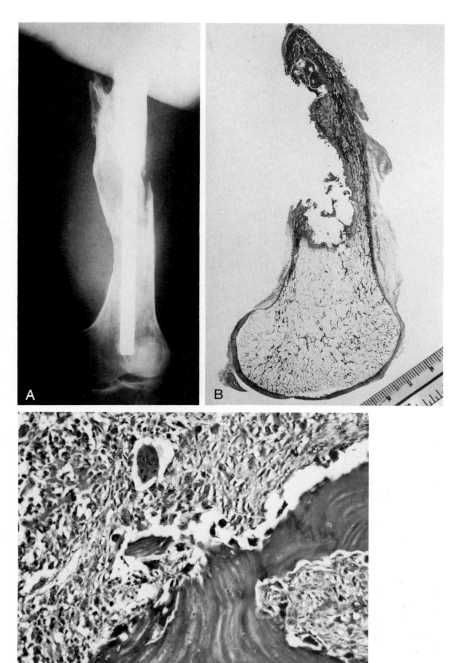

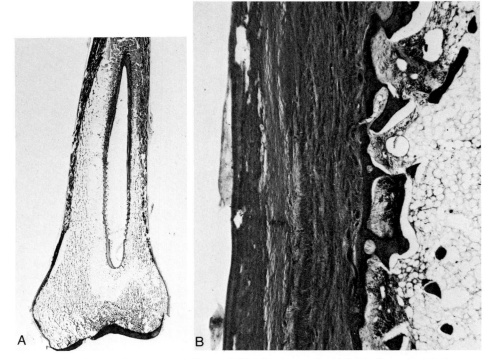

Figure 22–3. Fibrooseous sheath around an intramedullary rod. Metallic devices implanted in bone tend to become surrounded by a hypocellular fibrous membrane ("internal periosteum") and a thin border of bone ("internal cortex"). Both these features are evident in the whole mount section *(A)* and detailed view *(B)* of a distal femur in which a long intramedullary rod was in place for 1.5 years after pathologic fracture of the shaft.

The hypocellular fibrous sheath reflects an ischemic environment analogous to the "reactive interface" around bone infarcts. Sarcomatous change around metallic devices are very rare and require careful exclusion of a pre-existing neoplastic condition.

old of 1500r after which bone sarcomas are seen. Accidental introduction of radioactive elements into the environment is an increasing concern. Some nucleotides, such as plutonium and strontium, selectively seek bone.

An alarming incidence of postradiation sarcomas (Chan et al., 1979) and as much as 30 percent of latent residual round cell sarcomas have been described in cases of Ewing's sarcoma treated nonsurgically. These results and the long-term disability of heavily irradiated extremities have led to a reevaluation of the role of radiotherapy and surgery in managing primary lesions of this entity. Yet, relegation of patients with Ewing's sarcoma to non-surgical protocols continues with conviction not found in the early words of the originator: "I wish to emphasize the caution, that, while the diffuse endotheliomas of young subjects have proved uniformly susceptible to heavy radium packs and to repeated applications of roentgen ray, sufficient time has not elapsed to determine the final outcome of this treatment" (Ewing, 1922).

Inflammation

Osteomyelitis. In chronic osteomyelitis, whatever the cause, the walls of draining sinus tracks frequently become lined by a downgrowth of squamous epithelium from the skin and surrounded by cicatrix. Ongoing inflammation stimulates a hyperplastic response that may form an irregularly raised rim or mass at the point of drainage (Marjolin ulcer). Squamous cell carcinoma arises in 0.5 percent of chronic sinuses, usually more than 20 years after the initial infection or open fracture. Sinus track carcinomas are predominantly located in the lower extremity, arising twice as often adjacent to the tibia as to the femur. Malignant transformation is often signaled by a sudden change in longstanding symptoms, including pain, mass, bleeding, character of the discharge, and/or radiographic clues, especially progressive osteolysis superimposed upon the density of an otherwise chronic but stable process. The appearance of any of these should arouse suspicion and not be assumed part of the patient's infection. In suspected cases, biopsy should include tissue from multiple sites, especially from deep within the sinus. Biopsies around the rim of the draining sinus are almost predictably benign; the resultant false reassurance of "pseudoepitheliomatous hyperplasia" can delay diagnosis and treatment.

The borderline between atypical pseudoepitheliomatous hyperplasia and squamous cell carcinoma may be impossible to define or, at best, is arbitrary. Particularly problematic are those specimens in which only moderately atypical epithelial nests are mixed

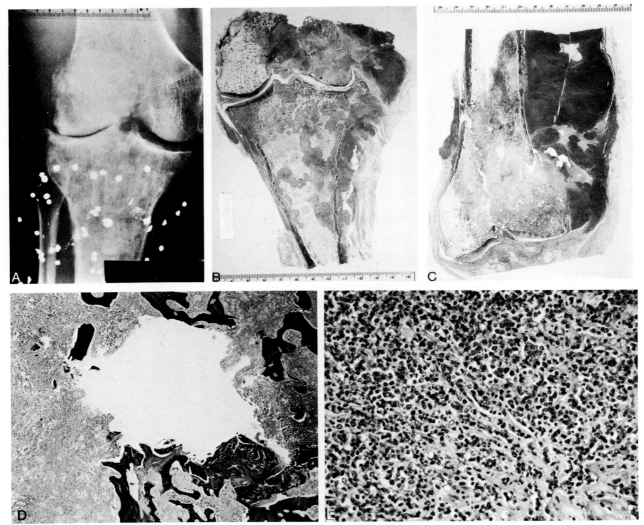

Figure 22–4. Histiocytic lymphoma arising in old gunshot wound. *A 64 year old man had been wounded in the knee by a shotgun blast 25 years previously. Recent knee pain and swelling in the thigh prompted x-ray studies.* A, Spherical and deformed lead shot is distributed in soft tissue and bone below the knee. A cancellous moth-eaten lytic pattern in the proximal tibia and distal femur is accompanied by erosion of the lateral femoral condylar cortex and intercondylar pathologic fracture. B, The whole mount histologic section reveals lymphoma filling the marrow space of the proximal tibia and extending into the lateral femoral condyle (right). The dark geographic areas inside the bone represent viable tumor cells; the paler staining internal areas are necrotic tumor. C, Spread around the joint capsule creates a large, soft tissue mass beside the femur. An oblique pathologic fracture beginning at the intercondylar notch extends as a jagged line through the metaphysis. A second oblique fracture line separates the lateral condyle along a diagonal, terminating in the intercondylar notch. D, This clear space within the cancellous bone of the tibia was occupied by a deformed lead shot, removed prior to processing. Toward the lower right corner are dark metallic fragments and corrosion products associated with new bone formation. The surrounding marrow is replaced by lymphoma. E, The marrow infiltrate consists of variably sized malignant lymphoid elements, lymphoblastic cells predominating.

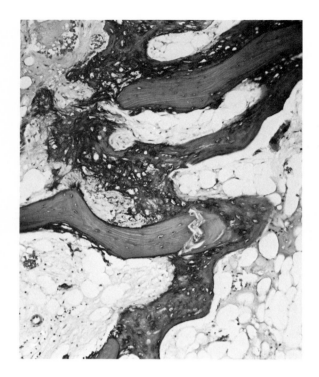

Figure 22–5. Radiation osteitis with microfracture. A 43 year old woman underwent femoral head resection and prosthetic replacement due to a pathologic subcapital fracture. A year and a half previously, the bone had received 3000 rads for metastatic carcinoma from the breast; mastectomy had been performed 9 years earlier. Crude-textured, irregularly cellular osteoid emerging from edematous, fibrotic fatty marrow is being applied to antecedent lamellar trabeculae. The center trabecula is crossed by a transverse microfracture. The most superficial deposits of radiation bone are smoother textured, as if the damage to normal turnover has been partially overcome. Whether this represents a primary injury to marrow mesenchyme, or relative hypovascularity due to irradiation, or a combination of these factors, is speculative.

with reactive and cancellous bone. Marked cellular atypicality, individual cell dyskeratosis, abnormal mitoses, and lymphatic permeation or vascular invasion favor malignancy. Final diagnosis must take into account all data, including clinical history and available radiographs, in addition to histologic criteria (Ragsdale, 1983).

The usual behavior of sinus tract carcinomas is indolent, as with de novo squamous cell carcinoma of the extremities. Amputation at an inadequate level may be followed by stump recurrence (Spjut et al., 1971). Regional lymphadenopathy may be due to inflammation, but tissue should be examined histologically to exclude regional node metastases, which are

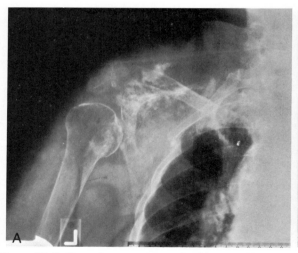
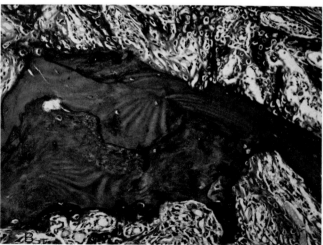

Figure 22–6. Postradiation sarcoma. *An 81 year old woman underwent "circumferential node irradiation" 10 years previously for infiltrating ductal breast carcinoma involving 6 of 14 axillary lymph nodes. Recently, shoulder pain and enlargement led to biopsy, followed by left forequarter amputation. A,* Radiographically, the epicenter of the sarcoma appears to be at the base of the achromion and scapular spine. Extensive osteolytic destruction is associated with small, cloudlike densities, some of which are in soft tissue beyond the bone outline. Rarefaction of the proximal humerus was due to extrinsic invasion by an aggressive spindle cell component of the tumor. The fractures of the second and third ribs, pulmonary fibrosis, and pleural thickening are additional sequelae to radiation. *B,* The original lamellar bone in the center of the tumor shows numerous surface resorption defects into which has been substituted crude, radiation-type bone that subsequently grades into hypercellular sarcomatous osteoid all around the periphery. This photomicrograph appears to show progressive stages of radiation osteitis into osteosarcoma.

reported in 10 to 20 percent of cases. Some individuals have developed distant metastases.

Prevention of sinus track carcinoma can be achieved by adequate treatment of the infection with drainage, sequestrectomy, removal of foreign bodies, exteriorization of the wound, and antibiotic therapy. Failure of draining sinuses to heal is an added indication to consider amputation, especially when the involved limb is non-functional and the patient's mobility is likely to be improved by prosthetic replacement and a good rehabilitation program.

Other neoplasms less commonly reported complicating chronic, draining osteomyelitis include basal cell carcinoma, adenocarcinoma, fibrosarcoma, osteosarcoma, hemangiosarcoma (Olmi and Rubbini, 1975) (Fig. 22–7), lymphoma, and plasma cell myeloma (Spjut et al., 1971).

Metabolic Factors

Constitutional factors, some of which may act through metabolic pathways, are variously associated with a

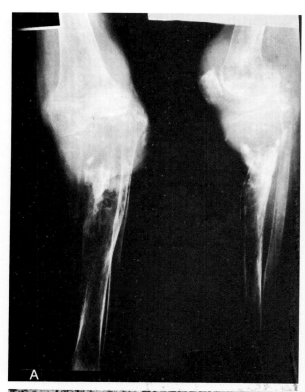
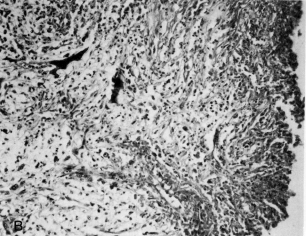
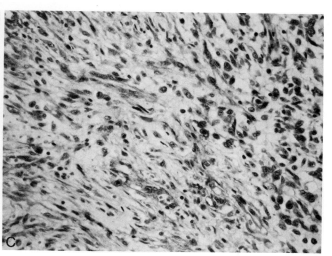

Figure 22–7. Chronic osteomyelitis complicated by angiosarcoma. *A,* Following many years of chronic osteomyelitis, marked osteolysis of the proximal tibia is superimposed on chronic reactive-reparative changes, including widening of the tibia contour. *B,* A diffuse infiltrate of neutrophils and other inflammatory cells in granulation tissue, plus partly resorbed bony spicules, indicates persistent active osteomyelitis. *C,* Rather pleomorphic epithelioid malignant cells in a fibrous background showing mitotic activity were found to contain factor VIII–related antigen by immunoperoxidase technique.

higher or lower incidence of bone sarcomas. These include bone growth (association of osteosarcoma with the pubertal growth spurt), sex (osteosarcoma more common in males, possibly related to greater bone growth), nutrition (abnormal carbohydrate metabolism associated with osteosarcoma, chondrosarcoma, and fibrosarcoma), familial and genetic factors (siblings with osteosarcoma, Ewing's sarcoma, or chondrosarcoma; extracranial osteosarcoma following retinoblastoma), and ethnic factors (Ewing's sarcoma virtually absent in blacks or Japanese). However, we are unaware of any direct linkage of specific metabolic bone diseases, such as rickets, osteomalacia, or scurvy, to secondary sarcomas.

Circulatory Factors

Infarct. Peculiarities of the vascular structure predispose bone to ischemic infarction. Because of the rigid cortical confines and internal modular construction (cancellous trabecular system), anything that increases the internal hydrostatic pressure will cause collapse of the only collapsible element, the vascular bed. The nomenclature of osteonecrotic lesions is based upon location: end of bone—*avascular necrosis* a term that evolved many years ago to distinguish "aseptic necrosis" from bone devitalized by osteomyelitis; metaphyseal/diaphyseal—*bone infarct*. Sarcomas can arise in relation to bone infarcts of known and unknown

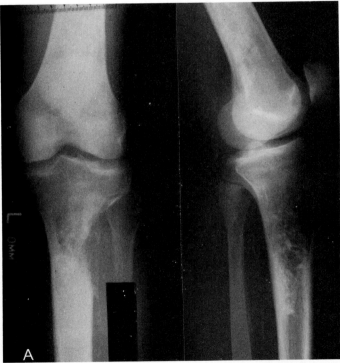

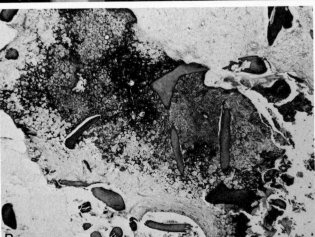

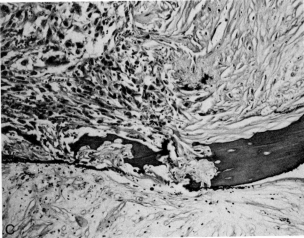

Figure 22–8. Sarcomatous change around a bone infarct. *A 63 year old black man sustained a tibial fracture when hit in the shin by an automatic door. A,* Lytic destruction of the proximal tibia is superimposed on irregular internal density. A similar lesion but without lytic change is situated in the distal femur. Note multiple calcified atherosclerotic plaques in the lower leg arteries. The patient's hemoglobin was normal and he had no exposure to hyperbaric pressure or steroids. *B,* The tumor was resected and replaced with a total knee prosthesis. A central area of dead fat and cancellous bone (lower left) retains the cell membrane outlines of dead fat cells. At the upper right is the hypovascular fibrous marrow of the reactive interface. Notice how the cancellous trabeculae remain unresorbed along the edge of the infarct, which passes diagonally from upper left to lower right. Within it are the mineralized outlines of necrotic fat cells with dystrophic mineralization in dense fibrous tissue. These changes explain the radiodense border around an infarct; centrally there is no change in density over extended periods of time. *C,* The secondary sarcoma (upper left) consists of pleomorphic cells, some with vacuolated cytoplasm reminiscent of an immature liposarcoma. The hypocellular ischemic environment of the reactive interface is the substratum of sarcomatous change. *The patient died with pulmonary and osseous metastases 12 months after surgery.*

etiology but are virtually unheard of in relation to avascular necrosis despite the many patients with necrotic femoral heads. The longer presence of bone infarcts in an occult asymptomatic stage may explain this. Even so, malignant change does not develop in the overwhelming majority of patients with bone infarcts (Dorfman, 1973). Malignancy arises in the reactive interface where hypocellular desmoplasia and ischemic bone is found. The commonest sarcoma is malignant fibroxanthoma (Fig. 22–8), but other patterns can also occur.

Paget's Disease. Since malignant neoplasia should be anticipated wherever accelerated cell activity is found, it is not surprising that Paget's disease of bone is associated with a substantial risk of malignant change. Even the lower estimate of 1 percent incidence of sarcoma in Paget's disease is likely to be high, since 3 percent of the general population over 40 years of age have Paget's disease and many are asymptomatic (Price, 1969).

The major long bones and limb girdles are most often affected by secondary sarcomas in Paget's disease (Fig. 22–9) (Huvos, 1983). Clinical evidence of metastatic spread at the time of diagnosis is common. Vertebral body lesions are especially likely to be metastatic from other sites. "Multicentric malignant change" actually represents bone-to-bone metastases. The commonest malignant types are osteosarcoma, spindle cell sarcoma, and malignant giant cell tumor. Other malignant types are uncommon but include chondrosarcoma, malignant fibroxanthoma (Fig. 22–10), and high-grade pleomorphic sarcoma. Paget sarcomas tend to be rapidly progressive with a median survival of about one year after diagnosis. Prolonged survival even with prompt amputation is unusual (Price, 1969; Huvos et al., 1983). Because most patients with Paget's disease are over 40 years of age,

Paget sarcomas substantially contribute to the second peak in bone sarcoma incidence appearing in the older age groups (Fraumeni, 1975).

Important radiographic signs of Paget's sarcoma in symptomatic patients include focal cortical lysis or fracture superimposed on the typical chronic, radiodense picture. Most Paget's sarcomas are obvious at the time of fracture or become clinically manifest within a year. An occult Paget sarcoma should be sought if osteosarcoma is found in an unusual location in an older adult, such as a cervical lymph node or subcutaneous nodule. Elevation of serum alkaline phosphatase parallels the extent of pagetic skeletal remodeling but may be extreme in those cases with secondary osteosarcoma.

Aneurysmal Bone Cyst. Those who believe in this entity as a primary lesion mostly regard it as a localized vascular disturbance in bone. We have abandoned use of the term aneurysmal bone cyst because of the wide variety of lesions to which it has been applied. Dr. Jaffe, who helped popularize the designation, subsequently regarded it a secondary change, engrafted on a variety of bone lesions which could be otherwise named (1962). The Memorial Hospital Group came to the conclusion that many of their so-called aneurysmal bone cysts were really other lesions (Biesecker et al., 1970). In most cases diagnostic histology (benign or malignant) is usually demonstrable if adequate material is obtained from the base of the lesion where the expansile component arises from bone. A particularly common antecedent is cystic change in a giant cell tumor. It is conceivable that a superimposed cystic change ("aneurysmal blow out") could obliterate an underlying antecedent, but most often the inability to demonstrate diagnostic histology is the result of inadequate sampling, explaining in part the 20 percent rate of recurrence after curettage. No

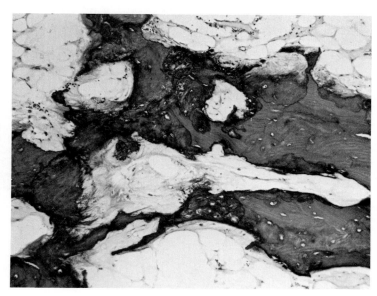

Figure 22–9. Unusually crude bone in Paget's disease. An 82 year old man died 6 months after symptomatic onset of a distal femoral sarcoma arising in Paget's disease. The autopsy specimen of the femur included areas showing unusually coarse-textured bone, not unlike that seen in radiation osteitis. It is possible that dysplastic areas such as this are a substratum for malignant change.

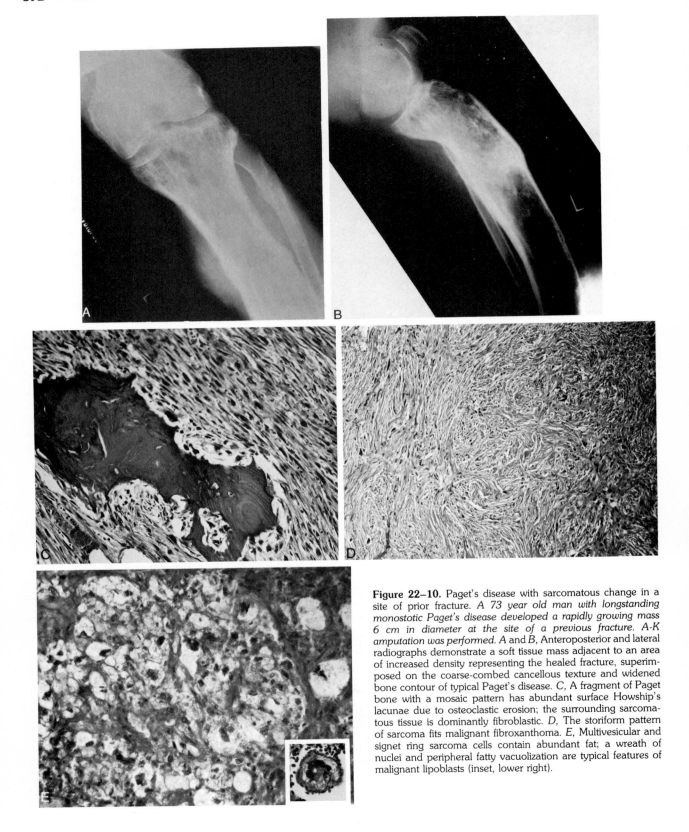

Figure 22–10. Paget's disease with sarcomatous change in a site of prior fracture. *A 73 year old man with longstanding monostotic Paget's disease developed a rapidly growing mass 6 cm in diameter at the site of a previous fracture. A-K amputation was performed. A and B, Anteroposterior and lateral* radiographs demonstrate a soft tissue mass adjacent to an area of increased density representing the healed fracture, superimposed on the coarse-combed cancellous texture and widened bone contour of typical Paget's disease. *C,* A fragment of Paget bone with a mosaic pattern has abundant surface Howship's lacunae due to osteoclastic erosion; the surrounding sarcomatous tissue is dominantly fibroblastic. *D,* The storiform pattern of sarcoma fits malignant fibroxanthoma. *E,* Multivesicular and signet ring sarcoma cells contain abundant fat; a wreath of nuclei and peripheral fatty vacuolization are typical features of malignant lipoblasts (inset, lower right).

example of malignant transformation of this "pseudo" entity will be presented, although sarcoma has arisen after lesions so diagnosed have been irradiated (Tillman et al., 1968).

Neuromechanical Adaptations

Examples of neuromechanical adaptations include individually unique modifications of bone shape that result from unusual or specific use and disuse patterns. We know of no examples of secondary sarcomatous change in this category.

Anomalies

Case after case verifies Codman's postulate: "repair of a congenital (anomalous) benign tumor (can) cause the advent of malignancy" (caption, Figure 5, p. 112, 1925). During the course of growth and remodeling, a great number of cells arise, function, and disappear; as a result various quantities of intra- and extracellular material are produced. Anachronistic persistence of cells involved in this activity gives rise to space-occupying residua that can enlarge (Fig. 22–11). Some give rise to secondary sarcoma, either directly from their cellular components (Fig. 22–12, and see

Fig. 22–16) or indirectly through involutional change (Fig. 12–13) or chronically accelerated turnover in their vicinity (see Fig. 22–18).

Chondromas. The cartilage category of anomalies, chondromas, is commonly encountered in orthopedic oncology and presents several morphologic configurations. Chondromas can be subclassified by location: cortical chondroma, centered within cortical bone; (sub)periosteal chondroma, beneath periosteum (perichondrium) on intact cortical bone; osteochondroma, in which lesional cartilage projects from bone on a broad base (sessile type) or stalk (pedunculated type) of bone built up through enchondral ossification; enchondroma, intramedullary. The radiograph is usually more helpful than histology in subclassification.

Periosteal Chondroma. The presence of a solid cortex beneath a developing cartilage mass favors periosteal chondroma. A minority of early periosteal chondromas may later evolve toward a more conventional osteochondroma configuration. The absence of significant enchondral ossification at their base helps separate periosteal chondromas from early sessile osteochondromas. If a periosteal chondroma is simply shelled out from beneath its capsule, recurrence is likely because the perichondrium may continue generating new chondroid substance.

The risk of sarcomatous change in a periosteal chondroma is predominantly in the direction of chon-

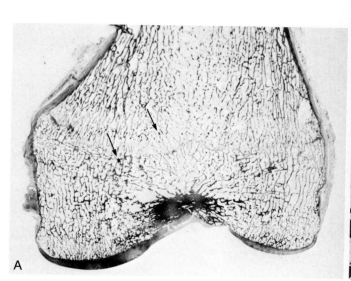
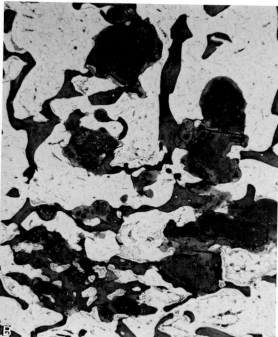

Figure 22–11. Closing growth plate with chondral remnants. *Distal femur of a 19 year old man. A,* The whole section shows remnants of the growth plate extending a few millimeters in from each cortex at the epiphyseal-metaphyseal junction. The arrows denote minute chondral remnants of growth plate cartilage illustrated at higher magnification in *B.* Also note the as yet imprecise integration of the epiphyseal and metaphyseal cancellous networks. *B,* A detailed view of benign hyalin cartilage remnants, any one of which could, through continued proliferation, enlarge to become an enchondroma.

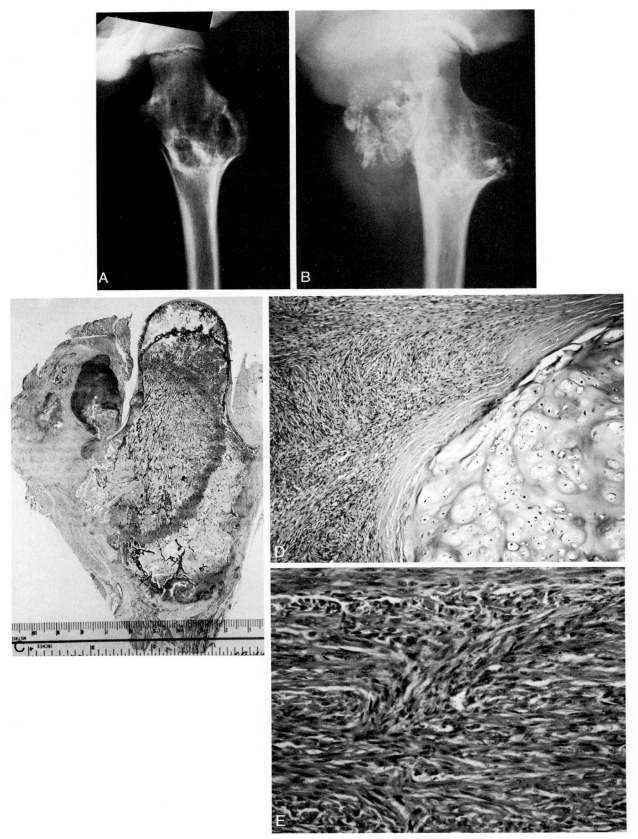

Figure 22–12. *See legend on opposite page.*

Figure 22–13. Osteochondroma with anachronistic stalk cartilage. *A 54 year old man complained of recent enlargement of a scapular lesion known to be present for 40 years. A bone scan uptake was "intense."* A, Within the large scapular lesion are patches of almost metallic density. The lobular periphery is typical of an osteochondroma, but unusual in the extent of deformity. B, A section from the surface shows a cartilage cap contacting extraosseous fat (upper right). The multiple tidemark lines are reminiscent of that beneath articular cartilage and bespeak fluctuations of cap thickness over time. In the marrow space beneath the cartilage cap are irregular cartilage matrix remnants surrounded by hypocellular fibrous tissue, reflecting incomplete enchondral removal of cartilage. C, Deeper within the marrow space are large islands of irregular hypocellular hyalin cartilage with increased hematoxylin uptake indicative of marked mineralization. Fifteen histologic sections were negative for malignancy. Hypermineralized anachronistic stalk cartilage is often associated with increased bone scan uptake and should not be mistaken for malignancy.

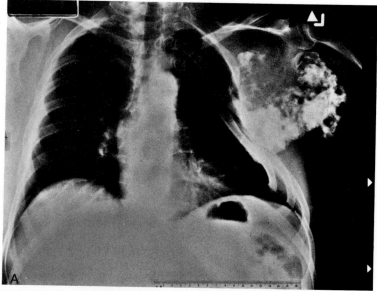

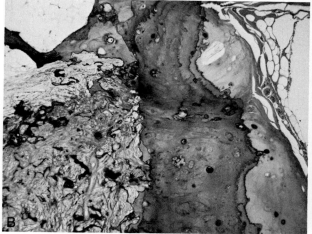

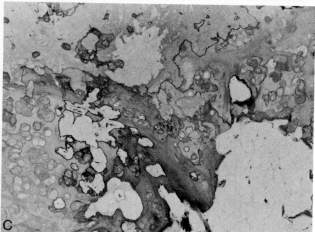

Figure 22–12. Sarcoma arising from the capsule of an osteochondroma. *A 16 year old youth complained of a few weeks of pain referable to a large sessile proximal femoral lesion known present for 7 years and previously biopsied (diagnosis: osteochondroma). A "typical osteochondroma" had also been excised years before from the distal femur.* A, An early radiograph shows the typical configuration of a sessile osteochondroma involving the intertrochanteric line. B, A film 6.5 years later, at the time of complaint of pain, indicates a medially projecting, partially mineralized lobular density superimposed on the lesser trochanter component of the antecedent osteochondroma. C, A large section from the disarticulation specimen shows loss of the bone cortex along the medial aspect of the proximal femur (left). From this area of cortical loss, a broad front of tumor invades across the intertrochanteric zone; only a 4 mm wide leading edge of the invading tumor remains viable, appearing as a crescentic band of darker staining. This medullary invasion correlates well with radiograph B where it matches the lytic loss of cancellous bone in the proximal femur. D, Benign hyalin cartilage of the osteochondroma cap (lower right) is covered by a thin fibrous capsule, the outer layers of which present abnormal cellularity. E, A detailed view of the cellular areas shows substantial variation in size, shape, and staining of the collagen-producing cells (fibrosarcoma).

drosarcoma and appears increased in the more proximal appendicular and axial skeleton. The degree of cytologic atypism required to confirm a diagnosis of malignancy is greater than that required of intramedullary cartilage lesions.

Osteochondromas. The incidence of malignant change in osteochondromas is probably overstated due to (1) the practice of "establishing" this diagnosis by measuring cap thickness rather than by correlating all data including histology, and (2) the ability of early stages of some parosteal sarcomas to mimic the structure of a small osteochondroma subsequently obscured by more obviously malignant growth.

The very low incidence of distant metastases in published cases of "chondrosarcoma" arising in osteochondromas (Garrison et al., 1982) contrasts with the usual behavior of sarcoma. Our experience suggests high-grade metastasizing (especially spindle cell) sarcomas arising from osteochondromas (Fig. 22–12) may actually outnumber true chondrosarcomas. Those with the hereditary multiple exostosis syndrome are at increased risk of having malignant change in proportion to the number of lesions, but each individual lesion is probably no more dangerous than a solitary osteochondroma.

A clinical suspicion of malignancy often comes up in regard to a certain peculiar variant of osteochondroma. In those where the maturing cartilage cap is incompletely removed by enchondral ossification, anachronistic chondroid accumulates in the bony stalk, like icebergs from the edge of a glacier, where it *excessively* mineralizes and casts almost metallic radiographic density (Fig. 22–13). The odd x-ray appearance is associated with increased activity on bone scan.

The following features favor parosteal sarcoma over malignant change of an osteochondroma.

Clinical: Acquisition of a totally new, progressively enlarging mass lesion in a patient beyond the growth years.

Radiographic: Indistinct outer periphery that grades imperceptibly from bony to soft tissue density with nothing resembling a subchondral bony plate beneath the cartilage cap.

Histologic: Closely-spaced, atypical, hyperchromatic spindle cells in the fibrous "capsule"; very gradual versus abrupt transition from atypical spindle cells in the "capsule" to cells in lacunae surrounded by cartilage matrix in the "cap"; persistence of close-spaced, atypical, hyperchromatic spindle cells between osseous trabeculae in the bony base or stalk; coarse-textured trabeculae that may have surface osteoid or bone that is lamellar; an abundantly convoluted outer cartilage layer that appears in large sections as multiple discontinuous chondro-osseous lobules.

At times the distinction between a chondro-osseous parosteal sarcoma and an osteochondroma undergoing malignant transformation becomes arbitrary.

Enchondromas. Well-circumscribed phalangeal enchondromas are rarely a diagnostic problem because of the well-publicized mitigation of histologic atypicality in acral location. In contrast, enchondromas of proximal long bones and limb girdles, especially if large, are liable to be designated as low-grade chondrosarcomas. In parallel with uterine leiomyomas, size alone is not a valid criterion of malignancy for cartilage tumors, since size does not necessarily equate with abnormal cellularity. More problematic are the enchondromas with limited areas of hypercellularity, atypia, and loose, watery-appearing matrix. It is generally easy to find a few binucleate chondrocytes in these tumors to satisfy one of the more popular conventional criteria of malignancy. In direct proportion to rendering malignant diagnoses based on the latter criterion alone, the survival figure for "chondrosarcoma" will be increased. Our experience with lesions composed predominantly of well-formed hyalin cartilage but with focal areas of loose, watery matrix and crowded cellularity parallels the literature: they have little or no capacity to metastasize without further change in histology (that is, increase in grade), can be cured by complete local removal, but tend to regrow locally if not completely removed, even years after surgery. Since the imminent probability of metastasis without treatment is part of the usual concept of malignancy, we usually code such cases as *active enchondromas.* Others prefer to call these "low-grade chondrosarcomas." In parallel with the trend started with ovarian tumors, there may be room for a "borderline" (active) category. The term "active" is useful to denote certain bone tumors which are prone to extensive local invasion, a propensity to recur and the likelihood for eventual aggressive behavior if not completely excised (Fig. 22–14).

Worrisome radiographic features associated with what otherwise looks like a benign enchondroma include: (1) lobular indentations along the endosteal cortical surface (endosteal scalloping); (2) periosteal reactions other than the solid type, especially thin lamellated and interrupted reactions; and (3) juxtacortical masses.

Awareness of *chondrosarcomatous change* of enchondromas (Fig. 22–15) is as old as the concept of chondrosarcoma itself (Phemister, 1930) and was identified in half of Lichtenstein and Jaffe's chondrosarcoma cases (1943). Nevertheless, this phenomenon remains controversial in the literature (Pritchard et al., 1980). Failure to verify this sequence seems mainly due to differences in interpretation of the more mature cartilage components, that is, antecedent benign enchondroma versus the low-grade component of a malignant tumor.

As indicated, we do not attach particular diagnostic importance to the finding of binucleate chondrocytes, since these are regularly seen in normal cartilage (articular, growth plate, costochondral, nasal septal, tracheobronchial, and ear), as well as in intra-articular loose bodies and osteochondroma caps. Binucleatism

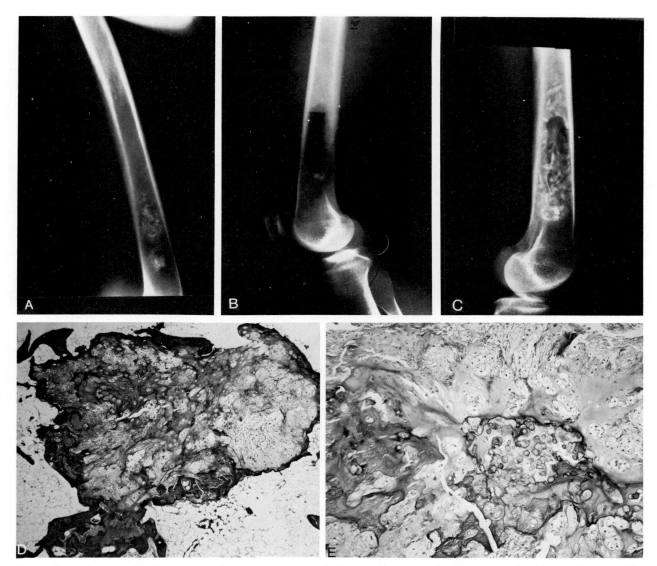

Figure 22–14. Active enchondroma, incomplete curettage biopsy. *A 43 year old man was found to have a distal femoral lesion on films taken for left thigh pain. A,* The ring-and-arc pattern plus grouped flocculent densities in the preoperative radiograph fit enchondroma; the clinical symptoms are suspicious for activity. *B,* The initial postcurettage radiograph indicates residual lesional density at the distal end. *C,* The cortical window was extended in both directions and additional curettage performed, followed by chemical cautery and autogenous iliac crest bone grafting; despite this, there is still residual cartilage matrix density at the distal extreme. This may have been undetectable without intraoperative view *B. D,* An enchondroma lobule is circumferentially bound by a rim of enchondral bone, an index of chronicity and stability. *E,* A lobule of enchondroma is hypocellular in comparison with the surrounding active enchondroma pattern with looser matrix texture. Comment: Intraoperative and postoperative radiographs are useful in assessing adequacy of removal.

as a criterion of malignancy is traced to Lichtenstein and Jaffe (1943). In point of fact, their reference actually lists small binucleated cells as one of five features "creating the picture of benignity." To favor a more aggressive chondroid lesion, it specified the double nuclei should be plump and show coarse hyperchromatism. Unfortunately, their emphasis on atypicality of the two nuclei is not always considered when this criterion is applied as a feature favoring chondrosarcoma.

Circumstantial evidence overwhelmingly supports the sarcomatous potential of enchondromas: (1) those cases where an extended radiographic sequence over many years initially shows a stable enchondroma, then superimposed osteolysis becomes associated with symptoms, and finally a radiographic lesion with obvious malignant features; (2) those cases of enchondroma, often with symptoms referable to the lesion, in which excessive variation in cell size, shape, and staining, cellular crowding and loose, watery matrix force recognition of at least focal malignant change ("sarcoma-in-situ"); (3) those cases of chon-

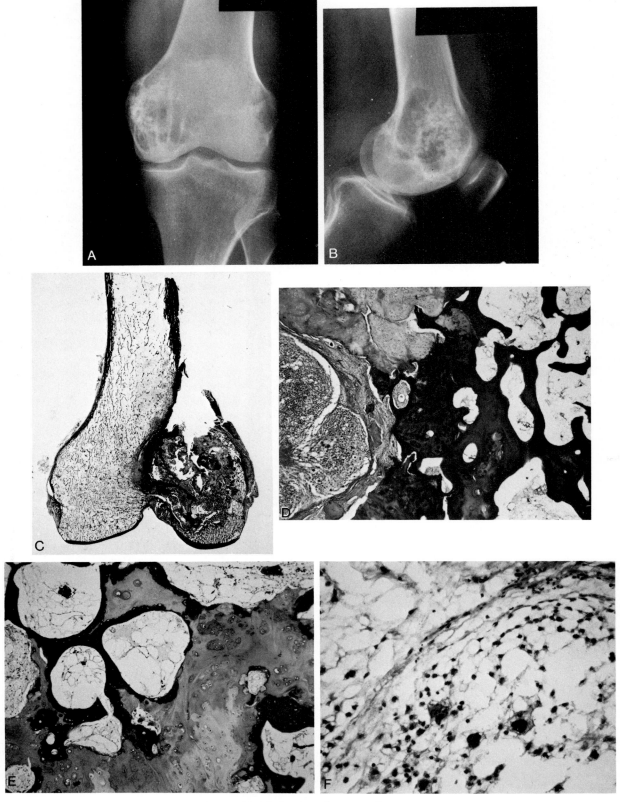

Figure 22–15. *See legend on opposite page.*

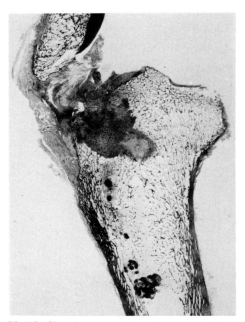

Figure 22–16. Chondrosarcomatous change of a discontinuous enchondroma. *A 61 year old man gave a history of occasional knee pain of 1 year's duration, leading to arthroscopy and biopsy. He had been unable to fully extend the knee for 4 years. A biopsy diagnosis of chondrosarcoma was followed by amputation.* In the dark area near the articular cartilage, the chondrosarcoma histology predominates over darker patches of benign hyaline cartilage and extends anteriorly into soft tissue. Additional enchondromatous nodules occur in the anterior tibial marrow space more distally. There were at least nine of these spatially separate benign chondroid nodules below the level of the chondrosarcoma, not apparent on clinical films or specimen x-ray films. An enchondroma may partially regress or enlarge. The multiple nodules in this tibia are deemed scattered remnants of what was initially a single large enchondroma that underwent substantial enchondral removal and ossification.

drosarcoma in proximity to enchondromatous foci scattered in the marrow space, presumably the remnants of a once continuous, larger enchondroma that underwent extensive enchondral removal (Fig. 22–16); and (4) the significant risk of sarcoma associated with enchondromatosis, with (Maffucci [Fig. 22–17] and without (Ollier) angiomas.

Evidence for a benign antecedent enchondroma can be marshaled from the radiograph and histology. The two density patterns seen with enchondromas, flocculent and rings and arcs, are sufficiently distinctive to permit radiographic separation from other focally

mineralized lesions with which they are often confused, for example, bone infarct (Sweet et al., 1981). Seeing such radiographic patterns, especially rings-and-arcs configuration, in a lesion histologically demonstrating chondrosarcoma is evidence for an antecedent enchondroma since the typically loose, watery matrix of unequivocal chondrosarcoma is reluctant to mineralize and unlikely to be rimmed by enchondral bone. Under these circumstances, histologic support for an antecedent enchondroma should always be sought, and, if absent, post-biopsy films should be reviewed to ascertain whether the apparent benign radiographic area was actually sampled. Histologic features supporting an antecedent enchondroma include broad areas of well-formed, hypocellular, hyalin cartilage; rims of enchondral bone on cartilage lobules; and hyalin cartilage cores in cancellous bone trabeculae near the epicenter of such a tumor in adults.

In patients over 50 years of age, proximal long bone enchondromas with substantial areas of loose-textured matrix and hypercellularity most likely represent low-grade sarcomatous transformations. However, it has become clear that chondromas in young patients can look histologically worse than they behave, probably because of the hormonal stimuli for growth. For this reason, such tumors in children may be tentatively considered as active enchondromas.

Enchondromas in the major proximal long bones and axial skeleton have a propensity for sarcomatous change. Ordinarily this is a process of slow acquisition of hypercellularity and loose matrix texture, eventually leading to a low-grade malignant pattern. Certain radiographic features, such as sclerotic margins and widened bone contour, and residual benign hyalin cartilage (enchondroma), usually persist as testimony to the sequence of events (Sweet et al., 1981). A definite incidence for malignant change is difficult to determine, especially from consultative material. However, benign antecedents in chondrosarcomas of adults are sufficiently common to recommend complete local removal of enchondromas in major long bones and the axial skeleton, when permitted by the patient's general medical condition.

High-grade spindle cell sarcomas arising in relation to antecedent enchondromas seem to appear in the literature as "dedifferentiated chondrosarcoma." The pre-existent benign component tends to be called

---

Figure 22–15. Chondrosarcomatous change of an enchondroma. *A 61 year old man complained of left leg discomfort for 3 months. A and B, P-A and lateral radiograph views indicate flocculent densities grouped in the medial condyle and surrounded by zones of lucency. C, A whole mount histologic section correlates with the films. The supracondylar cortical defect is the result of open biopsy that preceded amputation. D, Histology from the right margin of the condylar lesion shown in C presents a gradation from normal cancellous bone and marrow (extreme right) through enchondroma cartilage surrounded by enchondral bone (center), to active enchondroma (upper left), to overt chondrosarcoma (lower left). E, The benign enchondroma component can be recognized by well-formed hyalin cartilage of solid appearance and sparse cellularity, encased by enchondral bony rims. F, The chondrosarcoma component is recognized by loose, watery-appearing matrix, cell crowding, and extreme variation in cell size, shape, and staining.*

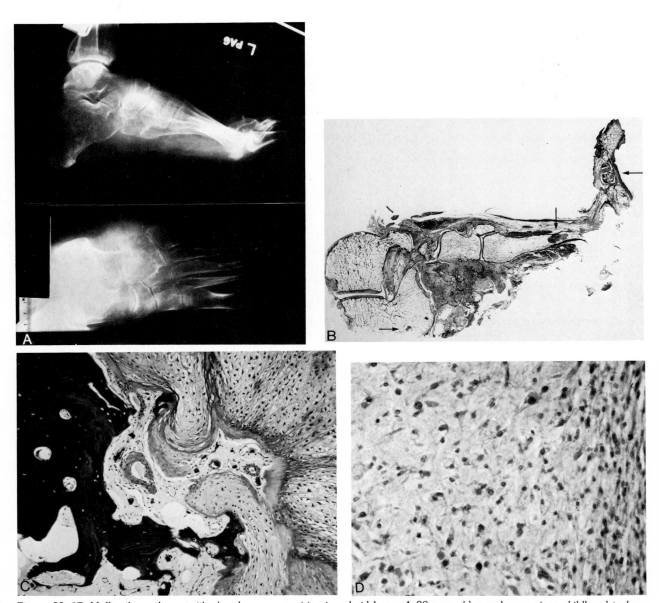

Figure 22–17. Maffucci's syndrome with chondrosarcoma arising in cuboid bone. *A 38 year old man known since childhood to have Maffucci's syndrome had multiple calcified enchondromata evident radiographically in the shortened and deformed right upper extremity and in scapulae and ribs. Cutaneous angiomas were obvious on the right arm, left lower leg, and chest. Progressive enlargement of the left foot had occurred in the past month. The area of swelling on the foot was biopsied and amputation performed.*

A, The lateral and oblique films of the foot show enlargement and cortical erosion of the cuboid. The oblique view indicates extension of a soft tissue mass from the lateral aspect of the bone. *B,* The whole mount section of the foot correlates well with the radiographs. The cuboid is entirely filled with cartilaginous tumor which has extended into soft tissue as multiple lobules. Several well-circumscribed benign enchondromas are evident in other bones (arrows). *C,* Toward the center of the cuboid is active-appearing, hyalin enchondroma cartilage populated by uniform chondrocytes. Multiple cement lines in adjacent trabeculae bespeak remodeling over a long period of time, further evidencing a benign antecedent. *D,* Around the periphery of central residual enchondroma are areas with loose matrix texture and closely spaced chondrocytes of quite variable size, shape, and staining; these are the hallmarks of chondrosarcoma.

Illustration continued on opposite page

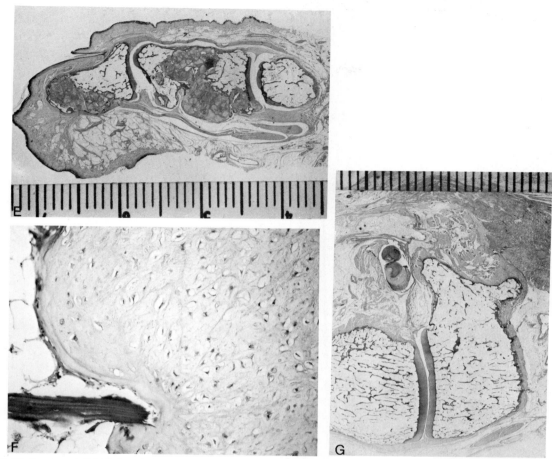

Figure 22–17. *Continued. E,* Middle and distal phalanges of a toe are distorted by enchondromas. It is more common for the enchondromas of the Ollier and Maffucci syndromes to extend to the subperiosteal position and form masses that bulge from the bone surface than for solitary phalangeal enchondromas to do this. *F,* A high power view of a benign enchondroma depicts more solid-appearing cartilage matrix and wider spacing of more uniform cells than in *C.* Despite this, note the pushing border connoting proliferative pressure, which impinges in lytic fashion on a medullary trabecula. *G,* Maffucci's syndrome is distinguished by enchondromas in combination with hemangiomas. In this view, laminated phleboliths occur within one of the anomalous vascular spaces beside the tarsal bones.

low-grade chondrosarcoma because of binucleated cells. Observers who recognize an underlying benign component in some of their cases (Mirra and Marcove, 1974) are in the minority. Even radiographic proof of the presence of a lesion for decades tends to be interpreted as supporting "low-grade malignancy" rather than a benign antecedent. High-grade spindle cell sarcomas can also be mislabeled "mesenchymal chondrosarcoma" and probably underlie the plethora of patterns in some cases labeled "primitive multipotential primary sarcoma of bone" (Hutter et al., 1966).

We believe these high-grade sarcomas arise from exuberant fibrovascular tissue involved with enchondral replacement around enchondromatous cartilage. The secondary malignancy can manifest any cellular pattern associated with this process, from undifferentiated spindle cells through vascular patterns to osteoid-secreting proliferations (Fig. 22–18), or may mimic metastatic carcinoma. In most cases, intercel-

lular collagen is scant; accordingly, the name "high-grade spindle cell sarcoma" is recommended.

Fat and Bone

Fibrous Dysplasia. Malignant change can develop in fibrous dysplasia with or without prior irradiation. It may be observed in monostotic as well as in polyostotic lesions, and occurs most often in the craniofacial region and in major long bones. The incidence of malignant change is less than 1 percent (Lichtenstein, 1977). Early as well as recent review articles (Huvos et al., 1972) agree this is a rare event.

More likely to be encountered are fibrous dysplasia variants that radiographically or histologically may be mistaken for malignancy. Rapid radiographic enlargement of benign lesions can occur. Alarming lucent defects predisposing to pathologic fracture may be found in films of otherwise typical fibrous dysplasia, and this is usually due to superimposed cystic change.

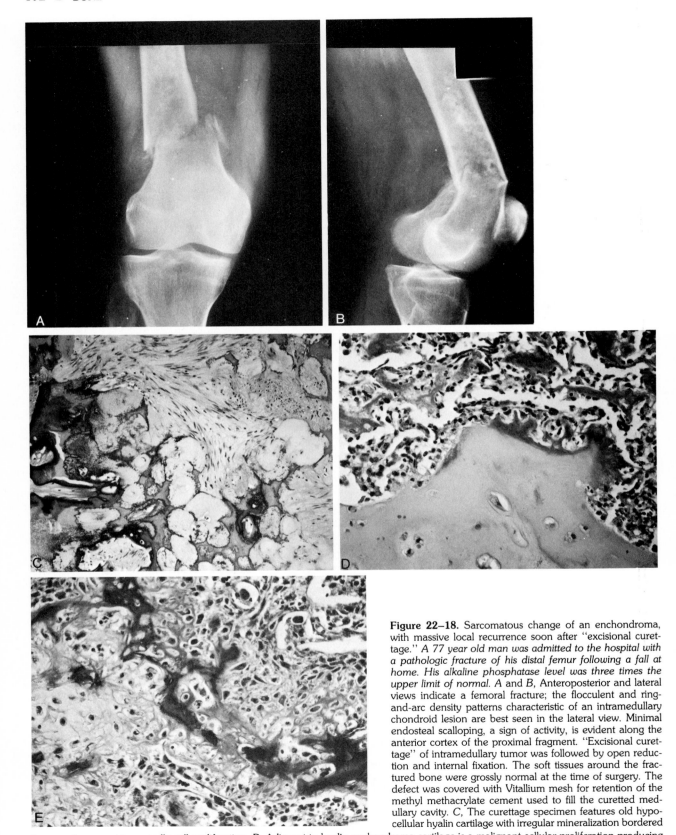

Figure 22–18. Sarcomatous change of an enchondroma, with massive local recurrence soon after "excisional curettage." *A 77 year old man was admitted to the hospital with a pathologic fracture of his distal femur following a fall at home. His alkaline phosphatase level was three times the upper limit of normal. A and B, Anteroposterior and lateral views indicate a femoral fracture; the flocculent and ring-and-arc density patterns characteristic of an intramedullary chondroid lesion are best seen in the lateral view. Minimal endosteal scalloping, a sign of activity, is evident along the anterior cortex of the proximal fragment. "Excisional curettage" of intramedullary tumor was followed by open reduction and internal fixation. The soft tissues around the fractured bone were grossly normal at the time of surgery. The defect was covered with Vitallium mesh for retention of the methyl methacrylate cement used to fill the curetted medullary cavity. C, The curettage specimen features old hypocellular hyalin cartilage with irregular mineralization bordered* by an active-appearing spindle cell proliferation. *D, Adjacent to hyalin enchondroma cartilage is a malignant cellular proliferation producing an osteosarcoma pattern. E, Farther away from the enchondroma lobules is a chondro-osseous sarcoma pattern.*

Illustration continued on opposite page

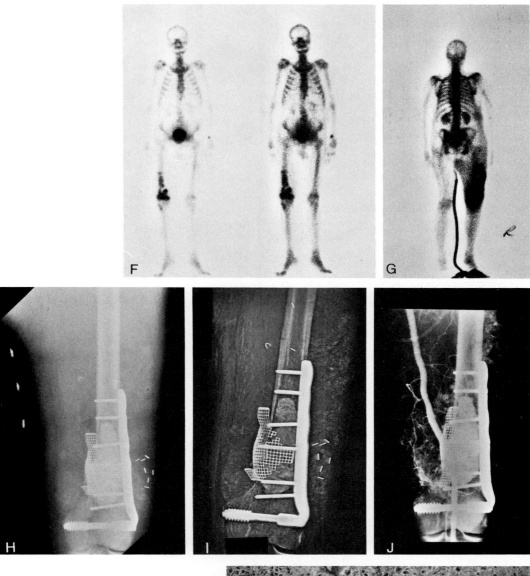

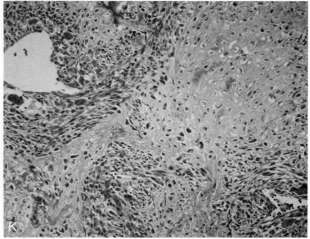

Figure 22–18. *Continued. F,* A bone scan 5 days after surgery indicates uptake corresponding to the operative area only. Five weeks after surgery, an 8 × 6 cm soft tissue mass was palpable in the thigh around the operative area; the patient's alkaline phosphatase level was now ten times the upper limit of normal. Rebiopsy indicated malignancy recurrent in the soft tissues *(K). G,* A repeat bone scan 3 months after the original operation shows extensive uptake of isotope in the soft tissues around the distal and midfemur. *H, I, and J,* Three different modalities depict partly mineralized sarcoma in soft tissue. Comparison of plane film *A* indicates that multiple small, cloudlike densities have appeared on both sides of the femur. The xerogram *(I)* shows these abnormal densities more clearly. The same areas correlate with abnormal vascular patterns in angiogram *J. K,* A biopsy of recurrent sarcoma in the thigh indicates its chondro-osseous pattern. *Comment: Curettage or piecemeal removal of a benign lesion with malignant change is likely to be followed by local recurrence.*

Associated sheets of plump fibrous dysplasia spindle cells suggest cyst formation occurs in the more proliferative, less cohesive stages of fibrous dysplasia. Coexistent reactive osteoid and abundant osteoclasts create one of the lesions easily mislabeled "aneurysmal bone cyst." Jaffe (1946) mentions the occasional occurrence of "congenital arteriovenous aneurysm" in instances of fibrous dysplasia.

Lesions combining the pattern of chondroma (enchondroma) and fibrous dysplasia are particularly problematic. "Islands of hyaline cartilage" are mentioned in the early works of both Jaffe (1946) and Lichtenstein (1938) on fibrous dysplasia, and in their paper under joint authorship (1942). Fibrous dysplasia having islands of cartilage can occur as solitary or polyostotic lesions in both females (with or without precocious puberty) and males. The proximal femur is the most common location for this combination, and it should not be mistaken for malignancy.

Sarcoma arising in fibrous dysplasia should be suspected when irregular lytic change and/or a periosteal reaction other than a shell or solid type is encountered. The secondary sarcomas include osteosarcoma, fibrosarcoma, spindle cell sarcoma, and malignant fibroxanthoma (Huvos, 1972).

Ossifying Fibroma. This term was pre-empted for a distinctive fibro-osseous lesion of the jaw (Montgomery, 1927) that some believe is a form fibrous dysplasia takes in this site (Jaffe, 1974). The term is rarely needed as a designation outside the cranialfacial skeleton. (See cortical fibrous dysplasia, below.) Jaw tumors of this type rarely undergo sarcomatous change.

Fibroxanthoma. The term "fibroxanthoma" under some circumstances is preferable to fibrous cortical defect or nonossifying fibroma. This is because it is often more descriptive and because the common focal ossification seen in these lesions presents a paradox of terms. The ossification derives from modulation of the lesional cells themselves. Usually the bone formed is scant and of a woven type, as in fibrous dysplasia, but with a less striking curvilinear trabecular array. At the other extreme, dense sclerotic patches are encountered having a mosaic histologic pattern as an indication of chronically accelerated remodeling activity (Fig. 22–19D). This is usually seen in a less cellular phase of adult lesions, often with substantial xanthoma cells and storiform desmoplasia. Occasional neutrophilic infiltration of such areas favors their formation through ischemic injury to become the seedbed of sarcomatous transformation.

Reports of malignant change of fibroxanthomas are so few (Bhagwandeen, 1966) that the popular view they are innocuous is rarely challenged. The secondary malignant patterns we have seen include malignant fibroxanthoma, spindle cell sarcoma, and fibrosarcoma; very rarely, osteosarcoma or other patterns are encountered.

Lipoma. It has become apparent that space-occupying lesions related to medullary fat are more com-

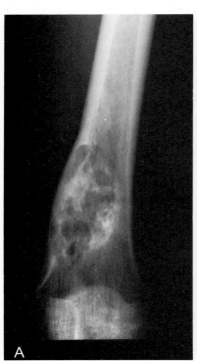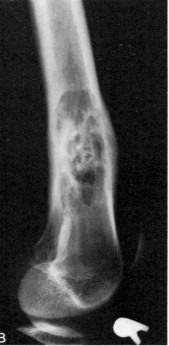

Figure 22–19. Fibroxanthoma with sarcomatous change. *A 44 year old man gave a 3.5 month history of pain in the right distal femur. A and B,* Radiographs indicate an old eccentric lesion with signs of recent change. Along the lobular contact with the medullary cavity is a zone of sclerotic density within the pre-existing border. Elsewhere, a great number of lucent patches have sharp lytic contact with cancellous bone and have deleted the cortex on the medial side; in place of the cortex, a lamellated periosteal reaction has been substituted. Also, note the indistinct, lobular, ground glass density component around the medial cortex beyond the lytic edge at the proximal end of this eccentric lesion. *C,* The curettage biopsy specimen reveals spindle and vacuolated cells arranged in a storiform pattern. The combination of benign xanthoma cells and fibroblasts fits with the eccentric metaphyseal location to establish the presence of an old fibroxanthoma. *D,* The sclerotic areas correlate with crude pseudo-Paget bone, the result of intralesional osteoblastic activity under moderately ischemic conditions. The foci filled with hypocellular fibrous tissue represent areas of osteoclastic removal that were not refilled with bone. *E,* The malignant areas that correlate with the lucent patches show plump malignant cells against a background of mixed inflammatory cells ("inflammatory malignant fibrous histiocytoma"). *F, The latter could easily be mistaken for malignant lymphoma on biopsy. A year and a half after amputation, the patient died 10 days after a craniotomy for cerebral metastases.*

Illustration continued on opposite page

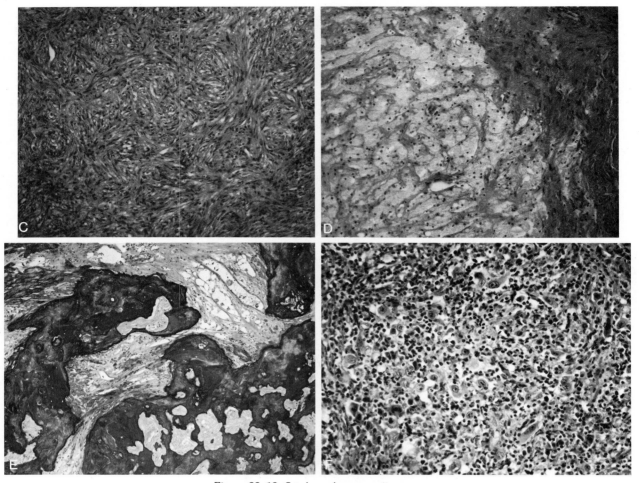

Figure 22–19. *See legend on opposite page.*

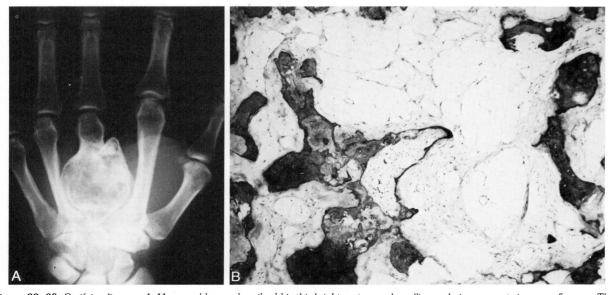

Figure 22–20. Ossifying lipoma. *A 41 year old man described his third right metacarpal swelling as being present since age 5 years. There was no history of fracture or local trauma.* A, The bone outline is widened by a mixed lucent and dense lesion; the cortical surface, reconstituted by periosteal apposition, forms a smooth outer contour. The radiographic appearance is benign. B, Biopsy revealed coarse bone arranged in trabeculae; some of this bone has an "ischemic" appearance. The intervening marrow fat presents a gradation between fibrous tissue, xanthoma cells, and large signet ring fat cells. Since the names of tumors should reflect cellular composition, ossifying lipoma was the diagnosis rendered.

405

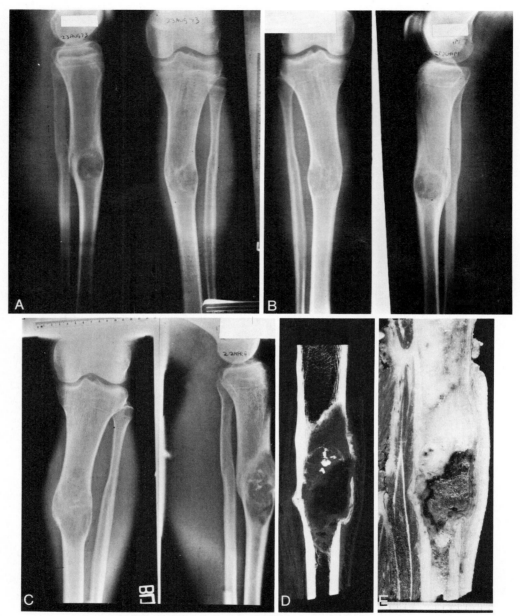

Figure 22–21. Ossifying lipoma complicated by osteosarcoma. *While running track, a 22 year old man fractured his left tibial shaft through a lucent lesion regarded by x-ray study as a "bone cyst." Treatment with a cast resulted in union, but slow enlargement of the area was noted over the next several years. Recently, after one month of pain in the left leg, he fell off a bicycle. Accentuated pain prompted x-rays (C), followed by biopsy and amputation. A,* A film taken 10 months after the original fracture shows a rounded, lucent area with focal internal densities, associated with widened bone contour. A healed fibular fracture is evident at the same level. *B,* Two years after the film shown in *A,* the lucent area has a more distinct sclerotic border. *C,* The film taken after the bicycle accident indicates substantial enlargement of the lucent area of the lesion. In the lateral view, irregular internal densities and an oblique fracture without displacement are seen. *D,* A specimen x-ray of an 8 mm thick longitudinal slab of the amputation specimen indicates that the internal densities lie just within the thin proximal sclerotic border that was overrun by invasive tumor extending proximally. The anterior cortex has been totally removed and an incomplete periosteal shell substituted. Pathologic fracture with buttressing callus is noted along the posterior cortex. *E,* (see Plate XX, Figure 22–21E). The gross photograph corroborates the observations made in the specimen radiograph. Note the residual golden-yellow lipoma tissue distally, the tan sarcoma extending proximally, and the hematoma-filled biopsy cavity centrally.

Illustration continued on opposite page

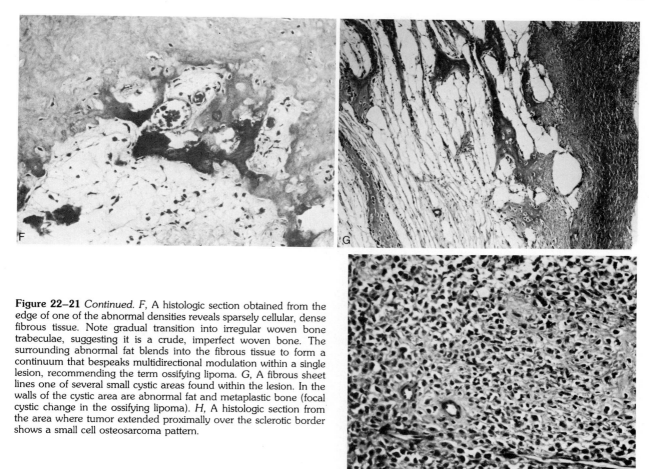

Figure 22–21 *Continued. F,* A histologic section obtained from the edge of one of the abnormal densities reveals sparsely cellular, dense fibrous tissue. Note gradual transition into irregular woven bone trabeculae, suggesting it is a crude, imperfect woven bone. The surrounding abnormal fat blends into the fibrous tissue to form a continuum that bespeaks multidirectional modulation within a single lesion, recommending the term ossifying lipoma. *G,* A fibrous sheet lines one of several small cystic areas found within the lesion. In the walls of the cystic area are abnormal fat and metaplastic bone (focal cystic change in the ossifying lipoma). *H,* A histologic section from the area where tumor extended proximally over the sclerotic border shows a small cell osteosarcoma pattern.

mon in bone than generally appreciated. This is in line with the incidence of lipomatous lesions in other body sites where adipose tissue is found, for example, subcutaneously. Intra-osseous lipomas commonly undergo cystic transformation resulting in either typical or unusual-appearing bone cysts (Johnson and Kindred, 1958). Not uncommonly there will be intralesional production of lamellar bone in a coarse cancellous pattern, which can mask the expected radiolucency, and also a coarsely textured, irregular, and hypocellular ("ischemic") bone leading to possible confusion with bone infarcts (Fig. 22–20). This and concurrent desmoplasia confer the same potential for sarcomatous change that both lesions share. An antecedent benign lipoma should be suspected from radiographic features, especially when a widened bone outline with central lucency and patchy density can be confirmed by prior x-rays (Fig. 22–21).

Polymorphic Fibrocytic Disease of Bone. Atypical ossifying fibrocytic lesions of the proximal femur are a common consultative problem. These odd, almost site-specific intertrochanteric lesions are frequently incidental findings. The radiographic appearance is distinctive and repetitive. Full-size lesions present as cone-shaped lucent defects in Ward's triangle with variable amounts of patchy central density and peripheral sclerosis. They typically extend distally to a few centimeters below the lesser trochanter where a medially sloping sclerotic border is seen (Fig. 22–22). The x-ray appearance is frequently confused with bone infarct, and this can be avoided if there is central density and widening of bone outline (Jaffe, 1972, Fig. 175 A, p. 681); the latter implies proliferative pressure that would not be expected in an infarct.

Biopsy often presents a complex mixture of tissue patterns defying a conventional designation. The presence of curvilinear trabeculae in the fibrous background of most cases suggests the possibility of a fibrous dysplasia variant. Furthermore, "typical" fibrous dysplasia at this site is not uncommon. However, many cases fail to demonstrate typical fibrous dysplasia–like features. Additional components include lipomatous fat, xanthoma cells (considered incompletely developed fat cells as in hibernomas), rounded cementum-like ossicles, crude pseudo-Paget bone with mosaic structure (centrally and along the radiodense border), and myxofibrous tissue, often with focal cystic change. Rarely there are enchon-

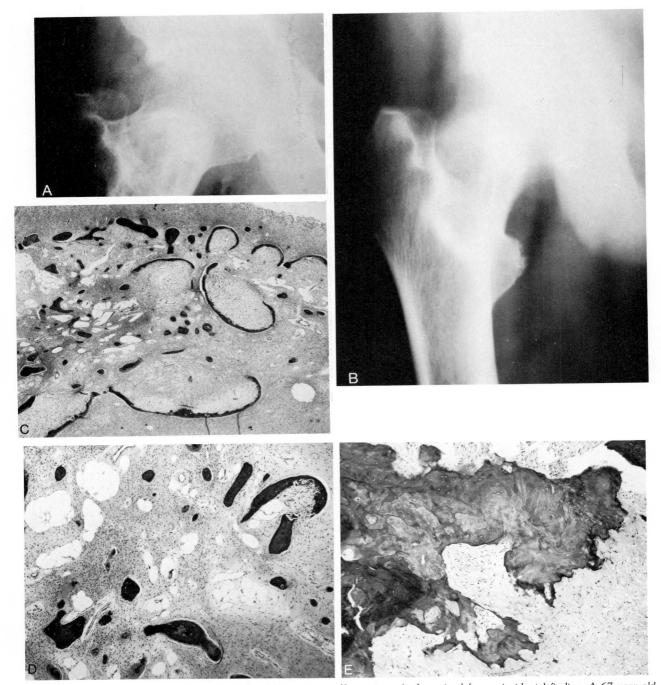

Figure 22–22. Polymorphic fibrocystic disease (liposclerosing myxofibrous tumor) of proximal femur, incidental finding. *A 67 year old man under care for cervical arthritis complained of vague stiffness in the lower back region and both hips. A proximal femoral lesion was discovered in the subsequent radiographs. A and B,* An intertrochanteric lesion is shown in plain film *A* and tomogram *B;* the predominantly lucent central area has focal densities. The periphery is marked by a sclerotic border which is cone shaped proximally and slants obliquely across the marrow space medially at the distal end. This is a repetitive configuration for this lesion. On bone scan, the lesion showed increased uptake. *C,* The curettage specimen shows round and crescentic ossicles in a myxofibrous background punctuated by islands of mature fat. *D,* The ossicle at the upper right is undergoing remodeling activity, accounting for increased uptake on the bone scan. This combination of elements is beyond current standard concepts of fibrous dysplasia, but all are mentioned in the classic description of Lichtenstein and Jaffe (1942). *E,* In some areas of the specimen, crude pseudo-Paget bone occurs within a hypocellular fibrous background; note the lytic component (below center) of smoldering, chronic remodeling activity that accounts for the plethora of cement lines.

droma-like foci of hyalin cartilage. All or only some of these may be seen in a given case and the complex gradation of histologic patterns makes it difficult to assign a simple designation. Should a single pattern dominate, then a specific diagnosis is possible. While all these patterns are mentioned in the original description of fibrous dysplasia (Lichtenstein and Jaffe, 1942), they go beyond current popular concepts of that entity. Accordingly, the term "polymorphic fibrocystic disease" seems more suitable. Alternatively, the more descriptive term "lipo-sclerosing myxo-fibrous tumor" (LSMFT) covers their quiltwork of tissue types that exceeds the usual fibrous dysplasia.

An attractive hypothesis is to regard these patterns as an interrelated spectrum derived from medullary fat or a medullary hamartoma. Their sclerotic borders suggest stability over many years. Others have gradually enlarged, leading to pain referable to stress-related infarctions along the femoral neck or sudden pathologic fracture.

Internal ischemic damage is followed by desmoplasia and this, in our opinion, predisposes to sarcomatous change. In other instances, malignancy appears to have arisen from progressive in-situ atypism of the lipomatous element. Malignant change should be carefully excluded when symptoms referable to such a lesion appear, especially in the later decades of life or when accompanied by focal lucent change in the radiograph. Remnants of the distinctive sclerotic border configuration and widened bone outline are not expected with a de novo sarcoma and alert one to the probability of a pre-existent benign lesion. With time, sequential x-rays in an untreated case will show the enlarging sarcoma obliterating the benign antecedent (Fig. 22–23). Nearly 10 percent of well over 100 AFIP cases of this entity were submitted with sarcomatous change, suggesting a high risk and perhaps the wisdom of appropriate early prophylactic treatment.

Cyst. The number of bone sarcomas on file arising in relation to bone cysts have more than tripled since four were reported by Johnson and Putschar (1962). Radiographic clues of an antecedent cyst include widened bone outline and remnants of sclerotic borders. Occasional cases have a complete radiographic sequence fully documenting the transition. Histologically, an antecedent cyst might be suspected when laminated sheets of dense, hypocellular fibrous tissue, thin planes of osteoid, and/or fibrin-like osteoid is found. None of these, however, is absolutely specific for bone cysts and a number of other benign antecedents can be focally cystic. Spindle cell sarcoma, chondrosarcoma, liposarcoma (Fig. 22–24) and round cell sarcoma (Fig. 22–25) can all arise in bone cysts.

"Juvenile Uncommitted Metaphyseal Tumor." There is a benign intra-osseous mass that defies conventional classification for which we use the term "juvenile uncommitted metaphyseal tumor." "Juvenile" refers to the patient's age, "metaphyseal" to

location and "uncommitted" to the fact that the lesion demonstrates many coexistent patterns in relatively equal amounts. The latter includes cyst, giant cell tumor, fibrous dysplasia, fibroxanthoma (nonossifying fibroma), osteoblastoma, and occasionally other patterns. Cases followed for a period of time generally resolve into a single dominant pattern as the lesion matures. The most common transition is to simple bone cyst; somewhat less common is a cystic type of giant cell tumor. Other transformations also occur. In a few instances, the patterns persist into adult life and instances of malignant change have been observed.

Vascular Anomalies

Hemangioma and Its Relation to Angioendothelioma and Angiosarcoma. The term angioma is applied to vascular channel-forming lesions composed of flattened endothelial cells. Beyond this, the literature is rather confusing as to the proper terminology for vascular tumors of bone; various meanings have been attached to the same words. For the purpose of this discussion, the term angioendothelioma is used for the group of vasoformative tumors midway in aggressive potential and histology between angioma and angiosarcoma, characterized by plumper endothelial and channel-forming cells (more "epithelioid") than angioma. Angiosarcoma differs by having solid cellular areas; the cells can be epithelioid, spindle-shaped, pleomorphic, or a mixture of these shapes.

We have encountered several cases which suggest a potential for some angiomas to progress over a period of years through a histologic spectrum to angioendothelioma and angiosarcoma (Fig. 22–26). This is not a totally new concept (Pulford, 1925). Others have noted this histologic spectrum (Volp and Mazabrand, 1982; Unni et al., 1971). Conversely, a number of observers have denied the concept of spontaneous malignant transition of angiomas (Aegerter and Kirkpatrick, 1964; Lichtenstein, 1977). Jaffe (1974) estimated the incidence of de novo sarcomatous change of an angioma as "almost never." Radiographic and histologic indications of a sclerotic border around the sites of aggressive-appearing tumors composed of sheets of angiosarcoma cells favor a prolonged, indolent (angioma) phase. Histologic support for angioma should be sought toward the periphery, with evidence of transition through hemangioendothelioma to angiosarcoma. The rarity of angiosarcoma following irradiation of a hemangioma (Lichtenstein, 1977) may reflect the vulnerability of endothelial cells to this treatment modality. Ultrastructural and immunoperoxidase studies are helpful in distinguishing the rare epithelioid angioendothelioma arising in bone (Tang, 1976) from metastatic carcinoma.

Cortical Fibrous Dysplasia and Its Relation to Adamantinoma. Intracortical fibrous dysplasia (Fig. 22–27) is found almost exclusively in the anterior cortex of the tibia, less commonly in the fibular shaft,

Text continued on page 415

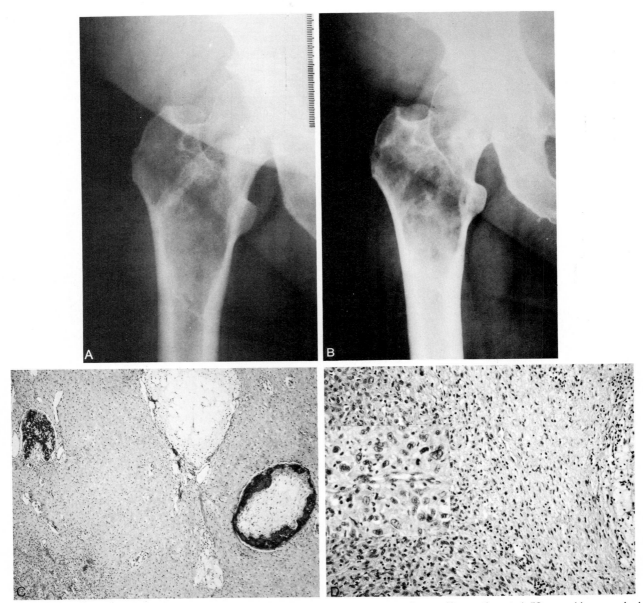

Figure 22–23. Polymorphic fibrocystic disease of bone (LSMFT) with transition into malignant fibroxanthoma. *A 53 year old woman had radiographs for persistent right hip pain, initally attributed to arthritis. A,* The initial radiograph of the proximal femur displays an intertrochanteric lesion with sclerotic margins. Proximally, the margin forms a cone-shaped density pointing to the femoral neck. Distally, the margin slopes medially. *B,* A follow-up film 4 months later indicates that a substantial portion of the sclerotic border at the base of the greater trochanter has undergone lytic destruction. The area was curetted and a metallic prosthesis installed. *C,* Crude crescent (upper left) and circular (right) ossicles emerge from a benign fibrous background with a focal (top central) patch of fat modulation. *D,* A zone of atypical hypercellularity (left) occurs near a patch of xanthoma cells (right); the higher magnification inset (left) indicates pleomorphism and mitotic activity.

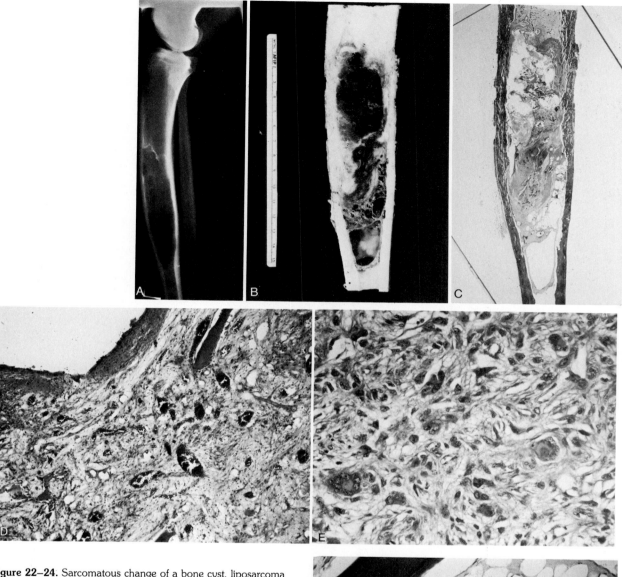

Figure 22–24. Sarcomatous change of a bone cyst, liposarcoma pattern. *A 17 year old youth complained of pain of 1 month's duration in the left tibia while playing basketball. Subsequently, he was lost to follow-up for 10 months. He returned with increased pain and observed that his left leg had become larger. Lower leg measurement documented a 2 cm circumferential increase compared with the initial evaluation. X-ray films had not changed appreciably during the interval. Amputation was performed after a biopsy confirmed malignancy.*

A, The lateral clinical film upon the patient's second presentation indicates a widened cortical outline. A lobular sclerotic border proximally suggests an antecedent benign lesion. The distal extreme is radiolucent with endosteal scalloping. *B,* Hemorrhagic tumor largely fills the lucent defect, as seen in a longitudinal cut through the gross specimen; residual bone cyst is at the distal extreme. *C,* A whole mount section shows the thin fibrous wall of residual bone cyst distally; the invasive edge of the sarcoma infiltrates through cancellous bone proximally. *D,* Well-vascularized cellular tumor occurs beside the cystic space. *E,* Multinucleated lipoblasts and vacuolated liposarcoma cells comprise the tumor. *F,* Abnormal fat consistent with intraosseous lipoma was observed in the nontumorous proximal tibia. This suggests the bone cyst originated from cystification of an intraosseous lipoma (Johnson and Kindred, 1958).

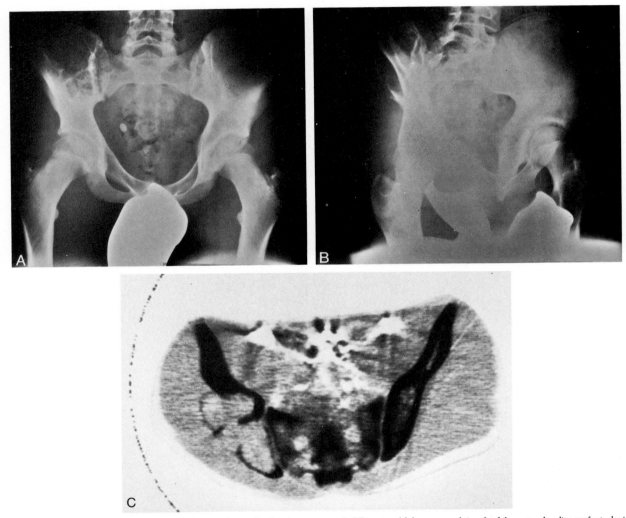

Figure 22–25. Round cell sarcoma arising in the wall of a bone cyst. *A 15 year old boy complained of low grade discomfort during activity.* A and B, Plain films depict an iliac wing lesion with a widened bone contour and a coarsely trabeculated bony shell. C, CT scan confirms that a trabeculated shell is responsible for the widened bone outline. *At open biopsy, the lesion was very vascular, producing 2 units of bleeding within 2 to 3 minutes. The surgeons rapidly curetted the "cyst" to its base with a total blood loss of 4 units. The scant curettage specimen (3 × 2 × 1 cm aggregate) testifies to the predomonantly cystic nature of the lesion.*

Illustration continued on opposite page

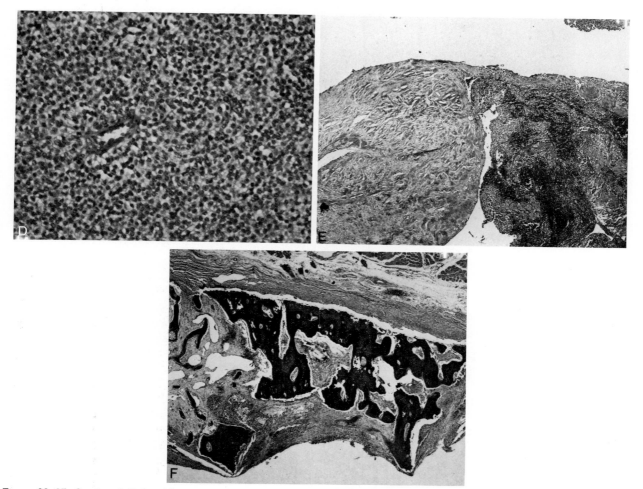

Figure 22–25. *Continued. D,* In addition to the fibrocystic pattern, a malignant round cell component with cytoplasmic PAS positivity is present. "Ewing sarcoma," while a tempting diagnosis based on histology alone, would ignore the radiographic and operative findings. *E,* A fibrous lining that fits unicameral bone cyst occurs on the left side; toward the right are sheets of malignant round cells seeming to have arisen within the fibrous wall. *F,* A histologic view of the trabeculated shell shows reactive periosteum (top) and the chamber of the cyst (bottom). Note the fibro-osseous lining typical of the wall of an antecedent unicameral bone cyst.

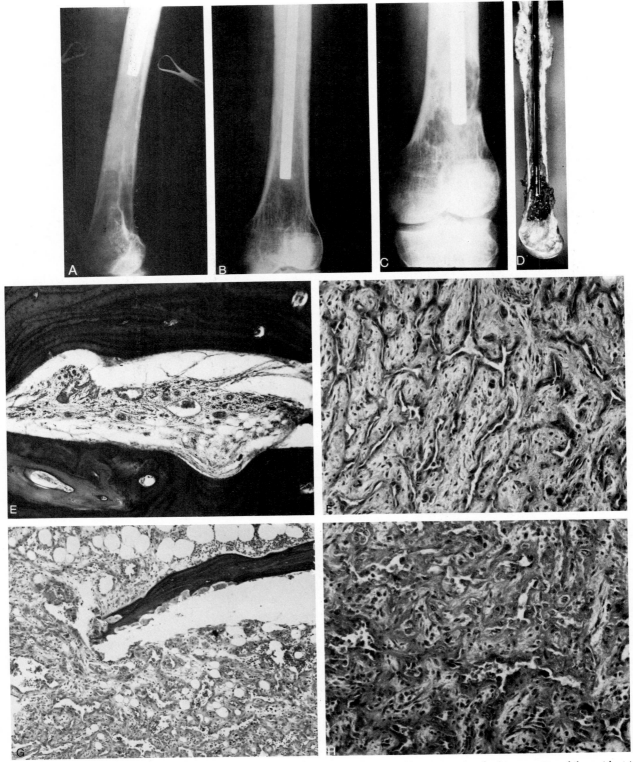

Figure 22–26. Evolution of angiosarcoma from an antecedent angioma. *A 58 year old man was involved in an automobile accident in 1955, during which he sustained a femoral shaft fracture. Internal fixation with a metallic rod was performed. A and B, Intraoperative radiographs perused for retrospective study include a lateral view during rod insertion with an area of lucency (A). The 1955 anteroposterior view (B) shows "corduroy cloth" coarsening of cancellous fabric, suggestive of an angioma in the distal femur at the point where the intramedullary rod came to rest. Knee pain began 14 years later at age 72. C, The 1969 x-ray film shows substantial osteolytic change around the tip of the rod and endosteal scalloping. Cortical fracture is evident on the lateral aspect near the tip of the rod. Amputation was performed after biopsy.*

Legend continued on opposite page

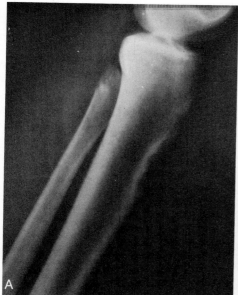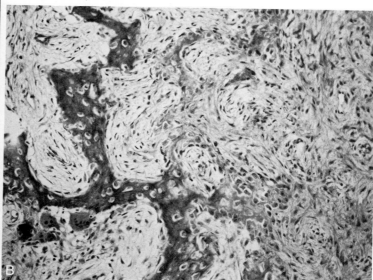

Figure 22–27. Cortical fibrous dysplasia. *A 14 year old girl gave a history of a slightly painful mass on the anterior surface of the tibia for 4 months. A,* A lobular sclerotic deep margin demarcates a lucent anterior intracortical defect from the medullary cavity. *B,* The fibro-osseous tissue of the lesion features gradual emergence of curvilinear woven bone trabeculae out of a fibrovascular background. Some tendency for osteoblastic alignment on the surface of the new bone is often encountered in these lesions, especially around the periphery near contact with normal bone. Note the active osteoclasts indicating ongoing internal remodeling.

and sometimes in both lower leg bones synchronously. Cases with sequential x-rays taken over a period of years illustrate the natural history of this initially intracortical process. The earliest appreciable stage is a focal intracortical lucency which enlarges, causing increased cortical width around the lucency. Continued enlargement subsequently leads to encroachment on the marrow space and a tendency for progressive deformity, including a palpable bulge of bone and/or actual bowing. Subtotal removal has been followed by local reformation of lucent defects filled with reformed lesional tissue. The advancing edge of an enlarging lesion is composed of proliferating fibrovascular tissue and for this reason is discussed as a "vascular anomaly." Active hyperemia drives osteoclastic resorption. Ossification in the form of fiber bone occurs subsequently. These lesions tend to slow down, usually stabilizing in size after puberty, but can cause substantial deformity.

Synonyms under which this lesion appears in the literature are osteofibrous dysplasia (Campanacci and Laus, 1981) and ossifying fibroma of long bone. The latter term is based on rigid adherence to the histologic criterion (Reed, 1963) that *any* amount of osteoblastic rimming excludes fibrous dysplasia (Goergen et al., 1977; Markel, 1978; Kempson, 1966; Schoenecker et al., 1981). This may be traced to Lichtenstein (1938) but is not mentioned in the article on fibrous dysplasia under joint authorship (Lichtenstein and Jaffe, 1942).

Since "osteoblastic rimming" may be found in the more mature areas of both monostotic and polyostotic (Albright type) of radiographically typical fibrous dysplasia in the tibia and elsewhere, this feature does not warrant a change of name, in our opinion. It may only reflect the modulatory consequence of greater stress in lower leg bones than is applied to fibro-osseous lesions in other bones. The term ossifying fibroma was pre-empted long ago for a distinctive lesion of the jaw (Montgomery, 1927) and is rarely needed for lesions outside the cranial skeleton.

We believe cortical fibrous dysplasia may represent

Figure 22–26 *Continued. D,* The gross findings correlate well with the radiograph *(C):* Hemorrhagic tumor surrounds the tip of the rod; a pathologic fracture separates the distal femur. Indolent tumor scallops the endosteal surface of the proximal fragment. *E,* Widely spaced benign vascular channels are surfaced by uniform, rather widely spaced benign endothelial cells (angioma). The surrounding bone has the appearance of having been under a chronic remodeling stimulus. *F,* In the more active areas, crowded hyperchromatic, more variable endothelial cells are confined to small channels separated by fibrous tissue (angioendothelioma). *G,* Angioendothelioma pattern surrounds a bone trabecula which is under osteoclastic attack; this correlates well with the lytic radiographic change. *H,* In areas of angiosarcoma, malignant endothelial cells are not restricted to vascular channels and form confluent sheets.

The early x-ray films (A and B) establish that the lesion had its beginning from a pre-existing lesion with radiographic features of an angioma present at the time of fracture. These and the spectrum of vascular tumor histology in the specimen pose an alternative to de novo angiosarcomatous change around a metallic device (Lichtenstein, 1977, p. 174.)

part of a related spectrum of fibrovascular anomalies spanning pseudoarthrosis of the tibia in infancy and adamantinoma in adults (Johnson, 1972). This is because coexistent areas of adamantinoma are found in some cases of cortical fibrous dysplasia, varying from a single high-powered perivascular field on one of many slides, through multifocal areas of emergence, to substantial areas of adamantinoma. Exceptional cases followed radiographically over an extended period of time have evolved into typical adamantinoma. However, diffuse adamantinomatous areas in patients under 20 years of age are somewhat unusual (Alguacil-Garcia et al., 1984), but the existence of such cases indicates that the fibrous dysplasia-like stroma commonly found in adamantinoma (Baker et al., 1954) is more than an insignificant histologic "look-alike" (Fig.

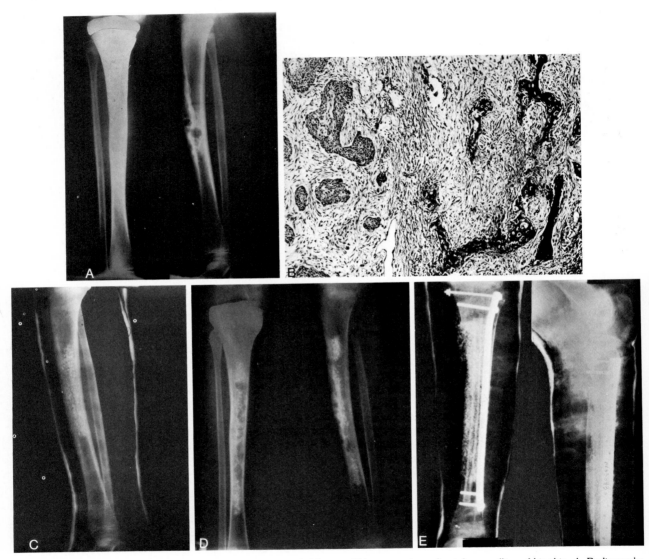

Figure 22–28. Cortical fibrous dysplasia with adamantinoma. *A 12 year old boy experienced painless swelling of his shin.* A, Radiographs reveal a midshaft anterior tibial lesion centered on the cortex, consisting of multiple lucent areas bound anteriorly by a smooth periosteal shell, and on the deep surface by a type I-A sclerotic border. The anterior cortex was excised, followed by curettage and bone grafting (bank bone). B, The specimen presents the combined histology of fibrous dysplasia (right) and adamantinoma (left). C, The postoperative radiograph indicates partial persistence of the original intracortical lucency at the proximal and distal extremes of the excision. These areas progressively enlarged and were curetted, followed by bone grafting 9 months after the original procedure. D, A follow-up film 1.5 months after the second operation shows fresh bone graft material at the proximal and distal extremes. Between, multifocal enlarging lucent areas in the original operative site have appeared. E, One year after the first procedure, the anterior and lateral tibial cortex was excised and replaced with a long screw plate and bone graft (fibular shaft and multiple bone chips). Pathologically, the lucencies contained cortical fibrous dysplasia tissue without evidence of adamantinoma, found only in the first specimen. *This case indicates that adamantinoma can arise within cortical fibrous dysplasia in the pediatric group, even when the underlying fibro-osseous lesion is still in a proliferative phase.*

22–28). Prominent intramedullary lytic defects super-imposed on the benign, intracortical, fibro-osseous radiographic picture can be a clue to adamantino-matous change, but commonly turn out to be filled with more cellular and actively proliferating cortical fibrous dysplasia.

The histogenesis of adamantinoma remains contro-versial. The name reflects the original theory of ectopic oral enamel anlage in the tibia. The tendency for adamantinoma cell nests to link up with vascular channels is counterbalanced by highly differentiated keratinizing squamous epithelium in the exceptional case. Electron microscopic studies have alternately favored epithelial origin and an angioblastic nature. Histochemical evidence of a vascular genesis (Chan-gus et al., 1957) has been countered by immunope-roxidase evidence: lack of Factor VIII–related antigen and presence of cytokeratin in the usual case. How-ever, the soft tissue tumor, epithelioid sarcoma, often has cytokeratin, and synovial sarcomas may show keratinizing squamous epithelium, yet no one postu-lates an epithelial origin for these mesenchymal tu-mors. Tumors differentiate toward recognizable char-acteristics of normal tissue; it is an unwarranted assumption that such characteristics necessarily inform us of the "cell of origin." Adamantinoma may be a biphasic neoplasm capable of differentiating along both mesenchymal and epithelial lines (Weiss and Dorfman, 1977).

Systemic Anomalies of Growth and Develop-ment. The most common diseases in this category can be arranged under three deficiencies: cartilage model substance for enchondral ossification— achon-droplasia; osteoid production—osteogenesis imper-fecta; and remodeling—osteopetrosis.

Of the above, only osteogenesis imperfecta has been implicated as a source for secondary sarcoma. It is the mild and "tarda" cases of osteogenesis imperfecta that survive infancy whose delicate bones are at increased risk of fracture. Trauma seems, on occasion, able to overcome the genetic compromise of osteoid production, and the resultant hypertrophic callus can simulate osteosarcoma (Fig. 22–29). Rare instances of true sarcoma with metastases are on record (Klenerman, 1967) (Fig. 22–30). For these and other sarcomas in this category of disease, the very low incidence makes it difficult to exclude coin-cidental occurrence.

Benign Neoplasms

Osteoblastoma

It has become apparent that not all osteoblastomas are benign. Rarely, a lesion originally diagnosed as a benign osteoblastoma may, over a period of years, transform into a metastasizing tumor. Several local

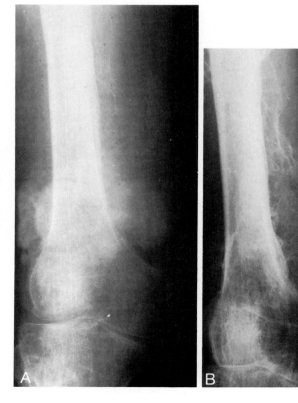

Figure 22–29. Osteogenesis imperfecta tarda with fracture and hypertrophic callus. *A 33 year old man with known osteogenesis imperfecta. A,* Lobular os-sific densities mimicking extraosseous extension of osteosarcoma surround a transverse pathologic frac-ture of the distal femur. *B,* A follow-up film taken 4.5 years after *A* indicates maturation of the callus into trabecular bone, proving its reactive nature (Coe-negracht, et al. 1958).

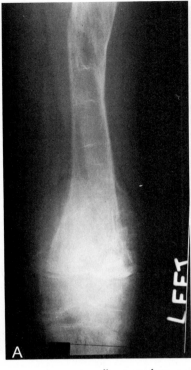
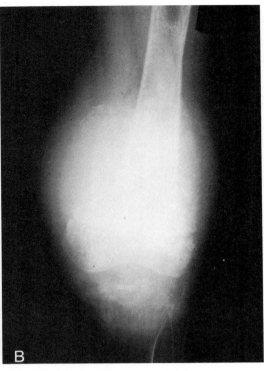

Figure 22–30. Osteogenesis imperfecta tarda with osteosarcoma. *A child known to have osteogenesis imperfecta developed distal thigh pain and swelling and eventual pulmonary metastases. A,* An initial film shows a radiodense endosteal metaphyseal process that extends out into the lateral soft tissues, creating a sunburst periosteal pattern and proximally situated Codman angles typical of osteosarcoma. *B,* A follow-up film taken 2.5 months after *A* indicates progressive enlargement and the destruction expected with malignancy.

recurrences usually antedate metastases. Radiotherapy seems to increase the chance of malignant change.

Locally aggressive osteoblastic tumors have been placed in four categories by Dorfman and Weiss (1984): (1) low-grade osteosarcomas that resemble osteoblastoma histologically, (2) rare osteoblastomas that undergo spontaneous transformation into osteosarcoma, (3) very rare osteoblastomas with "pseudosarcomatous histologic features" but a benign clinical course, and (4) (locally) aggressive osteoblastomas.

Group 1 lesions are osteosarcomas with trabeculated areas mimicking osteoblastoma. Radiographic review helps avoid this pitfall of histologically underestimating the tumor's malignant potential. Group 2 accommodates osteoblastomas that, after an interval of time and usually recurrence, or after radiotherapy, pursue a malignant course confirmed by metastasis. Group 3 lacks the cellularity, abnormal mitotic activity, and disorganized osteoid production of osteosarcoma; the extreme atypism is ascribed to "degenerative changes." Group 4 tumors are distinguished by epithelioid osteoblasts at least twice the size of ordinary tumor osteoblasts. These are equated with the "malignant osteoblastomas" of Schajowicz and Limos (1976).

Giant Cell Tumor

Beyond the three "types" of giant cell tumor (benign, active, and malignant), there are instances of apparent "malignant" transformation of the benign variety with (Fig. 22–31) or without (Fig. 22–32) prior radiotherapy. Some preponderantly "active" tumors

can have a few histologic foci consistent with early malignant change, completing a spectrum leading to those with substantial areas of overt malignancy. Local recurrence is a problem common to all three histologic subtypes.

Because radiation therapy appears to increase the risk of malignant transformation of benign giant cell tumors, its use should be discouraged for surgically approachable lesions. Biopsy-proven metastasizing giant cell tumors are extremely rare, probably under 1 percent. Cases where lung colonization preceded some form of surgery on the bone lesion are even rarer. This favors the view that at least in some cases spread to the lung is "passive," that is, by venous transportation of small bits of surgical debris. Tumor grade has been widely discredited as a reilable indicator of malignant potential. In part, this is because of the rare benign giant cell tumors that have given rise to one or a very few small pulmonary nodules. The tendency for the latter pulmonary nodules to remain small in size and to decrease in cellularlity while ossifying further separates this rare group from the standard concept of malignancy and salvages the general utility of histologic grade in prognostication.

Involutional changes, including the organization that follows focal infarction within giant cell tumors, tend to be followed by fibroblastic proliferation (often with a storiform pattern as dictated by the capillary arrangement) and xanthoma cell modulation. This gives rise to giant cell tumor "variants" with focal histologic similarity to fibroxanthoma (non-ossifying fibroma). Misdiagnosis is avoided by consulting the radiographs, which show giant cell tumors to be positioned toward the end of the bone and fibroxanthomas, which can

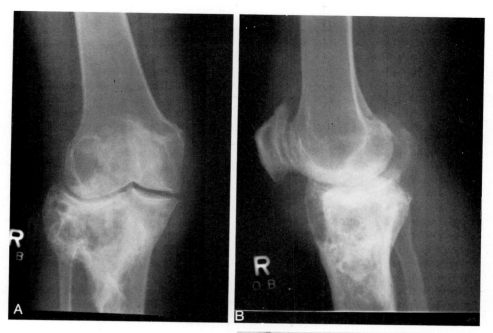

Figure 22–31. Sarcoma following radiation of a benign giant cell tumor. *Twenty years previously, a 45 year old woman had refused amputation for a locally recurrent benign giant cell tumor in the proximal tibia evident 2 years after primary curettage. Therefore, repeat curettage and radiotherapy were employed. One and one half years before radiographs A and B, the patellar tendon was avulsed at its tibial attachment and reattached without clinical suspicion of malignancy. More recently, two operations were performed for pain and swelling believed to be infection. Tissue samples established the presence of malignancy, and amputation was performed.*

A and *B*, Anteroposterior and lateral radiographs show old distortion of the tibial outline and a rim of irregular sclerosis (radiation osteitis) around central patches of lucency. *C*, An anteroposterior whole mount section of the amputation specimen displays the irregular trabecular arrangement and thickness in the midzone, correlating with the coarse sclerosis in the clinical films. Toward the proximal end of the bone is a hematoma-filled chamber from which malignant tissue had been evacuated during biopsy. An anterior soft tissue extension occurs at the upper right. *D*, This postradiation sarcoma presents extreme pleomorphism that, without the history, might bring to mind metastatic carcinoma. *E*, Bordering the tumor lucencies are areas of marrow fibrosis and coarse-textured osteoid (radiation osteitis); presumably the sarcoma arose from areas of relative ischemia like this.

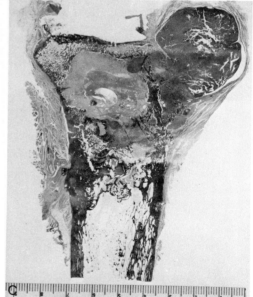

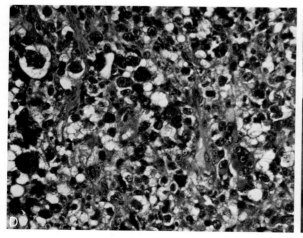

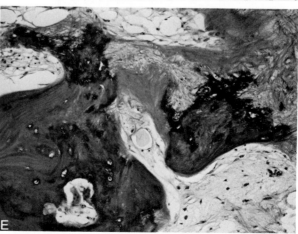

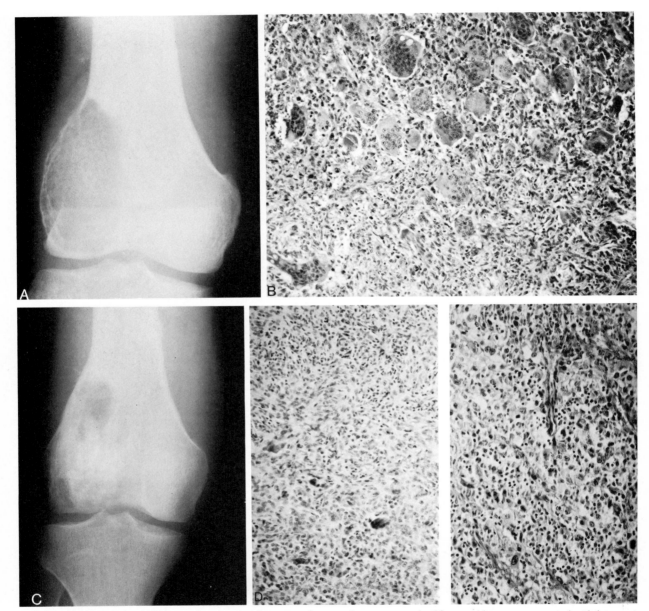

Figure 22–32. Benign giant cell tumor that recurs with sarcoma 9 years after curettage. *An 18 year old woman presented with knee pain.* A, The initial radiograph reveals an eccentric lucent lesion extending to the subchondral plate, with a lobulated periosteal shell replacing most of the lateral femoral condyle. B, "Excisional curettage" produced a benign giant cell tumor pattern. C, Nine years after curettage, a 5 month history of pain and swelling led to this radiograph showing a prominent lucent area at the proximal end of the prior surgical field. The density in the remainder of the old operative site represents bone graft. D, Tissue from the lytic area in C features active giant cell tumor histology (left) but also cellular pleomorphic sarcoma. The concurrence of these two patterns and the antecedent benign lesion establish a direct relationship rather than the possibility of a sarcoma arising in relation to incompletely incorporated bone graft material analogous to an infarct sarcoma. *Amputation was performed after 7020 rads of preoperative radiotherapy.*

be rich in giant cells, to be eccentrically situated in the metaphysis nearer the shaft. The notion of fibroxanthomatous changes in giant cell tumors nearly went out of existence following Jaffe and Lichtenstein's (1942) publication on "nonossifying fibroma" (fibroxanthoma) as their designation for cases previously regarded as "xanthic" (Ewing, 1942), "fibrous," or "healing" (Kolodny, 1927) variants of giant cell tumor. We agree with Ewing (1926) that giant cell tumors with fibroxanthomatous areas can be unusually aggressive, are more likely to recur, and are probably at increased risk for secondary change into a malignant fibroxanthomatous pattern.

"MULTICENTRIC" TUMORS

Two or more sites in the skeleton may be involved by tumor. Such occurrence may be divided into the following categories:

1. Synchronous versus metachronous involvement.

2. Synchronous versus dissimilar lesions: It should never be assumed that an adequate sample from one of several bone lesions accurately represents the histologic composition of all. A case radiographically resembling polyostotic fibrous dysplasia may actually be fibrous dysplasia in one bone and a bone cyst in another. Multiple fibroxanthomas suggest the wisdom of excluding coexistent neurofibromatosis, the cutaneous stigmata of which may not yet be fully expressed.

3. Anomaly versus neoplasm: Enchondromatosis may be considered a proliferative aberration of growth plate activity. Angiomatosis may have developmental origins with later hemodynamic inflation of the latent abnormal vascular beds, rendering them symptomatic and/or radiographically apparent.

4. "Multicentric" primary bone tumors versus bone-to-bone metastases.

Giant Cell Tumors. The problem of multiple synchronous benign giant cell tumors is in need of clarification.

Osteosarcoma

Osteosarcomatosis. In every case known to the authors, even those reported in literature as osteosarcomatosis of the "multiple synchronous" or "juve-

Table 22–1. **Representative Transitions by Disease Category**

Category	Benign	In-situ sarcoma or substratum for malignancy	Malignant
TRAUMA AND REPAIR	Radiation osteitis ⟶ Metallic prostheses ⟶	atypical cellular foci ⟶ hypocellular fibrous sheath ⟶	Postradiation sarcoma Sarcoma
INFLAMMATORY	Osteomyelitis ⟶	sinus tract atypicality ⟶ medullary cicatrix ⟶	Carcinoma Sarcoma
CIRCULATORY	Bone infarct ⟶ Paget's disease ⟶	reactive interface ⟶ cellular hyperactivity ⟶	Sarcoma Paget sarcoma
ANOMALY	Osteochondroma ⟶ Enchondroma ⟶ Fibrous dysplasia ⟶ Fibroxanthoma ⟶ Lipoma ⟶ Polymorphic fibrocystic disease (LSMFT) ⟶ Cyst ⟶ Hemangioma ⟶ Cortical fibrous dysplasia ⟶	ischemic changes in stalk thick cap ⟶ active enchondroma ⟶ atypical enchondral ossification at margin ⟶ ? ⟶ progressive atypism ⟶ ischemic desmoplasia ⟶ progressive atypism ⟶ ? ⟶ angioendothelioma ⟶ focal adamantinoma pattern ⟶	High grade sarcoma Chondrosarcoma High grade sarcoma Sarcoma Malignant fibroxanthoma Sarcoma Malignant fibroxanthoma Sarcoma Angiosarcoma Adamantinoma
NEOPLASIA	Osteoblastoma ⟶ Giant cell tumor ⟶	aggressive osteoblastoma ⟶ stromal cell atypism ⟶ plump atypical spindle cell zones ⟶	Osteosarcoma Malignant giant cell tumor Sarcoma

nile" type, one of the skeletal lesions has appeared more advanced, having the radiographic features of a primary bone sarcoma. We believe such cases represent multiple osseous metastases rather than true synchronous multicentric malignant change. The preferential localization of circulating tumor cells is understandable by field concepts: osteoblastic activity is normally dominant in metaphyseal segments and these "favored fields" are selectively colonized.

"Skip" Lesions. Discontinuous foci of sarcoma within the same bone or in multiple bones of one extremity also favors metastatic dissemination. These are rare.

Sarcomas Associated with Paget's Disease

We believe the so-called "multicentric malignant change" in Paget's disease represents polyostotic metastases from an original solitary Paget sarcoma. The presence of several advanced lesions at presentation is understandable in view of the virulence of these tumors and their metastatic localization in other pagetic bones being favored by increased vascularity.

Vascular Tumors

Angiosarcoma, with or without coexistent angioma and angioendothelioma components, is distinguished by the ability to present as multiple synchronous or rapidly metachronous lesions in a single extremity. Immunoperoxidase studies are of great help in separating this unusual syndrome from metastatic carcinoma, especially from the kidney.

Plasma Cell Dyscrasias

Multiple Myeloma. Monotypic immunoprotein synthesis implies rapid widespread dissemination from an original site of malignant mutation. The origin of this malignant process in well-vascularized marrow and the facility with which hematopoietic elements cross endothelial membranes explains rapid colonization of the skeleton.

Plasmacytoma. Most solitary plasma cell tumors eventually disseminate after the fashion of multiple myeloma. In some cases, a series of isolated well-circumscribed lesions appear over a period of many years.

CONCLUSION

Ideas of tumor origin must take into account radiographic sequences. With the passage of time, the histology of benign bone lesions can change (Table 22–1, page 421). The substratum of malignancy in benign bone lesions includes proliferating anomalous and dysplastic tissue, chronically accelerated cell turnover secondary to necrosis or injured tissue, hypocellular desmoplasia, and cystification.

References

Aegerter, E., Kirkpatrick, J. A.: Orthopedic Diseases, 2nd ed. Philadelphia, W. B. Saunders Co., 1964.

Alguacil-Garcia, A., Alonso, A., Pettigrew, N. M.: Case Reports. Osteofibrous dysplasia (ossifying fibroma) of the tibia and fibula and adamantinoma. Am. J. Clin. Pathol. 82:470–474, 1984.

Baker, P. L., Dockerty, M. B., Coventry, M. D.: Adamantinomas(so called) of the long bones. J. Bone Joint Surg. 36:704–720, 1954.

Bhagwandeen, S. B.: Malignant transformation of a non-osteogenic fibroma of bone. J. Pathol. Bacteriol. 92:562–564, 1966.

Biesecker, J. L., Marcove, R. C., Huvos, A. G., Mike, V.: Aneurysmal bone cysts. A clinicopathologic study of 66 cases. Cancer 26:615–625, 1970.

Campanacci, M., Laus, M.: Osteofibrous dysplasia of the tibia and fibula. J. Bone Joint Surg. 63A:367–375, 1981.

Chan, R. C., Sutow, W. W., Lindberg, R. D., Samuels, M. L., Murray, J. A., Johnston, D. A.: Management and results of localized Ewing's sarcoma. Cancer 43:1001–1006, 1979.

Changus, G. W., Speed, J. S., Stewart, F. W.: Malignant angioblastoma of bone; A reappraisal of adamantinoma of long bone. Cancer 10:540–559, 1957.

Codman, E. A.: In discussion of Bone Sarcoma Registry Case #185, AFIP Accession Number 600185, 1924.

Codman, E. A.: The nomenclature used by the Registry of Bone Sarcoma. Am. J. Roentgen. Rad. Ther. 13:105–126, 1925.

Coenegracht, D. J., et al.: Diafysaire aclasie, gecombineered met fragilitas ossium. Ned. T. Geneesk 102:II. 29, 1398, 1958.

Dorfman, H. D.: Malignant transformation of benign bone lesions, Seventh National Cancer Conference. Philadelphia, J. B. Lippincott, 1973, pp. 901–913.

Dorman, H. D., Weiss, S. W.: Borderline osteoblastic tumors: Problems in the differential diagnosis of aggressive osteoblastoma and low-grade osteosarcoma. Sem. Diag. Path. 1:215–234, 1984.

Ewing, J. A.: A review and classification of bone sarcomas. Arch. Surg. 4:485–533, 1922.

Ewing, J. A.: The classification and treatment of bone sarcoma. In Report of International Conference on Cancer. Bristol, John Wright and Sons, 1926.

Ewing, J. A.: Neoplastic Diseases, 4th ed. Philadelphia, W. B. Saunders Co., 1942.

Fraumeni, J. F., Jr.: Bone cancer: Epidemiologic and etiologic considerations. Front. Radiat. Ther. Oncol. 10:17–27, 1975.

Garrison, R. C., Unni, K. K., McLeod, R. A., Pritchard, D. J., Dahlin, D. C.: Chondrosarcoma arising in osteochondroma. Cancer 49:1890–1897, 1982.

Goergen, T. G., Dickman, P. S., Resnick, D., Saltzstein, S. L., O'Dell, C. W., Akeson, W. H.: Long bone ossifying fibromas. Cancer 39:2067–2072, 1977.

Hutter, R. V. P., Foote, F. W., Jr., Francis, K. C., Sherman, R. S.: Primitive multipotential primary sarcoma of bone. Cancer 19:1–25, 1966.

Huvos, A. G., Higinbotham, N. L., Miller, T. R.: Bone sarcomas arising in fibrous dysplasia. J. Bone Joint Surg. 54A:1047–1056, 1972.

Huvos, A. G., Butler, A., Bretsky, S. S.: Osteogenic sarcoma associated with Paget's disease of bone. Cancer 52:1489–1495, 1983.

Jaffe, H. L.: Fibrous dysplasia of bone. Bull. N.Y. Acad. Med. 22:588–604, 1946.

Jaffe, H. L.: Tumors and Tumorous Conditions of the Bones and Joints. Philadelphia, Lea and Febiger, 1958. (1974 reprinting)

Jaffe, H. L.: In discussion of Donaldson, W. F.: Aneurysmal bone cyst. J. Bone Joint Surg. 44A: 25–39, 1962.

Jaffe, H. L.: Metabolic Degenerative, and Inflammatory Diseases of Bones and Joints, Philadelphia, Lea and Febiger, 1972.

Jaffe, H. L., Lichtenstein, L.: Non-osteogenic fibroma of bone. Am. J. Pathol. 18:205–221, 1942.

Johnson, L. C.: A general theory of bone tumors. Bull. N.Y. Acad. Med. 29:164–174, 1953.

Johnson, L. C.: Congenital pseudoarthrosis, adamantinoma of long bone and intracortical fibrous dysplasia of the tibia (Abstr.). J. Bone Joint Surg. 54A: 1355, 1972.

Johnson, L. C., Kindred, R. G.: The anatomy of bone cysts (Abstr.). J. Bone Joint Surg. 40A:1440, 1958.

Johnson, L. C., Putschar, W. G. J.: Sarcomas arising in bone cysts. Virchows Arch. Pathol. Anat. 335:428–451, 1962.

Kempson, R. L.: Ossifying fibroma of the long bones. Arch. Pathol. 82:218–233, 1966.

Klenerman, L., Ockenden, B. G., Townsend, A. C.: Osteosarcoma occurring in osteogenesis imperfecta. Report of two cases. J. Bone Joint Surg. 49B:314–323, 1967.

Kolodny, A.: Bone sarcoma. The primary malignant tumors of bone and the giant cell tumor. Surg. Gynecol Obstet. 44 (Suppl.I):1–214, 1927.

Lichtenstein, L.: Polyostotic fibrous dysplasia. Arch. Surg. 36:874–898, 1938.

Lichtenstein, L.: Bone Tumors, 5th Edition. St. Louis, C. V. Mosby Co., 1977.

Lichtenstein, L., Jaffe, H. L.: Fibrous dysplasia of bone. Arch. Pathol. 33:777–816, 1942.

Lichtenstein, L., Jaffe, H. L.: Chondrosarcoma of bone. Am. J. Pathol. 19:553–589, 1943.

Madewell, J. E., Ragsdale, B. D., Sweet, D. E.: Radiologic and pathologic analysis of solitary bone lesions. Part I: Internal margins. Radiol. Clin. N. Amer. 19:715–748, 1981.

Markel, S. F.: Ossifying fibroma of long bone: Its distinction from fibrous dysplasia and its association with adamantinoma of long bone. Am. J. Clin. Pathol. 69:91–97, 1978.

Merkow, L. P., Frich, J. C., Jr., Slifkin, M., Kyreages, C. G., Pardo, M. Ultrastructure of a fibroxanthosarcoma (malignant fibroxanthoma). Cancer 28:372, 1971.

Mirra, J. M., Marcove, R. C.: Fibrosarcomatous dedifferentiation of primary and secondary chondrosarcoma. Review of five cases. J. Bone Joint Surg. 56A:285–296, 1974.

Montgomery, A. H.: Ossifying fibromas of the jaw. Arch. Surg. 15:30–44, 1927.

Newland, R. C., Harrison, M. A., Wright, R. G.: Fibroxanthosarcoma of bone. Pathology 7:203–208, 1975.

O'Brien, J. E., Stout, A. P.: Malignant fibrous xanthomas, Cancer 17:1445–1455, 1964.

Olmi, R., Rubbini, L.: Hemangiosarcoma developing in a chronic osteomyelitis of the tibia. Chir. Organi Mov. 61:765–768, 1975.

Otis, J., Hutter, R. V. P., Foote, F. W., Jr., Marcove, R. C., and Steward, F. W.: Hemangioendothelioma of bone. Surg. Gynecol. Obstet. 127:295–305, 1968.

Ozzello, L., Stout, A. P., Murray, M. R.: Cultural characteristics of malignant histiocytomas and fibrous xanthomas. Cancer 16:331–334, 1963.

Phemister, D. B.: Chondrosarcoma of bone. Surg. Gynecol. Obstet. 50:216–233, 1930.

Price, C. H. G., Goldie, W.: Paget's sarcoma of bone. J. Bone Joint Surg. 51B:205–224, 1969.

Pritchard, D. J. Lunke, R. J., Taylor, W. F.: Chondrosarcoma: A clinicopathologic and statistical analysis. Cancer 45:149–157, 1980.

Pulford, D. S., Jr.: Neoplasms of blood-lymph-vascular system with special relevance to endotheliomas. Ann. Surg. 82:710–727, 1925.

Ragsdale, B. D.: Case for diagnosis: Squamous cell carcinoma arising from a gunshot fracture. Milit. Med. 148:553–556, 1983.

Ragsdale, B. D., Madewell, J. E., Sweet, D. E.: Radiologic and pathologic analysis of solitary bone lesions. Part II: Periosteal reactions. Radiol Clin. N. Amer. 19:749–784, 1981.

Reed, R. J.: Fibrous dysplasia of bone. A review of 25 cases. Arch. Pathol. 75:480–495, 1963.

Schajowicz, F., Limos, C.: Malignant osteoblastoma. J. Bone Surg. 58B:202–211, 1976.

Schoenecker, P. L., Swanson, K., Sheridan, J. J.: Ossifying fibroma of the tibia. J. Bone Joint Surg. 63A:483–488, 1981.

Spjut, H. J., Dorfman, H. D., Fechner, R. E., et al.: Tumors of bone and cartilage. *In:* Atlas of Tumor Pathology, Fascicle 5, Second Series, Washington, D.C., Armed Forces Institute of Pathology, 1971.

Spjut, H. J., Fechner, R. E., Ackerman, L. V., Tumors of Bone and Cartilage. *In* Atlas of Tumor Pathology, Supplement to Fascicle 5, Second Series. Washington, D.C., Armed Forces Institute of Pathology, 1981.

Stout, A. P., Lattes, R.: Tumors of soft tissue. *In* Atlas of Tumor Pathology, Series 2. Washington, D.C., Armed Forces Institute of Pathology, 1967, pp. 38–52.

Sweet, D. E., Madewell, J. E., Ragsdale, B. D.: Radiologic and pathologic analysis of solitary bone lesions. Part III: Matrix patterns. Radiol. Clin. N. Amer. 19:785–814, 1981.

Tang, T. T., Zuege, R. C., Babbit, D. P., Blount, W. P., McCreadie, S. R.: Angioglomoid tumor of bone. J. Bone Joint Surg. 58:873–876, 1976.

Thompson, P. C.: Subperiosteal giant cell tumor. Ossifying subperiosteal hematoma—aneurysmal bone cyst. J. Bone Joint Surg. 36A:281–306, 1954.

Tillman, B. P., Dahlin, D. C., Lipscomb, P. R., Stewart, J. R.: Aneurysmal bone cyst: an analysis of ninety-five cases. Mayo Clin. Proc. 43:478–495, 1968.

Unni, K. K., Dahlin, D. C.: Premalignant tumors and conditions of bone. Am. J. Surg. Pathol., 3:47–60, 1979.

Unni, K. K., Ivins, J. C., Beabout, J. W., Dahlin, D. C.: Hemangioma, hemangiopericytoma, and hemangioendothelioma (angiosarcoma) of bone. Cancer 27:1403–1414, 1971.

Volp, R., Mazabrand, A.: Hemangioendothelioma (angiosarcoma) of bone: A distinctive pathologic entity with a predictable course? Cancer 49:727–736, 1982.

Weiss, S. W., Dorfman, H. D.: Adamantinoma of long bone. An analysis of nine new cases with emphasis on metastasizing lesions and fibrous dysplasia-like changes. Human Pathol. 8:141–153, 1977.

Yamamoto, T., Wakabayshi, T.: Bone tumors among the atomic bomb survivors of Hiroshima and Nagasaki. Acta Pathol. Jpn. 19:201–212, 1969.

PHILIP M. GRIMLEY
RONALD A. DeLELLIS

23 Multisystem Neuroendocrine Neoplasms

INTRODUCTION

The capacity of neoplasms to synthesize and secrete a variety of pharmacologically active peptides and other products has been recognized increasingly during the past three decades (Law et al., 1965; Odell and Wolfson, 1980; Oberg et al., 1982). At the same time, the ability of pathologists to define and classify such neoplasms has been amplified by successive advances in cytochemistry, electron microscopy, immunohistochemistry and molecular biology. As a result, new pathobiologic concepts and tumor groupings are emerging.

In this chapter we discuss groups of neoplasms which express "neuroendocrine" features. These neoplasms arise from phenotypically defined groups of normal cells or their progenitors in visceral organs or the peripheral nervous system. Despite diverse origins and anatomic sites of development, they nevertheless express biosynthetic functions characteristic both of neurons in the central nervous system and of classic endocrine cells. Hence, the blend-word "neuroendocrine" empirically describes these combined features.

The histopathologic manifestations of neuroendocrine cell proliferations include benign and preneoplastic hyperplasias, benign neoplasms, locally invasive neoplasms, and neoplasms with low or high metastatic potential. While some proliferations exhibit well-established familial patterns, most occur sporadically or show inconsistent familial patterns. In the present context of "incipient neoplasia," attention is directed to those neuroendocrine neoplasms which are often multicentric or which may involve multiple tissue systems with significant frequency. The latter may be preceded by proliferative stages that declare their presence symptomatically or biochemically and offer unique opportunities for early diagnosis and therapeutic intervention.

Operational Definition of Neuroendocrine Phenotype

The groups of cells exhibiting a common neuroendocrine phenotype or program (NE cells) are anatomically dispersed and histogenetically diversified. Operationally, they are defined as an interrelated entity on the basis of shared cytologic, biosynthetic, histochemical, and neuroregulatory characteristics (Pearse, 1969; Glenner and Grimley, 1974; Tischler et al., 1977; Polak and Bloom, 1979; DeLellis and Wolfe, 1981; Kissel et al., 1981). These common features and widespread distribution led to their description as a "diffuse (or dispersed) neuroendocrine system" (Polak and Bloom, 1979; DeLellis and Wolfe, 1981).

Groups of dispersed NE cells often are allied closely with autonomic nerve fibers or ganglia; and NE cells of the extra-adrenal paraganglia and other sites such as the anterior pituitary may be supported by glial, Schwann-like elements ("sustentacular" or "satellite" cells) (Grimley and Glenner, 1967, Blaivas et al., 1985). Like the terminals of autonomic nerves, many NE cells engage in amine precursor uptake and decarboxylation. This physiochemical characteristic led to the acronym "APUD" and generated Pearse's concept of an extended "APUD" system (Pearse, 1977; Pearse and Polak, 1978).

The biosynthetic products of NE cells include monoamines, regulatory peptides, and a host of common enzymes, structural proteins, and other substances:

1. The secretory products of NE cells are stored within relatively homogeneous cytoplasmic granules

---

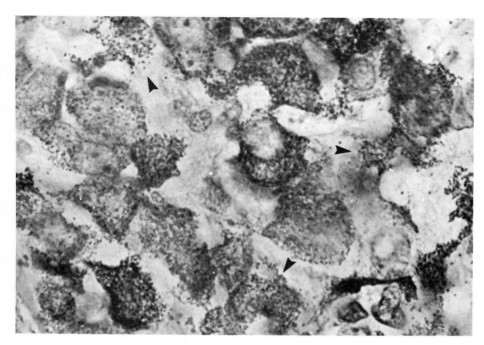

Figure 23–1. Paraffin section showing Grimelius silver reaction in NE cells of a paraganglioma. Numerous intensely stained granules are evident (arrowheads). ×1000.

of a size range near the limits of conventional light microscopic resolution (0.5–2 μM). These granules are highlighted by nonspecific argyrophil or argentaffin reactions with silver stains (Sevier and Munger, 1965; Grimelius, 1968) (Fig. 23–1). Ultrastructurally, the neurosecretory granules are membrane-delimited and their cores are electron-dense in osmicated tissues (Fig. 23–2). The latter is due to internal concentration of amines and associated nucleotides. The nucleotides also react intensely with uranyl ions (Richards and Da Prada, 1977; Payne et al., 1984).

2. The granule matrix contains a large proportion of acid-soluble proteins identified as *chromogranins* (O'Connor et al., 1983). These can be identified immunocytochemically with polyclonal or monoclonal antibodies (O'Connor et al., 1983; DeStephano et al., 1984; Wilson and Lloyd, 1984).

3. Neuroendocrine cells synthesize, store, and secrete monoamines and/or regulatory peptides (Table 23–1). Functions and structures of these molecules overlap those of neurohumoral mediators found in

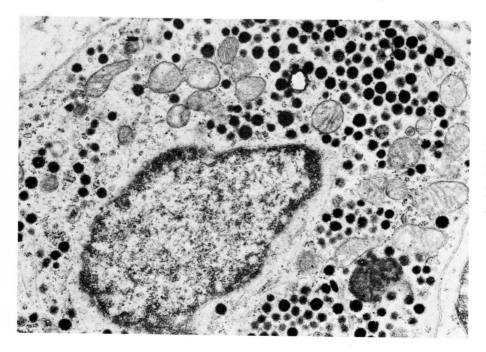

Figure 23–2. Ultrathin section of a paraganglion cell illustrating the abundant, relatively uniform, electron-dense cytoplasmic granules observed by electron microscopy. These are characteristic of the NE cell phenotype. ×26,000.

Table 23–1. Selected Examples of Some Biosynthetic Products Found in Multiple Groups of Neuroendocrine Cells

Monoamines
Epinephrine
Norepinephrine
Dopamine
Serotonin

Regulatory Peptides
Adrenocorticotropin (ACTH)
Calcitonin
Somatostatin
Vasoactive intestinal peptide (VIP)
Gastrin-releasing peptide (GRP)
Pancreatic polypeptide (PP)
Opiate peptides (encephalins)

Enzymes/Structural Proteins
Neuron-specific enolase (NSE)
Chromogranin A
Leu 7 membrane antigen
DOPA—decarboxylase
Histaminase
A2B5 antigen/tetanus toxin binding sites
Neurofilament and cytokeratin proteins

the central nervous system (Tischler et al., 1977; Snyder, 1980; Roth et al., 1982; DeLellis et al., in press). Distribution of the mediators is not anatomically compartmentalized and the same products may be identified in cells of different tissues and of separate embryologic origins: regulatory peptides such as vasoactive intestinal peptide (VIP), somatostatin, or a bombesin-like gastrin-releasing peptide (GRP) are detected in NE cells of the respiratory, gastrointestinal, or genitourinary tracts. Moreover, individual NE cells can produce multiple different peptides together with monoamines.

4. The biosynthesis of NE cell products is highly complex and subject to considerable microenvironmental influence. NE cells may produce multiple peptides derived from common biosynthetic precursors. For example, adrenocorticotropin (ACTH) is synthesized from a larger precursor, pro-opiomelanocortin (POMC) (Krieger, 1984). In the pituitary *pars anterior*, POMC is processed predominantly to a 16K N-terminal fragment, ACTH, and β-lipotropin. In the *pars intermedia*, ACTH and β-lipotropin are processed to yield α-MSH and β-endorphin related peptides, respectively. Another example is the recent work which demonstrated that alternative processing of RNA transcribed from the gene for calcitonin produced a related peptide (CGRP) and calcitonin (Rosenfeld et al., 1983). The CGRP is thought to function in nociception, ingestive behavior, and autonomic or endocrine gland modulation. Multiple genes may encode for identical or highly related neuroendocrine cell products; in pancreatic islet cells of fish, recombinant DNA techniques revealed two different messages for somatostatin. Finally, NE cells can be shown to synthesize similar or even identical products from

different biosynthetic precursors (Goldstein et al., 1979; Lewis et al., 1980).

5. The individual molecules synthesized by NE cells can exert multiple pharmacologic actions. They can act systemically (endocrine function) or locally on adjacent NE cells (paracrine function). Thus, they can influence hormonal secretory activity, microcirculatory dynamics, and other autonomic activities (Polak and Bloom, 1979; Snyder, 1980). The NE cell secretions also can modulate biosynthesis by adjacent NE cells (Larsson et al., 1979). Paracrine interactions of monoamines may explain how some groups of NE cells became uniquely specialized for chemoreception (Krammer, 1978). Stimulatory effects of NE cell regulatory peptides on cell division (Hanley, 1985) or of NE cell monoamines in the targeting of neurite growth (Scott et al., 1981; Stahlman and Gray, 1984; Meinertzhagen, 1985) have recently been suggested.

6. Many NE cells contain high levels of enolase with a gamma subunit characteristic of neural tissues (Schmechel, 1985). The enolase isoenzymes are products of three independent gene loci: alpha, beta, and gamma. The gamma gene is expressed almost exclusively by brain and neuroendocrine cells (Lloyd and Warner, 1984). This "neuron specific" enolase is present within the cytoplasmic compartment of NE cells and can be detected by monoclonal antibodies (Lloyd and Warner, 1984). Other monoclonal antibodies have been shown to react with plasma membrane constituents of NE cells. The monoclonal antibody A2B5 reacts with a ganglioside in the membranes of neurons, astrocytes, adrenal medullary cells, pheochromocytoma cells, and medullary thyroid carcinoma cells (Eisenbarth et al., 1982; Schnitzer and Schachner, 1982). Monoclonal antibody produced against a membrane immunogen of human lymphoblastoid cells and found in a subpopulation of natural killer lymphocytes (Leu 7) cross-reacts with plasma membrane antigens in myelin, NE cells, and cells of some neoplasms of NE phenotype (McGarry et al., 1983; Lipinski et al., 1983; Bunn et al., 1985). Recently, this antibody also was found to react with a constituent of the secretory granule matrix in normal and neoplastic adrenal medullary cells and other NE cell types (Adelman et al., 1985).

Ontogenetically, NE cells have been demonstrated to arise from neuroectoderm or gut-endoderm in embryologic experiments (Pearse and Polak, 1974; Andrew, 1976; Pictet et al., 1976; Sidhu, 1979). Moreover, they are also found in certain tumors of probable mesodermal derivation involving the female genital tract (Scully et al., 1984). The stable expression of an NE phenotype in disseminated cell populations of plural embryogenesis can be explained by convergent evolution (Roth et al., 1982). Cells with homologous biosynthetic and neuroregulatory capacities occur in invertebrates, so that phylogenetic recombinations and independent resorting of conserved genetic elements (Gilbert, 1985) could explain the homologies of regulatory peptide or monoamine synthesis in multiple vertebrate cell populations.

In summary, disseminated groups of cells of diverse origins exhibit an NE phenotype. They are biologically programmed to express a comparable spectrum of their genomic information. The range and level of biosynthetic expression in individual NE cells or groups of cells is variable and contributes to their physiologic diversity and functional adaptability. This, combined with topographic dispersion, evidently amplifies the ability of NE cells to help maintain nervous, vascular, and glandular homeostasis.

Neoplastic Expression of NE Phenotype

Well-differentiated neoplasms expressing NE phenotypic characteristics arise from NE cells or their precursors (Glenner and Grimley, 1974; Pearse and Polak, 1974; DeLellis and Wolfe, 1981; DeLellis et al., in press). Cells that are related by virtue of their neuroendocrine program can nevertheless differentiate from progenitors arising in any of the classic germ layers. Thus, cytologic, biosynthetic, or functional expression of a neuroendocrine phenotype in neoplasms may reflect only one aspect of a multipotent developmental capacity in otherwise unrelated stem lines. These neoplasms can secrete multiple, functionally active regulatory peptides (Baylin et al., 1970; White and Hickson, 1979; Olsen et al., 1982) or synthesize multiple substances with the immunoreactivity of NE cell regulatory peptides (Mukai et al., 1982; Hassoun et al., 1982) (Table 23–2).

Differentiated neoplasms of NE cell phenotype often are multicentric. They can be distributed widely in many tissues or organ sites, and complexes of frequently associated tumors may exhibit familial patterns (Ballard et al., 1964; Steiner et al., 1968; Kissel

Table 23–2. **Selected Examples of Immunoreactive Peptides Shared by Multiple Neuroendocrine Neoplasms**

Examples of Shared Peptides (recent references)
ACTH (Apple and Kreines, 1982; Gould et al., 1983; Grizzle et al., 1983)
Calcitonin (Hassoun et al., 1984; White and Hickson, 1979)
Somatostatin (Gould et al., 1983; Hassoun et al., 1984; Saito et al., 1982)
Vasoactive intestinal peptide (Gould et al., 1983; Mukai et al., 1982; Said and Faloona, 1975; Tischler et al., 1981)

Multiple Neoplasms Sharing Peptides Listed Above (locations)
Medullary carcinoma (thyroid gland)
Paragangliomas (adrenal medulla, extra-adrenal paraganglia)
Carcinoids (lungs, intestinal tract)
Oat cell carcinomas (lung)
Islet cell adenomas (pancreas)

et al., 1981). The latter are described more completely below. Oncopathologic observations of tumor complexes reinforce the logic for the operational grouping of cells or neoplasms expressing the NE phenotype despite distinct embryogenetic and histogenetic pathways (Hansen, 1976; Marchevsky and Dickman, 1979; Morris and Tymms, 1980; Griffiths et al., 1983).

Clinical Implications of Tumor NE Activity

The clinicopathologic implications of the modern concept of a common NE phenotype are gradually being assessed. Information concerning developmental associations, clinical manifestations, patterns of growth and biological behavior of neoplasms expressing NE functions or biosynthetic activities is an essential prerequisite to developing rational approaches for diagnostic screening, differential diagnosis, appropriate therapies, prognosis, and follow-up. For example, pulmonary small cell neoplasms of NE phenotype (oat-cell carcinomas) exhibit an aggressive metastatic behavior (Greco and Oldham, 1979; Gould et al., 1983) which is quite distinct from the leisurely expansion of neoplasms that arise from the adrenal medulla or extra-adrenal paraganglia (Melicow, 1977; Lack et al., 1979a, 1980).

Clinical presentations of NE cell neoplasms are remarkably variable. The potential for multicentricity and multisystem involvement always must be appreciated. This is most obviously exemplified by repetitive familial patterns in the multiple endocrine neoplasia (MEN) syndromes, but sporadic or familial cases with irregular or mixed patterns of tumors should not be overlooked. The possibility of synchronous or metachronous neoplasms in all such cases should encourage presymptomatic screening and early diagnosis of susceptible individuals. Obviously, these opportunities will increase in proportion to ambient levels of clinical suspicion. In particular, kindred studies in MEN have fostered greater awareness of the benefits of early detection of neuroendocrinologic abnormalities (Steiner et al., 1968; Baylin et al., 1970; Melvin et al., 1971; Gagel et al., 1975; Hamilton et al., 1978; Block et al., 1980).

Catecholamine secreting NE tumors may cause unexpected death as a result of hypertensive paroxysms (Steiner et al., 1968). Many neoplasms of NE cell phenotype are densely vascularized and some are associated intimately with major cardiovascular structures. When uncontrolled, local neoplastic infiltration can be life-threatening or complicate surgical therapy.

TOPOGRAPHIC SUBGROUPS OF NE CELLS

NE cells constitute a topographically diffuse system associated with neurovascular tissues or viscera of the head and neck, thorax, abdomen, retroperitoneum, and pelvis. In general, NE cells in separate anatomic locations would be difficult to distinguish cytologically and they often synthesize the identical or similar regulatory peptides (see Table 23–1). The principal physiologic activities nevertheless vary: for example, NE cells of the head and neck region may be specialized for chemoreception, NE cells of the gut may be involved in paracrine autonomic regulation, and NE cells of the adrenal medullae are active in systemic hormone secretion.

The major topographic subgroups of NE cells are distinguished empirically (Table 23–3) and include at least two germinal lineages: (1) NE cells derived from neuroectodermal or neural crest precursors and (2) NE cells derived from endodermal or mesodermal precursors in the pharyngeal pouches, foregut, bronchopulmonary tract, or genitourinary anlage. Diversity in the ontogeny and histogenesis of NE cell groups in separated anatomic regions may ultimately relate to predominant patterns of the morphology, clinicopathologic manifestations, and genetic associations of derivative neoplasms, but there are many overlapping features.

Paraganglion Cells. These NE cells are associated principally with cervical and mediastinal tissues of ontogenetic gill arch derivation, paravertebral autonomic ganglia, and elements of the visceral-autonomic ortho/parasympathetic nervous systems (Glenner and Grimley, 1974). Paraganglion cells occur as macroscopically cohesive units in the adrenal medullae (intra-adrenal paraganglia) and in major branchiomeric or paravertebral paraganglia (extra-adrenal paraganglia). In the walls of visceral organs, paraganglion cells are more diffusely distributed and typically associated with neural plexi or mural ganglia. They share a lineage from the neural crest in common with ventrally migrating neuroblasts and sympathicoganglioblasts (Glenner and Grimley, 1974). Thus, neoplasms of these several cell types often co-express biosynthetic and immunohistochemical features (Funato et al., 1982; Jaffe, 1982).

Thyroid Gland C Cells. The calcitonin producing C cells are found *within* the thyroid gland and follicles. Most studies have indicated an origin of C cells from the neuroectoderm or neural crest (see Andrew, 1976), but some recent observations suggest the possibilities of endodermal or combined endodermal/neural crest origins (Fernandes et al., 1982). A common association of C cell neoplasia (medullary carcinoma of the thyroid gland) with neoplasia of the intra-adrenal paraganglia (pheochromocytoma) has been interpreted in favor of a neural crest lineage (Pearse and Polak, 1974).

Merkel Cells. Merkel cells are present singly in the basal layer of the epidermis throughout the skin and in epidermal pads in the vicinity of hair follicles and other adnexa (Gould et al., 1985). Individual as well as groups of Merkel cells are intimately associated

Table 23–3. **Major Topographic Subgroups of Neuroendocrine Cells**

Location	NE Cells	Probable Source
Craniopharyngeal region	Anterior hypophysis	Neuroectoderm (neural ridge)*
	Cranial nerve paraganglia	Neural crest
Nasopharynx	Intravagal paraganglia	Neural crest
Cervical region	Branchiomeric paraganglia	Neural crest
	C-cells of thyroid gland	Neural crest
Superior mediastinum	Branchiomeric paraganglia	Neural crest
	Intravagal paraganglia	Neural crest
Anterior mediastinum	Thymic NE cells	Pharyngeal pouch*
Respiratory tract	Branchiomeric paraganglia	Neural crest
	Bronchopulmonary neuroepithelial bodies	Neural crest*
	Bronchopulmonary NE cells	Foregut endoderm*
Posterior mediastinum	Aorticosympathetic paraganglia	Neural crest
Abdominal viscera	Gastrointestinal NE cells	Gut endoderm
	Pancreatic islet cells	Pancreatic ductules
	Visceral-autonomic paraganglia	Neural crest
Retroperitoneum	Adrenal medullae	Neural crest
	Organs of Zuckerkandl	Neural crest
	Aorticosympathetic paraganglia	Neural crest
Genitourinary tract	Bladder intramural paraganglia	Neural crest
	Prostate gland NE cells	Hindgut endoderm*
	Female genital NE cells	Hindgut endoderm* Mesoderm*
Skin	Merkel cells	Neural crest*

*The precise embryologic origin of many of these cells is not certain.

with nerve terminals. Origin of these cells from dorsal neural crest precursors has been surmised from immunocytochemical, ultrastructural, and oncodevelopmental observations (Gould et al., 1985). Alternatively, it has been suggested that they could arise from neighboring keratinocytes. They are associated with melanocytes in the basal epidermis, contain regulatory peptides (Hartschuh et al., 1979), and give rise to sporadic carcinomas with some NE cell characteristics (Wick et al., 1983; Silva et al., 1984; Gould et al., 1985).

NE Cells of the Hypophysis. The concept of a phenotypic relationship of hypophyseal secretory cells to other groups of diffuse NE cells is controversial

(Kissel et al., 1981). Inclusion within the NE cell category is supported by associations of pituitary adenomas with multiple endocrine neoplasia (Levine et al., 1979). Putative NE cells in the anterior hypophysis probably originate from primitive neural tube or neural ridge precursors (Takor-Takor and Pearse, 1975), or from pharyngeal pouch lining cells and neural crest (Kissel et al., 1981).

Gastrointestinal and Pancreatic NE Cells. These NE cells appear during early differentiation of the gastroenteric pancreatic axis both in normal embryos (Andrew, 1976; Sidhu, 1979) and in teratomas (Bosman and Louwerens, 1981). There is additional pathobiologic evidence for an origin from pluripotential foregut precursors (Mukai et al., 1982; Dayal, 1983; Ichijima et al., 1985). The NE cells localize *within* the mucosa of the stomach or the intestine. In the pancreas, they form both the classic islets and extrainsular collections of hormonally active cells. Differences in the spectrum of regulatory peptide biosynthesis may be related to specific anatomic location (Bosman and Louwerens, 1981).

Bronchopulmonary NE Cells and Neuroepithelial Bodies. These NE cells are widely distributed within the bronchopulmonary system, both singly and as tight clusters, which have been referred to as "neuroepithelial bodies" (Stahlman and Gray, 1984; Tateishi and Ishikawa, 1985). They appear during first trimester differentiation of the fetal lung (Stahlman et al., 1985). Dual origins from neuroectoderm and from endoderm are suggested both by immunohistochemical studies and patterns of neoplasia (Bosman and Louwerens, 1981; Gould et al., 1983; Blobel et al., 1985; Manning et al., 1985).

Thymic NE Cells. These cells are evidently fetal remnants of third pharyngeal pouch derivation (Rosai et al., 1976).

Genitourinary Tract NE Cells. Intramural NE cells associated with neural plexi in the bladder or vagina probably represent visceral-autonomic paraganglia related to the sacral parasympathetic limb of the autonomic nervous system (Glenner and Grimley, 1974). It has been suggested that cells immunoreactive for somatostatin, recently found in the prostatic urethra and prostate gland, are probably of endodermal (perhaps hindgut) origin (Di Sant'Agnese and de Mesy Jensen, 1984). A mesodermal origin of genital tract NE cells must also be considered (Scully et al., 1984).

NE CELL NEOPLASMS

Neoplasms of NE cell phenotype occur sporadically and in familial patterns. Both environmental and genetic factors have been implicated in their pathogenesis and could explain the high frequency of multicentric-multisystem involvement. Recent findings suggest that a multidirectional histogenetic capacity of pluripotent precursors underlies the diversity in neoplastic expression of the NE phenotype.

Pathogenesis

Genetic Factors

Repetitive familial patterns of multicentric NE cell neoplasms or multisystem endocrine neoplasias with NE cell components are well recognized (Ballard et al., 1964; Steiner et al., 1968; Perreira and Hunter, 1980; Parry et al., 1982; Van Baars et al., 1982). Familial inheritance of susceptibility to NE cell neoplasia is most commonly transmitted in an autosomal dominant mode; however, there is considerable variation in penetrance both within single kindreds and between different kindreds. A female sex predominance has been noted in several types of syndromes involving NE cells and in some types of extra-adrenal paragangliomas (Glenner and Grimley, 1974; Lack et al., 1979b; Parry et al., 1982). This could be explained by sex-related differences in genetic penetrance (Van Baars et al., 1982). Evidence for autosomal dominant transmission was found in up to 7 percent of extra-adrenal paragangliomas, and familial intercarotid paragangliomas occurred ten years earlier than nonfamilial cases (Parry et al., 1982).

Cytogenetic studies have suggested a high rate of chromosomal instability in family members with a high rate of cancer, including those individuals with multiple endocrine neoplasia (MEN) syndromes (Hsu et al., 1981; Gustavson et al., 1983; Stevens and Moore, 1983). Using a high resolution banding technique, Van Dyke and co-workers detected consistent minor deletions in the short arm of chromosome 20 in patients with MEN type II (Babu et al., 1984). As in neural tumors (Whang-Peng et al., 1984), it is conceivable that chromosomal translocations lead to activation of oncogenes. Location on chromosome 20 of the *c-src* proto-oncogene which encodes for tyrosine kinase is therefore of interest (Babu et al., 1984). Further work will be necessary to determine the frequency of deletions in chromosome 20 and to ascertain their relevance to tumor development in MEN II syndromes.

In animals, brachycephalic breeds of male dogs are particularly susceptible to development of intercarotid or para-aortic paragangliomas (Hayes and Fraumeni, 1974). In addition to the role of dietary factors in development of C-cell neoplasms in bovines (Krook et al., 1969), there is a hereditary pattern of occurrence of C-cell and adrenal medullary neoplasia in certain bovine breeds (Sponenberg and McEntee, 1983). Spontaneous neoplasms of C cells occur in many rat strains, and detailed studies have revealed an age-related increase. Hyperplasia of C cells invariably precedes development of tumors, and comparative studies revealed a striking similarity to human familial medullary thyroid carcinoma (DeLellis et al., 1979). In the Long-Evans rat strain, the C-cell proliferative lesions are accompanied by a high frequency of diffuse and nodular hyperplasias of the adrenal medulla, anterior pituitary proliferative lesions composed predominantly of prolactin secreting cells, and parathyroid hyperplasia (Lee et al., 1982). Preliminary data support a role of genetic factors in the development of multiple NE neoplasms in rats. Pituitary nodules, for example, are more common in the WAG/Rij strain than in the BN/Bi strain. In F1 hybrids, the incidence of such nodules is intermediate. Similar data have been obtained concerning the incidence of C-cell tumors in the F1 hybrids of high and low incidence strains (Burek, 1978).

Environmental Factors

A role of chronic hypoxemia leading to compensatory hyperplasia of chemosensitive paraganglia (intercarotid bodies) and subsequent development of paraganglioma has been suggested both by clinical and veterinary studies. The chronic hypoxemia may be produced by high altitude (Edwards et al., 1972; Saldana, 1973; Arias-Stella and Bustos, 1976; Arias-Stella and Velacrel, 1976; Gaylis and Mieny, 1979), chronic pulmonary disease (Edwards et al., 1971, Lack, 1978), or congenital cyanotic heart disease (Bockelman et al., 1982). The adrenal medulla is also exquisitely sensitive to hypoxemia, and cyanotic cardiac malformations have been associated with pheochromocytomas (Folger et al., 1964).

Hyperplasia of parafollicular C cells is very common in bulls fed excess dietary calcium (Krook et al., 1969). In hamsters, hyperplasia of pulmonary neuroendocrine cells was induced experimentally by chemical carcinogens (Linnoila et al., 1984; Tateishi and Ishikawa, 1985).

Other Factors

In contrast to lymphomas and some carcinomas, the frequency and malignant potential of NE cell neoplasms are not overtly increased by suppression of cell-mediated immunity (Spees et al., 1983).

A role of nerve growth factor or other humoral factors in the pathogenesis of multiple mucosal neuromas associated with certain NE cell neoplasms has been considered (DeSchryver-Kecskemeti et al., 1983).

Multidirectional Neoplastic Expression and Multihormonality

Various cell types in the NE system give rise to a wide spectrum of neoplasms which maintain many of the phenotypic characteristics of their assumed normal progenitors. The use of ultrastructural, immunocytochemical, and cell culture techniques, has shown that these neoplasms frequently evidence manifold lines of divergent differentiation, in addition to the expected neuroendocrine features. For example, those neoplasms conventionally classified as bronchopulmonary NE tumors (that is, oat cell carcinoma, carcinoid, etc.) also can exhibit glandular or squamous differentiation (Sidhu, 1979; Gould et al., 1983). This phenomenon of multidirectional differentiation may become evident early in the development of a neoplasm, presumably reflecting characteristics present in the progenitor cells, or may occur later, perhaps reflecting characteristics acquired during neoplastic progression. In effect, NE tumors may be subclassified into those composed of nearly pure populations of NE cells, such as pheochromocytoma, and those with significant admixtures of non-NE cell types (DeLellis et al., 1984). Such mixed tumors could arise from indigenous NE cells or from pluripotent stem cells which normally retain the capacity to differentiate in the direction of NE or non-NE cells. Various factors might influence NE programming and expression of divergent phenotype (DeLellis et al., 1984).

Production of multiple hormones is one of the most common forms of multidirectional differentiation in NE tumors. When the hormones are identical to those produced by putative normal progenitor cells, they are designated *eutopic*. When the hormones are not produced by indigenous cells they are designated *ectopic*. This is a relatively arbitrary distinction, which depends in part upon the sensitivity of methods for detecting hormonal biosynthesis. For example, somatostatin messenger RNA can be detected in certain cortical neurons by in-situ hybridization, despite inability to detect immunoreactive somatostatin.

The phenomenon of multihormonality, whether eutopic or ectopic, occurs in most neuroendocrine neoplasms. Recent data supports the view that production of various peptide products is subject to microenvironmental modification. For example, clonal strains of cells obtained from rat medullary thyroid carcinoma produce both calcitonin and neurotensin in vitro (Zeytinoglu et al., 1983). The latter is normally found to be highly concentrated in the brain or terminal ileum. When the clonal carcinoma cells are repassaged in rats, the experimental tumors continue to synthesize calcitonin, but produce negligible amounts of neurotensin. The neurotensin production was renewed only in subsequent tissue culture. Along similar lines, Linnoila et al. (1981) showed that hyperplastic neuroepithelial bodies of hamster lungs contained the same biosynthetic products as their normal counterparts, yet these cells began to express ACTH immunoreactivity in vitro. Pulmonary NE cells contained several regulatory peptides, but only expressed the opiate peptide leu-encephalin after in vitro isolation.

The presence of NE cells in usual types of adenocarcinomas is being recognized with increased frequency. Application of silver impregnation techniques and antibodies specific for chromogranins led to the identification of NE cells in a significant proportion of colonic and pancreatic adenocarcinomas (Kay et al., 1985), and they can also be found in carcinomas of the gallbladder (Fig. 23–3) (Albores-Saavedra et al., in press), endometrium, and ovary (Scully et al., 1984).

Conversely, NE neoplasms of the gastrointestinal tract (carcinoids) or pancreas (islet cell tumors) often contain neoplastic subpopulations of mucus secreting or Paneth cells and thus exhibit mixed NE and non-NE differentiation (Sidhu, 1979; Mukai et al., 1982). Indeed, pancreatic islet cell tumors probably can arise from primitive duct epithelium (Dahms et al., 1976; Dayal, 1983), and some intestinal carcinoid tumors may actually arise from a multipotent crypt-base endodermal cell which can differentiate into all intestinal cell types. This view is supported by studies of teratoma differentiation (Bosman and Louwerens, 1981) and experiments utilizing cloned cells from experimental colonic carcinomas (Cox and Pierce, 1982). Reinjection of cloned cells from the carcinomas led to the development of tumors composed of all major intestinal epithelial cell types, including some composed almost exclusively of NE cells.

A common stem cell theory fails to explain the presence of NE cells in tumors which arise from tissues in which no indigenous progenitors are evident (Scully et al., 1984). In such instances, we may postulate genetic activation of an NE program during the process of neoplastic progression or under microenvironmental influences.

Multicentricity and Multisystemic Involvement

Multicentricity and multisystemic associations with other endocrine or neural tumors are striking biologic characteristics of many NE cell neoplasms. Multisystem NE cell tumor constellations typically involve either tissues of neuroectodermal lineage or tissues of foregut-endodermal lineage. Complex multisystem associations of neoplasms derived from tissues of both lineages are relatively rare (see below), but their very existence buttresses the holistic concept of an interrelated, diffuse NE cell system.

The origin of neural crest from neuroectoderm at the earliest stages of embryonic differentiation and the close association with epidermal placodes provide a spatial and temporal scenario for carcinogenic events to impact a number of developmentally interrelated but histogenetically distinct cells or tissues. Synchronous or metachronous development of multicentric-multisystem neoplasms within anatomically separated and sometimes ontogenetically diverse subgroups of NE cells could be explained by a single biochemical defect (Steiner et al., 1968; Andrew, 1976) or by a common susceptibility to carcinogenic factors at particular stages of phenotypic differentiation (Schimke et al., 1968). Early events could also account for the coincidences of NE cell neoplasms in tissues of neural crest ancestry with neuroblastoma, neurofibromatosis, ganglioneuromatosis, cerebellar or retinal hemangiomas, and mucosal neuromas (Avsare et al., 1982; Kissel et al., 1981; Griffiths et al., 1983; Hoffman et al., 1982; Hull et al., 1982; Machin, 1982; Sato et al., 1974; Schimke et al., 1968; Steiner et al., 1968).

Several investigators have proposed two-step mutational models in the pathogenesis of multicentric NE neoplasms (Knudson, 1971; Hermann, 1977; Baylin et al., 1978). This may be related to the many observations of hyperplastic or proliferative lesions preceding NE cell neoplasia in man (Wolfe et al., 1973; DeLellis et al., 1976; Carney et al., 1976; Melicow, 1977; Wolfe et al., 1980) and in experimental animals (Jubb and McEntee, 1959; DeLellis et al., 1979). In familial medullary carcinoma, Baylin et al. (1978) found that individual tumor nodules were monoclonal with respect to glucose-6-phosphate dehydrogenase isoenzymes, suggesting that they arose

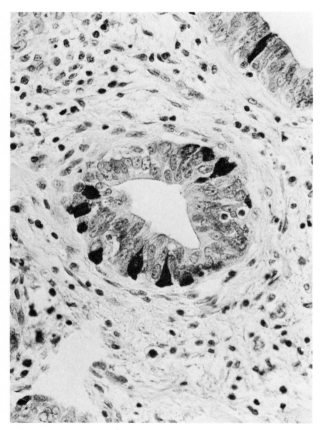

Figure 23–3. Intestinal-type adenocarcinoma of the gallbladder. Serotonin-containing cells are found among columnar cells. Peroxidase-antiperoxidase technique. (Courtesy of Drs. Albores-Saavedra and Henson.)

as a final monoclonal mutation from hyperplastic and polyclonal C cells. Hereditary neurofibromas appear to have a similar multicellular origin (Fialkow et al., 1971).

Preneoplastic Lesions

In familial forms of multiple neuroendocrine tumors, there is substantial evidence for a biologic progression from hyperplastic proliferative lesions to neoplasia, and the preneoplastic lesions may be detected serochemically. These findings tend to support proposed two-step mutational models of pathogenesis, but the evidence is incomplete and may not be relevant to all of the extra-adrenal paragangliomas. Moreover, our emphasis within the subject of "incipient neoplasia" reflects aspects of histopathology that differ from usual epithelial neoplasms: (a) Cytopathologic transitions from metaplasia or preneoplastic dysplasia to anaplasia and malignant behavior are difficult to prove histopathologically. (b) Cytologic grade is a limited predictor of biologic behavior and only some neoplasms of NE cell phenotype display the aggressively malignant potential of sarcomas or glandular carcinomas (i.e., small cell undifferentiated carcinomas). Thus, the concept of minimal lesions as applied to NE cell tumors has unique connotations.

Certain NE cell neoplasms clearly develop against a background of hyperplasia. The evidence is most striking in the familial syndromes of multiple endocrine neoplasia (MEN). In MEN type 1, both antral G-cell hyperplasia and islet cell hyperplasia may precede full clinical expression of the syndrome, allowing early serologic detection (Friesen et al., 1983). In MEN type 2, hyperplasia of parafollicular C cells precedes and is associated with the thyroid gland medullary carcinoma (Wolfe et al., 1973, 1980). A spectrum of C cell proliferative abnormalities and early stages of medullary carcinoma are illustrated in Figures 23–4 and 23–5. Similarly, adrenal medullary hyperplasia (Figs. 23–6 through 23–8) consistently precedes the development of intra-adrenal paragangliomas (pheochromocytomas) (Carney et al., 1976; DeLellis et al., 1976). The intra-adrenal hyperplasia evidently begins as a diffuse and nodular process, progressing to formation of discrete nodules (DeLellis et al., 1976, 1979). There was a non-uniform increase in distribution of the immunoreactive opiate-like pentapeptide identified as leu-enkephalin (Fig. 23–7B). Quantitative studies by DeLellis et al. (1976) suggested that some pheochromocytomas might actually represent exaggerated stages of atypical nodular hyperplasia. In a large series of sporadic cases of pheochromocytoma, Melicow (1977) reported several examples of 1 to 3 mm "chromaffin nodules" detected at autopsy. He surmised that these were predecessors of symptomatic pheochromocytomas.

In contrast to the observations cited above, morphologic patterns of cell growth in hyperplasia of the extra-adrenal paraganglia appear to differ significantly from the pattern in neoplasia: In hyperplastic paraganglia, both the chief cell (NE cells) and sustentacular cells (glial-type cells) or associated neural elements are found to proliferate (Lack, 1978; Jago et al., 1984; Fitch et al., 1985). In contrast, neoplasia of the extra-adrenal paraganglia is characterized by overwhelming growth of the chief cells (Grimley and Glenner, 1967; Robertson and Cooney, 1980). As in pheochromocytoma, increased leu-enkephalin reactivity may occur (DeLellis et al., 1983).

PATHOLOGIC CLASSIFICATIONS

The concept of multiple interrelated subgroups of dispersed NE cells with common phenotypic expression evolved over many decades and confronted historical views that individual endocrine functions were restricted to anatomically discrete components. The histopathologic and functional commonalities of NE cell neoplasms arising in diverse locations were often obscured by overlapping terminologies. Against this background, efforts to syndicate classification of all NE cell neoplasms with umbrella categories such as "APUDoma" or "neurocristopathy" (Pearse, 1969; Bolande, 1974; Pearse and Polak, 1974) represented important conceptual advances. Further, these nosologic generalizations proved particularly useful as pedantic constructs. Gradually, however, it has become evident that any rigid application of a unitary morphologic classification to all NE cell neoplasms is not clinically appropriate. The many NE cell neoplasms differ histogenetically, biologically, and in specific biochemical or biosynthetic activities. A valid nosology must recognize functional and prognostic diversity (Andrew, 1976; Sidhu, 1979; Skrabanke, 1980; Stevens and Moore, 1983).

In principle, neoplasms arising from any of the multiple tissues of neural crest lineage can be designated logically as "neurocristopathies" (Bolande, 1974). This categorization is indeed supported by pathobiologic evidence: constellations of developmental dysplasias can involve cells of more than one neural crest element in temporally concerted neoplastic processes (Schimke, 1980; Kissel et al., 1981; Hull et al., 1982; Zollinger and Hedinser, 1983). Nevertheless, neoplasms such as nevi or malignant melanomas, which conform to the formal definition of "neurocristopathy," do not meet all criteria for the NE cell phenotype. More obviously it is a misnomer to classify NE cell neoplasms clearly arising in tissues of foregut-endodermal histogenesis among the "neurocristopathies" (Schimke, 1980).

The above considerations lead us to advocate that regional-topographic and histogenetic information must be preserved in any nomenclature employed for clinical diagnostic and therapeutic classifications of NE cell neoplasms. The traditional designations such as

Text continued on page 439

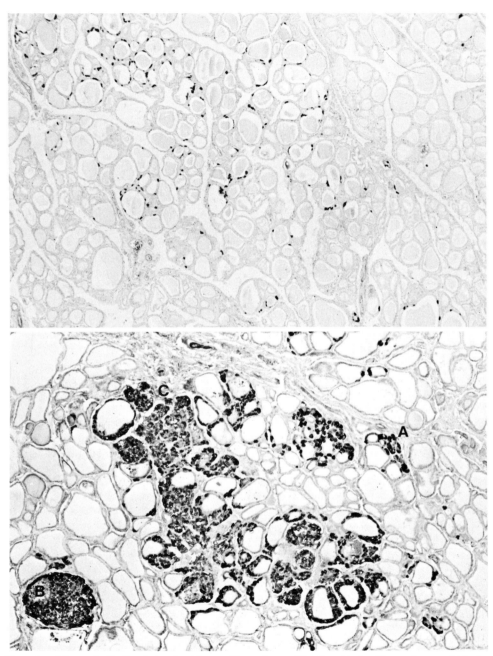

Figure 23–4. Normal and hyperplastic C-cells localized in paraffin sections of the thyroid gland by an immunohistochemical reaction for calcitonin (peroxidase-antiperoxidase technique). *Top,* Neonatal thyroid gland in which the C-cells are much more abundant than in adult glands and are concentrated along a hypothetical central axis in each lateral lobe. This section is from the junction of upper and middle thirds of a lobe. ×60. *Bottom,* Proliferative abnormalities of C-cells in a section of thyroid gland from a patient with familial medullary carcinoma. Note areas of diffuse hyperplasia *(A),* nodular hyperplasia *(B),* and early medullary carcinoma *(C).* ×60. (From DeLellis, R. A., and Wolfe, H. J.: Pathol Ann. *16* (part 2):25–52, 1981, with permission from Appleton-Century-Crofts.)

carcinoid tumor, paraganglioma, and medullary thyroid carcinoma are well recognized by pathologists and can be accompanied by a regional-topographic descriptor. For purposes of cataloguing and cross-indexing, parenthetic addition of the terms ''neuroendocrine tumor, functional'' or ''neuroendocrine tumor, non-functional'' might be particularly helpful. Eventually, development of more refined diagnostic categories with specific prognostic value will be based upon comprehensive morphologic analyses and integration of the clinical patterns of tumor development with profiles of functional or immunochemical biosynthetic expression.

HISTOPATHOLOGIC DIAGNOSIS

Conventional Histopathology

We have emphasized repeatedly that the cytologic and biochemical or biosynthetic interrelationships among normal or neoplastic NE cells transcend specific differences in ontogeny and histogenesis. Predominant histologic patterns of neoplasms arising in different topographic subgroups of NE cells can nevertheless be recognized by pathologists (Rosai et al., 1976). These histologic patterns may be correlated to histogenesis (Table 23–4) but often overlap. For example, a pattern of richly vascularized, compart-

mentalized cell nests or ''zellballen'' is typical of extra-adrenal paraganglion hyperplasia or well-differentiated extra-adrenal paragangliomas (Fig. 23–9); nevertheless, this pattern can sometimes be seen in intra-adrenal paragangliomas. A pattern of highly vascularized, ''syncytial'' cell sheets with relatively large, epithelioid cells characterizes most intra-adrenal paragangliomas (typical pheochromocytoma) (Fig. 23–10) but also can occur in extra-adrenal paragangliomas of the retroperitoneum, bladder (Fig. 23–10C), or other sites. Intermixture of ganglion cell or neuroblastic elements in paragangliomas may repre-

Table 23–4. **Predominant Histologic Patterns of Multicentric Neuroendocrine Cell Neoplasms and Associated Lesions**

Paraganglion NE Cells
  Paraganglion cell hyperplasia (''zellballen'')
  Paraganglioma (''zellballen'')
  Adrenal medullary hyperplasia, nodular or diffuse
  Paraganglioma, ''pheochromocytoma'' type (''syncytial'' epithelioid pattern)
  Paraganglioma with mixed ganglion cell or neuroblastic components

Bronchopulmonary NE Cells
  NE cell hyperplasia (tumorlets)
  Carcinoid patterns
  Small cell undifferentiated carcinoma (''oat cell'' or intermediate patterns)
  Paraganglioma (''zellballen'')

Gastrointestinal NE Cells
  Enterochromaffin cell-like hyperplasia (microcarcinoidosis)
  Carcinoid patterns
  Small cell undifferentiated carcinoma
  Paraganglioma, mixed gangliocytic type

Pancreatic NE Cells
  Nesidioblastosis
  NE (islet) cell tumor (varied patterns)
  Small cell undifferentiated carcinoma

Thyroid Gland NE Cells
  C cell hyperplasia
  Medullary (C cell) carcinoma (solid epithelial, carcinoid-like, or spindle cell)
  Small cell undifferentiated carcinoma (C cell type)
  Paraganglioma (''zellballen'')

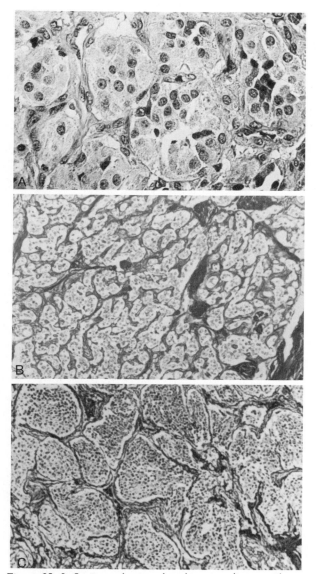

Figure 23–9. Sections of extra-adrenal paragangliomas with connective tissue stains highlighting the compartmentalized ''zellballen'' pattern. *A*, Cell nests illustrating uniformity of individual cells. ×250. *B*, Lower magnification of highly differentiated paraganglioma showing pattern of small compartments similar to that of a normal paraganglion. ×110. *C*, Another paraganglioma with a larger insular pattern similar to that of some gastroenteric NE cell tumors (see Fig. 23–11). ×110.

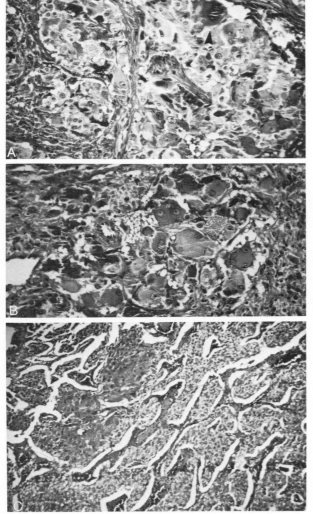

Carcinoid neoplasms arising in NE cells related to the gastrointestinal tract or NE (islet) cell tumors of the pancreas can display a range of organoid growth patterns reminiscent of normal pancreatic islet tissue, including a variety of trabecular, insular, gyriform, glandular, pseudoacinar, or medullary type patterns (see Dayal, 1983) (Fig. 23–11). Small cell undifferentiated carcinomas also can occur. Primary mediastinal carcinoids share similar histologic features (Wick et al., 1982).

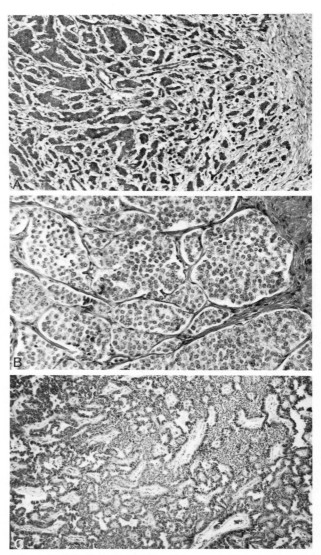

Figure 23–10. Sections of intra-adrenal paragangliomas and a paraganglioma of the bladder wall illustrating epithelioid and syncytial patterns typical of "pheochromocytoma." *A*, Syncytial sheets with irregular stromal demarcation and occasional giant pleomorphic cells (arrowhead). ×100. *B*, Plump epithelioid cells with relatively abundant cytoplasm compared with cells of other NE neoplasms. ×100. *C*, Bladder wall paraganglioma showing both syncytial cell sheets and compartmentalized regions similar to large "zellballen" (see Fig. 23–9). ×100.

sent a manifestation of multidirectional differentiation (see NE cell neoplasms above).

Bronchopulmonary neoplasms of NE cell phenotype display a variety of histologic patterns. Some hyperplasias or small intrapulmonary neoplasms have the "zellballen" pattern typical of extra-adrenal paragangliomas and are clinically benign. Larger bronchial or intrapulmonary neoplasms may show a range of carcinoid patterns, including a "spindle cell" variant (Ranchod and Levine, 1980; Mark and Ramirez, 1985). These tumors must be distinguished from small cell undifferentiated carcinomas with oat cell or intermediate patterns that indicate a poor prognosis.

Figure 23–11. Sections of NE cell tumors in the pancreas and colon with various islet or carcinoid patterns. *A*, Invasive islet cell tumor showing a trabecular pattern. Variation in thickness of trabeculae is considerable. ×100. *B*, Carcinoid tumor of colon showing large insular pattern. Compartments are larger and less regular than in paraganglioma "zellballen" (compare with Fig. 23–9). ×100. *C*, Same carcinoid tumor showing distinctive ribbon-like or gyriform pattern. This is also seen in some pancreatic NE cell tumors. ×100.

Neoplasms arising in C cells of the thyroid gland are perhaps the most pleomorphic NE cell tumors; areas of spindle, carcinoid, epithelioid, or small cell undifferentiated patterns often coincide within a single sample (Mendelsohn at al., 1980; Fenoglio et al., 1985). Association of these tumors with an amyloid stroma is common and supports the diagnosis (Fig. 23–12). Paraganglioma of the thyroid gland is rare.

Electron Microscopy

Advances in electron microscopy, cytochemistry, and immunohistochemistry within the past three decades have all reinforced the concept of a neoplastic NE cell phenotype. Ultrastructural analysis has been particularly important in demonstrating the cytologic commonality among widely dispersed NE cell groups and

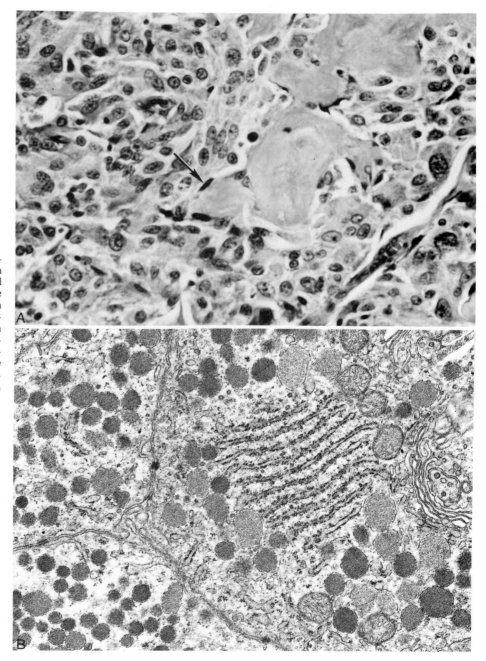

Figure 23–12. Illustrations of medullary thyroid carcinoma. *A*, Section showing typical pattern of solid cell sheets with epithelioid and spindle cells. Note amyloid accumulation (arrow). ×340. *B*, Electron micrograph of ultrathin section with membrane-bound secretory granules. There is considerable heterogeneity in size and electron density of the granules. Stacked endoplasmic reticulum is often noted in these cells. ×17,000.

in NE cell neoplasms regardless of origin (Glenner and Grimley, 1974; Payne et al., 1984). Normal NE cells exhibit cytoplasmic granules of Golgi origin with an electron-dense core (see Fig. 23–2). The granules tend to be uniform, within a size range of 0.5 to 2.0 µm, and react with uranyl salts at low pH (Payne et al., 1984). In both neoplastic and normal cells, the frequency of dense-core granules as observed in ultrathin sections can vary (e.g., Fig. 23–8), depending upon the phase of secretory activity or granule storage: release of granule contents occurs during their fusion with the plasma membrane.

NE cells of the paraganglion subgroup exhibit a rich innervation with cholinergic or adrenergic neural termini and close associations with Schwann-like sustentacular cells. Purified antibodies which react with a highly acidic calcium-binding polypeptide normally abundant in vertebrate neural tissues (S-100) also demonstrate the sustentacular cell elements of paraganglia (Ferri et al., 1982; Nakajima et al., 1982; Weiss et al., 1983; Blaivas et al., 1985). Bronchopulmonary NE cells exhibit close relationships to nerve fibers, but commonly display a polar asymmetry with apical microvilli (Stahlman and Grey, 1984). Neuroid cell processes with aligned neurotubules can be traced to NE cells in the extra-adrenal paraganglia (Grimley and Glenner, 1968) or the adrenal medulla (Fig. 23–8), and extension of paraganglion cell processes in response to nerve growth factor has been demonstrated in vitro (Tischler et al., 1980). Remarkably, neuroid features are shared by some NE cells of foregut-endodermal origin (Larsson et al., 1979).

Ultrastructurally, the normal relationships of paraganglionic NE cells to sustentacular cells and nerve fibers are usually lost in extra-adrenal paragangliomas, which represent a proliferation only of the primary NE cells (chief cells) (Grimley and Glenner, 1967; Robertson and Cooney, 1980). Monoclonal antibodies to the cell protein S-100 nevertheless show positive reactions in histologic sections of some paragangliomas and other NE cell tumors.

Immunohistochemistry

Immunohistochemistry has proved to be a powerful tool for identification of NE cells (e.g., Fig. 23–4). In general, high levels of immunoreactive neuron-specific enolase differentiate cells of NE phenotype from other endocrine epithelia (Schmechel, 1985; Johnson et al., 1985; DeLellis et al., in press). Very recently, it has been demonstrated that polyclonal or monoclonal antibodies to chromogranin, a soluble acidic protein which is found in the secretory granules of intra-adrenal paragangliomas, specifically cross-react with the granules in most cells of NE phenotype (that is, all paraganglia, gut-associated endocrine cells and pancreatic islet cells) (O'Connor et al., 1983; Wilson

and Lloyd, 1984; DeStephano et al., 1984). This may now prove to be another valuable aid in the differential diagnosis (Lloyd et al., 1984; Johnson et al., 1985; DeLellis et al., in press).

A broad spectrum of regulatory peptides and monoamines can be localized in normal NE cells by immunocytochemical techniques (see Table 23–1). Moreover, recent studies indicate a significant degree of heterogeneity in the expression of specific peptides within NE cells of a particular location, such as the adrenal medulla (DeLellis et al., 1983; Lloyd et al., 1984). As discussed previously (Introduction and Pathogenesis of NE Cell Neoplasms), the normal range of biosynthetic or functional expression of regulatory peptides is highly complex, and this complexity may be reflected or amplified in neoplasia resulting in both eutopic and ectopic hormone production. Thus, the biosynthetic profiles of NE neoplasms arising in tissues of neural crest or foregut-endodermal ancestry often overlap (see Table 23–2), and origin of a biosynthetically active neoplasm from a specific subset of NE cells cannot be ascertained solely on the basis of biochemical function or immunocytochemistry. Nevertheless, the biosynthetic profile as determined by immunochemistry can be very significant when correlated with clinical biochemistry and family history. Knowledge of the biosynthetic patterns is essential in planning prospective screening programs (Friesen et al., 1983), and further research should enable more specific classification of tumor constellations in conjunction with family studies.

Monoamine Cytochemistry

The catecholamine or serotonin content of NE cells can be differentiated with techniques of monoamine-induced fluorescence (De Lellis, 1971), immunocytochemistry (Verhofstad et al., 1983; Stahlman et al., 1985), or direct biochemical analysis of tumor tissue (Crowell, 1984), most recently including high-performance liquid chromatography. Catecholamine granules comprise a rich variety of distinctive matrix- or membrane-associated polypeptides, including specific biosynthetic enzymes (Angeletti et al., 1985), and immunoperoxidase techniques employing specific antibody to catecholamine-synthesizing enzymes have been developed for identification of the granules (Verhofstad et al., 1983).

Historically, the subgroups of paraneural NE cells producing abundant catecholamines (intra-adrenal and extra-adrenal paraganglia) were defined by the observation of a "chromaffin" reaction after fixation with dichromate solutions. A brown intracytoplasmic precipitate results from the oxidative polymers of monoamines with incorporated chromate salts. This led to the description "pheochromocytoma" for tumors of the adrenal medulla. At the same time, NE cells of the intestine were recognized by an "enterochromaffin'' reaction owing to the presence of serotonin. Although the chromaffin reaction is reproducible in cells with high concentrations of epinephrine or indol amines, its utility in diagnosis of NE cell tumors is limited by insensitivity and dependence upon immediate fixation of tissues in glutaraldehyde or a dichromate solution (Chambers et al., 1968). Cells of many normal extra-adrenal paraganglia and some neoplasms which produce or accumulate norepinephrine or dopamine fail to display a chromaffin product. Obviously, classification of neoplasms should not be based on such a limited cytochemical technique (Glenner and Grimley, 1974). Although the designation *pheochromocytoma* remains popular and typically refers to intra-adrenal neoplasms, it is technically synonymous with a *chromaffin-reactive paraganglioma*. In this context, we utilize *paraganglioma* as a generic term and specify *intra-adrenal paraganglioma* or *extra-adrenal paraganglioma* to avoid confusion.

EARLY CLINICAL AND LABORATORY DIAGNOSIS

NE cell neoplasms come to clinical attention for a variety of reasons: (a) palpation of a mass, (b) incidental detection of a mass on chest film or other radiograph, (c) signs of local expansion or infiltration, including nerve or vessel compression, pain, or hemorrhage, or (d) symptoms or signs of excessive or inappropriate secretion of polypeptide hormones.

Careful otorhinologic examination is essential to rule out jugulotympanic or intravagal paragangliomas of the nasopharynx. This should include cranial nerve and auditory tests.

Symptoms and signs related to increased or abnormal production of NE cell products can be very suggestive of the pathologic diagnosis, and excessive products may be secreted by hyperplastic lesions that precede neoplasia. The most frequent symptoms of hormonally active NE cell neoplasms include sweating, headache and palpitation/tachycardia related to excess catecholamine production (Melicow, 1977). Other important and overt signs can include watery diarrhea produced by excess vasoactive intestinal peptide (Verner-Morrison syndrome), hypoglycemia due to excess epinephrine or insulin, peptic ulcer related to excess gastrin (Zollinger-Ellison syndrome), and Cushing's syndrome due to excess ACTH. Overproduction of serotonin in the relatively rare carcinoid syndrome can lead to vasomotor, gastrointestinal, or cardiopulmonary disturbances, with flushing, nausea, vomiting, diarrhea, or asthmatic symptoms.

In the appropriate clinical settings, biochemical tests of serum or urine can be extremely valuable adjuncts for the diagnosis of NE cell neoplasms. These tests are not advocated as general screening tools: even with maximal levels of sensitivity and specificity, the predictive value remains <2 percent in the average population owing to an extremely low prevalence. The predictive value of serum or urine biochemical tests is significantly enhanced in family groups and other populations known to be at medically high risk (Oberg et al., 1982; Friesen et al., 1983). Thus, recognition of genetic or developmental factors predisposing to the pathogenesis of NE cell tumors deserves primary emphasis both for presymptomatic screening or provocative testing of subjects at suspected risk and in follow-up or management of patients with manifest disease.

Paragangliomas which secrete catecholamines are estimated to occur in 0.04 to 0.2 percent of Americans with diastolic hypertension. These include intra-adrenal paraganglioma (90 percent of cases) and the rarer forms of functional extra-adrenal paraganglioma (10 percent of cases). Thus, the total U.S. prevalence of functionally active paragangliomas approaches 40,000 cases (Gambino, 1982). Symptoms and laboratory findings related to excessive catecholamine production are by far the most common evidence of such tumors. At least one symptom in the triad of sweating, headache, and palpitation or tachycardia is found in more than 99 percent of cases (Bravo and Gifford, 1984). Laboratory screening must include a battery of *24-hour* urine biochemistries: metanephrines, vanillylmandelic acid (sequential degradation products of norepinephrine or epinephrine), and free catecholamines. Results of these 24 hour tests vary owing to differences in the tumor cell levels of catechol-O-methyl transferase and monoamine oxidase, which are involved in the sequential catabolic steps, so only one of the tests may be positive. Plasma catecholamines measured in fasting patients can be the most sensitive and specific test for excess catecholamine production; and pretreatment with clonidine to suppress physiologic catecholamine elevation in apprehensive or stressed patients increases the specificity (Bravo and Gifford, 1984). In patients with familial pheochromocytomas related to multiple endocrine neoplasia, an increase in the ratio of epinephrine to norepinephrine may be an early sign of adrenal medullary hyperplasia (Gagel et al., 1975; Hamilton et al., 1978).

Diagnostic radiography is a major tool in confirming the diagnosis of catecholamine-secreting neoplasms and fixing their locations. In conjunction with radiography, fine needle aspiration biopsy (Berge et al., 1976) may prove useful as a diagnostic tool, especially if combined with immunocytochemistry. Ultrasound examination of the cervical region (Gooding, 1979) combined with chest films and computed axial tomography of the thorax and abdomen provides a thorough screen for multicentric paragangliomas. Chest films are essential to rule out extra-adrenal paraganglioma of the heart base or posterior mediastinum (Reed et al., 1978). High-resolution abdominal

CT scan can even resolve increases in size of the adrenal medullae. The medullary tissue is normally concentrated in the head and body of the gland, so that expansion of the tail can be an early sign of hyperplasia/neoplasia (Brennan, 1985; DeLellis et al., in press).

Skeletal scanning and radionuclide scintigraphy are valuable adjuncts for diagnosis or staging of NE cell tumors (Veldman et al., 1980). A new radiopharmaceutical reagent, [131 I]*meta*-iodobenzylguanidine, concentrates in adrenergic vesicles and is retained for days (Sisson et al., 1981). Increased experience with this scintigraphic technique and computer axial tomography may lead to earlier detection of suspected catecholamine-secreting NE cell neoplasms in extra-adrenal locations (e.g. Ruijs et al., 1978).

MULTICENTRIC NEOPLASMS

Multicentric neoplasms of NE cell phenotype may develop within any of the families of paraganglia, or within NE cells of the gastrointestinal-pancreatic axis or the bronchopulmonary tract. Such tumors may be familial and display an autosomal dominant pattern of inheritance.

Paragangliomas

Extra-adrenal paraganglia are grouped empirically into major anatomic "families": branchiomeric-intravagal, aortico-sympathetic, and visceral-autonomic (Table 23–5). Solitary or multicentric paragangliomas may arise in any of these families. Overall, 90 percent of paragangliomas arise within the adrenal medullae and up to 10 percent are bilateral. Extra-adrenal para-

Table 23–5. Major Families of Extra-Adrenal Paraganglia and Sites of Paragangliomas

Family	Sites of Paragangliomas
Branchiometric/Intravagal	Jugulotympanic (middle ear)
	Nasopharyngeal (ganglion nodosum)
	Intercarotid (carotid bodies)
	Laryngeal
	Intrathyroid
	Aortico-pulmonary (superior mediastinum)
	Coronary-interatrial (heart base)
Aortic-Sympathetic	Intrathoracic paravertebral
	Retroperitoneal
	Organs of Zuckerkandl
Visceral-Autonomic	Gastroduodenal
	Porta hepatis
	Genitourinary
	Cauda equina

ganglia allied to anatomic structures of branchial arch ontogeny (branchiomeric paraganglia) or associated with the vagus nerve are the next most common sites of paragangliomas. Intercarotid paragangliomas are bilateral in up to 5 percent of cases and often associated with extra-adrenal paragangliomas in other locations (see below). Thus, the clinically important anatomic regions for detection of paragangliomas include jugulotympanic, intercarotid, mediastinal, and retroperitoneal.

Mediastinal supra-aortic or aortico-pulmonary paragangliomas may be associated with the atrial walls, the base of the heart or the great vessels, or the paravertebral sympathetic trunk (Olson and Salyer, 1978; Gallivan et al., 1980; Johnson et al., 1985). In a large series of neural tumors of the thorax, paragangliomas represented 4 percent of cases (Reed et al., 1978). Lack et al. (1979b) reviewed 36 published cases. Retroperitoneal paragangiomas are probably more common than mediastinal cases (Glenner and Grimley, 1974; Melicow, 1977; Lack et al., 1980).

Laryngeal, nasopharyngeal, and intrathyroid paragangliomas are relatively rare (Glenner and Grimley, 1974; Lack et al., 1979a). Least frequently, paragangliomas occur in visceral locations supplied by orthosympathetic or craniosacral parasympathetic elements: the orbit, duodenum, hepatic ducts, bladder wall, genitourinary tract, or cauda equina.

Multicentric extra-adrenal paragangliomas typically involve the intercarotid paraganglia and one or more additional extra-adrenal sites (for example, jugulotympanic, intravagal, or aortico-pulmonary paraganglia). In such cases, intercarotid paragangliomas are often bilateral (Wilson, 1970; Pereira and Hunter, 1980), but multiple ipsilateral tumors also occur (Kahn, 1976; Nicholas and Orsini, 1982). Other combinations of extra-adrenal paragangliomas occur in the thorax and abdomen (Steiner et al., 1968; Lack et al., 1979b; Bogdassarian and Lotz, 1979; Gallivan et al., 1980; Hoffman et al., 1982). Cases of disseminated extra-adrenal paragangliomatosis are well documented (Karasov et al., 1982), and may be associated with Carney's triad of gastric leiomyosarcoma and pulmonary chondroma (Carney, 1983). In a retrospective series of intercarotid paragangliomas, synchronous multicentric cases constituted less than 5 percent (Farr, 1980); however, the true incidence of multicentricity, including metachronous cases, probably would be higher in directed prospective studies (e.g., Revak et al., 1971).

Surprisingly, the concurrence of extra-adrenal and intra-adrenal paraganglioma is relatively infrequent (Sato et al., 1974), although multicentric paragangliomas often involve the remnant organ of Zuckerkandl (Glenner and Grimley, 1974; Melicow, 1977). Multicentric intra-adrenal or extra-adrenal paragangliomas can also be associated with developmental diseases of the CNS: hemangioblastomas (Hoffman et al., 1982; Hull et al., 1982; Steiner et al., 1968) or neurofibromatosis (Avsare et al., 1982; Griffiths et al., 1983; Hoffman et al., 1982; Kissel et al., 1981; White and Hickson, 1979; Zollinger and Hedinser, 1983).

Association of extra-adrenal paragangliomas with multiple endocrine gland neoplasias was noted in a Mexican family (Larraza-Hernandez et al., 1982). Other families with a high frequency of isolated or multiple paragangliomas have been reported (Parry et al., 1982; Van Baars et al., 1982), and there is an increased incidence of bilateral intercarotid paragangliomas in familial cases (Wilson, 1970; Glenner and Grimley, 1974; Pereira and Hunter, 1980). *Obviously, the finding of a paraganglioma in one anatomic site must always alert the clinician to the possibility that other paragangliomas are present already or will appear subsequently.*

Functional differentiation of paragangliomas with excess production of catecholamines is uncommon outside of the adrenal medulla or aortico-sympathetic paraganglia of the thorax or abdominal retroperitoneum; however, intercarotid, jugulotympanic, or intrathoracic paragangliomas sometimes produce symptoms or signs related to excess catecholamines (Glenner and Grimley, 1974; Melicow, 1977; Crowell et al., 1982). The clinical effects, discussed earlier, can include hypertension, sweating, and palpitations. Intraoperative or postoperative hypotension are serious risks for which the surgeon and anesthesiologist must be prepared in every case, *regardless of overt signs or symptomatic expression.* Preoperative testing for urinary catecholamines and metabolites is essential. Epinephrine may be the predominant catecholamine in pheochromocytoma or paragangliomas of the abdominal retroperitoneum. Paragangliomas of other sites usually secrete an excess of norepinephrine and have been reported in the thorax, intercarotid, and jugulotympanic regions. Rare cases of functional paragangliomas secreting biologically active calcitonin (White and Hickson, 1979), or ACTH (Apple and Kreines, 1982; Grizzle et al., 1983), have been reported and immunoreactive somatostatin (Saito et al., 1982) or VIP may be detected in tumor cells (Tischler et al., 1981). Clinical indications of biologically active serotonin in rare paragangliomas (Farrior et al., 1980) remain to be confirmed by serum or tissue analyses.

Extra-adrenal or intra-adrenal paragangliomas are highly vascularized and therefore well visualized by radiography after injection of radiocontrast material. Histopathologic diagnosis is not usually difficult, but differentiation from hemangiopericytoma, clear cell renal carcinoma, or epithelioid meningiomas of the spinal roots can pose a diagnostic challenge. In the mediastinum, paraganglioma may be difficult to distinguish from thymic carcinoid tumors (Rosai et al., 1976).

Local growth of paragangliomas is typically indolent with a natural evolution over several years. As discussed above (Preneoplastic Lesions), both sporadic and familial intra-adrenal paragangliomas can evidently be preceded by nodular hyperplasia (DeLellis et al., 1976; Melicow, 1977). Melicow (1977) found that 17 of 107 intra-adrenal paragangliomas were clinically silent and detected incidentally during laparotomy or autopsy. Asymptomatic extra-adrenal paragangliomas are a potentially grave problem in the retroperitoneum, where masses may not be detected before local extension, vascular invasion, or metastasis defy surgical excision (Lack et al., 1980; Gallivan et al., 1980). Extra-adrenal paragangliomas in confined locations, such as the middle ear, paranasal sinuses, vagal nerve trunks, or paravertebral sulcus, may produce neurologic signs or symptoms relatively early. Functional paragangliomas of the thorax (up to 48 percent of cases) or the abdominal retroperitoneum (up to 25 percent of cases) may also be detected early if any signs related to excess catecholamine secretion are promptly recognized.

Local infiltration of extra-adrenal paragangliomas can be insidious and very dangerous if major vessels or the heart base or atrial walls (Johnson et al., 1985) are involved. The situation is most analogous to basal cell carcinoma, where initial wide excision is imperative. Local infiltration of paraganglioma can be restrained by irradiation (Spector et al., 1975; Gaylis and Mieny, 1977), but this is probably due to induction of fibrosis rather than specific cytotoxicity (Spector et al., 1975). Thus far, chemotherapy has not proved successful (Soeprono and Hodgkin, 1983).

Overall, the metastatic potential of paragangliomas is less than 10 percent, but up to 30 percent of cases with lymph node metastasis have been reported in some series (Gaylis and Mieny, 1977; Lack et al., 1980). In a given case metastatic potential generally cannot be gauged on the basis of cytologic criteria. Most tumors, including those which metastasize, fail to exhibit dramatic cytologic atypia. On the other hand, cases in which sections display numerous mitoses or enlarged atypical nuclei are statistically more likely to metastasize. The incidence of systemic malignancy is evidently highest in mediastinal or retroperitoneal paragangliomas (Lack et al., 1980; Olson and Salyer, 1978), with relatively large mass at the time of detection. Systemic metastases often involve bones of the skull, vertebrae, or pelvis and the lungs. Immediate extirpation of metastatic nodules is optimal, since recurrence may be very slow and some patients are essentially cured (Soeprono and Hodgkin, 1983). *Obviously, it is essential to distinguish synchronous or metachronous occurrence of multiple paragangliomas from true metastasis.*

Gastroenteric and Pancreatic Neoplasms

NE cell neoplasms of the gastroenteric tract are often multicentric (Kissel et al., 1981; Brennan, 1983), and intrapancreatic NE cell neoplasms are nearly always multicentric and associated with a generalized nesidioblastosis or islet cell hyperplasia (Dahms et al., 1976; Mukai et al., 1982). Multicentric NE cell neoplasms of the gastroenteric tract typically exhibit a carcinoid-islet cell pattern, sometimes with focal mucin production. In the upper intestinal tract, tumors with mixed patterns of paraganglioma, ganglioneuroma, and carcinoid-islet cell tumor may occur (Reed et al., 1977).

Multicentric enteric carcinoids occur rarely in repetitive heredito-familial patterns (Moertel and Dockerty, 1973; Dayal et al., 1983). Associations with neurofibromatosis, intra-adrenal paraganglioma or small cell pulmonary carcinomas also are rare, but noteworthy with respect to interrelationships of the diffuse NE cell system (Hansen et al., 1976; Griffiths et al., 1983; Morris and Tymms, 1980).

Lack of early signs unfortunately results in a high incidence of hepatic metastasis (Brennan, 1985), and symptoms of pain, nausea, or vomiting may be the presenting evidence of enteric carcinoids. The classic carcinoid syndrome with vasomotor, cardiac, and pulmonary complications manifests after metastasis and occurs in 10 percent of small bowel cases (Brennan, 1985).

Bronchopulmonary Neoplasms

Bronchopulmonary NE cell neoplasms may present as paragangliomas, carcinoid tumors, or small cell undifferentiated ("oat cell") tumors (Greco and Oldham, 1979; Gould et al., 1983; Levine et al, 1979; Ranchod and Levine, 1980). Multicentric paragangliomas are typically minute and incidental autopsy or surgical findings. Clinically, they are not significant (Ichinose et al., 1971). Carcinoid or small cell anaplastic tumors are typically isolated and present with symptoms of cough, weight loss, dyspnea, chest pain, or hemoptysis. They are usually single central or peripheral lesions on x-ray. Small cell tumors have often metastasized by the time of diagnosis. While these tumors may synthesize a variety of regulatory peptides and other substances (Gould et al., 1983), specific genetic or environmental risk factors remain to be elucidated before screening by immunoassay can be appropriately targeted. Rare associations of pulmonary small cell neoplasms with other neoplasms of NE cell phenotype are of theoretical interest (Berg et al., 1976; Hansen et al., 1976; Morris and Tymms, 1980).

MULTISYSTEM NEOPLASMS

In addition to their multicentric character, neoplasms of NE cell phenotype can involve NE cell subgroups of both neuroectodermal-neural crest and foregut-endodermal ancestry in diverse tissues. Such *multisystem* constellations most frequently include the intra-adrenal paraganglia (adrenal medullae), C cells of the thyroid gland, and NE cells of the pancreatic islets and the anterior hypophysis. They often include proliferative non-NE lesions of the parathyroid or thyroid glands. Repeated tumor patterns (Table 23–6) characterize these "multiple endocrine neoplasia" syndromes (MEN, types I to III), and familial susceptibility is transmitted in an autosomal dominant mode (Ballard et al., 1964; Steiner et al., 1968).

The multisystem associations of neoplasms related to NE cells of different embryonic lineages strongly support concepts of developmental and functional linkages. Nevertheless, the specific pathologic factors underlying the predominant patterns of multisystem tumors remain obscure.

Three major categories of MEN with NE cell neoplasms are currently recognized, and designated types I, IIA (or II), and IIB (or III). As shown in Table 23–6, locations of the tumors in each subcategory of MEN, with many overlaps.

MEN Type I

This entity was recognized by Wermer (1954) and is inherited as an autosomal dominant with penetrance of up to 80 per cent. Multisystem proliferative lesions or neoplasms typically involve the anterior hypophysis, parathyroid glands, and pancreatic islets. The parathyroids are more commonly involved and nodular parathyroid hyperplasia may be the common underlying abnormality.

The clinical expression of MEN type I is variable and depends upon familial patterns and the activity of specific endocrine tissues which are initially involved. Signs related to parathyroid, pancreatic neuroendocrine cell, or pituitary gland hyperactivity may predominate. Evidence of diffuse or nodular parathyroid gland hyperplasia can be the earliest sign and warrants persistent screening for identification of further neuroendocrine abnormalities in the pancreas or pituitary (Majewski and Wilson, 1979; Van Heerden et al., 1983).

Pancreatic disease is associated with multifocal proliferations of islet neuroendocrine cells or their ductal precursors (nesidioblastosis). Approximately one third of lesions are predominantly beta cell and capable of insulin production (Ballard et al., 1964). The non-beta cell lesions are heterogeneous and capable of secreting multiple clinically active eutopic or ectopic peptides (Heitz, 1984). The symptoms of pancreatic disease may be related to excess insulin with hypoglycemia, uncontrolled gastrin production with intractable peptic ulcers (Zollinger-Ellison syndrome), excess VIP and watery diarrhea (Verner-Morrison syndrome), or overproduction of glucagon and the glucagonoma syndrome (Fig. 23–13).

Pituitary lesions, either hyperplasias or defined adenomas, occur in up to two thirds of patients with MEN type I. These may result in pituitary insufficiency or syndromes secondary to pituitary hormone excess. So-called chromophobe adenomas were most fre-

Table 23–6. **Neuroendocrine Cell Neoplasms: Spectrum of Multisystem Associations**

Location	Multiple Endocrine Neoplasia (MEN)				Mexican Family	Carney Triad
	I	*IIA (II)*	*IIB (III)*	*Mixed**		
Pituitary	adenoma			——— adenoma ———		
Parathyroid	——— hyperplasia/adenoma ———			——— hyperplasia ———		
Thyroid follicular cells	——— (hyperplasia/adenoma) ———				papillary carcinoma	
C-cells		——— hyperplasia/carcinoma ———				
Broncho-pulmonary	(carcinoid)			oat cell carcinoma		chondroma
Stomach	antral G-cell hyperplasia				leiomyoma	leiomyosarcoma
GI tract	(carcinoid)		ganglioneuroma	carcinoid		
Pancreas	islet cell hyperplasia/ adenoma/carcinoma			islet cell adenoma adenoma		
Adrenal cortex medulla	(hyperplasia/adenoma)	——— hyperplasia/pheochromocytoma ———		pheochromocytoma		
Extra-adrenal paraganglia	(intravagal paraganglioma)	——— (paragangliomas) ———		——— paraganglioma ———		

*Based upon combined observations of Berg et al., 1976; Doumith et al., 1982; Griffiths et al., 1983; Morris and Tymms, 1980; and Nathan et al., 1980.

quent in early studies of MEN type I (Ballard et al., 1964), but many of these probably represent sparsely granulated prolactin-secreting tumors (see DeLellis et al., in press). Galactorrhea-amenorrhea syndrome may be associated with prolactin-secreting adenoma in MEN type I (Levine et al., 1979).

In recognized MEN type I families, annual screening of kindred has included serum calcium and radioimmunoassay for parathyroid hormone to detect early parathyroid lesions and radioimmunoassay for gastrin to detect early islet cell hyperactivity at all ages between 10 and 65 (Lynch et al., 1979; Brennan, 1985). More recent studies show that serum levels of pancreatic polypeptide also can be useful in family screening (Oberg et al., 1982; Friesen et al., 1983). Serum tests for elevation of prolactin or other pituitary gland hormones may prove useful in detecting early proliferative lesions or adenomas (Oberg et al., 1982) and guide radiographic follow-up of the sella region.

MEN Type IIA (II)

This entity is characterized by medullary thyroid carcinoma, pheochromocytoma, and parathyroid neoplasms. The repetitive pattern of thyroid carcinoma and pheochromocytoma was recognized by Sipple (see Sapira et al., 1965). Hyperparathyroidism occurs in a high proportion of patients and is related to diffuse or nodular hyperplasia of the parathyroid glands (Van Heerden, 1983). Serum calcium and parathormone elevations often precede evidence of the thyroid disease (Melvin, 1974). Inheritance of MEN type IIA is governed by an autosomal dominant trait with high penetrance and variable expression (Steiner et al., 1968).

Medullary carcinoma of the thyroid gland is of C-cell origin, and typically accompanied or preceded by C-cell hyperplasia (Wolfe et al., 1973; Block et al.,

1980) (Fig. 23–4). These tumors synthesize multiple immunoreactive polypeptides and produce a characteristic amyloid stroma. Calcitonin and histaminase are typical markers and can be detected immunocytochemically (Mendelsohn et al., 1978, 1980) (Fig. 23–4). This aids in histopathologic differentiation of spindle cell, small cell, and giant cell anaplastic variants (Mendelsohn et al., 1980; Fenoglio et al., 1985).

Calcium and gastrin are calcitonin secretagogues and high-risk kindred can be effectively screened for evidence of C-cell hyperplasia or medullary carcinoma by a provocative pentagastrin test (Block et al., 1980; Brennan, 1985). The increase of serum calcitonin may be proportional to tumor bulk (Block et al., 1980). Serum histaminase was formerly useful for family screening (Baylin et al., 1970). Diarrhea related to vasoactive intestinal peptide was noted in up to 32 percent of patients with thyroid medullary carcinoma (Said and Faloona, 1975), and serotonin or ectopic ACTH can also be produced (Steiner et al., 1968; Block et al., 1980). In one case, excess serotonin production resulted in carcinoid syndrome (Moertel et al., 1965).

Pheochromocytoma is bilateral in 70 per cent of cases of MEN type IIA. Paroxysms associated with pheochromocytoma were often fatal (Steiner et al., 1968), so that lifetime surveillance for adrenal medullary hyperplasia or neoplasia is considered essential. Gagel et al. (1975) and Hamilton et al. (1978) advocate monitoring the urinary epinephrine/norepinephrine ratio (also see Clinical and Laboratory Diagnosis, above).

Medullary carcinomas of the thyroid gland are malignant and capable of metastasis. Cervical or mediastinal lymph nodes, lungs, and liver are common secondary sites. Tumors are bilateral in 80 percent of familial cases, and total thyroidectomy may be appropriate (Block et al., 1980).

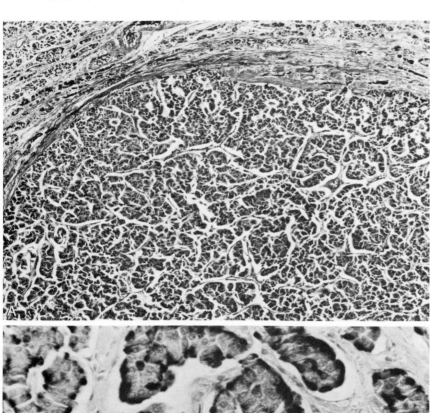

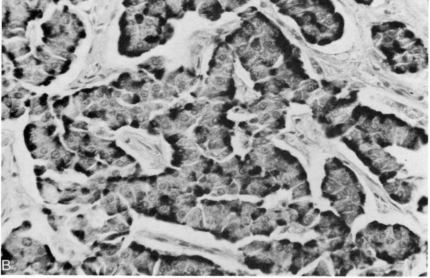

Figure 23–13. *A,* An endocrine pancreatic neoplasm found in a 68-year-old man, who also had a prolactin-producing pituitary adenoma and an aldosterone-producing tumor of the adrenal cortex. *B,* Most tumor cells of the pancreatic tumor contain immunoreactive glucagon, which is concentrated along the basal portion of the cytoplasm. Peroxidase-antiperoxidase technique. (Courtesy of Dr. Albores-Saavedra.)

MEN Type IIB (III)

This syndrome was recognized by Williams and Pollack (1966). Clinically and pathologically, there are close parallels to MEN type IIA, but the genetic trait is separate and distinct. The identical clinical and laboratory surveillance measures discussed for MEN type IIA apply, except that parathyroid disease is rare. The major distinction of MEN type IIB is the development of multiple mucosal neuromas, intestinal ganglioneuromatosis, and dysfunctional obstipation (Schimke et al., 1968; DeSchryver-Kecskemeti et al., 1983). The clinical and radiologic presentation may resemble Hirschsprung's disease, but the histologic pattern is a massive dysplasia of the myenteric plexus rather than aganglionosis. Elevated nerve growth stim-

ulating activity may occur (DeSchryver-Kecskemeti et al., 1983). Patients may also exhibit a Marfanoid habitus and other musculoskeletal abnormalities (Carney et al., 1981).

Mixed MEN Syndromes

Mixed syndromes in which a well-recognized component of one MEN type is present in combination with elements of a second type have been reported (see Table 23–6).

Kindreds with pancreatic islet cell tumors occurring together with adrenal medullary neoplasms have been reported by several groups, and genetic studies have demonstrated a probable autosomal dominant mode of inheritance (Carney et al., 1980; Nathan et al.,

1980; Hull et al., 1979). Pituitary adenomas have also been reported in association with paragangliomas (Blumenkopf and Boekelheide, 1983), and at least some of these patients have had parathyroid disease with associated hypercalcemia (Anderson et al., 1981). Cases of pituitary adenoma with otherwise typical MEN type II or type III have also been described, and it is of interest that pituitary adenomas composed of prolactin-secreting cells occur commonly in association with C-cell and adrenal medullary proliferations in Long-Evans rats (Lee et al., 1982). Association of pituitary prolactinoma, adrenal aldosteronoma, gastric schwannoma, and colonic adenomatosis may represent another variant of MEN syndrome (Doumith et al., 1982).

Duodenal carcinoids have been associated with neurofibromatosis and pheochromocytomas, and it also has been suggested that this association represents a distinct MEN syndrome (Griffiths et al., 1983). In these cases, the carcinoid tumors were composed predominantly of cells synthesizing somatostatin (Griffiths et al., 1983; Dayal et al., 1985).

SUMMARY OF RECOMMENDATIONS FOR EARLY DIAGNOSIS AND TREATMENT OF NE CELL NEOPLASIAS

It is essential for pathologists and clinicians to appreciate the multicentric character of NE cell neoplasms and their potential for multisystem involvement.

While the majority of neoplasms are sporadic or solitary examples, diagnosis of any NE cell tumor obligates careful clinical evaluation and selective laboratory testing to exclude additional synchronous or metachronous lesions. The relatively high frequency of hyperplasias or neoplasms secreting catecholamines dictates particular attention to symptoms and signs of catecholamine excess, and the appropriate battery of laboratory tests. Obviously, accurate pathologic diagnosis underlies family counseling and prospective screening of kindred.

The pathologist's observations also contribute to prompt and effective clinical management of NE cell tumors. In view of the variable histologic patterns, precise attention to the gross location and organ relationships of each tumor is of major importance in assigning classification. In addition to conventional processing, representative tissue samples should be retained frozen for biochemical, immunocytochemical, or cytochemical studies and retained in glutaraldehyde for electron microscopy.

The predilection of NE cell tumors to invade or metastasize is often related to bulk. Prompt and complete surgical excision of NE cell neoplasms remains the treatment of choice and reduces risks of vascular or cardiac invasion, compression or obstruction of vital structures, and metastasis with systemic spread.

PROSPECTIVE DEVELOPMENTS

The increasing availability of monoclonal antibodies for immunocytochemical localization of NE cell biosynthetic products, including specific enzymes, monoamines, regulatory peptides or granule proteins, opens exciting prospects for more functional histopathologic classifications and direct correlations with clinical symptomatology or serum immunoassays. In recognized familial constellations of NE cell tumors, serum screening for specific regulatory peptides or monoamines is well established, but clearer definition of associated tissue biosynthetic profiles would eventually strengthen both the clinicopathologic classifications and the ability to predict biological behavior.

The improved facility of immunocytochemistry also suggests that it would be timely to explore the potential of fine needle aspiration in conjunction with noninvasive radiographic modalities for more rapid diagnosis of suspected neoplasms expressing NE features. Earlier recognition of retroperitoneal masses and other NE cell neoplasms in hazardous locations could accelerate elective surgery.

In principle, the specific familial patterns of some multisystem tumors eventually could be linked to restriction fragment length polymorphisms of the patient's DNA in normal cells. Restriction endonuclease fragmentation of DNA combined with blot hybridization mapping has lately been employed in the prenatal diagnosis of hemoglobinopathies and the presymptomatic diagnosis of Huntington's chorea (Gusella et al., 1983). Once appropriate molecular probes are identified, the approach pioneered by Gusella and coworkers will enable detection of asymptomatic individuals in selected families at high risk for neuroendocrine lesions. As a practical matter, DNA screening is unlikely to replace current biochemical screening modalities in the near future, and there also are many examples of familial multicentric or multisystem neoplasias with unrecognized patterns of recurrence. A careful family history will always remain paramount and examination of asymptomatic kin must be considered as a prophylactic adjunct in all new cases of NE cell neoplasia.

References

Adelman, L. S., Wolfe, H. J., DeLellis, R. A., Mobtaker, H., Tischler, A. S.: Immunologic cross-reactivity between human neural neuroendocrine and T-lymphocyte antigen. J. Neuropathol. Exp. Neurol. 44:316, 1985.

Albores-Saavedra, J., Nadji, M., Henson, D. E.: Intestinal-type adenocarcinoma of the gallbladder. A clinico-pathologic and immunocytochemical study of seven cases. Am. J. Surg. Pathol., in press.

Anderson, R. J., Lufkin, E. G., Sigenore, G. W., Carney, J. A., Sheps, S. G., Silliman, Y. E.: Acromegaly and pituitary adenoma with pheochromocytoma: A variant of multiple endocrine neoplasia. Clin. Endocrin. 14:605–612, 1981.

Andrew, A.: APUD cells, apudomas and the neural crest. S. Afr. Med. J. 50:890–898, 1976.

Angeletti, R. H., Nolan, J. A., Zaremba, S.: Catecholamine storage vesicles: Topography and function. Trends Biochem. Sci. 10:240–243, 1985.

Apple, D., and Kreines, K.: Cushing's syndrome due to ectopic ACTH production by a nasal paraganglioma. Am. J. Med. Sci. 283:32–35, 1982.

Arias-Stella, J., Bustos, F.: Chronic hypoxia and chemodectomas in bovines at high altitudes. Arch. Pathol. Lab. Med. 100:636–639, 1976.

Arias-Stella, J., Valcarcel, J.: Chief cell hyperplasia in the human carotid body at high altitudes. Physiology and pathologic significance. Hum. Pathol. 7:361–373, 1976.

Avsare, S. S., Prabhu, S. R., Vengsarkar, U. S., Manghani, D. K., Dastur, Darab K.: Von Recklinghausen's disease with a malignant meningeal, cerebral and optic nerve tumour and bilateral vagal schwannomas. J. Neurolog. Sci. 54:427–443, 1982.

Babu, V. R., Van Dyke, D. L., Jackson, C. E.: Chromosome 20 deletion in human multiple endocrine neoplasia types 2A and 2B: A double-blind study. Proc. Natl. Acad. Sci. USA 81:2525–2528, 1984.

Ballard, H. S., Frame, B., Hartsock, R. J.: Familial multiple endocrine adenoma–peptic ulcer complex. Medicine 43:481–516, 1964.

Baylin, S. B., Beaven, M. A., Engelman, K., Sjoerdsma, A.: Elevated histaminase activity in medullary carcinoma of the thyroid gland. N. Engl. J. Med. 283:1239–1244, 1970.

Baylin, S. B., Hsu, S. H., Gann, D., Smallridge, R., Wells, S.: Inherited medullary thyroid carcinoma: A final monoclonal mutation in one of multiple clones of susceptible cells. Science 199:429–431, 1978.

Berg, B., Biorklund, A., Grimelius, L., Ingemansson, S., Larsson, L-I., Stenram, U., Akerman, M.: New pattern of multiple endocrine adenomatosis. Chemodectoma, bronchial carcinoid, GH-producing pituitary adenoma and hyperplasia of the parathyroid glands, and antral and duodenal gastrin cells. Acta Med. Scand. 200:321–326, 1976.

Blaivas, M., Lloyd, R. V., Wilson, B. S.: Distribution of chromogranin and S-100 protein in normal and abnormal adrenal medullary tissues. Lab. Invest. 52-8A, 1985.

Blobel, G. A., Gould, V. E., Moll, R., Inchul, L., Huszar, M., Geiger, B., Franke, W. W.: Coexpression of neuroendocrine markers and epithelial cytoskeletal proteins in bronchopulmonary neuroendocrine neoplasms. Lab. Invest. 52:39–51, 1985.

Block, M. A., Jackson, C. E., Greenawald, K. A., Yott, J. B., Tashjian, A. H., Jr.: Clinical characteristics distinguishing hereditary from sporadic medullary thyroid carcinoma. Treatment implications. Arch. Surg. 115:142–148, 1980.

Blumenkopf, B., Boekelheide, K.: Neck paraganglioma with a pituitary adenoma. Case report. J. Neurosurg. 57(3):426–429, 1982.

Bockelman, H. W., Arya, S., Gilbert, E. F.: Cyanotic congenital heart disease with malignant paraganglioma. Cancer 50:2513–2517, 1982.

Bogdasarian, R. S., Lotz, P. R.: Multiple simultaneous paragangliomas of the head and neck in association with multiple retroperitoneal pheochromocytomas. Otolaryngol. Head Neck Surg. 87(5):648–652, 1979.

Bolande, R. P.: The neurocristopathies: A unifying concept of disease arising in neural crest maldevelopment. Hum. Biol. 5:409–429, 1974.

Bosman, F. T., Louwerens, J-W. K.: APUD cells in teratomas. Am. J. Pathol. 104:174–180, 1981.

Bravo, E. L., Gifford, R. W. Jr.: Pheochromocytoma: Diagnosis, localization and management. N. Engl. J. Med. 1298–1303, 1984.

Brennan, M. F.: Cancer of the endocrine system. In: DeVito, V. T., Jr., Hellman, S., Rosenberg, S. A. (Eds.), Cancer: Principles and Practice of Oncology, 2nd Ed. Philadelphia, Lippincott, 1985.

Bunn, P. A., Linnoila, I., Minna, J. D., Carney, D., Gazdar, A. F.: Small cell lung cancer, endocrine cells of the fetal bronchus, and other neuroendocrine cells express the leu-7 antigenic determinant present on natural killer cells. Blood 65:764–768, 1985.

Burek, J. D.: Pathology of aging rats. West Palm Beach, Florida, CRC Press, 1978, pp. 29–53.

Carney, J. A.: The triad of gastric epithelioid leiomyosarcoma, pulmonary chondroma, and functioning extra-adrenal paraganglioma: A five-year review. Medicine 62:159–169, 1983.

Carney, J. A., Bianco, A. J., Jr., Sizemore, G. W., Hayles, A. B.: Multiple endocrine neoplasia with skeletal manifestations. J. Bone Joint Surg. 63:405–410, 1981.

Carney, J. A., Go, V. L., Gordon, H., Northcutt, R. C., Pearse, A. G. E., Sheps, S. G.: Familial pheochromocytoma and islet cell tumor of the pancreas. Am. J. Med. 68:515–521, 1980.

Carney, J. A., Sizemore, G. W., Sheps, S. G.: Adrenal medullary disease in multiple endocrine neoplasia, type 2. Pheochromocytoma and its precursors. Am. J. Clin. Pathol. 66:279–290, 1976.

Chambers, R. C., Bowling, M. C., Grimley, P. M.: Glutaraldehyde fixation in routine histopathology. Arch. Pathol. 85:18–30, 1968.

Cox, W. F., Pierce, G. B.: The endodermal origin of the endocrine cells of an adenocarcinoma of the rat. Cancer 50:1530, 1982.

Crowell, W. T., Grizzle, W. E., Siegel, A. L.: Functional carotid paragangliomas. Biochemical, ultrastructural and histochemical correlation with clinical symptoms. Arch. Pathol. Lab. Med. 106:599–603, 1982.

Dahms, B. B., Lippe, B. M., Dakake, C., Fonkalsrud, E. W., Mirra, J. M.: The occurrence in a neonate of a pancreatic adenoma with nesidioblastosis in the tumor. Am. J. Clin. Pathol. 65:462–466, 1976.

Dayal, Y.: Endocrine cells of the gut and their neoplasms. In: Norris, H. T. (Ed.), Pathology of the Colon, Small Intestine and Anus. New York, Churchill Livingstone, 1983, pp. 267–302.

Dayal, Y., Tallberg, K., DeLellis, R. A., Wolfe, H. J.: Duodenal carcinoids in patients with and without neurofibromatosis: A comparative study. Lab. Invest. 52:18A, 1985.

DeLellis, R. A.: Formaldehyde-induced fluorescence technique for the demonstration of biogenic amines in diagnostic histopathology. Cancer 28:1704–1708, 1971.

DeLellis, R. A., Nunnemacher, G., Bitman, W. R., Gagel, R. F., Tashjian, A. H., Jr., Blount, M., Wolfe, H. J.: C-cell hyperplasia and medullary thyroid carcinoma in the rat. Lab. Invest. 40:140–154, 1979.

DeLellis, R. A., Tischler, A. S., Lee, A. K., Blount, M., Wolfe, H. J.: Leu-enkephalin-like immunoreactivity in proliferative lesions of the human adrenal medulla and extra-adrenal paraganglia. Am. J. Surg. Pathol. 7:29–37, 1983.

DeLellis, R. A., Tischler, A. S., Wolfe, H. J.: Multidirectional differentiation in neuroendocrine neoplasms. J. Histochem. Cytochem. 32:399, 1984.

DeLellis, R. A., Wolfe, H. J., Gagel, R. F., Feldman, Z. T., Miller, H. H., Gang, D. L., Reichlin, S.: A morphometric analysis in patients with familial medullary thyroid carcinoma. Am. J. Pathol. 83:177–196, 1976.

DeLellis, R. A., Wolfe, H. J.: The polypeptide hormone-producing neuroendocrine cells and their tumors. Meth. Achiev. Exp. Pathol. 10:190–220, 1981.

DeLellis, R. A., Dayal, Y., Tischler, A. S., Lee, A. K., Wolfe, H. J.: Multiple endocrine neoplasia (MEN) syndromes: Cellular origins and interrelationships. In press.

DeSchryver-Kecskemeti, K., Clouse, R. E., Goldstein, M. N., Gersell, D., O'Neal, L.: Intestinal ganglioneuromatosis. A manifestation of overproduction of nerve growth factor. N. Engl. J. Med. 308:635–639, 1983.

DeStephano, D. B., Lloyd, R. V., Pike, A. M., Wilson, B. S.: Pituitary adenomas. An immunohistochemical study of hormone production and chromogranin localization. Am. J. Pathol., 116:464–472, 1984.

DiSant'Agnese, P. A., de Mesy Jensen, K. L.: Somatostatin and/or somatostatinlike immunoreactive endocrine-paracrine cells in the human prostate gland. Arch. Pathol. Lab. Med. 108:693–696, 1984.

Doumith, R., deGennes, J. L., Cabane, J. P., Zygelman, N.: Pituitary prolactinoma, adrenal aldosterone producing adenomas, gastric schwannoma and colonic polyadenomas: A possible variant of multiple endocrine neoplasia (MEN) type I. Acta Endocrinol. 100:189–195, 1982.

Edwards, C., Heath, D., Harris, P.: The carotid body in emphysema and left ventricular hypertrophy. J. Pathol. 104:1–13, 1971.

Edwards, C., Heath, D., Harris, P.: Ultrastructure of the carotid body in high-altitude guinea-pigs. J. Pathol. 107:313–316, 1972.

Eisenbarth, G. S., Walsh, F. S., Nirenberg, M.: Monoclonal antibody to a plasma membrane antigen of neurons. Proc. Natl. Acad. Sci. USA 76:4913–4917, 1979.

Farr, H. W.: Carotid body tumors: A 40-year study. CA-A Cancer Journal for Clinicians 30:260–265, 1980.

Farrior, J. B., III, Hyams V. J., Benke, R. H., Farrior, J. B.: Carcinoid apudoma arising in a glomus jugulare tumor: Review of endocrine activity in glomus jugulare tumors. Laryngoscope 90:110–119, 1980.

Fenoglio, C. M., Uribe, M., Grimes, M., Feind, C.: Medullary carcinoma of the thyroid gland: Clinical, pathologic and immunohistochemical features with review of the literature. Lab. Invest. 52:21A, 1985.

Fernandes, B. J., Bedard, Y. C., Rosen, I.: Mucus-producing medullary cell carcinoma of the thyroid gland. J. Clin. Pathol. 78:536–540, 1982.

Ferri, G-L., Probert, L., Cocchia, D., Michetti, F., Marangos, P. J., Polak, J. M.: Evidence for the presence of S-100 protein in the glial component of the human enteric nervous system. Nature 297:409–410, 1982.

Fialkow, P. J., Sagebiel, R. W., Gartler, S. M., Rimoin, D. L.: Multiple cell origin of hereditary neurofibromas. N. Engl. J. Med. 284:298–300, 1971.

Fitch, R., Smith, P., Heath, D.: Nerve axons in carotid body hyperplasia. Arch. Pathol. Lab. Med. 209:234–238, 1985.

Folger, Jr., G. M., Roberts, W. C., Mehrizi, A., Shah, K. D., Glancy, D. L., Carpenter, C. C. J., Esterly, J. R.: Cyanotic malformations of the heart with pheochromocytoma. A report of five cases. Circulation 29:750–757, 1964.

Friesen, S. R., Tomita, T., Kimmel, J. R.: Pancreatic polypeptide update: Its roles in detection of the trait for multiple endocrine adenopathy syndrome, type I and pancreatic polypeptide-secreting tumors. Surgery 94:1028–1037, 1983.

Funato, M., Fujimura, M., Shimada, S., Takeuchi, T., Kozuki, K., Iida, Y.: Rapid changes of serum vasoactive intestinal peptide after removal of ganglioneuroblastoma with watery-diarrhea-hypokalemia-achlorhydria syndrome in a child. J. Pediat. Gastroenterol. Nutr. 1:131–135, 1982.

Gagel, R. F., Melvin, K. E. W., Tashjian, A. H., Jr., Miller, H. H., Feldman, Z. T., Wolfe, H. J., DeLellis, R. A., Cervi-Skinner, S., Reichlin, S.: Natural history of the familial medullary carcinoma-pheochromocytoma syndrome and the identification of preneoplastic stages by screening studies: A five-year report. Trans. Assoc. Am. Phys. 88:177–191, 1975.

Gallivan, M. V. E., Chun, B., Rowden, G., Lack, E. E.: Intrathoracic paravertebral malignant paraganglioma. Arch. Pathol. Lab. Med. 104:46–51, 1980.

Gambino, R.: Laboratory diagnosis of pheochromocytoma. Lab Report for Physicians 4:75–79, 1982.

Gaylis, H., Mieny, C. J.: The incidence of malignancy in carotid body tumors. Br. J. Surg. 64:885–889, 1977.

Gilbert, W.: Genes-in-pieces revisited. Science 228:823–824, 1985.

Glenner, G. G., Grimley, P. M.: Tumors of the extra-adrenal paraganglion system (including chemoreceptors), Fascicle 9, Atlas of Tumor Pathology (2nd series), Armed Forces Institute of Pathology, Washington, D. C., 1974.

Goldstein, A., Tachibana, S., Lowney, L. I., Hunkapiller, M., Hood, L.: Dynorphin (1–13), an extraordinarily potent opioid peptide. Proc. Natl. Acad. Sci. USA 76:6666–6670, 1979.

Gooding, G. A. W.: Gray-scale ultrasound detection of carotid body tumors: report of 2 cases. Radiology 132:409–410, 1979.

Gould, V. E., Linnoila, R. I., Memoli, V. A., Warren, W. H.: Biology of disease. Neuroendocrine components of the bronchopulmonary tract: hyperplasias, dysplasias, and neoplasms. Lab. Invest. 50:519–537, 1983.

Gould, V. E., Moll, R., Moll, I., Lee, I., Franke, W. W.: Neuroendocrine (Merkel) cells of the skin: hyperplasias, dysplasias, and neoplasms. Lab. Invest. 52:334–353, 1985.

Greco, F. A., Oldham, R. K.: Small-cell lung cancer. N. Engl. J. Med. 301:355–358, 1979.

Griffiths, D. F. R., Williams, G. T., Williams, E. D.: Multiple endocrine neoplasia associated with von Recklinghausen's disease. Br. Med. J. 287:1341–1343, 1983.

Grimelius, L.: A silver nitrate stain for α_2-cells in human pancreatic islets. Acta Soc. Med. Ups. 73:243–270, 1968.

Grimley, P. M., Glenner, G. G.: Histology and ultrastructure of carotid body paragangliomas: Comparison with the normal gland. Cancer 20:1473–1488, 1967.

Grimley, P. M., Glenner, G. G.: Ultrastructure of the human carotid body. A perspective on the mode of chemoreception. Circulation 37:648–665, 1968.

Grizzle, W. E., Tolbert, L., Pittman, C. S., Siegel, A. L., Aldrete, J. S.: Corticotropin production by tumors of the autonomic nervous system. Arch. Pathol. Lab. Med. 108:545–550, 1983.

Gusella, J. F., Wexler, N. S., Conneally, P. M., Naylor, S. L., Anderson, M. A., Tanzi, R. E., Watkins, P. C., Ottina, K., Wallace, M. R., Sakaguchi, A. Y., Young, A. B., Shoulson, A. B., Bonilla, E., Martin, J. B.: A polymorphic DNA marker genetically linked to Huntington's disease. Nature 306:234–238, 1983.

Gustavson, K.-H., Jansson, R., Oberg, K.: Chromosomal breakage in multiple endocrine adenomatosis (types I and II). Clin. Genet. 23:143–149, 1983.

Hamilton, B. R., Landsberg, L., Levine, R. J.: Measurement of urinary epinephrine in screening for pheochromocytoma in multiple endocrine neoplasia type II. Am. J. Med. 65:1027–1032, 1978.

Hanley, M. R.: Neuropeptides as mitogens. Nature 315:14–15, 1985.

Hansen, O. P., Hansen, M., Hansen, H. H., Rose, B.: Multiple endocrine adenomatosis of mixed type. Acta. Med. Scand. 200:327–331, 1976.

Hartschuh, W., Weihe, E., Buchler, M., Helmstaedter, V., Feurle, G. E., Forssmann, W. G.: Met-enkephalin-like immunoreactivity in Merkel cells. Cell Tissue Res. 201:343–348, 1979.

Hassoun, J., Monges, G., Giraud, P., Henry, J. F., Charpin, C., Payan, H., Toga, M.: Immunohistochemical study of pheochromocytomas. An investigation of methionine-enkephalin, vasoactive intestinal peptide, somatostatin, corticotropin, β-endorphin, and calcitonin in 16 tumors. Am. J. Pathol. 114:56–63, 1984.

Hayes, H. M., Fraumeni, J. F.: Chemodectomas in dogs: Epidemiologic comparisons with man. J. Natl. Cancer Inst. 52:1455–1458, 1974.

Heitz, P. U.: Pancreatic endocrine tumors. In: Kloppel, G., Heitz, P. U. (Eds.), Pancreatic Pathology. Edinburgh, Churchill Livingstone, 1984, pp. 206–232.

Hermann, J.: Delayed mutation model: Carotid body tumors and retinoblastoma. In: Mulvihill, J. J., Miller, R. W. (Eds.): Genetics of Human Cancer. New York, Raven Press, 1977, pp. 417–437.

Hoffman, R. W., Gardner, D. W., Mitchell, F. L.: Intrathoracic and multiple abdominal pheochromocytomas in Von Hippel-Lindau disease. Arch. Intern. Med. 142:1962, 1965.

Hsu, T. C., Pathak, S., Samann, N., Hickey, R. C.: Chromosome instability in patients with medullary carcinoma of the thyroid. J.A.M.A. 246:2046–2048, 1981.

Hull, M. T., Roth, L. M., Glover, J. L., Walker, P. D.: Metastatic carotid body paraganglioma in Von Hippel-Lindau disease. An electron microscopic study. Arch. Pathol. Lab. Med. 106(5):235–239, 1982.

Hull, M., Warfel, K. A., Muller, J., Higgins, J. T.: Familial islet cell tumors in von Hippel-Lindau disease. Cancer 44:1523–1526, 1979.

Ichijima, K., Akaishi, K., Toyoda, N., Kobashi, Y., Ueda, Y., Matsuo, S., Yamabe, H.: Carcinoma of the pancreas with endocrine component in childhood. Am. J. Clin. Pathol. 83:95–100, 1985.

Ichinose, H., Hewitt, R. L., Drapanas, T.: Minute pulmonary chemodectoma. Cancer 28:692–700, 1971.

Jaffe, N.: Biologic vagaries in neuroblastoma. In: Pochedly, C. (Ed.), Neuroblastoma, Clinical and Biological Manifestations. New York, Elsevier Biomedical, 1982, pp. 293–309.

Jago, R., Smith, P., Heath, D.: Electron microscopy of carotid body hyperplasia. Arch. Pathol. Lab. Med. 108:717–722, 1984.

Johnson, T. L., Lloyd, R. V., Shapiro, B., Sisson, J. C., Beierwaltes, W. H.: Cardiac paragangliomas: A clinicopathologic study of four cases. Lab. Invest. 52:31A, 1985.

Jubb, K. V., McEntee, K.: The relationship of ultimobranchial remnants and derivatives to tumor of the thyroid gland in cattle. Cornell Veterinarian 49:41–69, 1959.

Kahn, L. B.: Vagal body tumor (nonchromaffin paraganglioma, chemodectoma, and carotid body-like tumor) with cervical node metastasis and familial association. Cancer 38:2367–2377, 1976.

Karasov, R. B., Sheps, S. G., Carney, J. A., van Heerden, J. A., deQuattro, V.: Paragangliomatosis with numerous catecholamine-producing tumors. Mayo Clin. Proc. 57:590–595, 1982.

Kay, D., DeLellis, R. A., Dayal, Y., Lloyd, R. V., Duggan, M. A., Tallberg, K., Sternberg, S. S., Wolfe, J. H.: Ductal adenocarcinomas of the pancreas with neuroendocrine cells: An immunohistochemical study. Lab. Invest.: In press.

Kissel, P., Andre, J. M., Jacquier, A.: The neurocristopathies. New York, Masson Publishing, U.S.A., Inc., 1981, p. 262.

Knudson, A. G., Jr.: Mutation and cancer: Statistical study of retinoblastoma. Proc. Natl. Acad. Sci. USA 68:820–823, 1971.

Krammer, E. B.: Carotid body chemoreceptor function: Hypothesis based on a new circuit model. Proc. Natl. Acad. Sci. USA 75:2507–2511, 1978.

Krieger, D. T.: Pituitary ACTH hyperfunction: Physiopathology and clinical aspects. In: Cormani, F., Muller, E. E. (Eds.), Pituitary Hyperfunction: Pathophysiology and Clinical Aspects. New York, Raven Press, 1984, pp. 221–234.

Krook, L., Lutwak, L., McEntee, K.: Dietary calcium, ultimobranchial tumors and osteoporosis in the bull. Am. J. Clin. Nutr. 22(2):115–118, 1969.

Lack, E. E.: Hyperplasia of vagal and carotid body paraganglia in patients with chronic hypoxemia. Am. J. Pathol. 91:497–516, 1978.

Lack, E. E., Cubilla, A. L., Woodruff, J. M.: Paragangliomas of the head and neck region. Human Pathol. 10:191–218, 1979a.

Lack, E. E., Cubilla, A. L., Woodruff, J. M., Lieberman, P. H.: Extra-adrenal paragangliomas of the retroperitoneum. A clinicopathologic study of 12 tumors. Am. J. Surg. Pathol. 4:109–129, 1980.

Lack, E. E., Stillinger, R. A., Colvin, D. B., Groves, R. M., Burnette, D. G.: Aortic-pulmonary paraganglioma. Report of a case with ultrastructural study and review of the literature. Cancer 43:269–278, 1979b.

Larraza-Hernandez, O., Albores-Saavedra, J., Benavides, G., Krause, L. G., Perez-Merizaldi, J. C., Ginzo, A.: Pituitary adenoma, multicentric papillary thyroid carcinoma, bilateral carotid body paraganglioma, parathyroid hyperplasia, gastric leiomyoma, and systemic amyloidosis. Am. J. Clin. Pathol. 78:527–532, 1982.

Larsson, L-I., Goltermann, N., DeMagistris, L., Rehfeld, J. F., Schwartz, T. W.: Somatostatin cell processes as pathways for paracrine secretion. Science 205:1393–1395, 1979.

Law, D. H., Liddle, G. W., Scott, Jr., H. W., Tauber, S. D.: Ectopic production of multiple hormones (ACTH, MSH and gastrin) by a single malignant tumor. N. Engl. J. Med. 273:292–296, 1965.

Lee, A. K., DeLellis, R. A., Blount, M., Nunnemacher, G., Wolfe, H. J.: Pituitary proliferative lesions in aging male Long-Evans rats. A model of mixed multiple endocrine neoplasia syndrome. Lab. Invest. 47:595–682, 1982.

Levine, J. H., Sagel, J., Rosebrock, G., Gonzalez, J. J., Nair, R., Rawe, S., Powers, J. M.: Prolactin-secreting adenoma as part of the multiple endocrine neoplasia—type I (MEN-I) syndrome. Cancer 43:2492–2496, 1979.

Lewis, R. V., Stern, A. S., Kimura, S., Rossier, J., Stein, S., Udenfriend, S.: An about 50,000 dalton protein in adrenal medulla: A common precursor of [met] and [leu]-enkephalin. Science 200:1450–1461, 1980.

Linnoila, R. I., Becker, K. L., Silva, O. L., Snider, R. H., Moore, C. F.: Calcitonin as a marker for diethylnitrosamine-induced pulmonary endocrine cell hyperplasia in hamsters. Lab. Invest. 51:39–45, 1984.

Linnoila, R. I., Netesheim, P., DiAugustine, R. P.: Lung endocrine-like cells in hamsters treated with diethylnitrosamine: alterations in vivo and in cell culture. Proc. Natl. Acad. Sci. USA 78:5170, 1981.

Lipinski, M., Braham, K., Caillaud, J-M., Carlu, C., Tursz, T.: HNK-1 antibody detects an antigen expressed on neuroectodermal cells. J. Exp. Med. 158:1775–1780, 1983.

Lloyd, R. V., Shapiro, B., Sisson, J. C., Kalff, V., Thompson, N. W., Beierwaltes, W. A.: An immunohistochemical study of pheochromocytomas. Arch. Pathol. Lab. Med. 108:541–544, 1984.

Lloyd, R. V., Warner, T. F.: In: DeLellis, R. A. (Ed.), Advances in Immunohistochemistry. New York: Masson Publishing, Inc., 1984, pp. 127–140.

Lynch, H. T., Lynch, P. M., Albano, W. A., Edney, J., Organ, C. H., Lynch, J. F.: Hereditary cancer: Ascertainment and management. Cancer—A Journal for Clinicians 29:216–232, 1979.

Machin, G. A.: Histogenesis and histopathology of neuroblastoma. In: Pochedly, C. (Ed.), Neuroblastoma, Clinical and Biological Manifestations. New York, Elsevier Biomedical, 1982, pp. 195–231.

Majewski, J. T., Wilson, S. D.: The MEA-I syndrome: An all or none phenomenon? Surgery, 475–484, 1979.

Manning, J. T., Ordonez, N. G., Rosenberg, H. S., Walker, W. E.: Pulmonary endodermal tumor resembling fetal lung. Report of a case with immunohistochemical studies. Arch. Pathol. Lab. Med. 109:48–50, 1985.

Marchevsky, A. M., Dikman, S. H.: Mediastinal carcinoid with an incomplete Sipple's syndrome. Cancer 43:2497–2501, 1979.

Mark, E. J., Ramirez, J. F.: Peripheral small-cell carcinoma of the lung resembling carcinoid tumor. Arch. Pathol. Lab. Med. 109:263–269, 1985.

McGarry, R. C., Helfand, S. L., Quarles, R. H., Roder, J. C.: Recognition of myelin-associated glycoprotein by the monoclonal antibody HNK-1. Nature 306:376–378, 1983.

Meinertzhagen, I. A.: Serotonin-containing cell charged with growth cone arrest. Nature 313:348–349, 1985.

Melicow, M. M.: One hundred cases of pheochromocytoma (107 tumors) at the Columbia-Presbyterian Medical Center, 1926–1976. A clinicopathological analysis. Cancer 40:1987–2004, 1977.

Melvin, K. E. W.: The paraneoplastic syndromes associated with carcinoma of the thyroid gland. Ann. N.Y. Acad. Sci. 230:378–390, 1974.

Melvin, K. E. W., Miller, H. H., Tashjian, A. H., Jr.: Early diagnosis of medullary carcinoma of the thyroid gland by means of calcitonin assay. N. Engl. J. Med. 285:1115–1119, 1971.

Mendelsohn, G., Bigner, S. H., Eggleston, J. C., Baylin, S. B., Wells, S. A., Jr.: Anaplastic variants of medullary thyroid carcinoma. Am. J. Surg. Pathol. 4:333–341, 1980.

Moertel, C. G., Dockerty, M. B.: Familial occurrence of metastasizing carcinoid tumors. Ann. Intern. Med. 78:389–390, 1973.

Moertel, C. G., Beahrs, O. H., Woolner, L. B., Tyce, G. M.: "Malignant carcinoid syndrome" associated with noncarcinoid tumors. N. Engl. J. Med. 273:244–248, 1965.

Morriss, T. A., Tymms, D. J.: Oat cell carcinoma, pheochromocytoma and carcinoid tumors—multiple APUD cell neoplasia—a case report. J. Pathol. 313:107–115, 1980.

Mukai, K., Grotting, J. C., Greider, M. H., Rosai, J.: Retrospective study of 77 pancreatic endocrine tumors using the immunoperoxidase method. Am. J. Surg. Pathol. 6:387–399, 1982.

Nakajima, T., Watanabe, S., Sato, Y., Kameya, T., Hirota, T., Shimosato, Y.: An immunoperoxidase study of S-100 protein distribution in normal and neoplastic tissues. Am. J. Surg. Pathol. 6:715–727, 1982.

Nathan, D. M., Daniels, G. H., Ridgway, E. C.: Gastrinoma and phaeochromocytoma: is there a mixed multiple endocrine adenoma syndrome? Acta Endocrinol. 93:91–93, 1980.

Nicholas, G., Orsini, M. A.: Simultaneous ipsilateral carotid body and vagal paraganglioma. Otolaryngol. Head Neck Surg. 90:246, 1982.

Oberg, K., Walinder, D., Bostrom, H., Lundqvist, G., Wide, L.: Peptide hormone markers in screening for endocrine tumors in multiple endocrine adenomatosis type I. Am. J. Med. 73:619–630, 1982.

O'Connor, D. T., Burton, D., Deftos, L. J.: Chromogranin A: Immunohistology reveals its universal occurrence in normal polypeptide hormone producing endocrine glands. Life Sciences 33:1657–1663, 1983.

Odell, W. D., Wolfsen, A. R.: Hormones from tumors: Are they ubiquitous? Am. J. Med. 68:317–318, 1980.

Olson, G. A., Olson, R. D., Kastin, A. J., Coy, D. H.: Endogenous opiates: Peptides (Fayetteville) 3:1039–1072, 1982.

Olson, J. L., Salyer, W. R.: Mediastinal paragangliomas (aortic body tumor). A report of four cases and a review of the literature. Cancer 41:2405–2412, 1978.

Parry, D. M., Li, F. P., Strong, L. C., Carney, J. A., Schottenfeld, D., Reimer, R. R., Grufferman, S.: Carotid body tumors in man: Genetics and epidemiology. J. Natl. Cancer Inst. 68:573–578, 1982.

Payne, C. M., Nagle, R. B., Borduin, V.: Methods in laboratory investigation. An ultrastructural cytochemical stain specific for neuroendocrine neoplasms. Lab. Invest. 51:350–365, 1984.

Pearse, A. G. E.: The cytochemistry and ultrastructure of polypeptide hormone-producing cells of the APUD series and the embryologic, physiologic and pathologic implications of the concept. J. Histochem. Cytochem. 17:303–313, 1969.

Pearse, A. G. E.: The diffuse neuroendocrine system and the APUD concept. Related "endocrine" peptides in brain, intestine, pituitary, placenta, and anuran cutaneous glands. Med. Biol. 35:115, 1977.

Pearse, A. G. E., Polak, J. M.: The diffuse neuroendocrine system and the APUD concept. In: Bloom, S. R. (Ed.), Gut Hormones. Edinburgh, Churchill Livingstone, 1978, p. 33.

Pearse, A. G. E., Polak, J. M.: Endocrine tumours of neural crest origin: neurolophomas, apudomas and the APUD concept. Med. Biol. 52:3, 1974.

Pereira, D. T., Hunter, R. D.: Familial multicentric non-chromaffin paragangliomas: A case report on a patient with glomus jugulare and bilateral body tumors. Clin. Oncol. 6(3):273–275, 1980.

Pictet, R. L., Rall, L. B., Phelps, P., Rutter, W. J.: The neural crest and the origin of the insulin-producing and other gastrointestinal hormone–producing cells. Science 191:191–192, 1976.

Polak, J. M., Bloom, S. R.: The diffuse neuroendocrine system. Studies of this newly discovered controlling system in health and disease. J. Histochem. Cytochem. 27:1398–1400, 1979.

Ranchod, M., Levine, G. D.: Spindle-cell carcinoid tumors of the lung. A clinicipathologic study of 35 cases. Am. J. Surg. Pathol. 4:315–331, 1980.

Reed, J. C., Hallet, K. K., Feigin, D. S.: Neural tumors of the thorax: Subject review from the Armed Forces Institute of Pathology. Radiology 126:9–17, 1978.

Reed, R. J., Daroca, P. J., Jr., Harkin, J. C.: Gangliocytic paraganglioma. Am. J. Surg. Pathol. 1:207–216, 1977.

Revak, C. S., Morris, S. E., Alexander, G. H.: Pheochromocytoma and recurrent chemodectomas. Radiology 100:53–54, 1971.

Richards, J. G., DaPrada, M.: Uranaffin reaction: a new cytochemical technique for the localization of adenine nucleotides in organelles storing biogenic amines. J. Histochem. Cytochem. 25:1322, 1977.

Robertson, D. I., Cooney, T. P.: Malignant carotid body paraganglioma: Light and electron microscopic study of the tumor and its metastases. Cancer 46:2623–2633, 1980.

Rosai, J., Levine, G., Weber, W. R., Higa, F.: Carcinoid tumors and oat cell carcinoma of the thymus. Pathol. Annual 11:201–226, 1976.

Rosenfeld, M. G., Amara, S. G., Birnberg, N. C., Mermod, J-J., Murdock, G. H., Evans, R. M.: Calcitonin, prolactin and growth hormone gene expression as model systems for the characterization of neuroendocrine regulation. Recent Progr. Horm. Res. 39:305–351, 1983.

Roth, J., LeRoith, D., Shiloach, J., Rosenzweig, J. L., Lesniak, M., Havrankova, J.: The evolutionary origins of hormones, neurotransmitters, and other extracellular chemical messengers. N. Eng. J. Med. 306:523–526, 1982.

Rujis, J. H. J., van Waes, P. F. G. M., deHaas, G., Hoekstra, A., Mulder, P. H. M., Veldman, J. E.: Screening of a family for chemodectoma. Radiologia Clin. 47:114–123, 1978.

Said, S. E., Faloona, G. R.: Elevated plasma and tissue levels of vasoactive intestinal polypeptide in the watery diarrhea syndrome due to pancreatic, bronchogenic and other tumors. N. Engl. J. Med. 293:155–160, 1975.

Saito, H., Saito, S., Sano, T., Kagawa, N., Hizawa, K., Tatara, K.: Immunoreactive somatostatin in catecholamine-producing extra-adrenal paraganglioma. Cancer 50:560–565, 1982.

Sapira, J. D., Altman, M., Vandyk, K., Shapiro, A. P.: Bilateral adrenal pheochromocytoma and medullary thyroid carcinoma. N. Engl. J. Med. 273:140–143, 1965.

Sato, T., Saito, H., Yoshinaga, K., Shibota, Y., Sasano, N.: Concurrence of carotid body tumor and pheochromocytoma. Cancer 34:1787–1795, 1974.

Scarpelli, D. G.: Multipotent development capacity of cells in the adult animal. Lab. Invest. 52:331–332, 1985.

Schimke, R. N.: The neurocristopathy concept: fact or fiction. In: Evans, A. E. (Ed.), Advances in Neuroblastoma Research, Proceedings of the 2nd Symposium on Advances in Neuroblastoma Research held in Philadelphia, 1979. Vol. 12. Progr. Cancer Res. Ther. 1980, p. 344.

Schimke, R. N., Hartmann, W. H., Prout, T. E., Rimoin, D. L.: Syndrome of bilateral pheochromocytoma, medullary thyroid carcinoma and multiple neuromas. A possible regulatory defect in the differentiation of chromaffin tissue. N. Engl. J. Med. 279:1–7, 1968.

Schmechel, D. E.: γ-Subunit of the glycolytic enzyme enolase: Nonspecific or neuron specific? Lab. Invest. 52:239–242, 1985.

Schnitzer, J., Schachner, M.: Cell type specificity of a neural cell surface antigen recognized by the monoclonal antibody A2B5. Cell Tissue Res. 224:625–636, 1982.

Scott, S. A., Cooper, E., Diamond, J.: Merkel cells as targets of the mechanosensory nerves in salamander skin. Proc. R. Soc. Lond. B211:455–470, 1981.

Scully, R. E., Aguirre, P., DeLellis, R. A.: Argyrophilia, serotonin and peptide hormones in the female genital tract and its tumors. Int. J. Gynecol. Pathol. 3:51–70, 1984.

Sevier, A., Munger, B. C.: A silver method for paraffin sections of neural tissue. J. Neuropathol. Exp. Neurol. 24:130–135, 1965.

Sidhu, G. S.: The endodermal origin of digestive and respiratory tract APUD cells: Histopathologic evidence and a review of the literature. Am. J. Pathol. 96:5–20, 1979.

Silva, E. G., Ordonez, N. G., Lechago, J.: Immunohistochemical studies in endocrine carcinoma of the skin. Am. J. Clin. Pathol. 81:558–562, 1984.

Sisson, J. C., Frager, M. S., Valk, T. W., Gross, M. D., Swanson, D. P., Wieland, D. M., Tobes, M. C., Beierwaltes, W. H., Thompson, N. W.: Scintigraphic localization of pheochromocytoma. N. Engl. J. Med. 305:12–17, 1981.

Skrabanek, P.: APUD concept: Hypothesi or tautology? Medical Hypotheses 6:437–440, 1980.

Snyder, S. H.: Brain peptides as neurotransmitters. Science 209:976–983, 1980.

Soeprono, F. F., Hodgkin, J. E.: Metastatic chemodectoma with multiple nodular lesions. CA—A Cancer Journal for Clinicians 33:98–99, 1983.

Spector, G. J., Compagno, J., Perez, C. A., Maisel, R. H., Ogura, J. H.: Glomus jugulare tumors: Effects of radiotherapy. Cancer 35:1316–1321, 1975.

Spees, E. K., Katz, R. S., Sandles, L., Light, J. A., Zachary, J. B., Williams, G. M.: APUD system neoplasms in renal transplant patients. Surgery 94:501–507, 1983.

Sponenberg, D. P., McEntee, K.: Pheochromocytomas and ultimobranchial (C-cell) neoplasms in the bull: Evidence of autosomal dominant inheritance in the Guernsey breed. Vet. Pathol. 20:396–400, 1983.

Stahlman, M., Gray, M. E.: Ontogeny of neuroendocrine cells in human fetal lung. I. An electron microscopic study. Lab. Invest. 51:449–463, 1984.

Stahlman, M. T., Kasselberg, A. G., Orth, D. N., Gray, M. E.: Ontogeny of neuroendocrine cells in human fetal lung. II. An immunohistochemical study. Lab. Invest. 52:52–60, 1985.

Steiner, A. L., Goodman, A. D., Powers, S. R.: Study of a kindred with pheochromocytoma, medullary thyroid carcinoma, hyperparathyroidism and Cushing's disease: multiple endocrine neoplasia, type 2. Medicine 47:371–409, 1968.

Stevens, R. E., Moore, G. E.: Inadequacy of APUD concept in explaining production of peptide hormones by tumours. Lancet 1:118–119, 1983.

Takor-Takor, T., Pearse, A. G. E.: Neuroectodermal origin of avian hypothalamo-hypophyseal complex: the role of the ventral neural ridge. Embryol. Exp. Morphol. 34:322, 1975.

Tateishi, R., Ishikawa, O.: The effect of N-nitrosobis(2-hydroxypropyl) amine on pulmonary neuroepithelial cells in Syrian golden hamsters. Am. J. Pathol. 119:326–335, 1985.

Tischler, A. S., Dichter, M. A., Biales, B., Greene, L. A.: Neuroendocrine neoplasms and their cells of origin. N. Engl. J. Med. 296:919–925, 1977.

Tischler, A. S., DeLellis, R. A., Biales, B., Nunnemacher, G., Carabba, V., Wolfe, H. J.: Nerve growth factor-induced neurite outgrowth from normal human chromaffin cells. Lab. Invest. 43:399–409, 1980.

Tischler, A. S., Lee, A. K., Nunnemacher, G., Said, S. I., DeLellis, R. A., Morse, G. M., Wolfe, H. J.: Spontaneous neurite outgrowth and vasoactive intestinal peptide-liked immunoreactivity of cultures of human paraganglioma cells from the glomus jugulare. Cell Tissue Res. 219:543–555, 1981.

Van Baars, F., Cremers, C., van den Brock, P., Geerts, S., Veldman, J.: Genetic aspects of nonchromaffin paraganglioma. Human Genet. 60:305–309, 1982.

Van Heerden, J. A., Kent, R. B. III, Sizemore, G. W., Grant, C. S., ReMine, W. H.: Primary hyperparathyroidism in patients with multiple endocrine neoplasia syndromes. Surgical experience. Arch. Surg. 118:533–536, 1983.

Veldman, J. E., Mulder, P. H. M., Ruijs, S. H. J., deHaas, G., van Waes, P. F. G. M., Hoekstra, A.: Early detection of asymptomatic hereditary chemodectoma with radionuclide scintiangiography. A possibility for family screening and surveillance. Arch. Otolaryngol. 106:547–552, 1980.

Verhofstad, A. A. J., Steinbusch, H. W. M., Joosten, H. W. J., Penke, B., Varga, J. Goldstein, M.: Immunocytochemical localization of noradrenaline, adrenaline, and serotonin. In: Polak, J. M., Van Noorden, S. (Eds.): Immunocytochemistry. Practical Applications in Pathology and Biology. Bristol, Boston, 1983, pp. 143–168.

Weiss, S. W., Langloss, J. M., Enzinger, F. M.: Value of S-100 protein in the diagnosis of soft tissue tumors with particular reference to benign and malignant Schwann cell tumors. Lab. Invest. 49:299–308, 1983.

Wermer, D.: Genetic aspects of adenomatosis of endocrine glands. Am. J. Med. 16:363–371, 1954.

Whang-Peng, J., Triche, T. J., Knutsen, T., Miser, J., Douglass, E. C., Israel, M. A.: Chromosome translocation in peripheral neuroepithelioma. N. Engl. J. Med. 311:584–585, 1984.

White, M. C., Hickson, B. R.: Multiple paragangliomata secreting catecholamines and calcitonin with intermittent hypercalcemia. J. Roy. Soc. Med. 72(7):532–535, 1979.

Wick, M. R., Carney, J. A., Bernatz, P. E., Brown, L. R.: Primary mediastinal carcinoid tumors. Am. J. Surg. Pathol. 6:195–205, 1982.

Wick, M. R., Goellner, J. R., Scheithauer, B. W., Thomas J. R., III, Sanchez, N. P., Schroeter, A. L.: Primary neuroendocrine carcinomas of the skin (Merkel cell tumors). Am. J. Clin. Pathol. 79:6–13, 1983.

Williams, E. D., and Pollack, D. J.: Multiple mucosal neuromata with endocrine tumours; A syndrome allied to von Recklinghausen's disease. J. Pathol. Bacteriol. 91:71–80, 1966.

Wilson, B. S., Lloyd, R. V.: Detection of chromogranin in neuroendocrine cells with a monoclonal antibody. Am. J. Pathol. 115:458–468, 1984.

Wilson, H.: Carotid body tumors: Familial and bilateral. Ann. Surg. 171:843–848, 1970.

Wolfe, H. J., DeLellis, R. A., Jackson, C. E., Greenawald, K. A., Block, M. A., Tashjian, A. H. Jr.: Immunocytochemical distinction of hereditary from sporadic medullary carcinoma. Lab. Invest. 42:161–162, 1980.

Wolfe, H. J., Melvin, K. E. W., Cervi-Skinner, S. J., Al Saadi, A. A., Juliar, J. F., Jackson, C. E., Tashjian, A. H., Jr.: C-cell hyperplasia preceding medullary thyroid carcinoma. N. Engl. J. Med. 289:437–41, 1973.

Zeytinoglu, F. N., Gagel, R. F., DeLellis, B. A., Wolfe, J. H., Tashjian, A. H., Jr., Hammer, R. A., Leeman, S. E.: Clonal strains of rat medullary thyroid carcinoma that produce neurotensin and calcitonin: functional and morphological studies. Lab. Invest. 49:453, 1983.

Zollinger, R., Hedinger, C.: Pheochromocytoma and sympathetic paraganglioma. 2. Combination with typical associated diseases. Familial occurrence. Schweiz Med. Wochenschr. 113(31–32):1086–1092, 1983.

Index

Note: Numbers in *italics* refer to figures; numbers followed by t refer to tables.